Lifestyled

jovis

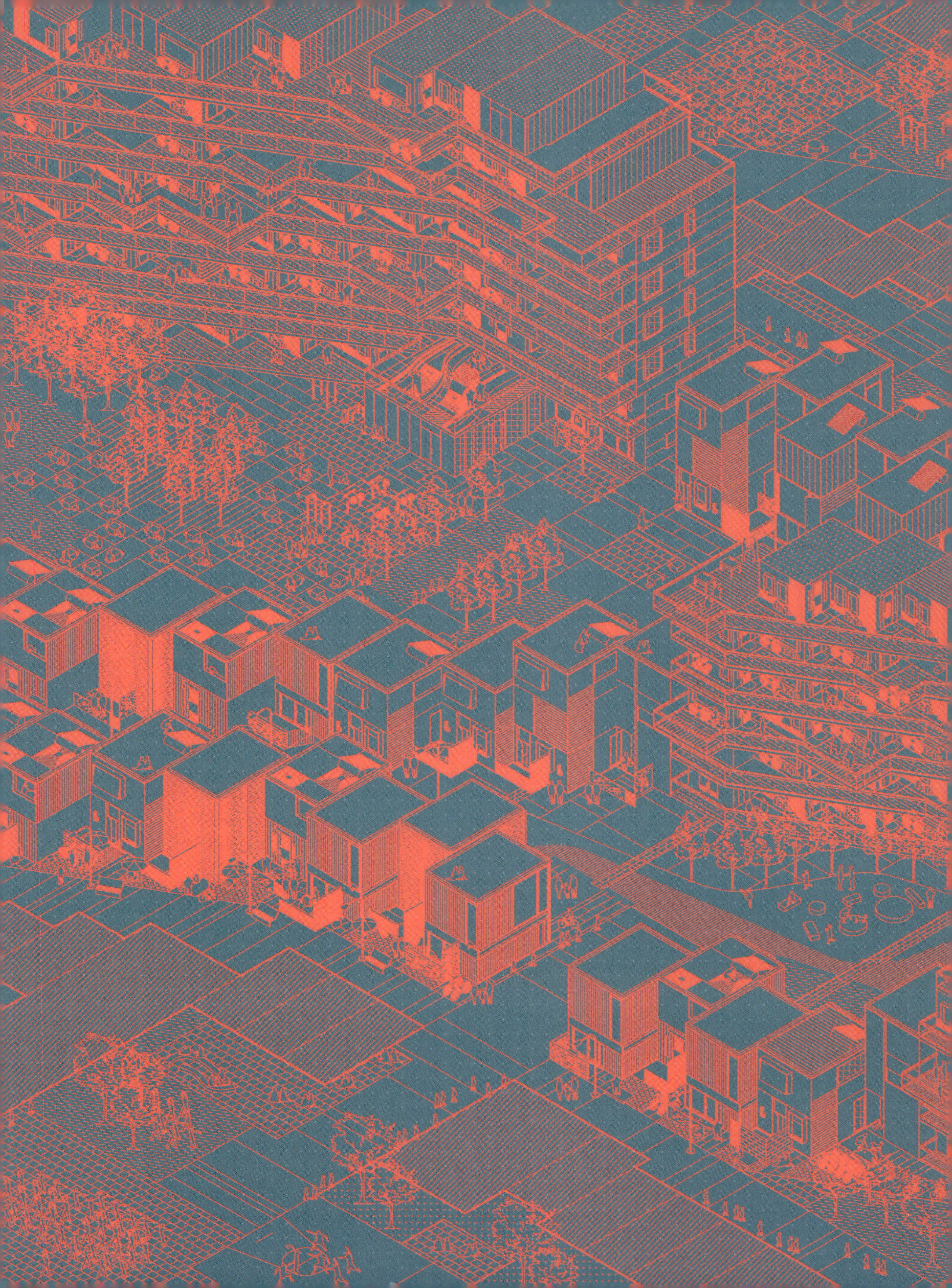

Lifestyled
Health and Places

David Mah and
Leire Asensio Villoria

jovis

Imprint

Cover: Lifestyled Studio Design Drawing by Justin Kollar and Ali Karimi

Copy-editing: Justin Kollar
Proofreading: Justin Ross, Berlin
Design and setting: David Mah, Leire Asensio Villoria and Justin Kollar
Printing and binding: DZS GRAFIK d.o.o., Ljubljana

Bibliographic information published by the Deutsche Nationalbibliothek
The Deutsche Nationalbibliothek lists this publication in the Deutsche Nationalbibliografie; detailed bibliographic data are available on the Internet at http://dnb.d-nb.de

jovis Verlag GmbH
Kurfürstenstrasse 15/16
10785 Berlin

www.jovis.de

jovis books are available worldwide in selected bookstores. Please contact your nearest bookseller or visit www.jovis.de for information concerning your local distribution.

ISBN 978-3-86859-422-5

For Lucas Asensio-Mah.

Contents

Lifestyled - China-Town

Preface

The research presented in this book is part of a broader research initiative developed through the Health and Places Initiative (HAPI) at Harvard University in Cambridge, Massachusetts. Founded in 2013, HAPI consists of multi-disciplinary groups involving faculty and researchers from both Harvard's Graduate School of Design and the T.H. Chan School of Public Health. This initiative has been engaged with investigating the scope and possibilities for creating healthier places in the future. The ambition of HAPI, as a whole, is to create a forum for understanding the multiple issues that cities face in light of rapid urbanization and an aging population worldwide. Through the coordinated work of different research subgroups within the initiative, the project is invested in developing templates for alternative models of urban development, with particular emphasis on their impact on health and aging.

Much of the work presented within this book was generated by the Prototypes group, a subgroup within HAPI that was established to focus specifically on the development of research on health and place through design. The HAPI Prototypes group was led by the authors and editors of this book: Leire Asensio Villoria and David Syn Chee Mah. The group's primary focus has been on the development of design models and processes that inform or guide readers in the ways that health concerns may be embedded within the main set of design considerations and parameters which organize urban neighborhoods in China.

The research work, writings, and interviews that follow aim to elaborate on the topic of health and the environment for a lay design audience and to offer design research findings and prototypes of healthy neighborhood models for readers invested in the thoughtful development of our urban environments. This book aims to deliver considerations of history, discussions on current challenges, as well as projections for the future. By addressing these challenges with a simultaneously reflective and projective drive, the book aims to raise questions, or offer insights, as to how the ongoing investigation into the relationships between health and place may evolve.

The prototypes research focuses specifically on addressing, through design, a number of important, emerging, place-based public health challenges currently unfolding or anticipated to be significant problems in the coming decades. The design research is specifically situated in China, and concentrates on health at the neighborhood scale within the country's second and third tier cities. The deliberate focus on China was indicated by its massive scale of urban and social transformation, offering a situation where research into healthier models for cities could provide strategies of imminent and immediate utility. However, many of the issues facing China today can be seen as concerns shared by many others in contexts where contemporary public health has global consequences as well as influence. While not always applicable in every circumstance, the issues and proposals offered through the research within this book are intended to provide insights that may spark conversation and reflection on similar issues in other situations.

The book is composed of three main sections. The first section, Public Health and the Design of the Built Environment, focuses on a more general discussion of the relationship between health and place that includes contributed essays by members of the GSD HAPI group, Ann Forsyth and Laura Smead, as well as interviews with leading researchers within the fields of public health, Dr. Ichiro Kawachi and Dr. Gary Evans.

Collectively, a series of essays and a detailed description of the HAPI Prototypes design research project form the second section: The Chinese Superblock. A more context specific series of essays by Peter Rowe with Har Ye Kan and Yu Yifan explicates the history of the Chinese Superblock (the "site" of research) and charts some of the contemporary challenges surrounding existing residential neighborhoods in China. This series is bundled together with an essay by the book's editors on the methods and theoretical positions adopted by the research team with regards to design research to support a detailed overview of the process and findings developed through a sustained investigative project completed by the HAPI Prototypes Group between 2014 and 2016.

The final section showcases the premise and background research, as well as the projects developed in an advanced graduate option studio offered at Harvard's Graduate School of Design in the fall of 2014. The studio was designed to speculate on models for residential neighborhood models for China that foreground public health issues. Contextual concerns surrounding the changing conceptions of collective life, approaches towards the management of the environment, relevant national policies, and the different residential types that have emerged in China are elaborated on in this section in order to provide readers an insight into the specific milieu which the projects are seeking to address.

Acknowledgments

This book emerged from a sustained investment of effort and energy over a period spanning between 2014 until 2016. We benefited greatly from the support, conversations, and feedback from many friends and colleagues. We would like to thank Professors Ann Forsyth and Peter Rowe of HAPI, and Harvard's GSD for giving the HAPI Prototypes team the space and support for developing the projects and book. The help and dedication of our research assistants and associates are also greatly appreciated and we are particularly grateful to Justin Kollar along with Xinhui Li, Bingjie Shi, Wen Wen, Elizabeth Wu, Han Yang and Yujun Yin.

We would also like to thank Dean Mohsen Mostafavi for his consistent support throughout the research project and studio. We are also very thankful to friends and guests who very graciously gave their time to offer comments and feedback in various reviews and discussions including Farshid Moussavi, Dr. Ichiro Kawachi and Dr. Ann Lusk of the Harvard School of Public Health, Dr. Gary Evans of Cornell University, Professor Yu Yifan of Tongji University, Inaki Abalos, Bing Wang, Laura Smead, and Emily Salomon.

Major funding for this research project was provided by Charoen Pokphand Group Co. Ltd.

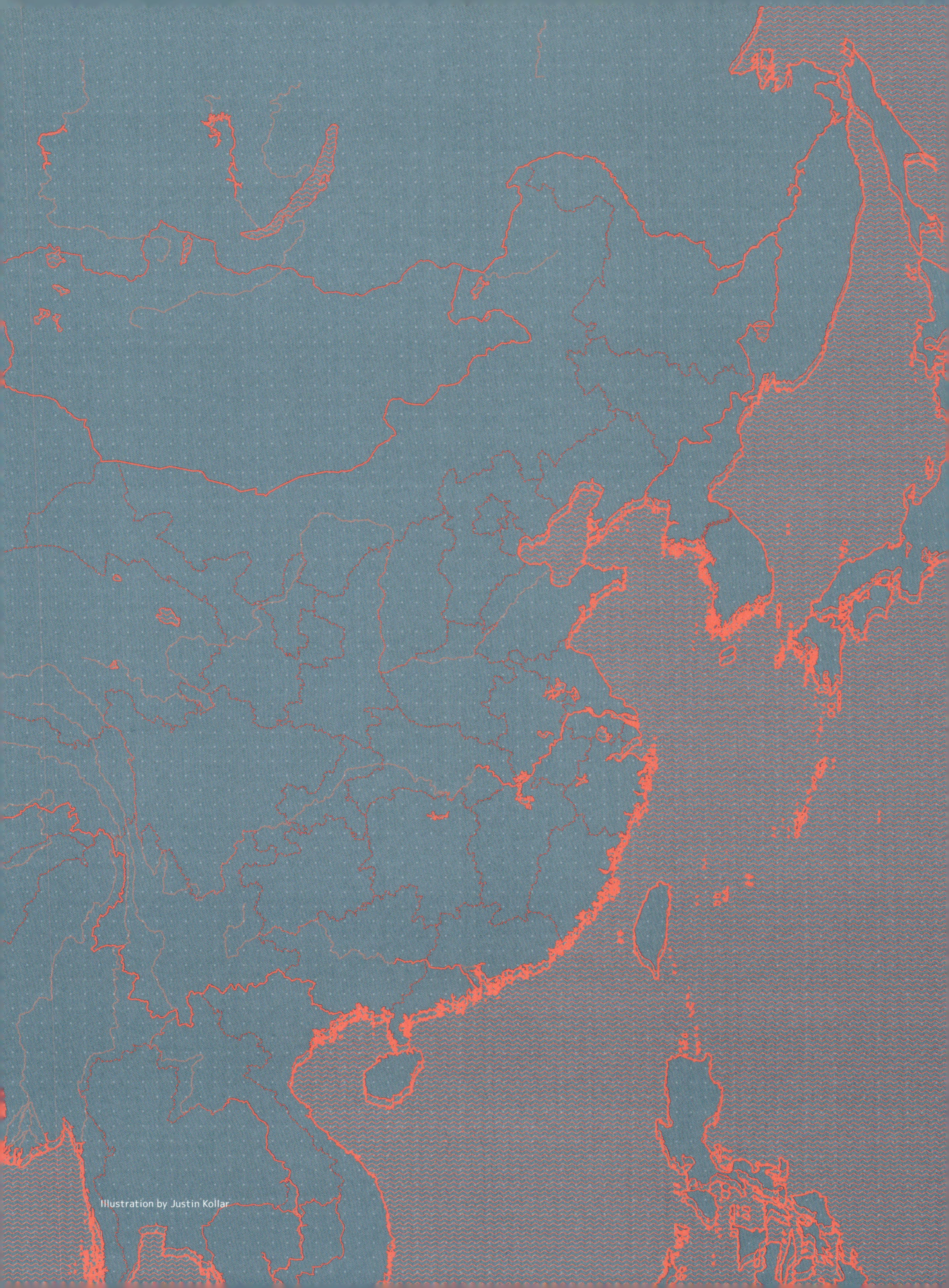

Illustration by Justin Kollar

Public Health and the Design of the Built Environment

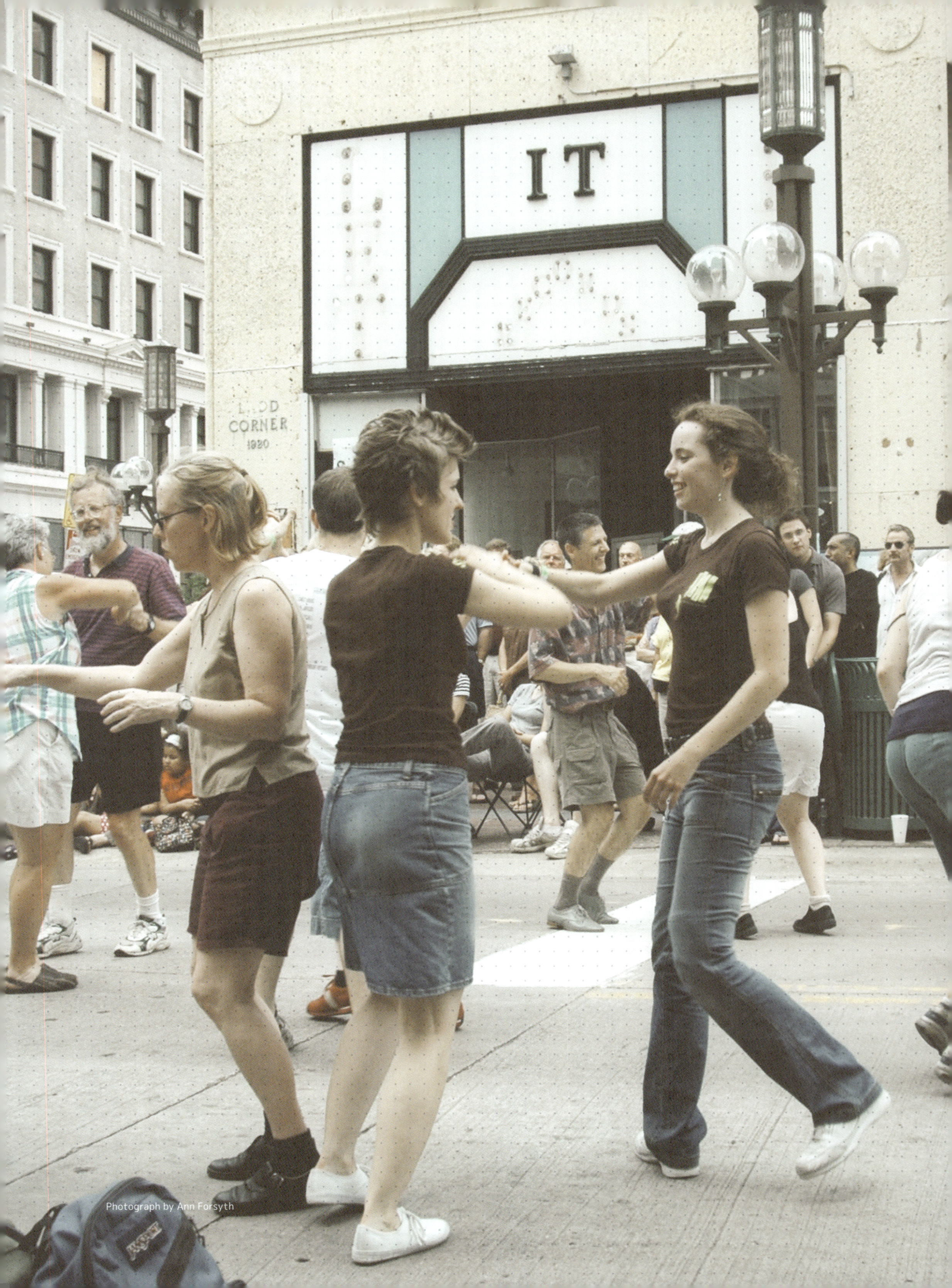

Photograph by Ann Forsyth

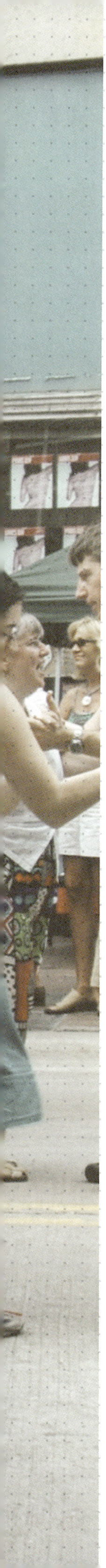

Chapter 1

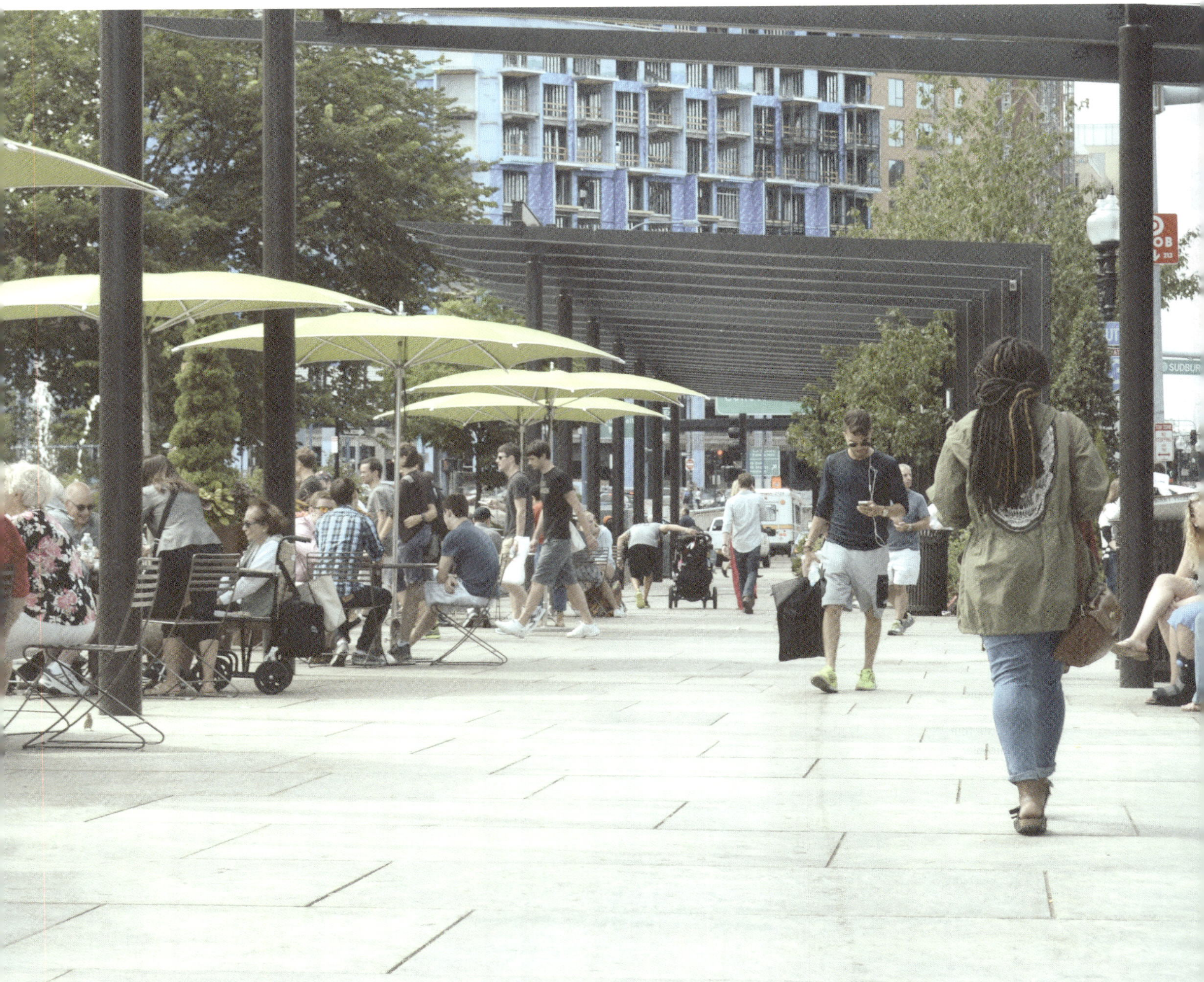

Photograph by Justin Kollar

Lifestyled – Health and Places
Introduction
Leire Asensio Villoria + David Mah

The contextual issues surrounding health have always been important considerations. The relationship between health and place has a persistent history of association where the quality and nature of the built environment have long been seen to play an important role as one of the contextual determinants of health. In parallel to an investment in the study of the compositional (individual influences), a number of public health trends have provoked a more recent resurgence in the contextual (environmental influences) approaches towards addressing these wider concerns. The built environment and the kinds of life practices that it enables have become a focus for the public health fields due to the perceived inadequacy of relying on compositional factors alone to comprehend and address contemporary and emerging public health issues. Given that place and the way that it is organized or designed is recognized as being a potentially significant influence for fostering healthy lifestyles and the well-being of its populations, it has become imperative for designers to engage with the relationship between health and place. This book is intended primarily for readers from the design field who wish to study this connection. It is structured to provide considerations of past, present, and future concerns that have, currently impacted, and are likely to impact in the future, the way that the built environment has been, is, or will be designed.

To offer the reader an immediate and tangible frame of reference for the issues and work presented in this book, a number of key contemporary public health concerns are introduced here. As a consequence of the urgency and scale associated with these considerations, the issues that have been addressed by the research work are the same ones that have captured the public imagination. Furthermore, these are issues that have the capacity to affect the ways in which we live out our lives, or more specifically alter our lifestyles. These concerns range from the prevalence of what are known as lifestyle diseases to the global demographic shift towards a rapidly aging population and the impacts that our mismanagement of the environment have on our own collective health.

Key Contemporary Public Health Concerns: Chronic Diseases

In the nineteenth to early twentieth centuries, much of the preoccupation and immediate focus of public health revolved around acute and contagious diseases. The Cholera, Typhoid and Tuberculosis epidemics had a dramatic, and typically, devastating effect on the burgeoning urban populations of the time. Both design and public health's preoccupation with these illnesses were born of necessity.

Unfortunately, in many parts of the world, these illnesses still exist as real and present challenges and the embedding of basic sanitary infrastructure and practices in human conurbations remains an important and greatly needed operation. The design professions have a long history of engagement with these concerns and were significantly transformed by the hygiene movement and its associated reform campaigns during the rapid industrialization and urbanization of the west during the nineteenth to early twentieth centuries.[1]

Globally, however, chronic or "lifestyle" diseases are emerging as one of the most significant health issues of our time. This aggregation of largely preventable diseases, associated with lifestyle choices, has been described by the World Health Organization as an invisible epidemic. The WHO estimates that 60% of all deaths in the world can be attributed to chronic diseases.[2] The assumption that these so-called "lifestyle" diseases are illnesses of prosperity, limited primarily to developed countries is misplaced. In fact, a far greater number of chronic disease deaths in the world occur in low and middle income countries, signaling a major global public health concern.[3]

1 See the chapter; "Environments, Populations and Health" for a longer discussion on this topic.

2 The WHO lists the four main non communicable or chronic diseases as cardiovascular diseases, chronic respiratory diseases and diabetes as well as cancers.

3 The mortality, morbidity, and disability rate attributed to the major chronic diseases currently account for almost 60% of all deaths and 43% of the global burden of disease. By 2020, the contribution of chronic disease is expected to rise to 73% of all deaths and 60% of the global burden of disease. Moreover, 79% of the deaths attributed to these diseases occur in the developing countries. (World Health Organization)

Figure 1 Prevalence of diabetes in the chinese population.

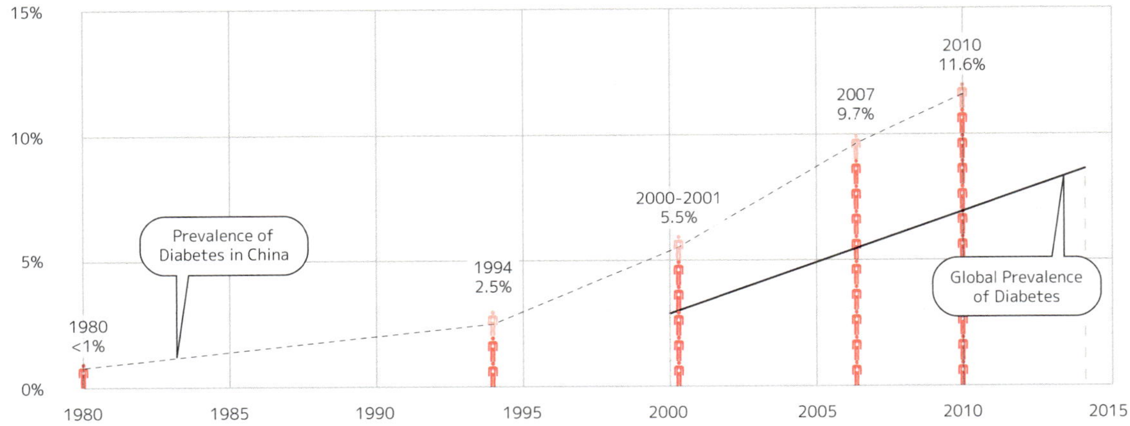

Source: Journal of the American Medical Association, 2013, Survey

4 The Lancet 2014, 716. It is also projected in the referenced article that non-communicable diseases make up 70% of the total disease burden for China.

5 World Health Organization (Department of Measurement and Health Information, 2010)

6 WHO cancer fact sheet.

7 Xu et al. 2013.

When considering the specific case of China, over 80% of the countries' current mortality rate is said to be a consequence of non-communicable diseases.[4] Cardiovascular disease alone is the leading cause of death worldwide and according to a study by the Chinese Society of Cardiology, China can attribute over 40% of total deaths every year[5] to cardiac illnesses, a rate more than double that of typical European countries. Furthermore, the WHO projects annual cardiovascular events in China to surge by 50% with trends in diabetes, cholesterol, blood pressure, and smoking contributing a projected 23% increase.

Cancer, another major chronic disease, is also recorded to have steadily increasing global rates with predictions that prevalence of the disease will rise by 70% over the next two decades.[6] China has suffered one of the highest rates of increase contributing to 27% of the world's total cancer deaths, and this trajectory is expected to continue.

In addition to cancer and cardiovascular diseases, diabetes is also emerging as a significant global problem with forecasts for it to become the seventh leading cause of death by 2030. However, it has already emerged as a much more acute concern in China, with an alarming prevalence that exceeds the global averages. According to a 2010 survey for diabetes in the country, it was found that close to 12% of adults or 114 million people,[7] (roughly equivalent to Nigeria's total population), suffer from diabetes with type II diabetes being pervasive. These numbers suggest that China may have the largest population of diabetes sufferers in the world.

In parallel to this pattern, an unexpected surge in worldwide obesity has also evolved into a major worldwide health challenge. At a global scale, obesity has been recognized as a pandemic, by the WHO. This inflammatory disease defies assumptions of its association with prosperity alone, where as it currently presents a significant concern for both developed and developing countries. The growth

Figure 2 Obese population in China as compared to the population of the UK.

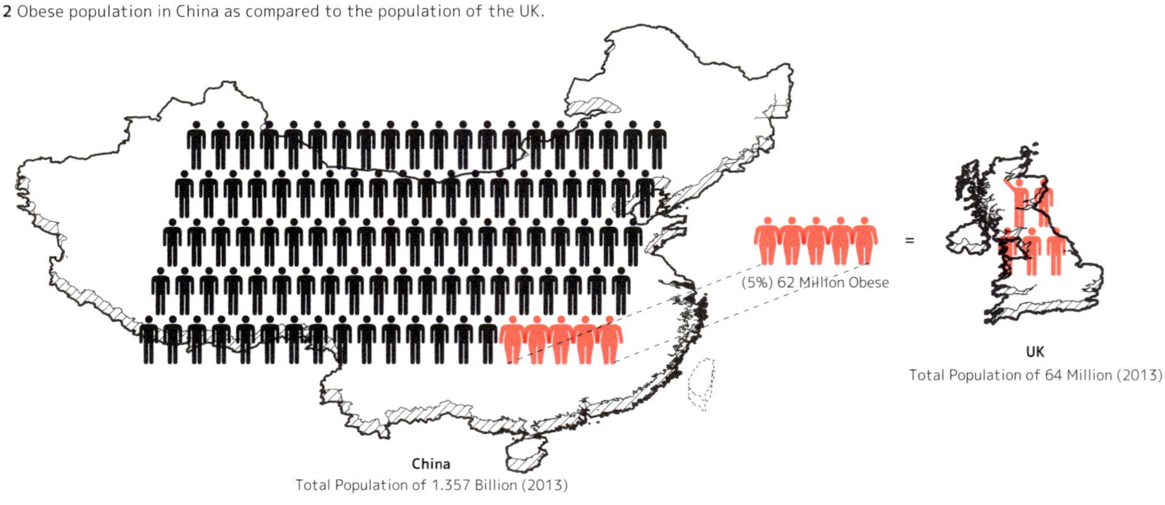

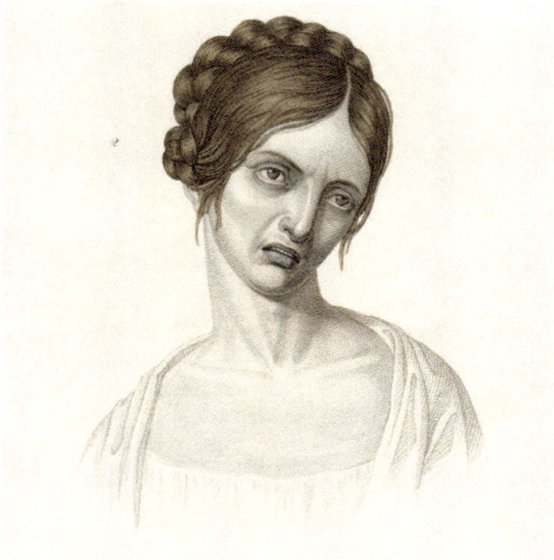

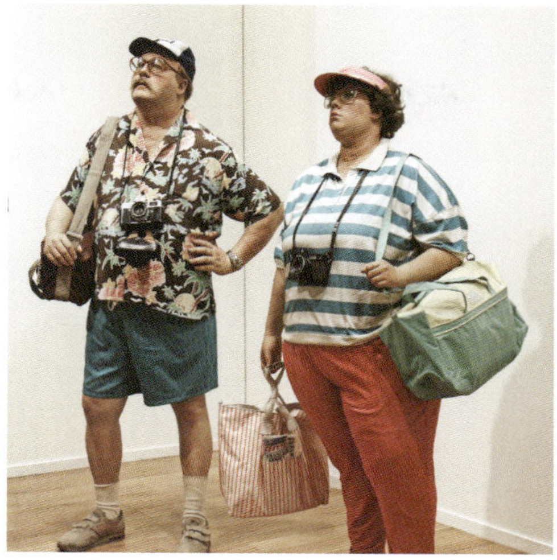

Figure 3 (Left) A young woman depicted after contracting cholera in the first European epidemic in 1831.

Figure 4 (Right) Tourists II, Duane Hansen, 1988. Courtesy Van de Weghe Fine Art, New York.

in the global population of overweight or obese individuals from 857 million in 1980 to 2.1 billion in 2013, indicates that the problem has rapidly expanded to affect nearly 30% of the total global population. Although type II diabetes, a prevailing concern in China, is linked to obesity, when taking a cursory glance at general numbers related to obesity incidence in the country, it would appear that, statistically speaking, it doesn't pose a significant problem. According to the WHO 2011 Global Database on Body Mass Index, China is among the countries with the smallest proportion of its population affected with a less than 5% obesity rate. However, given the size of China's population, this translates to roughly 62 million people, a population approximately equal to that of the United Kingdom, making it the country with the second largest number of affected individuals in the world. Even more significant is the rapid growth in the obesity rate for children, where young boys suffer a rate double to those of adult males with an overall overweight/obesity rate of 23%. Out of a survey of 188 countries, children in China were found to have had the fourth fastest growth in obesity rates between 1980 and 2013.[8]

8 All data on obesity rates from Marie Ng, PhD. et al. 2014.

Within this short summary of the main public health challenges posed by chronic illnesses, we clearly see their current and projected impact on the global population. These trends are anticipated to persist if little is done to address the modifiable risks that lead to many of these diseases. Modifiable risks for the major chronic diseases are common and include poor diet, physical inactivity, tobacco use, and environmental factors such as pollution. In addition to any number of strategies such as public education campaigns promoting physical activity or healthy eating and increasing taxes on cigarettes for instance, the design and planning of our built environments is also a crucial factor in addressing chronic diseases. Key among the concerns related to the built environment are the careful cultivation of physical activity and food environments, as well as providing the appropriate infrastructure or places that may contribute

Figure 5 Population in China with type II diabetes compared to the population of Nigeria.

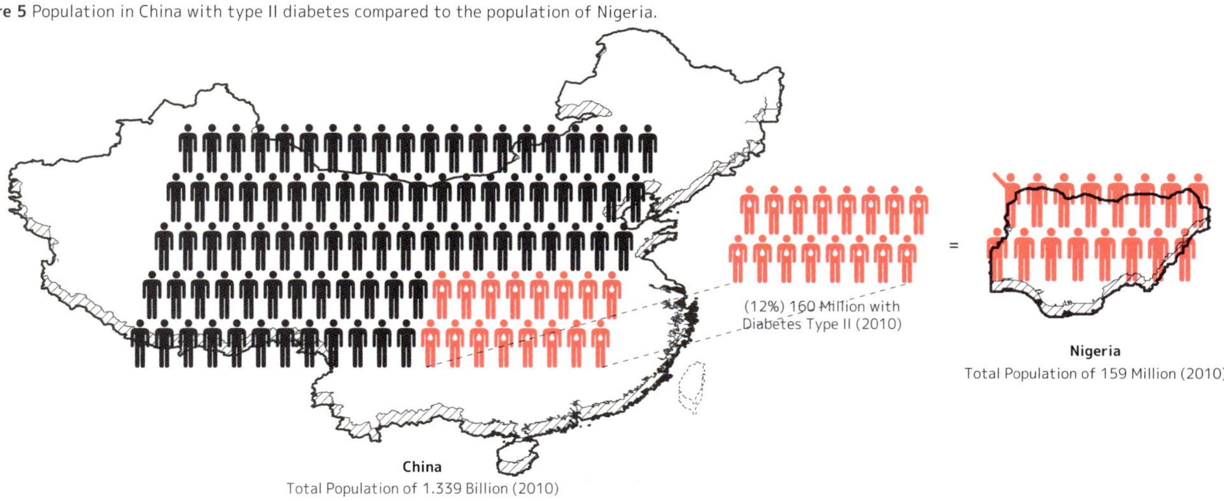

Figure 6 Contribution of chronic disease to the mortality, morbidity, and disability rates.

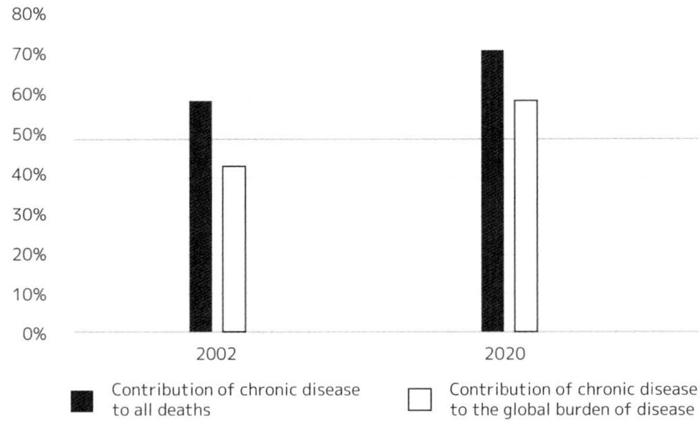

Source: The World Health Report 2002: Reducing Risks, Promoting Healthy Life, WHO, 2002

to improving the quality of life of its citizens. Architecture, planning, and landscape architecture have all contributed significantly to the ways in which the built environment affords improvements in people's lifestyles (with the converse also being true where the physical environment can also be a barrier to healthier living). If indeed chronic diseases can be considered as being partially a consequence of modifiable practices in people's lifestyles, the spaces and places within which they carry out their daily lives are significant influences in facilitating this.

In China, the current modifiable risk factors that are commonly contributing to the steady increase in chronic diseases include the changes in the food environment and shifting dietary habits coupled with the rise in physical inactivity as the workforce changes. Clearly the great social, economic, and environmental changes that China has been undergone area a significant underlying factor. Also important is the lack of emphasis, until recently, in preventative care, where as most effort had been given to treating the final stages of a disease. Even more significant for designers, the WHO identifies the nature and patterns of urbanization as potential accomplices in the rise of chronic or lifestyle diseases, stating that "city living can impose certain limitations on the way in which people live, and restricts their opportunities to be healthy."

The pervasiveness of lifestyle diseases has brought with it tension between advocates for the social and individual responsibilities for health. The growing argument for promoting personal responsibility is partially based on the notion that these illnesses are brought on by people's bad choices. This contentious issue has been used to argue against egalitarian healthcare or more specifically to make individuals liable for their own behavior. This recognition of illness associated with choices is reflected in the move by some insurance companies to penalize individuals who engage in what are deemed as risky lifestyle choices such as smoking.[9]

The emphasis in preventative medicine resonates with the concept and practices of biopolitics,[10] where the governance and management of risks facing a population's health and productivity is proliferated through strategies of prevention. Biopolitics is regularly and periodically disseminated so that it may become embedded within accepted social practices leading to self-monitoring and self-regulation. It aims to minimize the actual direct engagement of the disciplinary, or in the case of healthcare, curative care practices. In this case, control over a population through preventive medicine is manifested through the identification of "*potentials for sickness*" and a subsequent "*transfer of responsibility and agency to the patient*."[11]

However, studies have suggested that the practice of healthy lifestyles may not always be associated with personal choice, particularly in light of the evidence that the majority of these modifiable risks are more prevalent within poorer socioeconomic groups. This evidence suggests that there may in fact be unequal access to the choices that enable healthy practices such as healthy diets and physical exercise. The mandate of public health has typically been associated with an equitable and collective approach

9 See for instance Stoller-Conrad 2012.

10 Wallenstein 2009. Also see Michel Foucault's Lectures at the College De France between 1977 – 1979. Giles Deleuze's notion of societies of control, elaborated in his 1990 essay; "Postscripts on Societies of Control" converges with Foucault's concept of biopolitics in its explication of contemporary models of governing as control mechanisms that operate in a dispersed, "smooth" manner, diverging from Foucault's earlier work on disciplinary societies.

11 Wallenstein 2009, 37.

Figure 7 Population aged 60 or over: world and development regions, 1950-2050.

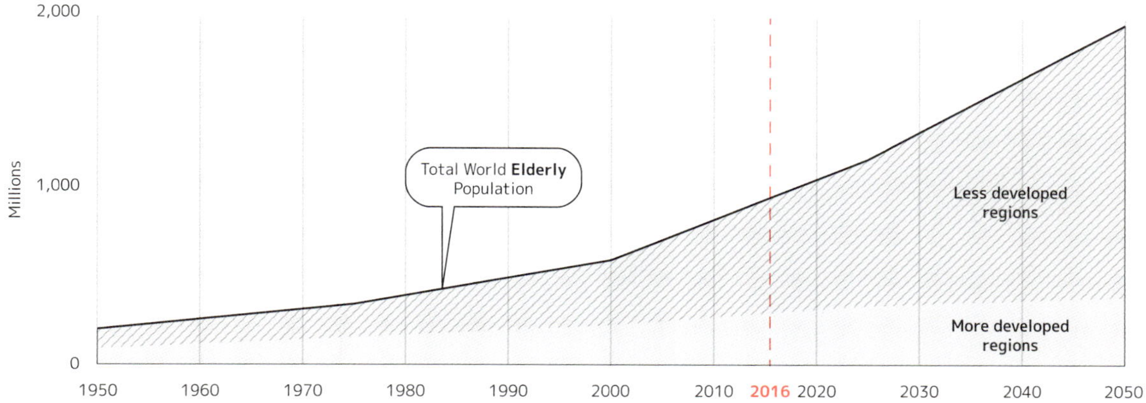

Source: World Population Aging: 1950-2050, the United Nations, 2013

towards healthcare and as a result, this recognition of the inequalities in access to healthy life practices has encouraged consideration of the environmental (social, physical etc) determinants of health.

> "Personal control, socially supportive relationships, and restoration from stress and fatigue are all affected by properties of the built environment." (Dr. Gary Evans)

The desire for a balance between individual and social responsibility for health has prompted the adoption of ecological perspectives on public health, emphasizing "the reciprocal relationships between people and their environments."[12] A growing interest in the capacity for the physical environment to provide "healthy defaults" or "nudges,"[13] coming from the public health and behavioral economics fields, offers designers some insight into the ways in which we may engage with the promotion of healthier, more active lifestyles. Can we organize our environments to offer healthy options as the easier default? Or by making them desirable and engaging, is it possible to stimulate people to adopt more active and vital life practices?

Ongoing research on the psychological effects of the built environment that affect the mental well-being of its occupants is another emerging body of knowledge that offers some insight into the affective capacities of places.[14] Equally significant is the mounting interest in the social determinants of health,[15] where there is a burgeoning recognition that supportive social relationships and networks are important influences on health. The realization by the public health and design fields, that place and the physical environment influences these factors, provides avenues through which we as designers may further our contribution to the arena of public health and move it beyond the approaches of sanitation and hygiene established during the Modern period.

Aging Populations

The aging of the global population is a trend that most of the countries in the world are facing; the global proportion of people aged sixty years or over has gone from 9.2% in 1990 to 11.7% in 2013, with forecasts for it to reach 21.1% by 2050. In actual numbers, this represents a growth from 841 million people in 2013 to a projected 2 billion elderly people in 2050.[16] Of this elderly population, two thirds live in the developing world, with this proportion forecasted to be close to 80% by 2050.

The anxiety caused by this shift towards an older population is rooted in the understanding that this may have major social and economic consequences by creating dramatic imbalances in the old-age support ratios (the relationship between the numbers of working-age adults per elderly person in the population). Anticipated support as well as pressure on the health infrastructures of many countries is expected to go hand in hand with this tendency. This pressure is exacerbated by the associated likelihood for chronic disease incidence and disability to rise even further in old age as it is a key unmodifiable risk for these conditions.

12 Minkler 1999, 121-141.

13 See Thaler 2008.

14 For an example of this, see the work of Dr. Gary Evans. In particular his article "The Built Environment and Health" in the Journal of Urban Health, as well as the interview with Dr. Evans in this publication.

15 For an example of this, see the work of Dr. Ichiro Kawachi. His books on *Neighborhoods and Health* offer a balanced consideration of social health factors being influenced by contextual as well as compositional factors. For more information see his book edited with Lisa Berkman; *Neighborhoods and Health: An Overview*, as well as the interview with Dr. Kawachi included in this publication.

16 Figures from a report released by the United Nations in 2013 entitled, World Population Aging 1950-2050.

Figure 8 Proportion of population aged 60 or over in China.

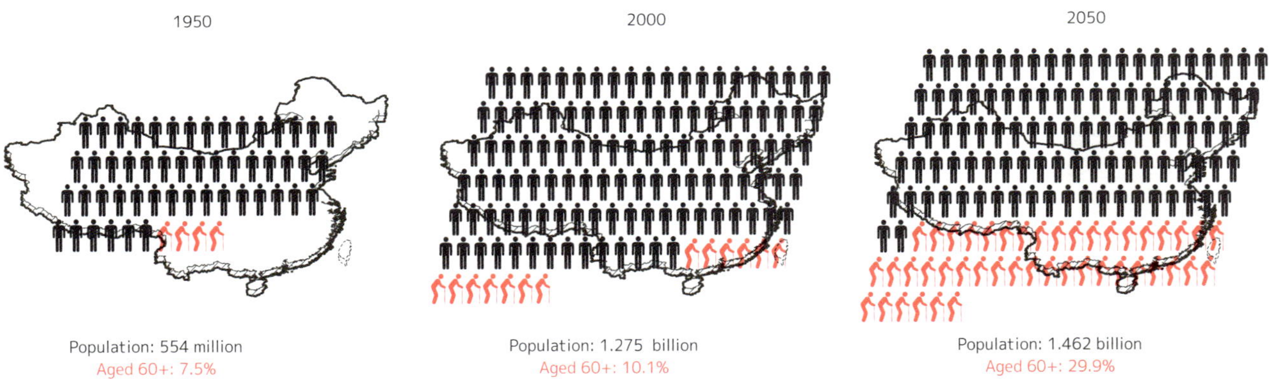

Source: World Population Aging: 1950-2050, the United Nations, 2013

Sensitivity to environmental pressures on health is also elevated amongst the elderly population, making the consequences of climate change, environmental disasters, and pollution likely to have a more acute effect on public health as a result. It is also fair to assume that much of this growing elderly population will be economically vulnerable as well; the UN's 2013 report on the elderly population estimates that poverty amongst this demographic group in some developing countries is often higher than that of the population as a whole. This presents a major challenge especially within countries with inadequate social safety nets.

On the flipside, in some countries, with strategies to safeguard the income security of the elderly through such efforts as actively integrating a generally older population in the workforce, there is a growing capacity for elderly people to live independently (alone or with their spouse only). In many countries, they have been found to be financially independent through their own labor income or savings, earnings from assets, and through public transfers.[17] In many developed countries, this expansion of the elderly demographic is also creating a new range of lifestyle groups associated with what has been called the "third age." The third age is a term coined by British sociologist, Peter Laslett which refers to the "fulfillment period"[18] of life, where old age is viewed as an opportunity for travel, further education and (for those who have access or may afford it), a generally pleasurable lifestyle of leisure.

This demographic shift has also been recognized as a significant market opportunity, where people aged over sixty were estimated to have spent more than $8 trillion worldwide, this is likely to grow to $15 trillion by 2020. Studies have found that in the US, people aged fifty and over possess 80% of the country's financial assets and account for half of its discretionary spending.[19] In the UK, 35% of this same age bracket own 75% of the country's total wealth.[20] With this economic clout together with a strong political lobby[21] the aged have the growing capability to greatly influence many major public issues. They also have the ability to impact the built environment, where strategies for facilitating aging in place within existing neighborhoods or the construction of new models for age-friendly or exclusively elderly communities (exemplified perhaps in the most extreme cases by Sun City, Arizona, a thirty-eight square kilometer retirement community) can drive the transformation of how neighborhoods are planned or renovated.

Following on from this, public health's preoccupations may no longer be restricted to ensuring or safeguarding a productive population. Rather than optimizing conditions for productivity, the focus may instead be on facilitating leisure and social opportunities. To enable the development of healthy, supportive social environments could even more prominently influence the construction and renewal of cities. Compounded with this is the need to make cities more inclusive and accessible to different levels of physical ability, with many building codes and universal design or accessibility rules in some countries becoming even more rigorous. All of these factors combined, have the potential to augment the built environment and design practice in significant ways.

17 Ibid

18 Laslett 1991

19 Figures from a report conducted by the global management consultancy firm, AT Kearney, "Understanding the Needs and Consequences of the Aging Consumer."

20 Figures from the building society and mortgage lender; Abbey.

21 The increase in proportion of elderly people can result in strong lobbies. This can be seen particularly in the lobbying of governments for healthcare and income security an example of which can be seen recently in Canada where partly as a result of lobbying, the government allocated $11,000 per person aged 65 and over (in contrast with $20,00 per person under 45) for healthcare in its 2015 budget.

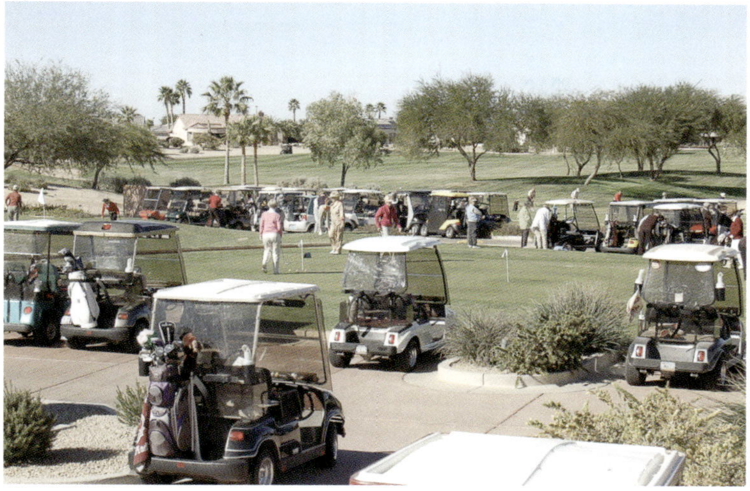

Figure 9 Sun City, Arizona

When looking specifically to China, in the year 2000 the population of individuals sixty-five years and older was close to 90 million, with it expected to be well over 300 million by 2050. Much of this can be attributed to the success of public health initiatives that have contributed to the extended longevity of its population (where the average life expectancy has increased from forty years in 1950 to seventy years now). However, the age imbalance has given rise to the 4-2-1 phenomena with a reverse pyramid of burden of four grandparents to two parents and finally to one grandchild.

Within traditional Chinese Confucian values of filial piety, there is an expectation that the younger generations are obligated to be responsible for the care of their older generations. This is not only a family responsibility, but also a legal obligation since 2013 when the Chinese National Council made filial piety a law. Named the Rights and Interests of Elderly People, the law requires children to regularly visit and care for their elderly parents. There are of course significant changes in China's social practices as a result of its massive economic and urban transformation that undermine traditional family values and obligations. Such changes range from mass urban migration and the decline in traditional co-residence due to the changes in housing to the unrealistic burdens on younger generations resulting from the aforementioned 4-2-1 phenomena. Without this traditional familial support, it is unclear how the elderly may be cared for given that there has not been an effective transition to institutionalized living (institutionalized living for the elderly in China is merely 1-2% of the total elderly population).[22]

22 Gu et al. 2007, 871-83

In addition to increased longevity, one of the catalysts for the aging population in China can also be attributed to the one-child policy enacted in 1980. In 2013 the one-child policy was relaxed, however the number of couples who have chosen to apply for this privilege has been surprisingly low (only 7% of those eligible have since applied). The possibility of persistent fertility rates at below replacement levels add to the general anxiety that China may face a population decline; some have projected that within a 150-year period (1950 to 2100), China's population will grow to 1.4 billion and then subsequently decline to 500 million.

It is clear that as designers we will need to rethink the approaches and assumptions embedded in current design processes. One way to reconsider our design approach may be to look at the subjects and images that have come to symbolize health and have been used in framing design choices in health.

One of the most emblematic figures in the history of Modern architecture and urbanism can be seen in the young, virile boxer depicted in Le Corbusier's hanging gardens, sketched in 1928 for his Algiers housing project. The ideal of health is personified by a solitary, young, athletic man, punishing himself to attain and display his physical fitness in an airy, bright, and open yet clearly private and discrete court in the sky.

Skip ahead fifty years to 1978 and Madelon Vriedensorp's illustration in Rem Koolhaas' book, *Delirious New York*: "A Machine for Metropolitan Bachelors" depicting metropolitan bachelors eating oysters nude on the ninth floor of the Manhattan Downtown Athletic Club with boxing gloves. A much more hedonistic illustration of health, the image is a celebration of a "metropolitan lifestyle."[23] The

23 See *AD (Architectural Design)*, OMA Special Issue. 1975.

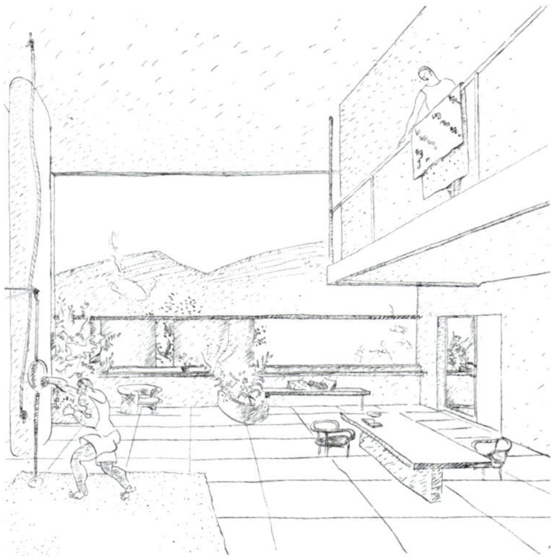

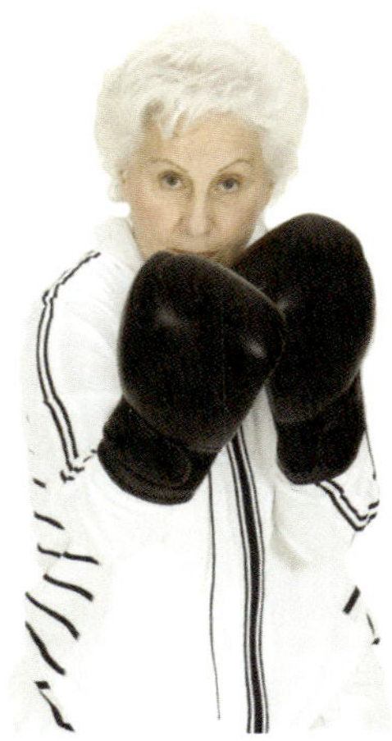

Figure 10 (Top, Left) Le Corbusier's sketch of apartment with a boxer 1928, © F.L.C. / ADAGP, Paris / Artists Rights Society (ARS), New York 2016.

Figure 11 (Top, Right) Elderly "third age" boxer. Stefano Valle © 123RF.com.

drawing is also significant for its location within an interior that envelopes a "culture of congestion" that supports the serendipitous juxtaposition of activities portrayed in this image. But again, the avatars for this lifestyle, just like Le Corbusier's image, are fit, young men associated with boxing, a sport so visceral and violent that it is perceived to be exclusive to youth.

In light of trends such as the aging population where the contemporary subject may no longer be just the young, our urban environment may not be appropriately framed by a project that is guided by any singular lifestyle but should broaden its constituency towards a complex agglomeration of diverse subjects. Both Le Corbusier and Koolhaas' boxers could very well be protagonists in the contemporary city, together with a multitude of other subjects; women, children and even third age boxers included. What is evident is the need for the built environment to enable and support the lifestyles of many different actors and to accept a scenario of the city not just as a site of growth and production but one that acknowledges the importance for it to also be the site for leisure as well as active inclusive social communication or interaction.[24]

24 For a discussion on the value of social interaction in health and in particular for the elderly, see the interview with Dr. Ichiro Kawachi in this book.

Healthy Environments

Equating the health of the environment with human health has been widely accepted as common sense, where everything from the environmental movement to major slum clearance campaigns of the past have all been motivated in part by this association. A range of significant events throughout history offer us insights into the ways that the health of the environment can have significant consequences for the health of populations.

Perusing the following timeline included in this book, we are able to see many instances where the communication of this association has captivated the public imagination. Rachel Carson's; *The Silent Spring*, Al Gore's *An Inconvenient Truth* and Chai Jing's *Under The Dome* are just a small number of popular films and books that have brought to light, the issues surrounding the negative impact of certain human activities on the environment and its subsequent effect on our health.

If we also look back at the evolution of a city emblematic of the west's rapid industrialization and urbanization period, we can see the impact of events such as the 1666 Great Fire of London, the 1858 Great Stink as well as The Great Smog of 1962 on mobilizing change in the ways that we organize the environment to ensure the health and safety of the population. Out of these three events emerged England's early building codes, a massive sanitation infrastructure building campaign, and the Clean Airs Act, all measures that would contribute significantly to public health and the transformation of the physical environment.

It is clear that pollution persists as a significant risk to human health today and that the mandate for carefully considering the ways in which we configure the built environment should also be maintained.

In many countries currently experiencing the culmination of rapid urbanization and industrialization, we can see that this has had an acute impact on the health of its populations. The elevated rates of respiratory and heart diseases as well as cancer in China can be partially attributed to the increases in industrialization and its associated pollution. The phenomena of cancer villages in China are another indicator of the great public health problem that is posed by an environment damaged by industry. Even more significant is the finding in the 2010 Global Burden of Diseases, Injuries, and Risk Factors Study published in The Lancet, that air pollution in China accounted for the premature deaths of 1.2 million of its citizens.

In addition to industrial activity, the impact of our lifestyles on the levels of pollution can also be considerable. Dramatic elevations in pollution and emissions can be brought about by changes in lifestyles, even more so in circumstances where large populations rapidly transform their lifestyles and economic circumstances. One of the more prevalent ways to study the impact of our lifestyles and human activity on environmental health has been through the measure of carbon emissions and carbon footprints as an indicator of our impact on climate change. The hazards to human health from climate change include the projected increases in extreme climatic events (heat waves and droughts), incidences of natural disasters (flooding and sea level rise) along with the exacerbation of smog. Despite being regarded primarily as a cause of larger, global problems, carbon dioxide emissions and concentrations have recently been identified as also posing a significant localized problem that can have a more immediate effect on human health. Based on a 2008 study by Stanford University professor of engineering; Dr. Mark Jacobson, carbon dioxide was found to affect health and life expectancy more acutely in areas where it is concentrated and emitted locally.

It would be fair to conclude that much of the environmental health concerns in China, when using carbon emissions as a gauge, should then be addressed by a range of measures that are often beyond the purview of designers, such as regulating industrial practices and promoting renewable, clean energy. At face value, the individual lifestyles of the Chinese population are not the main contributors to pollution per se. Based on a recent study, simply measuring household carbon production, Chinese household emissions are considerably lower than the United States. In the United States, household emissions make up 40% of the total carbon discharge, significantly more than in China, and similarly its per capita emissions are five times higher.[25] Yet China is estimated to have the highest carbon emissions in the world. Like the West's rapid urbanization in the nineteenth and early twentieth centuries, the bulk of the responsibility for environmental degradation is attributed to industrial practices.

25 Glaeser and Kahn 2010.

However, while China's pollution is largely associated with the intensity and types of industrial activity it hosts, urbanization or the planning of the built environment does contribute to the pollution of the atmosphere in ways which can affect human health more directly. Part of this link between environmental and human health and urbanization and the lifestyles it promotes is facilitated by current urbanization practices that privilege private automobile use as the dominant mode of transportation for its population. Policies and planning practices that favor sprawl have been prevalent in China's recent development. While automobile use in China may be seen to have a comparatively smaller impact than industry on carbon emissions, the associated particulate-based pollution have a significant impact on the rise in respiratory illnesses as well as cancer. By carefully reconsidering the prevailing urban models and practices in China that support sprawl, we may potentially offer an environment that facilitates other lifestyles beyond the ones prescribed by normative models of development. The reorganization of typical design defaults for our neighborhoods and cities may offer the possibility of a healthier lifestyle that reduces the impact our lives have on the environment, and through a feedback loop, improve our own collective health.

While the direct effects of the environment on human health are a pressing concern, a healthy place in today's terms would also need to broaden to encapsulate the affordances[26] that the built environment may allow for nurturing social and mental health. While addressing pollution and emissions are of great importance, any proposed reconfiguration of the physical environment in the name of health needs to also take into account the quality of life of its population as much as hygiene and clean air. As designers, we need to meet the challenge to address the wider considerations of the notion of health set down by the

26 Affordances relate to the opportunities and constraints that the built environment provides for certain behavior or lifestyle practices. See the interview with Dr. Gary Evans in this book for a more detailed definition of this term.

World Health Organization's definition of the term which encapsulates the physical, social, and mental well-being. The effect of the built environment on mental well-being and on enabling the building of social networks and capital are all matters that designers would have to consider when offering proposals for models of healthy places.

Lifestyled

All of the contemporary and emerging public health issues discussed here signal an opportunity for designers of the built environment to affect health by considering the links between places and lifestyles. How can we as designers impact or influence lifestyle practices? An ecological approach is one that takes into account the interconnected or relational links between places and the environment with people and the ways they may live their lives. This offers us the possibility to enable opportunities for healthier lifestyles by constructing and choreographing the built environment. Even more significantly, beyond encouraging and enabling healthy life practices, as designers, we will benefit from resolving how attaining and maintaining health can be seen as less of a punitive measure. Being healthy can sometimes be regarded as a process of self-discipline and self-sacrifice. However, our challenge as designers, is to reinterpret healthy life practices as opportunities to enrich both the individual and collective quality of life through the enhancement of our shared built environment.

Through this book, we hope to elaborate on the opportunities offered to designers in engaging with public health not simply as obligation but as a means to deepen our own disciplines and professions. This book is divided into three specific sections, starting with a series of essays, interviews with renowned public health researchers, and timelines that offer a general discussion on the relationship between health and place. More specifically, it presents an account of the impacts that the collaboration between the design and public health fields have had on our built environments to date and offers projections for the future. A second section offers more situated and context-specific elaborations on the Chinese situation, and in particular, the typical Chinese superblock as a model of a neighborhood (the "site" of the research work). Finally the results of the design research projects, prototypes and models of block configurations that embed health considerations, are showcased and discussed with relevant essays on important themes associated with the work. This also involve elaborations on the value and methods pursued in deploying design as a form of research, an ambition that the HAPI design prototypes group is deeply invested in pursuing.

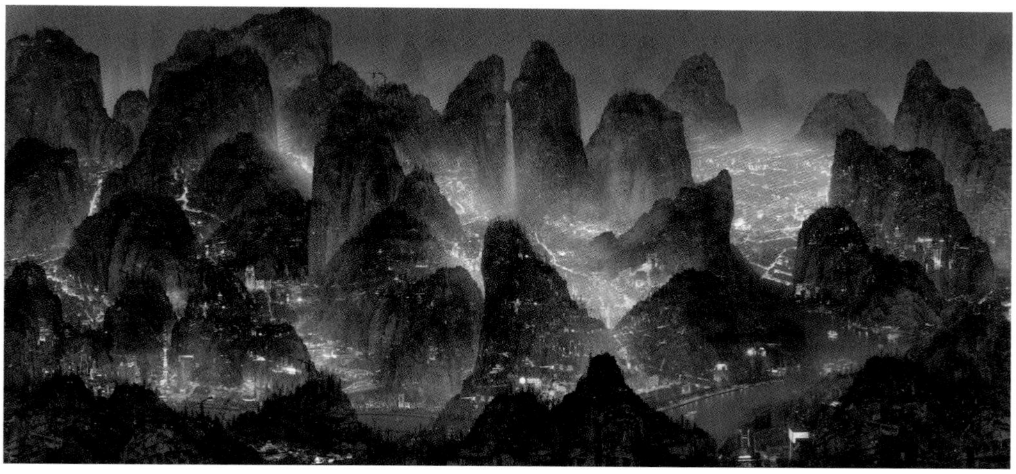

Figure 12 (Left) Yang, Yongliang, 2012, "The Moonlight—the landscape without night".

Figure Credits

Figure 3, *A young woman of Vienna who died of cholera, depicted four hours before death*, 1831, coloured stipple engraving, Wellcome Library, London. Creative Commons Attribution 4.0 International.

Figure 4, Hansen, Duane 1988, *Tourists II*, sculpture. Courtesy Van de Weghe Fine Art, New York.

Figure 9, Muslin, Nancy 2015, Sun City Grand, photograph. http://nancymuslin.com/active-adult-communities/sun-city-grand/.

Figure 10, Le Corbusier 1928, *Boxing in the Hanging Gardens of a Collective Apartment*, sketch, © F.L.C. / ADAGP, Paris / Artists Rights Society (ARS), New York 2016.

Figure 11 Valle, Stefano *Elderly 'third age' boxer*, photograph. © 123RF.com.

Figure 12, Yang, Yongliang, 2012, 'The Moonlight—the landscape without night,' *The Moonlight*, © Yang Yongliang.

References

AD (Architectural Design), OMA Special Issue, 1975, John Wiley & Sons, Ltd, London.

AT Kearney 2013, 'Understanding the Needs and Consequences of the Ageing Consumer,' Accessed 07 August 2015. https://www.atkearney.com/documents/10192/682603/Understanding+the+Needs+and+Consequences+of+the+Aging+Consumer.pdf/6c25ffa3-0999-4b5c-8ff1-afdca0744fdc,

Editorial, 30 August 2014, 'Obesity: A Growing Threat to Health in China,' *The Lancet* 384 (9945), p. 716.

Evans, Gary 2003 December, 'The Built Environment and Mental Health,' *The Journal of Urban Health* 80 (4), pp. 536-555.

Foucault, Michel 2007, *Security, Territory, Population: Lectures at the Collège de France 1977-1978*, Michel Senellart, François Ewald, Alessandro Fontana, and Arnold I. Davidson (eds.), transl. Graham Burchell, Palgrave Macmillan, London.

Foucault, Michel 2008 *The Birth of Biopolitics: Lectures at the Collège de France, 1978-1979*, Michel Senellart, François Ewald, Alessandro Fontana, and Arnold I. Davidson (eds), transl. Graham Burchell, Palgrave Macmillan, London.

Glaeser, Edward L and Kahn, Matthew E. 2010, 'The Greenness of Cities: Carbon Dioxide Emissions and Urban Development,' *Journal of Urban Economics*.

Gu, Danan; Dupre, Matthew E.; and Liu, Guangya 2007, 'Characteristics of the Institutionalized and Community-Residing Oldest-Old in China,' *Social Science and Medicine* 64 (4), pp. 871-83.

Journal of the American Medical Association, 2013 Survey.

Kawachi, Ichiro and Berkman, Lisa (eds) 2003, *Neighborhoods and Health: An Overview*, Oxford University Press, New York, p. 29.

Laslett, Peter 1991, *A Fresh Map of Life: The Emergence of the Third Age*, Harvard University Press, Cambridge, MA.

Marie Ng, PhD. et al. 2014 August 30– September 5, 'Global, regional, and national prevalence of overweight and obesity in children and adults during 1980–2013: a systematic analysis for the Global Burden of Disease Study 2013,' *The Lancet* 384 (9945), pp. 766–781.

Minkler, Meredith, DrPH 1999 February, 'Personal Responsibility for Health? A Review of the Arguments and the Evidence at Century's End,' *Health Education & Behavior* 26 (1), pp. 121-141.

Stoller-Conrad, Jessica 2012 August 10, 'Yoga on Commission: More Employers Pay for Good Habits,' *NPR*, Accessed 07 August 2015. http://www.npr.org/sections/health-shots/2012/08/10/158506049/yoga-on-commission-more-employers-pay-for-good-health-habits.

Thaler, Richard H.; Sunstein, Cass R. 2008, *Nudge: Improving Decisions about Health, Wealth, and Happiness*, Yale University Press, New Haven, CT.

Wallenstein, Sven-Olov 2009, *Biopolitics and the Emergence of Modern Architecture*, Princeton Architectural Press, New York.

World Health Organization 2010, Department of Measurement and Health Information.

World Health Organization Cancer Fact Sheet. http://www.who.int/mediacentre/factsheets/fs297/en/

United Nations Report 2013, World Population Aging 1950-2050.

Yu Xu; Wang Limin, He Jiang, et al. 2013, 'Prevalence and Control of Diabetes in Chinese Adults,' *Journal of the American Medical Association* 310(9), pp. 948-959.

A Timeline of Public Health and the Built Environment

Ann Forsyth, Leire Asensio Villoria, David Mah, Har Ye Kan, Justin Kollar, Xinhui Li + Han Yang

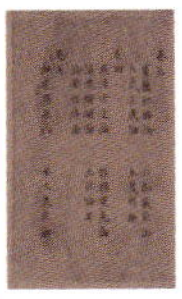

200BC Huangdi Neijing
Dated to between the late Warring States period (475-221 BC) and the Han period (206 BCE-220 CE), Huangdi Neijing has been researched and studied by various scholars for more than two millennia and treated as the fundamental doctrinal source for Chinese medicine.

5BC Airs, Water, and Place
Written by Hippocrates, it was the first written record of a rational approach to health and medicine that encouraged the study of local environemnts and climates in order to understand their effects on human health.

1423 The First Lazaret, Italy
Founded in Venice, on a small island adjoining the city.

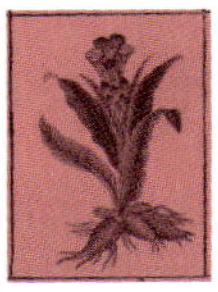

1578 Compendium of Materia Medica
Known as Bencao Gangmu, it is the most complete and comprehensive traditional Chinese medical book.

1683 Microorganisms
First seen and described by Dutch naturalist Antonie van Leeuwenhoek because of the development of the microscope.

1710 Quarantine Act, UK
Due to the rapid spread of diseases such as plague, cholera, and yellow fever through ships.

1799 Philadelphia Lazaretto
The first quarantine hospital in the United States

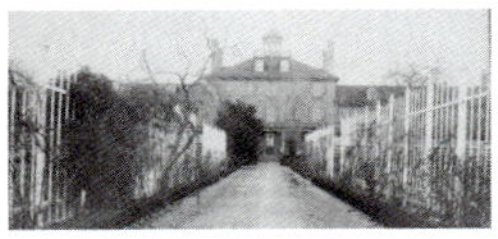

1844 The Condition of the Working Class in England
by the German philosopher Friedrich Engels, a study of the industrial working class in Victorian England.

1843 Supplementary Report
The formation of the Health of Towns Association and the creation of various city-based branches followed rapidly. These national and local movements contributed to the passing of the Public Health Act 1848.

1842 Chadwick's Report, UK
An Inquiry into the Sanitary Conditions of the Labouring Population of Great Britain.

1832 Right to Light Law, UK
A form of easement in English Law that gives a long standing owner of a building with windows a right to maintain a level of illumination.

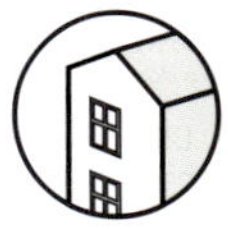

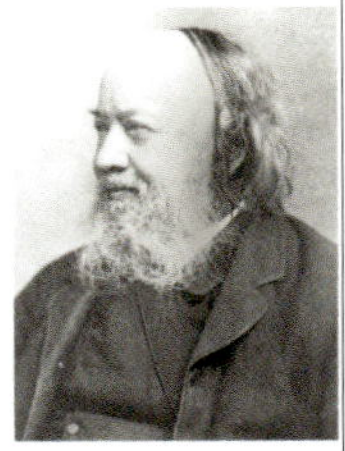

1810 1830

Prior to 1800...

Industrial cities
World population reaches 1 billion
Transit emerges

1800 1820 1840

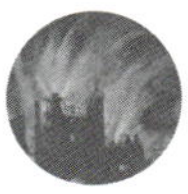

1666 Great Fire of London, UK
the densely built timber housing fostered its rapid spread.

The Rebuilding of London Act of 1666
Drawn up by Sir Matthew Hale, it was the first significant building regulation. The rebuilding of the city regulated fire resistance capacity for housing and authorized the City of London Corporation to reopen and widen roads.

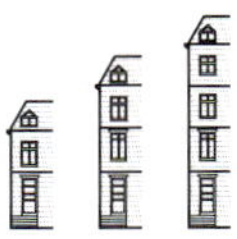

The Rebuilding of London Act of 1670
This particular Act extended the powers to enlarge streets and also ordered the rebuilding of St Paul's Cathedral.

1663 Quarantine, Colonial America
The establishment of a quarantine in New York City to control a smallpox outbreak.

1300s "Quarantine", Italy
"Quarantine" means "forty days" in the Venetian dialect. In order to prevent diseases related to the Black Death, ships and people were required to be isolated for 40 days before entering the city of Dubrovnik in Croatia.

China-related Events

China-related Events

1830s Introduction of Western Medicine to China
by Christian missionaries

1817 First Cholera Pandemic
This far-reaching pandemic swept through Asia and Europe and caused many deaths.

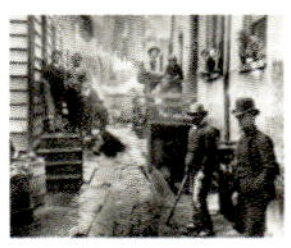

1825 First Slum
As the so-called Five Points in New York City evolved in to a large urban settlement, it is believe to be the first slum in the world history.

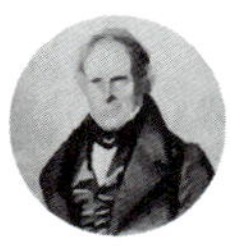

1826 Louis Rene Villerme, France
For the first time in the history, the relation between annual mortality rates across neighborhoods and the poverty and wealth patterns were demonstrated in his classic 1826 study, which contradicts the Hippocratic doctrine.

1829 Second Cholera Pandemic
It swept through Asia, Europe and Americas through various means of travel. Cholera caused more deaths than any other diseases in the 19th Century.

1845 Great Fire of New Yor
The fire destroyed 345 buildings in Lowe Manhattan and led to the enactment of th nation's first comprehensive building code 185

1846 Lariboisière Hospi
Built by Pierre Gauthier following the second cholera pande which had reached Paris in 1832, the hospital was an exampl the new emphasis on hygienic practices in hospi

The abridged history of health and place elaborated here, places significant moments in the history of the fields of public health and design (as well as their moments of convergence) into a timeline format. It organizes notable developments within a visual layout that invites the reader to study their place in time while also allowing for the possibility of recognizing overall or period-specific patterns. The timeline is intentionally open-ended, neglecting to categorize these events into discrete classifications, so that a number of possible readings may be gathered from scanning the information.

47 American Medical Association

ded as a national professional medical organization, its mission "promote the art and science of medicine for the betterment he public health, to advance the interests of physicians and patients, to promote public health" etc.

1848 Sanitary Ramblings: Being Sketches and Illustrations of Bethnal Green, UK

by Hector Gavin

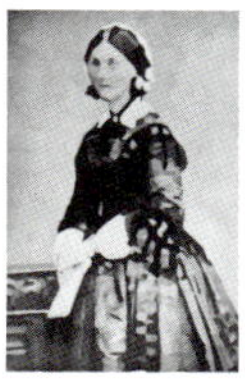

1848 Local Boards, UK

By arranging the supply of water, sewage, drainage, cleansing, paving, and environmental health regulation under a single body—the local board, the Public Health Act of 1848 tried to improve the sanitary conditions in urban areas of England and Wales. Local boards existed from 1848 to 1894 and became urban districts afterwards.

1863 Notes on Hospitals

Nightingale published 'Notes on Hospitals' in 1863, which included hospital design principles such as natural light, air, landscape, attention to diet, and a cleanly sanitary environment to create a better healing environment.

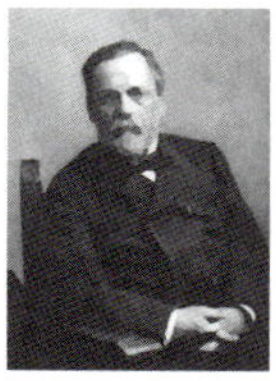

1864 Pasteurization

A process that lowered and eliminated pathogenic microbes for longer preservation times of food commodities.

1862 Thames Embankment, UK

1865 St. Thomas's Hospital, UK

Built between 1861 and 1865, St. Thomas's Hospital in London was designed by H. Currey and was the first to implement Nightingale's principles.

1860s Metropolitan Railway, UK

Catalyzed the spread of urban living. The line eventually extended as far as more than 50 miles (80 km) from Baker Street and the center of London.

1880s Bacteria

Robert Koch's discovery of the transmission of disease by bacteria.

1880s Pullman, USA

The designer of the Pullman sleeping car, George Pullman, founded a company town, Pullman, for his workers.

1875 Public Health Act, UK

It was passed to improve urban living conditions, and curb the spread of many diseases such as cholera and typhus.

1860s Emerald Necklace, USA

Designed by Frederick Law Olmsted to connect Boston Common to Franklin Park

1889 Poverty Maps of London

by Charles Booth

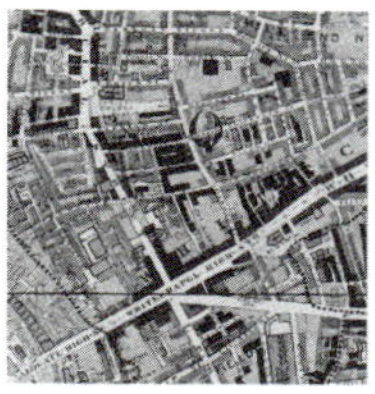

1889 Hull House, USA

Founded by by Jane Addams and Ellen Gates Starr for recently arrived European immigrants in Chicago.

1890 How the Other Half Lives, USA

By Jacob Riis, documenting squalid living conditions in New York City slums in the 1880s.

1893 Chicago World's Fair, USA

The exposition was one influence leading to the rise of the City Beautiful movement.

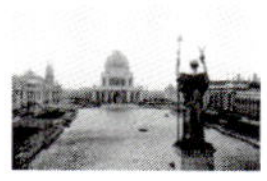

1894 Habitation à bon marché (HBM), France

This popular type of accommodation originated from the Siegfried Act of 30 November 1894 which created the name of HBM ("cheap houses") encouraging the provision of housing at subsidized prices with a tax exemption.

1895 Henry Street Settlement, USA

Founded in 1893 by Progressive reformer and nurse Lillian Wald. Its established one of New York City's first off-street playgrounds.

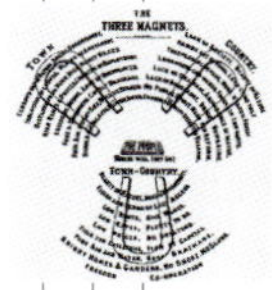

1898 Garden City Movement

Initiated by Sir Ebenezer Howard in UK, it promoted "planned, self-contained communities surrounded by greenbelts, containing proportionate areas, of residences, industry and agriculture".

1899 The Philadelphia Negro, USA

W.E.B. Du Bois's Seventh Ward Map

1850 — 1870 — 1890

early suburbs

72% UK pop. in urban areas

automobiles invented

urban reform (housing, settlements, parks)

city beautiful/municipal art

city practical/efficient government

16 cities with 1 mill+ pop.

1860 — 1880 — 1900

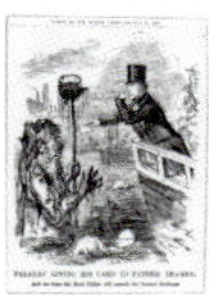

1858 Great Stink, UK

Because of the deteriorating and inadequate sewer system that discharged directly at the Thames, the Great Stink happened in July and August when hot weather aggravated the smell of "untreated human waste and industrial effluent."

1854 Cholera Outbreak Map, UK

The Broad Street cholera outbreak is best known for the physician John Snow's study of the outbreak and his discovery that cholera is spread by contaminated water.

1853 Haussmannization of Paris

The vast public works program commissioned by Emperor Napoléon III began.

1850 The Shattuck Report, USA

Report of the Sanitary Commission of Massachusetts

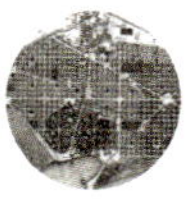

1850 United States of America Entacts Its First Comprehensive Building Code

1850s Ildefons Cerda, Spain

Survey of Barcelona's Old City Center

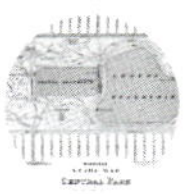

1850s Central Park, USA

by Frederick Law Olmsted and Calvert Vaux

1873 M. leprae

Discovered by G. H. Armauer Hansen in Norway, it is the first bacterium to be identified as causing disease in humans.

1872 American Public Health Association

1871 Great Chicago Fire, USA

1870s Ferdinand Julius Cohn, Germany

His classification of bacteria into four groups based on shape (sphericals, short rods, threads, and spirals) is still in use today. He is one of the founders of modern bacteriology and microbiology.

1869 Riverside, IL, USA

the first planned community in the US, designed in 1869 by Calvert Vaux and Frederick Law Olmsted.

1867 First Tenement House Act, USA

required fire escapes for each suite and a window for every room.

1867 Prospect Park, USA

by Frederick Law Olmsted

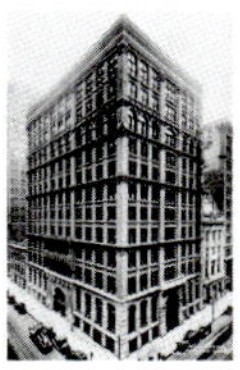

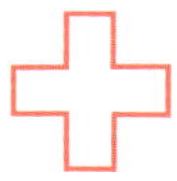

1904 China Red Cross

The Red Cross Society of China was founded as the "Shanghai International Red Cross Committee."

1905 Shanghai City Council

Under this new municipal administration, "a determined attempt was made to provide for welfare and primary education. There was a vigorous program, characterized by an extensive use of regulatory law, to improve the physical environment, to modernize customs and ways of thought, and to create a society that was healthier, safer, more efficient, and more humane."

1907 Typhoid Mary, USA

She is believed to be "the first person in the United States identified as an asymptomatic carrier of the pathogen associated with typhoid fever."

1885 Rabies Vaccines

Almost all human cases of rabies were fatal until a vaccine was developed by Louis Pasteur and Émile Roux.

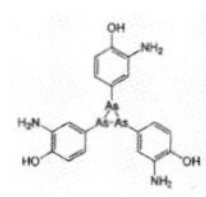

1908 Arsphenamine

It is the first effective treatment for syphilis and the first modern chemotherapeutic agent

1884 Home Insurance Building, USA

the world's first skyscraper, by William Le Baron Jenney

One such evaluation or categorization of these events is offered by Professor Ann Forsyth in her essay in this book, "When Public Health and Planning Closely Intersect (Five Moments, Five Strategies)." Forsyth rearranges key moments in the timeline into a series of different strategic approaches to health and place, through the lens of the planning discipline. She recognizes and acknowledges other possible categorizations, including the difference in significance afforded to these same key moments in history from the medical and public health field.

1917 Peking Union Medical College

Funded by the Rockerfeller Foundation PUMC provided the base for educating the new elite in Western medicine.

1921 Public Health Department

"Established at PUMC with the aim of providing epidemiological data and a focus for population based health care."

1923 Toward an Architecture, France
by Le Corbusier

1920 Rio de Janeiro
Rio de Janeiro documented its first slum in 1920 census.

1920s "Coughs and Sneezes Spread Diseases"
The memorable slogan originated in the 1920s in Europe to curb tuberculosis and influenza

1925 Plan Voisin, France
by Le Corbusier

1931 Villa Savoye, France
Designed by Le Corbusier, the villa is representative of the bases of modern architecture.

1932 Paimio Sanatorium, Finland
by Alvar Aalto

1935 Villa Girasole, Italy
by Angelo Invernizzi

1941 CIAM Athens Charter

1946 Centers for Disease Control and Prevention, USA

1934 London City Council
The first formal proposal "to provide a reserve supply of public open spaces and of recreational areas and to establish a green belt or girdle of open space."

1947 Town and Country Planning Act, UK
All further national urban developments were required to incorporate green belts.

1934 New Life Movement
Set up by Chiang Kai-shek and his wife, the Movement emphasized the Confucian and Methodist notion of self-cultivation and correct living and prescribed proper etiquette for every aspect of daily lives.

1948 World Health Organization
Dr. Szeming Sze, a delegate from China, was among the delegates who supported establishing an international health organization during the the 1945 United Nations Conference on International Organization.

1956 Federal Highway Act, USA

1949 Patriotic Health Campaign
A social movement in China, which declared war on the four pests "flies, mosquitoes, mice and sparrows" and persists until now.

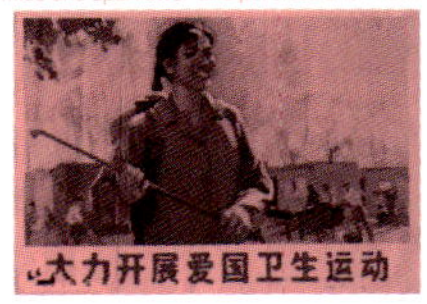

1949 Ministry of Health
One of the earliest ministries under The Central People's Government Administration Council

1954 Polio Vaccine

1956 Clean Air Act, UK

Design With Nature McHar

1969 National Environmental Policy Act, US
required additional documents including environmental impact statement (EIS) "projects proposed on federal lands or projec proposed by federal agencies or any projec that are or will be federally finance

1960 Cidade de Deus, Brazil
part of the policy to remove favelas from the center of Rio de Janeiro and settle their inhabitants in the suburbs.

1961 Zoning Resolution
Revised the 1916 Resolution. FAR was used instead of setback rules Ideas of privately owned public space emerged.

1962 Silent Spring
by Rachel Carson

1964 First Surgeon General's Report on Smoking and Health

1964 Traffic Towns, UK

1910 — R.O.China · WWI · influenza pandemic · first national city planning conference · neighborhood planning ideas · Corbusier, F. L. Wright visions — 1920 — 1930 — New Deal — 1940 — WWII · wartime planning · proliferation of automobile · New Towns/metropolitan plans — 1950 — P.R.China · R.O.China (Taiwan) · suburbanization · urban renewal · highway planning — Great Leap Forward · advocacy planning/community design · comprehensive/general plans · fair housing — 1960 — Sino-Soviet Split · Cultural Revo

1921 Hagerstown MD, USA
Periodic Standardized Health Surveys

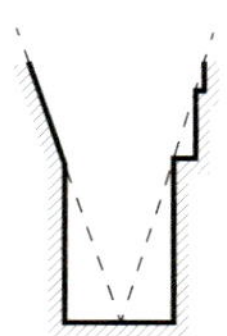

1916 Zoning Resolution, USA
Adopted in New York City in order to regulate the constructions of massive buildings that might prevent light and air from reaching the streets below.

1910 Forest Hills Gardens, USA

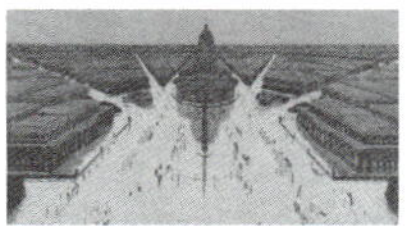

1909 Plan of Chicago, USA
Known as the Burnham Plan, the 1909 Plan of Chicago "recommended an integrated series of projects including new and widened streets, parks, new railroad and harbor facilities, and civic buildings."

1909 Wisconsin Planning Enabling Legislation, USA

1930 Villa Tugendhat, Czech Republic
by Ludwig Mies van der Rohe

1930s Traffic Calming, UK

1929 City of Tomorrow and Its Planning, France
by Le Corbusier

1929 Lovell Health House, USA
by Richard Neutra

1928 Zonnestraal Sanatorium, Netherlands
by Johannes Duiker and Bernard Bijvoet

1928 Penicillin Discovered

1926 Campaign to Protect Rural England, UK
Formed by Sir Patrick Abercrombie to "limit urban sprawl and ribbon development."

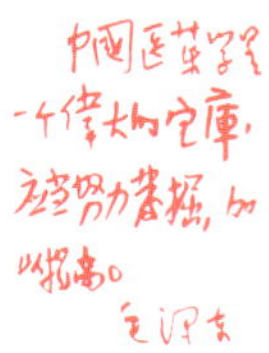

1950 Traditional Chinese Medicine
In 1950, Chairman Mao Zedong promoted Chinese medicine and claimed it was due to the political necessity.

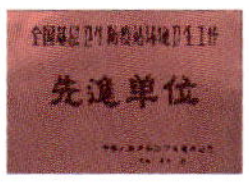

1950s EPSs
Originated in the Soviet Union, the epidemic prevention stations (EPSs) spread all over the country.

1950 Balanikov
"First create a major traffic route or a square, for example Tiananmen Square, already full of historic significance, for the purpose of parades both military and domestic and also for national day celebrations. This will further increase it's significance. The square therefore should be the centre of the city."

1951 Caoyang Xincun (Caoyang New Village)
"The first residential area in Shanghai or even nationwide designed specifically for factory workers." Caoyang was designed with one tenth of its land devoted to public facilities. It was also the first to offer water closets in the apartments.

1965 Barefoot Doctors
Minimally trained farmers worked as village health workers after the Rural Reconstruction Movement in 1930s. The system was further developed after Mao's speech in 1965.

1958 "Danwei"
New constructions took place throughout the surrounding area of the City of Beijing.

"Tugai"
A social movement in where land was taken from the rich and given to government or local groups.

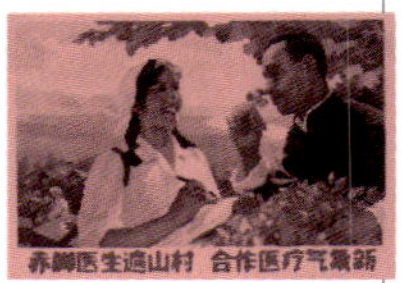

1966 Smallpox Campaign
WHO and the Centers for Disease Control began the worldwide smallpox eradication campaign in Africa

1957 Plan for Brasilia
by Lucio Costa

1967 Columbia MD, New Town, USA

1960 GIS
the world's first true operational GIS in Ottawa, Ontario, Canada

1952 Great Smog, UK
4000 deaths, 100,000 ill

1965 "New Venice Hospital"
by Le Corbusier

1952 Unité d'habitation
a modernist residential housing design principle developed by Le Corbusier

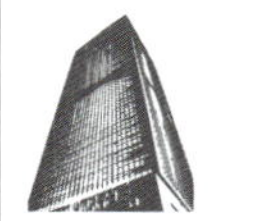

1958 Seagram Building, USA

1958 Urban Growth Boundary
The first in USA was established in Fayette County, Kentucky.

1952 Lever House, USA
by Gordon Bunshaft, Natalie de Blois

It is the possibility of multiple readings that motivates the configuration of this graphic.
This timeline is followed by a number of essays and interviews that elucidate, in more detail the past, present, and possible futures of the meeting between health and place concerns from the fields of architecture, planning, and public health.

1970s Cleveland Policy Plan, USA

1970 Environmental Protection Agency, USA
After 1970, major environmental legislations passed.

1974 Karen Silkwood, USA

1974 De Drie Hoven, Netherlands
by Herman Hertzberger

1974 Expanded Programme on Immunization
by WHO

1980 857 million
overweight or obese individuals worldwide

1981 AIDS Identified

1988 Kentlands Development, USA

1988 State Environmental Protection Administration

1989 Environmental Protection Law
Revised in 2014 with more strict measures

1986 Bureau of Land Administration
It was established in the same year that the Land Administration Law was passed, which legalized the private use of state-owned land by private companies and individuals.

1992 Regulations on Managing and Urban Appearance and Environmental Cleanliness
Revised in 2011

万科 让建筑赞美生命

1992 Vanke – City Garden
A series of real estate development emphasizing lower density and more open space that helped Vanke became the world's largest real estate developer.

1999 European Spatial Development Perspective

1990 BREEAM
Building Research Establishment Environmental Assessment Methodology. An UK method of assessing, rating, and certifying the sustainability of buildings.

88%
Dayuans (danweis' land) accounted for 88% of total land use in Beijing in the 90s. Many of their privileges still exist because of the political influence danweis had.

Code for Classification of Urban Land Use and Planning Standards of Development Land (GBJ137-90)

9.2% (841 million)
of world population over sixty years old

2000 Erin Brockovich

Fifth National Population Census
Population aged sixty-five and over was 88 million, 6.96% of the total population.

100 million / 26 million
100 million people were reported to suffer from high blood pressure and 26 million with diabetes.

2001 924 million
the total number of slum dwellers in the world, about 32% of the world's total urban population.

Ecological Residential Neighborhood Development and Technical Guidelines

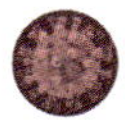

2002 SARS Outbreak
7,082 of the 8,096 cases were in China (including Hong Kong and Macau SARs). "Public health" became a focus of the government.

Revision of Code of Urban Residential Areas Planning & Design

2003 Avian Influenza H5N1 Outbreak in Asia

2010 Sixth National Population Census
Population aged 65 and over was 118.8 million, 8.87% of the total population. 13.26% were aged 60 or over.

2011 Basically Insured
More than 95% of the population has basic health insurance.

Code for Classification of Urban Land Use and Planning Standards of Development Land (GB50137-2011)

2012 PM2.5
MEP began to conduct PM2.5 monitoring in all major cities.

2013 "Cancer Villages"
China's Ministry of Environmental Protection acknowledges the existence of "cancer villages" in its twelfth five year plan.

2.1 Billion
overweight or obese individuals worldwide

11.7%
of world population over sixty years old

2015 Under the Dome (film)
By Chai Jing. Air pollution in China accounted for 1.2 million premature deaths of its citizens (2010 Global Burden of Diseases, Injuries, and Risk Factors Study)

2050 300 million
population over sixty-five

79.2 years
life expectancy

1.38 billion
total population

2050 21.1% (2 billion)
of world population over sixty years old

1990 — 2010

environmental/open space planning; crisis/environmentalism; Defensible Space; Cleveland Policy Plan; economic reforms; smallpox eradicated; special economic zones; PCs; one-child policy; the "Posts" (-fordism, -modernsim, etc.); Healthy Cities Program, WHO; Chernobyl Disaster; GIS; Internet; Healthy People Campaign; Kobe Earthquake; Kyoto Protocol; Human Genome Project; sustainability; Hong Kong SAR; UN Millennium Development Goals; security/disaster planning; Bilbao effects; Council for European Urbanism; 500 cities with 1 mill+ pop.; "Three Represents"; "harmonious society"; Sichuan Earthquake; swine influenza; 50%+ urban pop. worldwide; 7 billion world pop.; Tohoku Earthquake and Tsunami; MERS Outbreak; Ebola Outbreak; PM2.5 Interim Target-1; 8 billion world pop.; after 2030...; pop. peak

1980 — 2000 — 2020

…8 Reform and Opening
…introduction of a market economy and privatization.

1980 Regulation on Norm and Quota in Urban Planning

1982 City-led Development

1983 Environmental Protection Became a State Policy

1984 Water Pollution Prevention and Control Law

1987 Ju'er Hutong Courtyard Housing
As an innovative new approach to Beijing urban renewal, the Ju'er Hutong Project restored and improved the traditional courtyard housing without complete demolition of the historic but dilapidated houses. The project also "seeks to bring about a new approach to the funding and planning of housing provision within historic cities."

1980s China–Cornell–Oxford Project
The project conducted observational studies in rural China and 6,500 people across sixty-five counties were examined and compared regarding their diets, lifestyle, and disease prevalence (excluding causes of death such as accidents).

1989 China Health and Nutrition Survey

1990 Americans with Disabilities Act

1991 Real Estate Market
New land legislation gave the danweis an incentive to hand their accumulated excesses of land either back to the state, to developers, or to develop the vacant plots themselves, prompting increased land-use efficiency in existing danwei owned areas.

1993 LEED USGBC

1994 Tax Reform
The central government introduced a tax assignment system to increase the central government's share of the tax revenue. Local government began to look for revenue through the sales of land-use rights, which resulted in the land bidding processes and the expropriation of rural land.

1994 Code of Urban Residential Areas Planning & Design

1995 Maggie's Centres, UK
a network of drop-in centres in Great Britain, which aim to help anyone who has been affected by cancer.

1996 RPA's Third Regional Plan, USA

1999 Downsview Park Competition Entry, Canada
by Field Operations

2000 National Health City
evaluated and awarded by the National Patriotic Health Movement Committee Office

2004 New Cooperative Medical Scheme in Rural China

2005 Urbanization
Rural residents now can settle in the city via official channels.

Jianwai SOHO: mixed-used open neighborhood
Code for Design of Civil Buildings

2006 "An Inconvenient Truth" - Al Gore

Residential Building Code
Evaluation Standard for Green Building

Vanke – Langrun Garden
Ecological residential neighborhood and Green Building certified neighborhood

2007 Obese Kids
According to the Ministry of Education, 8% of ten to twelve-year-olds in China's cities are considered obese and an additional 15% are overweight.

2008 Chronic Diseases
28.3%/17.1% of residents in urban and rural areas.

MEP
The Ministry of Environmental Protection (MEP) became a cabinet-level ministry.

2009 Linked Hybrid by Steven Holl

2030 Diabetes
Diabetes is emerging as a significant global problem with forecasts for it to become the seventh leading cause of death.

Cancer
Cancer, another major chronic disease, is recorded to have also steadily increasing global rates with projections for it to increase by 70% over the next two decades. China has suffered one of the highest rates of increase with 27% of the world's cancer deaths and this trajectory is projected to continue.

2020 $15 Trillion
Spending of population over sixty years old worldwide

2020 "A New Center"
Beijing Tongzhou Government Center Citywide population less than 23 million in 2020; 15% decrease of downtown population

1 Billion
Chinese cities will contain more than 1 billion people.

248 Million
17% of the population will be over 60.

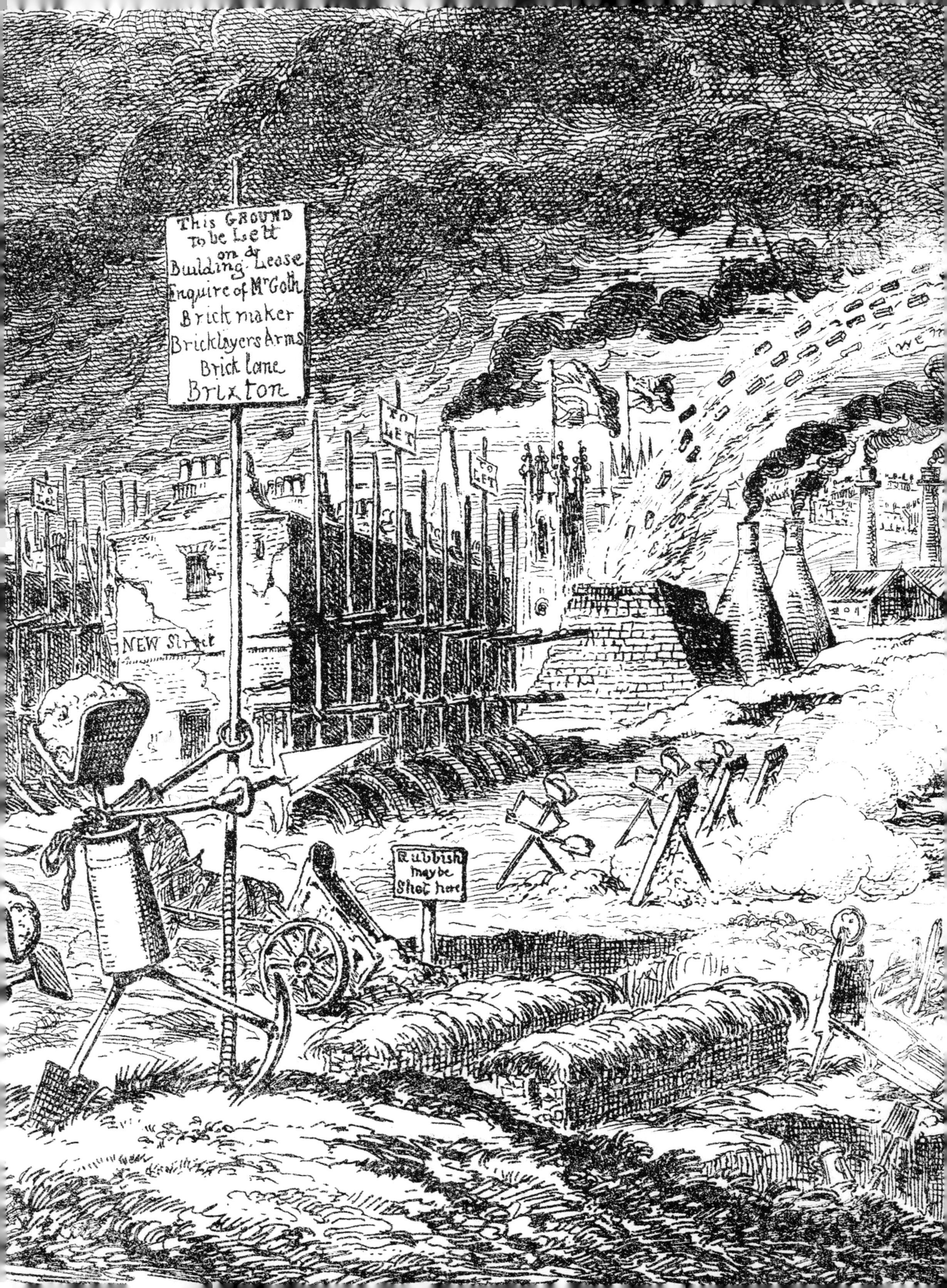
This GROUND
To be Lett
on a
Building Lease
Enquire of Mr Goth
Brickmaker
Bricklayers Arms
Brick lane
Brixton
TO LET
TO LET
TO LET
TO Let
NEW Street
Rubbish
may be
Shot here

Environments, Populations, and Health
Learning from (Modern) Health and Place
Leire Asensio Villoria + David Mah

Foundations

The relationship between the health of a population and their environment (or place) can appear to be self-evident. It would seem apparent that place should bear considerable effect on the well-being and health of its occupants. As a consequence of this obvious affiliation, formal associations between the design fields engaged in the definition of our built environment and public health can also be said to have a well-established historical legacy.

For the public health and medical field, the physical environment has frequently been an area of deep concern and focus. This investment in exploring the links between health and the environment can be seen to enjoy a recurring significance, even from as early as what can be described as the inception of western medicine.

More specifically, Airs, Waters, and Places written by Hippocrates in the fifth century BCE offered the first written record of a rational approach to health and medicine that, in the particular case of endemic diseases, encouraged the study of the local environment and climate in order to understand its effects on human health. The book was one of the first systematic and scientific attempts to describe causal relationships between the environment and well-being, clarifying what already existed as common yet intuitive wisdom.

While the physical environment was established as a focus for early western medicine, conversely concerns for the collective health of the public also played a role in the foundation of western architecture. For architecture, place (and more specifically, the towns and cities that have come to constitute the environments for large human populations), and its relationship to health has been a consistent emphasis. An approach to the laying out of cities expounded by Vitruvius in the sixth chapter of his book De Arquitectura offers an early example of the interest in the management of the relationship between the configurations of towns and cities with the well-being of its citizens:

Excerpts from the sixth chapter highlight the value Vitruvius attributed towards the sensitive organization of towns and their streets in favorable relation to different prevailing winds. In the chapter, Vitruvius would go on to describe, in detail, the development of a systematic process for determining the layout of a hypothetical city based on eight principal wind directions. For him, the morphology of towns and cities was to be considered in relation to the various climatic factors so as to allay their potential effects on human health.

> "When the walls are set around the city, there follow the division of the sites within the walls and the laying out of the broad streets and the alleys with a view to aspect. These will be rightly laid out if the winds are carefully shut out from the alleys. For if the winds are cold they are unpleasant; if hot, they infect, if moist, they are injurious."

From these early foundational narratives for western medicine and architecture, we can surmise that the intertwining of human health and place has enjoyed a long-standing association. Beyond these beginnings, the exchanges and dialogue between these fields has since persisted to frequently wield influence over the motivations and practice of each respective discipline.

Throughout various moments in history, the design fields have found health concerns to be a strong catalyst for invention, where the urgency and immediacy associated with addressing the health of human

Figure 1 (Left) March of bricks and mortar, George Cruikshank, 1843.

populations has greatly motivated the advancement of the quality of the built environment. The creation of countless innovations for the built environment are all indicators of the great inventive drive provoked by various public health concerns, which have exerted considerable influence over the shaping of the public, institutional, and domestic spaces of the city as well as the lifestyles of its citizens.

Modern Public Health and Design

The rapid modernization and industrialization of the west, during the nineteenth through to the mid-twentieth centuries, saw one of the most significant periods in the convergence between public health concerns and the actors who came to shape the built environment. It would also see the institutionalization of both the architecture and public health fields with the establishment of official bodies overseeing the training and practice of these professions. As a consequence, design strategies that would evolve from the application of public health and social concerns as important considerations in the planning of the built environment, would be deployed in a highly systematic manner and would go on to affect the city on an unprecedented scale.

For a balanced sense of the potentially vital effect that the association between the design fields and public health may still yield, we may look back to the ways that its previous convergences had exerted an acute influence over aspects of urban, landscape, and architectural design. A general understanding of the motivations and concerns associated with modern public health and its formalization during this period, offer us an insight into the forces that influenced the design disciplines' corresponding turn towards the scientific and rational.

The institutional origins of modern public health was greatly influenced by positivism or utilitarianism and the presumptions of a scientific approach towards the study and reform of cities and human populations. The philosophical and ethical underpinnings of modern public health are exemplified by the notable nineteenth century public health and social reformer, Sir Edwin Chadwick's own sympathy towards the political and social ideas of the early philosophers of utilitarianism: John Stuart Mill and Jeremy Bentham. Chadwick's significance in the foundation of modern public health can be attributed to his role in defining and overseeing the report, "The Sanitary Condition of the Laboring Population (1842) which would go on to motivate the constitution of the Public Health Act in England of 1848, institutionalizing public health in England.

The influential works of Sir John Snow and John Graunt exemplify the general scientific and objective emphasis in modern public health from this period. These two figures would bring into focus the operative capacity for utilizing scientific techniques such as mapping and statistics as methods for studying and improving larger population and urban patterns. Both events offer a clear exemplar of a systematic impulse in the study and monitoring of urban populations in service of what was seen as the greater public good. These also isolate two key practices that would form the basis for a number of public health's core and associated disciplines, notably epidemiology and environmental health.

In 1854, Sir John Snow's deductive mappings of East London were instrumental in the isolation of the contaminated water source responsible for an outbreak of cholera in that population. Beyond this technical facility, it was also important for its contribution towards an understanding and validation of disease based on germ theory, something that would reorient public health efforts towards sanitation rather than the widely accepted miasma theory of the time. As we will see, scientific mapping would offer both an operative or instrumental technology as well as a larger polemical device for advancing the agenda of the hygiene movement.

In addition to mapping, the hygiene movement was also advanced by the work of John Graunt, who together with William Petty, undertook what would be one of the earliest exercises in census and statistical studies, forming the basis for the field of demography. Its particular area of investigation was the study of London's mortality rolls and was a very early example of a study that would foreshadow the foundation of epidemiology.[1] The formalization of epidemiology itself, which still persists as one of the basic sciences of public health today, came much later in 1838 when William Farr, who, as the Compiler

1 With its shared foundations, epidemiology and demography have since developed as different disciplines with specific methodologies and areas of focus. However both share political arithmetic and statistical analysis of populations and health factors in their methodologies.

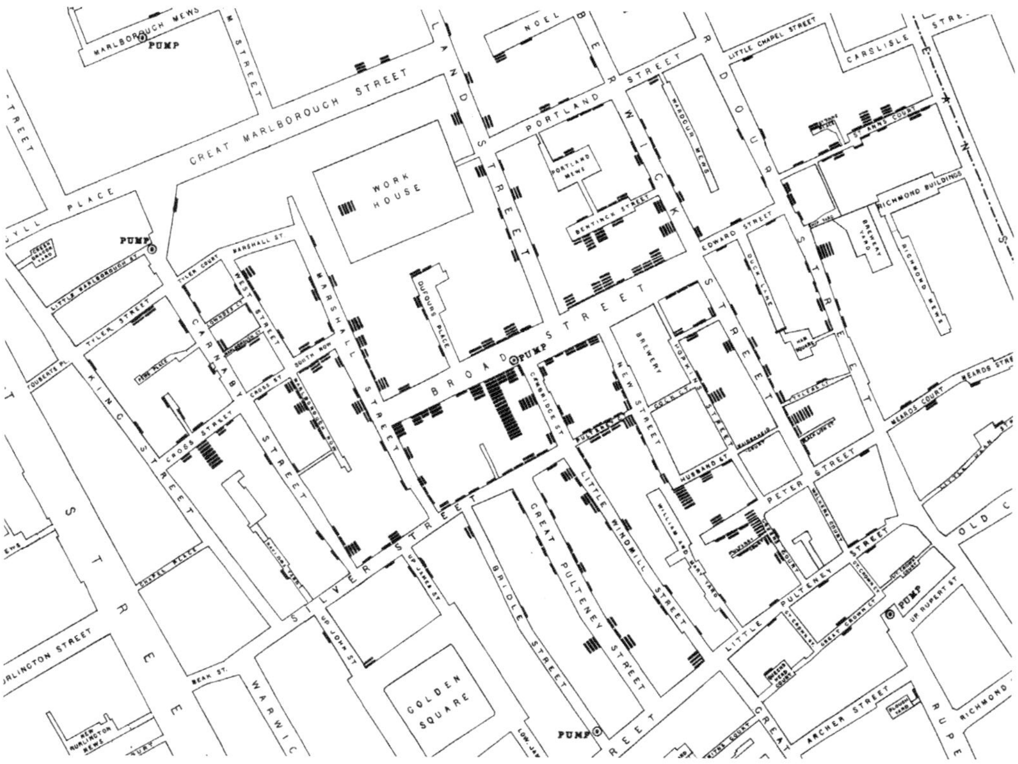

Figure 2 (Left) Map of East London cholera outbreak (1854) Sir John Snow.

of Abstracts to the General Register Office in England, would adopt the instrumentality of demography as an investigative practice in light of the cholera epidemics that emerged during the nineteenth century.

The long-standing perceived efficacy and widespread utilization of demography, epidemiology as well as scientific mapping in modern public health, can be linked to various moments when a prevailing civic interest in health and environmental crises mandated the deployment of a systematized understanding of the situation. Amongst other things, the struggle of managing the unprecedented scale of modern urban populations and cities demanded new health and governing apparatuses. This was addressed most effectively through the consolidation of scientific practices and knowledge to intervene in the various challenges of the time, from the excessive infant mortality rate, epidemic or contagion containment, and managing the incidence of endemic diseases. The elaboration of protocols and techniques for the systematic and scientific monitoring of populations and the environment would offer one of the most effective technologies to achieve this.

Science, Hygiene, and the City

> "We would like science to be free of war and politics. At least, we would like to make decisions other than through compromise, drift and uncertainty. We would like to think that somewhere, in addition to the chaotic confusion of power relations, there are rational relations... To this end we have created, in a single movement, politics on one side and science and technoscience on the other... We have to give evidence that "science" and "society" are both explained more adequately by an analysis of the relations among forces and that they become mutually inexplicable and opaque when made to stand apart." [2]

As articulated by Latour's book on Pasteur,[3] the processes of formulation and dissemination of the sciences are often entangled with the practice of power relations and politics. The varied political and social agendas that underpin the development and promotion of scientific knowledge offer a more nuanced understanding of the dissemination of scientific developments within society.

Significant for the ascendancy of the scientific method, in the period described by Latour, was the

2 Latour 1988, 5–7 Latour's book offers a revision and re-reading of what has been called Modernity by revisiting the political circumstances and relationships that underpinned the development and dissemination of the sciences. This is also expanded on in his book *We Have Never Been Modern.*

3 Ibid.

perception of its indisputability, and as a corollary; its instrumentality as leverage in the health reform campaigns associated with the hygiene movement. Latour's work on Pasteur situates this process within the context of the support, promotion, and subsequent adoption of bacteriology or germ theory by these reform movements.

Pasteur's work and bacteriology in general, while providing scientific legitimacy for sanitation, emerged within the overall milieu of the hygiene movement, gaining significance and inertia through its alliance with and investment by the already politically active hygiene movement. The hygiene movement's efficacy and public recognition prior to Pasteur's discovery in medicine has been recognized as already significant in itself. However, prior to the widespread promotion of bacteriology, the previously all-encompassing and broad nature of the hygiene movement was the reason for its sometimes skeptical or ambivalent reception by the general public, as it failed to present a strong focus or target. The capacity for the general fear of contagion to focus public interest in reform was not enough by itself and mobilizing public consensus for hygiene needed to be provoked by other means.

In addition to bacteriology, epidemiology and demography would also play a significant role in promoting the mandate for the transformation of the city in accordance with health and hygiene concerns. The statistical work of the nineteenth century French public health official Louis-René Villermé would make the argument for the association between health and wealth. His 1828 study of mortality rates and area-based economic data illustrated the correlation between economic classes and health, highlighting for the first time, the importance of social factors in the determination of health. This would induce the convergence between health and social reform movements with parallel motivations in England spurred on by Hector Gavin's 1848 survey of the neighborhoods of the working classes; "Sanitary Ramblings." Beyond the recognition of the social determinants of health, this also brought into focus the great threat to the labor force posed by contagions and epidemics. The threat to human capital would compel the philanthropic and industrialist classes to view hygiene and public health as a major economic concern for them, adding momentum to the large scale campaigns for the transformation of working class neighborhoods and the implementation of sanitary infrastructure in the city.

While bacteriology or germ theory offered the indisputable mandate for sanitation and hygiene by isolating a significant causal factor for the disease; microbes, the means for constructing scientific "evidence," through instruments such as surveys, also served to provide the evidence of the associations between health, social and economic concerns. These would be persuasive instruments that would building consensus for larger reform campaigns and agendas. This would provide the hygiene movement with the legitimacy to consolidate and extend its influence even more forcefully over every aspect of life, including the redefinition of the manner in which the design disciplines approach the articulation of the built environment.

Biopolitics

As a result of the risks associated with the sheer scale of urbanization and the unprecedented concentrations of populations unfolding during this period, other means of governance would also emerge. This would result in the appearance of a liberal and rational approach to governing the city and its populations which the philosopher Michel Foucault identifies as "Biopolitics."

The biological life of the population would pose "a profound source of worries that require the invention of new techniques and forms of knowledge able to probe the depths of this new bios."[4] The biopolitical governing of large populations would operate by identifying as well as mitigating large potential risks as a means to ensure the general health and productivity of its population. Significant to this is the study of collectives of humans as statistical categories or populations. This would facilitate the formation of new forms of knowledge on populations that would be based ostensibly on scientific and rational methods.

4 Wallenstein 2009, 10

"In this emerging formation of knowledge, new questions pose themselves; how do people live, how is their domicile structured, what is their hygienic and medical status, how do they mate, under what conditions does the family become happy and when does it turn into a source of diseases?"[5]

5 Ibid., 11.

In addition to the emergence of the study of its citizens as populations, biopolitics, as a means of governing, would also promote the conceptualization of the city as an "environment." Populations and environments would be monitored and represented objectively through epidemiology, mapping, and surveys. Together with an associated concern for the contagion of acute diseases, this boosted the deployment of "a general medicalization of urban space."[6]

6 Ibid., 12.

Inevitably, this would also augment the design fields engaged in the definition of the built environment. In his book, Sven Olov Wallenstein,[7] heavily influenced by the late works of Michel Foucault, outlines the specific effects that the practice of Biopolitics and the imperatives of hygiene would have on the emergence of Modern Architecture. Most significantly is a shift from architecture's representational role as an art, to its emphasis on function and the ways in which it may devise novel organizations (or a reconsideration) of existing institutions and ways of living. Foucault describes the formation of theÉcole des Ponts et Chaussées as a significant event in this transformation for architecture, where these institutions would facilitate "the emergence of polytechnicians" as the organizers of the new social space.

7 Wallenstein 2009. See also Michel Foucault's Lectures at the College De France between 1977 – 1979 published in *Security, Territory and Population* and *The Birth of Biopolitics*.

Engineered Urbanization: the Birth of Modern Planning

In addition to the immediate material consequences of addressing sanitary needs and the management of disease within towns and cities, one of the more significant impacts on the art and science of city-making can be exemplified by the birth of the theory and practice of modern planning. The influence of the hygiene movement and the influence of the social and health reforms of the nineteenth century contributed significantly to its emergence. In literal terms, the application of scientific planning principles that would come to be associated with modern urbanization had a significant role in the transformations of a large number of cities in the 19th century, ranging from Haussmann's restructuring of Paris to the construction of new models of public space and infrastructure in London, (an example being the construction of London's Embankment along the Thames as a result of the city's major public works implementation of a modern sewage system). It would also extend through the twentieth century, influencing the urban practice of the Modernists, with Le Corbusier's visionary plans being amongst the most emblematic and contentious. These urban practices emerged out of the public health concerns of the time regarding urban contagion, and most notably the epidemics of cholera and typhoid, while these modern planning practices offered a new vision for how the city may be reorganized to accommodate a new modern society.

The general enthusiasm for scientific methods of the time would also see a parallel in architectural and urban practices where the adoption of operative tools such as statistical analysis, functionalism, and scientific mapping, would also contribute significantly towards a reorientation of the design fields invest in its role as an applied sciences. It would herald a new practice of city making that would come to be aligned with the applied science of engineering. We can see this through the particular case of one of the originators of the theory and practice of urbanization: Ildefons Cerdà.

Barcelona's 19th century extension, the Eixample (or Ensanche), is an emblematic instance of modern planning that also illustrates a general theory of urbanization developed by the civil engineer; Ildefons Cerdà. The concept of urbanization was developed and defined by Cerdà through a multi-volume collection: *The General Theory of Urbanization*, that would set the theoretical and operational basis for the deployment of a massive enlargement of Barcelona's territorial extension. Highly systematic approaches to the definition of many of the constituent parts of the city as well as the relationships between these urban elements, were developed for their eventual proliferation and implementation in the Eixample. Mathematical associations that defined the building to open space ratios are a clear indication

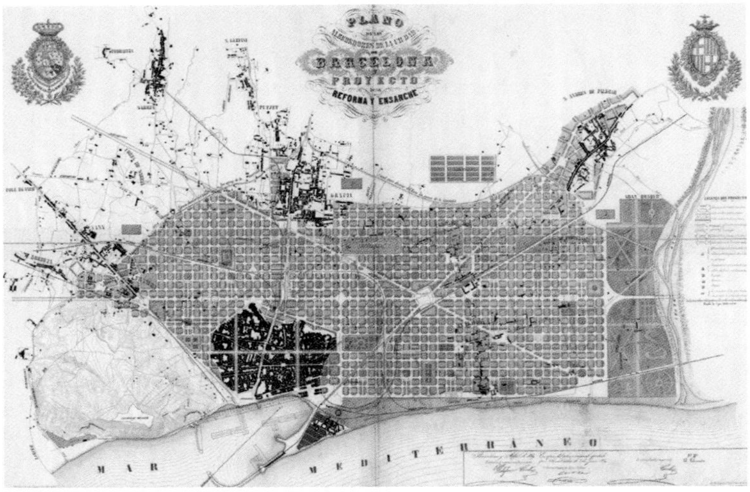

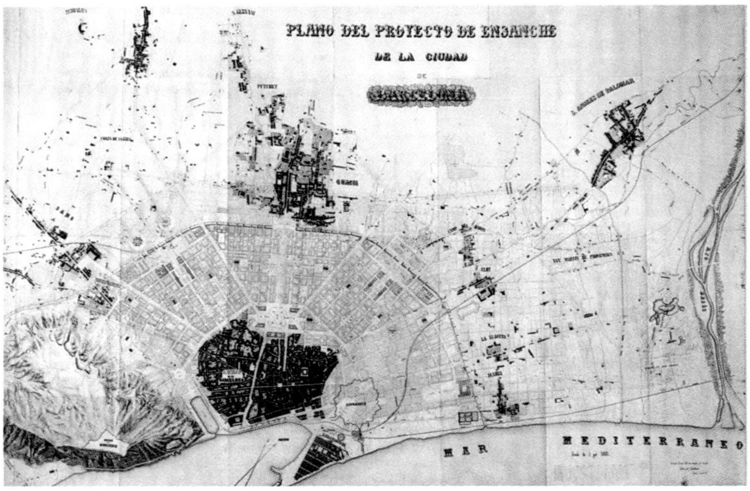

Figure 3 (Top Left) Original plan of the extension of Barcelona (1859), Ildefons Cerdà.

Figure 4 (Bottom Left) Eixample map of Barcelona (1859) Antoni Rovira.

of the ambition for precision and control over the quality of the built environment. These ratios were informed by factors that were observed to contribute to population health, such as access to sunlight, open spaces, and the promotion of appropriate ventilation through the urban fabric.

Cerdà, clearly motivated by the concerns of the hygiene movement, preceded his work on the plan by undertaking surveys of the social, environmental, and health conditions of the existing medieval and Roman urban fabric of Barcelona. He would make use of scientific analysis to deliver a study of the existing conditions of Barcelona's older neighborhoods offering a rational and scientific account of the physical aspects of these areas and proving their inadequacy as environments for human health. These conclusions formed the pretext for his engineered proposals which were motivated by the need to dramatically improve the urban environment of its population and, more importantly, to offer this in an equitable manner. The public open spaces and streets within the plan were dimensioned to allow for generous exposure and openness to light and air, providing what was seen as a healthy environmental condition for the city's public. The existing old city core of Barcelona was considered by Cerdà to be the antithetical model of his projected city with its congested, dense, and poorly ventilated streets, environments which he associated with incubators of disease. Cerdà's proposal developed a counterpoint between the proposed extension and the existing fabric, deliberately offering an isotropic expression for the city in distinction to the intricacy and irregularity of the old city. His adoption of the grid was also a conscious attempt to both accommodate and communicate the idea of an egalitarian city. Cerdà used the plan as a representation of his ambitions for accommodating a modern, healthy democratic society in contrast to the inequity characterized by the chaos of the medieval core of Barcelona's old city. The plan not only needed to be developed through rational methods but would also need to express rationality.

The full political and social circumstances that gave rise to the development and implementation of Cerdà's Eixample—and its subsequent implementation and augmentation as a built city—are perhaps too lengthy to describe in full detail here. However, it is important to consider the perceptions and conventions of the time that motivated the push for alternative designs for the extension to replace Cerdà's.

The debate over the plan for the extension became an instrument of a larger professional and political struggle to control the development and shaping of the city, bringing the professional bodies of architects and engineers into conflict. An early attempt to usurp the adoption of Cerdà's plan emerged with the promotion of the architect Antoni Rovira's alternative proposal for the extension in 1859. Rovira adopted an artfully composed radially arrayed arrangement, and his plan centered on the existing Barcelona city core, using it as the focal point of the composition. Cerdà, however, used the old city as reference rather than a focal point. Cerdà's plan offered regularity as an alternative to differentiated fabrics, coherent circulation schemes in place of congestion, a calibrated relationship between building mass and open space as opposed to uncontrolled concentration, and a predictable means of growth instead of haphazard accumulation. From both proposals we can discern the difference in emphasis for architects and engineers of the time; where Rovira's proposal could be described as an exercise in composing elements into a careful arrangement, we may regard Cerdà's plan as being engineered for performance more than being artfully composed.

What is significant about the contrast between these two proposals and the larger professional struggle is a perception at the time of engineering, with its foundations in applied sciences, as being in opposition to an architectural profession mired in service to patrons from the aristocratic and landowner classes. Engineering was seen as exemplifying the more modern and democratic profession with science and technology as its instruments in service of wider public concerns and for delivering public infrastructure and urban systems, a sentiment that would temper much of the later polemical work of twentieth century modernism.

Public Health and the Birth of Landscape Architecture

The establishment of landscape architecture as a profession and discipline is closely tied to the work and biography of Frederick Law Olmsted. It's distinction from the older gardening tradition can be found in the new modern role for cultivating landscapes in the city as spaces for the public. The oeuvre of leading figures from the gardening tradition such as Andre Le Notre and Capability Brown can be characterized by their primary engagement in the composition of private gardens and estates for privileged patrons. Though landscape architecture may inherit many formal and compositional traits from this older tradition, its mandate in modern times would be defined by the manner in which it would deploy this art to articulate and organize the public spaces for the city. Olmsted was one of the significant figures in the foundation of landscape architecture and would contribute to the definition of the public role for landscape architecture with Central Park, NY being among his most emblematic models for metropolitan public landscapes.

A part of landscape architecture's foundational history that is often overlooked is Olmsted's brief three-year career as a public health official. During the Civil War, as general secretary of the United States Sanitary Commission, Olmstead conducted surveys and evaluations of Union army camps. During a brief resignation from his role as chief architect of Central Park in 1861, Olmsted was engaged by the Unitarian minister and President of the United States Sanitary Commission and reformer, Henry Whitney Bellows. His reports on the camps and health of the soldiers betrayed his experiences as a landscape designer by directing focus on to the physical aspects of the camps. The inadequate drainage, waste disposal, poor ventilation, and subsequent flooding within the camps would be linked by Olmsted to a negative effect on the health and morale of the soldiers.[8] This period spent focused on public health would offer Olmsted a view onto the deployment of scientific methods for the study and transformation of the built environment and undoubtedly strengthened his alliances with the wider hygiene movement's campaigns.

8 Fisher 2010.

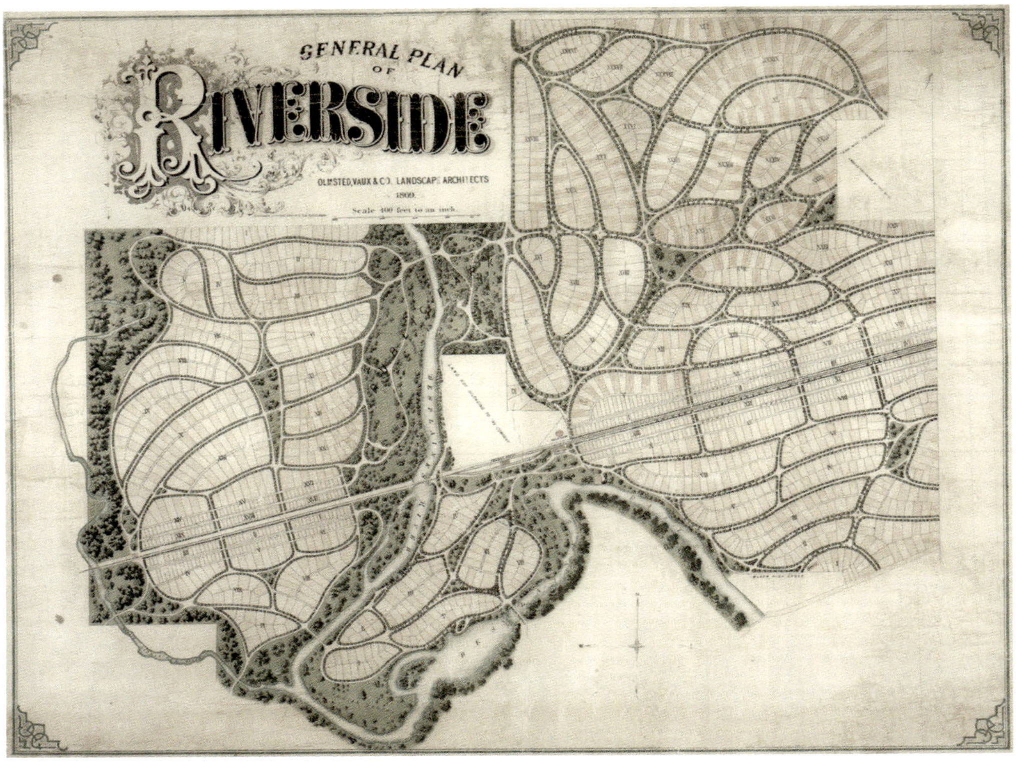

Figure 5 (Left) Riverside, Chicago plan (1868) Frederick Law Olmsted.

It is evident that Olmsted's dalliance with public health also had an influence on his ideas on the value and role of public spaces for the city. It seems that Olmsted recognized the applicability of public health concerns as a way to frame the conceptualization of public landscapes. He would oversee the development of urban spaces that provided naturalistic respite from the congested urban environment while promoting and making visible, collective forms of active recreation as a shared and accessible public experience for its citizens.

While open, public green parks would be adopted as a panacea to the ills incubated by the metropolis, Olmsted would also return to landscape as an operative medium for cultivating the more private realm of residential environments. This culminated the design and layout of a suburban community in Riverside, Chicago. Here he exemplified his model for appropriate living environments, where the general arrangement of the plan would be driven by landscape concerns and constraints and equate the abundance and health of the natural environment with the health of its population. Morphological strategies were be influenced by the natural (albeit relatively flat) topography and watershed using landscape as the means for addressing open space patterns and coordinating plotting. The generous open space pattern would involve the preservation of the floodplain and riverbanks while ensuring that recreational spaces would be integrated within the overall plan. This approach would manifest itself even at the detail of street intersections where Olmsted would deliberately arrange streets to meet at acute angles, creating awkward plots at their junction. These plots, difficult for development, would subsequently be reserved for open green spaces, ensuring a consistent buffer as well as safeguarding a finer grain of open spaces for the plan. Significantly, this project would also allow us to see the translation and transposition of many strategies and features common to his public park spaces into a residential community. The careful elaboration of the domestic and private realm with concepts and techniques developed for public parks represent Olmsted's interest in promoting forms of living that profit from the health benefits of shared, open green spaces.

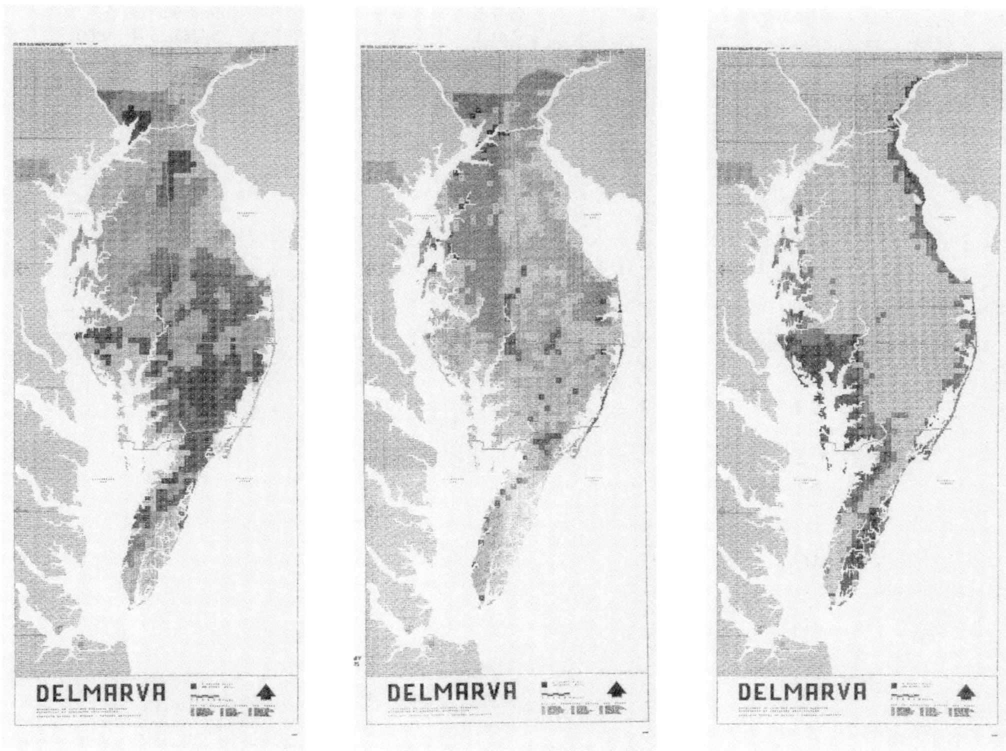

Figure 6 (Left) Maps made by an early model of GIS software: SYMAP representation developed by Carl Steinitz, 1967.

Landscape and Mapping

Landscape architecture as a discipline would later evolve to integrate scientific mapping into its core disciplinary concerns. The persistent influence of cartography on the discipline would assume an apotheosis with its convergence with the fields of geography and ecology. Streams within landscape architecture aggressively articulated a scientific position aimed at expanding their influence to ecological planning at wider regional and territorial scales. Ian McHarg's promotion of mapping techniques in service of a more nuanced approach to regional planning, explicitly assimilating natural systems considerations, would be significant for the establishment of a scientific legitimacy for the discipline of landscape architecture and would contribute to the field of planning in general. Amongst the many concerns that shaped and motivated this momentum has been a concern for safeguarding ecological or environmental health, with an assumption of its value for human populations. This inclination would persist, with the discipline's enthusiastic adoption of computational cartographic methods (GIS); the motivation to represent the natural and urbanized world with what is assumed as higher degrees of granularity and precision, resonates with the faith invested in scientific mapping by the public health field.

Form Follows Well-being

The pervasive realignment towards the scientific would also have its impact on architecture, with key Modern polemicists such as Le Corbusier arguing for the ascension of the figure of the engineer as representative of the new Modern design ethos, in opposition to what was seen as the drained stylistic canons burdening the architects of the time. This sentiment, while most forcibly campaigned for by the twentieth century Modernists, already exerted its influence on the profession and discipline in the 1800s with the establishment of a model pedagogy for the education of architects based on type developed by Jean Louis Durand at the Ecole Polytechnique in France. This approach offered a model of practice and training for architects that did away with much of the dogma attached to prescribed aesthetic and compositional rules and would open up architectural design to many different formal possibilities.

The elevation of function, or performance, as the main determinant of design followed the dissolution of established compositional and stylistic rules and was a consequence of the assumption of an almost linear causality between form and function. This opened up the definition of the built environment to technocratic drivers, which, on the one hand gained legitimacy through their association with a seemingly scientific method and on the other, was intended to make the deliberation on the design of the built environment more accessible to a wider public. Modern architecture aimed to invite wider public engagement by addressing the definition of the institutions and living spaces of a new, modern society through what was seen as generally more accessible discussions on the accommodation and expression of their functions rather than through their representation via symbols. Rather than recapitulating the codes and symbolism inherited from older traditions and styles, Modern architecture would establish a new design language to communicate a novel expression for this emerging society through function. Architecture would be transformed by a Neue Sachlichkeit (new objectivity) or Functionalism, which would go on to offer performance both as a means (and at times as an alibi) for its expression.

The influence of Mediterranean vernacular and an interpretation of the machine aesthetic on the development of the formal language of Modern Architecture has been assimilated into the main narrative of the history of architecture as a profession and discipline. In addition, the formal innovations in Modern Architecture have also been attributed to any number of other determinants ranging from the radical transformation of historical types and influences from prevailing avant-garde art movements such as cubism to the opportunities offered by innovations in construction. In parallel to these stylistic or technological influences, much of modern architecture's early agenda was influenced by the wider social reform movements of the time, (of which the hygiene movement was a vital part). The influence of these factors is perhaps less acknowledged for its impact on the development of a Modern architectural style (the International Style) despite its conspicuous role in the discourse of Modern Architecture. In fact many of modern architecture's tropes and its seminal projects can be associated with, and even be said to have been shaped by, the entwined health and social concerns of the time.

As described in the paper "The Medical Body in Modern Architecture" delivered by Beatriz Colomina at the Anybody conference of 1996,[9] "not only did modern architects emphasize health and exercise, their architecture was understood that way. The buildings became unconsciously identified with the healthy body."[10] Colomina would go on to describe a range of architectural elements that embodied many of the architectural traits associated with Modern Architecture, which she would equate with an attempt to address the inhibition of tuberculosis, a considerable public health concern during the early twentieth century. "Sunlight, ventilation, exercise, roof terraces, hygiene, and whiteness," in principle most of LeCorbusier's five points of architecture, from roof gardens operating as sun terraces to the piloti operating as the means to remove the living spaces from the humidity of the ground, can in some way be traced to an attempt to construct new environments for the practice of a healthier lifestyle.[11] Beyond the seminal projects of early Modernism that were models for new healthcare buildings and treatments (such as Alvar Aalto's Paimo Sanatorium and its rooftop terraces for sun therapy) what is also significant in the text is the description of a medicalization of domestic spaces with the exact same characteristics.

Beyond the more conventional and canonical Modern projects, other significant examples that demonstrate this novelty spurned on by health span the wide spectrum between the mechanically revolving Villa Girasol, a house by the engineer Angelo Invernizzi that would physically rotate to align itself with the sun's path to the work of Richard Neutra, as described by Sylvia Lavin in her book, *Form Follows Libido*.[12] Through Lavin's description of the architectural work of Neutra in respect to his preoccupations with psychiatry and the then emerging theories of psychoanalysis, we are offered an example of the deliberate implantation of mental health and well-being concerns into the physical fabric of Neutra's domestic spaces.

Neutra's interests in the notion of mood being influenced by architecture would motivate him to articulate architectural elements, that he believed had the capacity to induce different moods in its occupants. These elements and design features would be propagated throughout his projects, generating many formal, material and ambient qualities for his architecture.

9 Colomina 1997.

10 Ibid, p. 230.

11 Ibid.

12 Lavin 2004.

Within the wider discussion of transformations to the discipline and practice of architecture, the interest in the affective dimensions of the designed environment can be located in the shift described by Olov Wallenstein, from a symbolic or representational art to one that claims to cultivate its expression through the immediate ways in which occupants may sense and be affected by architecture as a bodily experience.

This would be an architecture that was thought to be based less heavily on representational signs and instead be the spaces and ambient environments that affect the physiology of its occupants, hence endowing it with the potential to influence both the physical and psychological well-being of its occupants. What is clear from this cursory survey of the influence of health concerns on Modern architecture is the great impact it had on the evolution of architectural practice and discourse through the opportunities it offered for architects to devise innovative and novel architectural organization and expression.

Reflections — Misgivings

Despite all the good that may be claimed for the influence of public health on the emergence of modern architecture, landscape architecture, and planning, it is clear that any contemporary enthusiasm for the convergence between health and the design of the built environment would benefit from reflection. Rather than replicate established practices and theories inherited from the convergence between Modern design and public health, it would be prudent to address the renewed exigency for approaching health and place with a more nuanced or balanced view.

Resonating with Latour's arguement for the entwining of social, cultural, and political concerns with the sciences, the reconsideration of the tendency to artificially divide cultural from scientific matters allows for the possibility of broadening the manner in which designers of the built environment may contribute towards health and place. The definition offered by the WHO in 1946[13] expands the realm of health from an exclusively scientific concern centered on medicine to one that introduces social issues and considerations. This contributes to a general understanding of the determinants of health to be multi-level influences. Upon revisiting some events in the long history of the relationship between health and place, we can see the repercussions of either unconscious or surreptitious convergences between social, political, and scientific agendas that have given both fields pause for thought. Another pertinent lesson from the perceived failures of this period is that the multi-level or multi-faceted nature of the determinants of health confound the engagement with public health solely through the design of the built environment. This reconsideration of the history of design of place and health allows for the recognition of the limits of the impact of built environment as a medium for health reform, and conversely, for the recognition of the vulnerabilities in the design disciplines of an uncritical acceptance of public health directives. Certainly by undertaking a more nuanced view of history, the possibility for misconstrued translations between the disciplines or other inadvertent effects to arise out of such experimentation is recognized.

13 In 1946, the Constitution of the World Health Organization defined health as "a state of complete physical, mental, and social well-being and not merely the absence of disease or infirmity." Preamble to the Constitution of the World Health Organization as adopted by the International Health Conference, New York, 19-22 June, 1946; signed on 22 July 1946 by the representatives of 61 States (Official Records of the World Health Organization, no. 2, p. 100) and entered into force on 7 April 1948.

There have been many moments in the history of architecture and planning where a junction with public health had offered the design fields an acute sense of optimism for the capacity of design to deal with wider public concerns. But upon reflection, these have also often been moments when the discipline and profession had subsequently lost confidence as well as agency in affecting these matters. Many have interpreted these as pointed lessons as to why architecture should be, at the very least ambivalent of the efficacy of its ability to deliver on its wider public ambitions solely through the design of the physical. It can also be assumed that public health agendas for design have been indiscriminatingly accepted as inherently positive and exemplifying the moral or ethical high ground for architecture and design's purpose. History offers many moments where this incontrovertible notion has proven to be suspect.

An example of this can be illustrated by revisiting the Hippocratic text, "Airs, Waters, and Places," described earlier in order to trace some of its subsequent influences. While the book offered one of the first records of a scientific approach towards health and medicine, the theories explicated in the book on the relationship between health and place, can also be seen as promoting an underlying environmental determinism that assumes a formative role for place in not just the physical but also the mental nature of a population.

> "When the soil is rich, soft and well-watered and where surface water is drunk, which is warm in summer and cold in winter, and where the seasons are favorable, you will find the people fleshy, their joints obscured, and they have watery constitutions... In addition, such people are, for the most part, cowards. They are easy-going and sleepy, clumsy craftsmen and never keen or delicate."[14]

14 Hippocrates as cited in Wear 2008.

This environmental determinism occupies an important role in underpinning a general conceit that aligns place and climate with the moral and cultural characteristics of a population. From bolstering modern concepts of nationalism to providing often misguided moral imperatives to many health and social reform movements such as those in England during the Victorian era, the Hippocratic text's influence has been shown by some historians to be more chequered and complex than may be assumed at first.[15]

15 Ibid.

> "Morals reformed—health preserved—industry invigorated, instruction diffused—public burthens lightened—Economy seated, as it were, upon a rock—the gordian knot of the Poor-Laws are not cut, but untied—all by a simple idea in Architecture!"[16]

16 Bentham 1843, 39.

During the nineteenth and up until the mid-twentieth centuries, when the construction of large swathes of England's built environment operated as design and public health experiments, these initiatives which were mandated by the indisputability of the "sciences," were commonly usurped and exploited for other social and political agendas. Like the environmental determinism underlying "Airs, Waters, and Places," the drive for slum and rookery clearance by the reformers of Victorian England was informed by the assumed pairing between physical environment and its capacity to shape the physical and moral health of its populations. In order to offer a diagnosis for the population's health problems, voluminous surveys and studies were undertaken to examine, and subsequently critique the existing conditions of the neighborhoods of the urban poor. The descriptions of the living conditions and an assumed causal link between these environments and the circumstances of the urban poor would be the basis on which much of the proposed health and social reforms would be justified. Hector Gavin's 1848 survey of Bethnal Green's slums in London, "Sanitary Ramblings," Charles Booth's Descriptive Maps of London Poverty would act as the lightning rods that would focus Victorian reformers and philanthropists towards what was to be a major exercise in slum clearance. The descriptions of the spatial conditions of these neighborhoods then came to be associated with the social and health maladies ascribed towards the residents in these surveys. The congestion, complexity, and intricate nature of the material condition

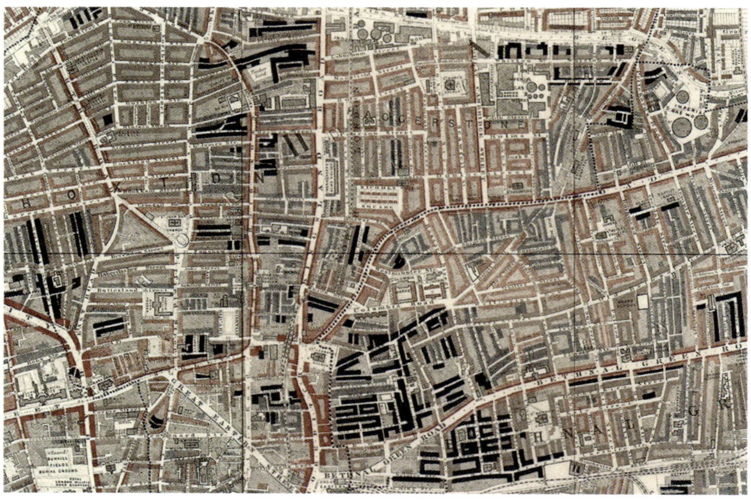

Figure 7 (Left) Portion of descriptive maps of London poverty, Charles Booth, 1892.

of these environments were often elaborated and exaggerated in these texts to impress upon the general public; the efficacy of clearance and rebuilding rather than renovation. As in many instances throughout history, the perceived moral and corporeal ills of these surveyed populations was seen to be reflected and incubated in the physical fabric of the slums and rookeries themselves, the results of a haphazard aggregation of abandoned mansions and hovels. Their spatial intricacy and overcrowding, their lack of hierarchy or differentiation between private and public spaces, and the ambiguous nature of these spaces were seen to be the root of the problem.

> "The Descriptive Maps of London Poverty joined the physical pattern of the city to the social and moral condition of its inhabitants with an unprecedented, methodical boldness, and confirmed that the chronically poor and dangerous classes tended to congregate in distinct enclaves with a noticeable different pattern from the rest of the city...The discernible differences at the scale of the city between layouts consistent with morality and layouts conducive to brutality could be compared with differences, equally self-evident, at a smaller scale. Thus architecture—in its broader social perspective, beyond the territory marked out for it by art—could be interpreted as a physical geography of moral conditions...."[17]

17 Evans 1997, 100-101.

The shared strategy by many Modern reformers throughout the nineteenth and early twentieth centuries was this careful construction and consequent adoption of formal disorder and incoherence as the symptoms of pathological environments that would come to be typified most tangibly by older medieval architecture and urban fabrics. A clear campaign against an assumed model of disorder and congestion was pursued, against which reformers would offer strict organization and order as a panacea and a disciplinary device. Countless design strategies emerged as innovations in the planning and ordering of the built environment as a consequence of this aggressive turn towards coherence and order. Amongst these were the deployment of discrete, separated land use or Euclidean zoning and an often simplistic understanding of Functionalism which would come to act as the defaults and standards for the general profession and discipline.

Sir Edwin Chadwick's friendship and philosophical sympathy with Sir Jeremy Bentham contributed to their shared belief in the role of the physical environment as a technology to discipline society. Beyond Bentham's own deliberations on the design of corrective institutions through his work on the Panopticon, investment in the the notion of architecture operating as a mechanism for social and health reform broadened the corresponding focus of the built environment from the design of institutional buildings to the restructuring of domestic environments. If, in fact, health reform were to be motivated both by environmental determinism and a mandate to correct the moral disposition of impoverished populations, the restructuring of the way in which these populations live through the organization of their life spaces (both public and private) would appear to be manifest.

A notable byproduct of this sensibility is exemplified by the model houses for four families of 1851 developed by Henry Roberts under the influence of the social and health reformer, Sir Edwin Chadwick.[18] This example of collective housing was intended to operate as the model dwelling for the relocation campaigns of the urban poor from the rookeries. In distinction to the blurring of public and private as well as the general ambiguity of its spatial and programmatic hierarchy within the slums, the design proposed a very strict separation of public circulation and private units, with the corridor becoming a very clearly articulated element in itself. This together with a clear organization of the interior of the family units to ensure a clear separation between the respective spaces of each family member from the more public rooms would prioritize a very private sensibility of domesticity in reaction to what reformers saw as the irrational ambiguity of the spaces that the urban poor were living in.

18 Ibid.

This would go on to elevate a highly private and compartmentalized idea of domesticity as a standard and default for future practice. It is also a model of domesticity that, as described by Robin Evans in relation to the Victorian slum clearance campaigns, was motivated by the privileging of what were idealizations of middle class values and lifestyles as the benchmark for restructuring the lives of the

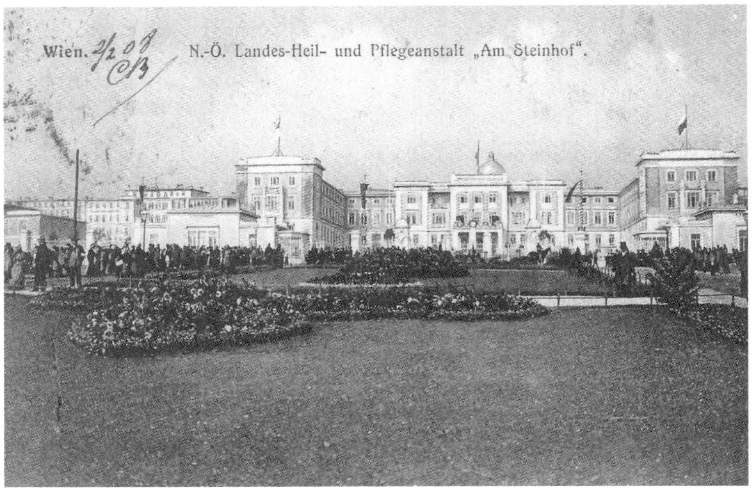

Figure 8 (Left) Postcard of Am Steinhof, 1908. developed by Otto Wagner, 1907.

urban poor. For all intents and purposes, the ideal middle class lifestyle or family was the subject that the relocated urban poor were expected to aspire to and assimilate into their own lives, with the provision of these domestic organizations operating as the mechanisms to enable this transformation.

The pervasiveness of the focus on domesticity in public health influenced reform campaigns included the reverse corollary with its use as the curious model adopted for many institutional transformations. A more humane and morally correct setting for the treatment of mental health would be adopted from the aristocratic and emerging bourgeois domestic sensibilities of the time. Interestingly, domestic settings associated with privileged lifestyles would be utilized in a number of models for hospitals such as the 1907 Am Steinhof sanatorium by Otto Wagner near Vienna which adopted the organization and qualities of an aristocratic manor. William Tuke's retreat at York of 1796, was exemplary of a humane model of a mental health institution which deliberately did away with the preceding institutional models based on discipline and incarceration. Instead, it constructed a setting more akin to a stately manor; a domestic environment that was expected to better facilitate the treatment of its patients.

While some precedents, such as the retreat at York, may have offered successful models , we would of course come to see many of these assumptions to be misplaced. The imposition of idealized models did not always have the desired effect. In the cases of the rookery or slum clearance and relocation campaigns, while physical circumstances may have been improved, often social capital and the support networks of the relocated populations would be dismantled by such efforts. This imposition of living arrangements based on middle class ideals would, in many instances, fail to translate to the working classes. Also to the horror of the reformers, ways were often found to reinstate the social practices and living arrangements targeted for reform within their new environments.

The infamous Pruitt Igoe episode that took place from 1954-1972, has been elevated in the public imagination to symbolize the obliteration of confidence in the efficacy of Modern public housing. As another more recent example of the failure of slum clearance campaigns it was also more generally associated with the failure of High Modernism in relation to its social ambitions. This widely accepted conclusion has been described by Katherine Bristol in her article, "The Pruitt Igoe Myth"[19] as a failed opportunity for learning as it persisted in placing the responsibility for the project's failure on its design. The Modern architectural organization and features were routinely demonized as the scapegoats for the failures of the social ambitions of the projects.

This narrative fails to outline what deeper and significant problems related to race politics and institutionally sanctioned segregation that plagued the project had culminated to undermine much of the social and public health ambitions for these large scale public housing projects. The combination of redlining practices[20] and a corresponding policy that would advocate "white flight" to the newly constructed suburbs, contributed to the disinvestment in many of America's city centers as well as a

19 See Bristol 1991.

20 Beginning with the National Housing Act of 1934 and the establishment the Federal Housing Administration (FHA), 'redlining' was the practice of restricting services to areas based on ethnic or racial makeup. See Zenou and Boccard 2000.

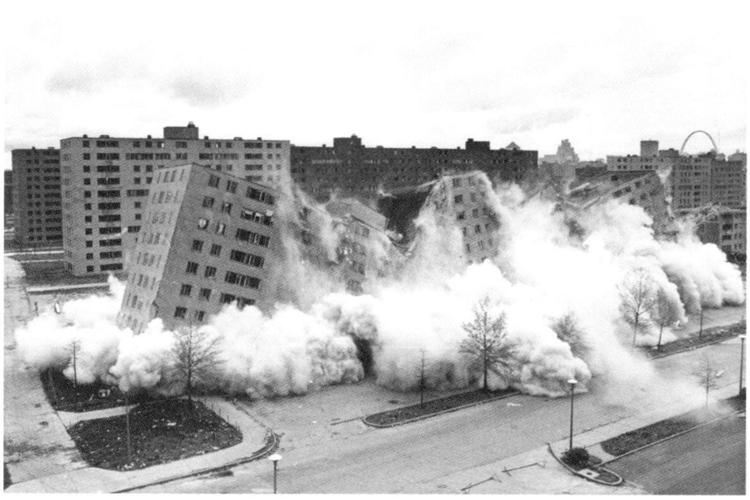

Figure 9 (Left) Aerial photograph of Pruitt-Igoe housing complex collapsing.

pattern of segregation. Paired with other imposed rules and restrictions on the living arrangements of the residents of Pruitt Igoe, the design of the built environment can be seen as only one of the many factors that would lead to its perceived failure. Given the reality of the complex set of influences, it is perhaps conceivable that the built environment may have had a very minor role in the outcomes here or even that its potentially positive effects were undermined by a misalignment with the policies of the time.

Nevertheless, the cumulative effect of many of these perceived failures of the Modern Movement contributed to a shift in focus within the architectural discipline away from a commitment to social and health reform which also saw a parallel discrediting or waning of interest in contextual factors for the public health field. However, what these examples best illustrate is less the failure or insignificance of design and the physical environment in determining well-being, but rather the more nuanced recognition of the confluence of many levels of influence over the constitution of a neighborhood or community's health. Despite being an important component, health is rarely delivered comprehensively through the definition of place and the built environment alone. The factors affecting health are as much associated with compositional factors as it is with contextual ones. What this revisionist view on the convergence between the designs of the built environment in relation to public health offers is the possibility of rehabilitating design's ambitions for contributing to human well-being with a tempered understanding of its capacities and effects.

Projections

Following the implementation of major sanitation measures and improvements to the built environment that came about as a result of the success of the hygiene movement, much of the focus in public health shifted away from the physical environment. However the public health field has recently reignited its interests in place or contextual factors after a long period of bias towards the study of the compositional. This turn has in part been influenced by the recognition that compositional factors alone are not sufficient to explain or address emerging public health concerns such as the obesity epidemic and the challenges posed by the rapid urbanization of the developing world. The mounting significance of chronic and lifestyle diseases as a major public health concern has also contributed to the corresponding growth in the focus on the ways in which the environment can impact our capacity to make appropriate health choices.

A renewal in optimism for the collaboration between the design fields and public health would do well to be informed by a balance between reflection and projective momentum. A momentum that for the design fields has waned since the apparent discrediting of the Modern movement. Both fields could adopt the notion offered by Bruno Latour of the interrelationship between science and culture, where a consciousness of the amalgamation of the rational with the political and social should operate as the basis for any reading of what we generally understand as wider public concerns. We may practice a more nuanced and conscious sensibility towards the elaboration and framing of matters of concern as a prelude to engagement.[21]

21 See Latour 2004.

It is a predicate that for ostensibly rational and scientific approaches the unconscious or deliberate masking of political and cultural motivations is not sufficient. Any novel design approach would benefit from an awareness of the capacity for external issues to affect health outcomes by place that may be beyond the typical purview and practices of the design fields. This emphasizes the value of being mindful of how design interventions may more effectively contribute to health outcomes by expanding its tools and approaches. Our tools may broaden to encapsulate an understanding of policy, to engage the multiple actors involved (the network of constituents and stakeholders), and to consider the effect of time on our interventions. In other words' it would require us to always situate our engagement within a network of actors and things.

To influence wider issues of public concern, there is a need to acknowledge that rational explanation or an investment in facts alone is not sufficient. Politics can be said to be fueled equally by beliefs and opinions. While epidemiology, demography, and mapping can still persist in informing our decisions and strategies, the link between health and the environment is one of the most direct ways in which we may see the intricate convergence of science and politics. The effects of polluting our common environment on human health and produces a complex series of associations spanning from scientific debate to the tangible effects it has on personal narratives of the allficted. With this awareness, designers are confronted with the question of how to make design practices and interventions aimed at healthier places captivate and mobilize multiple audiences today.

The cognizance of health's multi-level influences also promotes the efficacy of addressing these issues through a collaboration and conversation between diverse disciplines. Within the public health field itself, there is a recognition of the efficacy in addressing collective health concerns armed with varying expertise. This is also a view shared in many discussions within the design fields in relationship to addressing the contemporary challenges of the built environment. Whether this result in multi- or inter-disciplinary approaches, it is clear that the ability to address and evaluate the multi-level influences that affect wider matters of concern cannot conceivably be carried by any single discipline. An equal investment in the borderlands between disciplines and a commitment in disciplinary specificity may offer us a series of valuable practices that would involve a more deliberate attentiveness to the ways that the dialogue and translation between diverse knowledge is achieved.

As designers we would also profit from the reconsideration of precedents in relationship to their unfolding and subsequent evolution over time. This would involve a sensitivity to the ways in which these projects had undergone transformation or adaptation and also an understanding of the forces that mobilized their conception, delivery, and successive modifications. Lessons from the study of exemplars as time-worn places rather than idealized models encourage us to anticipate or allow for various scenarios of transformation that may contribute to the robustness of our interventions. Recently some revisionist readings of Modernism's success in delivering on its social ambitions has brought into focus a number of projects that offer designers lessons on the beneficial effect that evolution over time may have for the nurturing of socially active and healthy neighborhoods.[22] Reflecting on these lessons, rather than relying solely on the formulation of ideal and visionary master plans, the pragmatic investment in frameworks, guidelines, bylaws, and mutable systems may allow designers to expand the ways in which we imbue place with the capacity for supporting the emergence of healthy neighborhoods.

22 In addition to Katherine Bristol's text on Pruitt Igoe, a study of the PREVI Experimental Housing project in Lima, Peru, three decades after its construction by EquipoArquitectura adds to the growing literature on a revisionist view of Modernism's social impact. See Time Builds!, 2008, EquipoArquitectura, Gustavo Gili, Barcelona, Spain. For a reconsideration of the Eixample by Cerdà as it has evolved over time, see Mah David, 2014, The Eixample Example in Berrizbeitia Anita, 2014, Urban Landscape (Critical Concepts in Built Environment), Routledge, London, UK.

Part of the urgency in addressing the physical environment in public health is influenced by the realization that the notion of our collective health can no longer be neatly compartmentalized into national boundaries. In fact, with many of the waves of contagion seen in the nineteenth century having their origins in the migration of various carriers (both human and non-human) which were mobilized by the burgeoning international trades of the time, we can see that compartmentalization has never truly been possible. Public health challenges are often global concerns and this broadening of scope means that problems facing many parts of the world related to environmental issues were thought to have been eliminated in the developed world are now matters of concern for all of us. Adding to this is the massive urbanization in the developing world, unfolding at a rate that has no historical precedent in scale or speed. This process that is effectively transforming our common global biosphere, signals the urgency for us to deliberate on how we may contribute to a shared knowledge and series of practices that may inform how a response to these challenges may be leveraged to deliver well-being and health in an equitable manner to a wider global public.

Figure Credits

Figure 1, George Cruikshank, 1829, The March of Bricks and Mortar, *Scraps and Sketches*, etching, © 2016 Malcolm Warrington

Figure 2, Snow, Sir John; Cheffins C.F. lithograph, Southhampton Buildings, London, England, 1854 in *John Snow. On the Mode of Communication of Cholera, 2nd Ed*, John Churchill, New Burlington Street, London, England. Accessed 13 January 2016, http://matrix.msu.edu/~johnsnow/images/online_companion/chapter_images/fig12-5.jpg.

Figure 3, Cerdà, Ildefons 1859, *Original plan of the extension of Barcelona*, Museu d'Historia de la Ciutat, Barcelona. Public Domain. Accessed 13 January 2016, https://commons.wikimedia.org/wiki/File:Ensanche_-_eixample_-_Barcelona.jpg

Figure 4, Rovira, Antoni 1859, *Eixample map of Barcelona*, image, Museu d'Historia de la Ciutat, Barcelona. Public Domain. Accessed 13 January 2016, https://upload.wikimedia.org/wikipedia/commons/1/13/EixampleBCN-projecteRovira.jpg

Figure 5, Olmsted, Vaux, and Co., Landscape Architects. 1869. *General Plan of Riverside*. Olmsted Lithograph Collection. Olmsted Job #607 Riverside, Illinois. Chicago: Chicago Lithographing Co. Courtesy of the United States Department of the Interior, National Park Service, Frederick Law Olmsted National Historic Site

Figure 6, Steinitz, Carl 1967, *Computer Mapping and the Regional Landscape*. Harvard University. Laboratory for Computer Graphics and Spatial Analysis.

Figure 7, Charles Booth, 1892, Descriptive map of London poverty, 1889 (south-eastern sheet) Life and labour of the people in London Wellcome Library, London. Wellcome Images, http://wellcomeimages.org, Copyrighted work available under Creative Commons Attribution only licence CC BY 4.0

Figure 8, Am Steinhof, 1908, postcard. Public Domain. Accessed 13 January 2016, https://commons.wikimedia.org/wiki/File:19080202_wien_am_steinhof.jpg.

Figure 9, *Pruitt-Igoe Collapses*, United U.S. Department of Housing and Urban Development Office of Policy Development and Research. Public Domain. Accessed 13 January 2016, https://commons.wikimedia.org/wiki/File:Pruitt-Igoe-collapses.jpg

References

Bentham, Jeremy 1843, *The Works of Jeremy Bentham, vol. 4 (Panopticon, Constitution, Colonies, Codification) [1843]*. John Bowring (ed.), Liberty Fund, Inc., p. 39. http://oll.libertyfund.org/titles/1925.

Bristol, Katharine May 1991, 'The Pruitt-Igoe Myth,' *Journal of Architectural Education* (Association of Collegiate Schools of Architecture), pp. 163–171.

Colomina, Beatriz 1997, 'The Medical Body in Modern Architecture,' *Anybody*, Cynthia Davidson (ed.). MIT Press, Cambridge, Massachusetts, London, England.

Evans, Robin 1997, 'Rookeries and Model Dwellings: English Housing Reform and the Moralities of Private Space,' *Translations From Drawing to Building and Other Essays*, The Architectural Association Publications, London, pp. 100 – 101.

Fisher, Thomas November 2010, 'Frederick Law Olmsted and the Campaign for Public Health,' *Places Journal*. https://placesjournal.org/article/frederick-law-olmsted-and-the-campaign-for-public-health/.

Foucault, Michel 2007, *Security, Territory, Population: Lectures at the Collège de France 1977-1978,* Michel Senellart, François Ewald, Alessandro Fontana, and Arnold I. Davidson (eds), trans. Graham Burchell, Palgrave Macmillan, London.

Foucault, Michel 2008, *The Birth of Biopolitics: Lectures at the Collège de France, 1978-1979,* Michel Senellart, François Ewald, Alessandro Fontana, and Arnold I. Davidson (eds), trans. Graham Burchell, Palgrave Macmillan, London.

Latour, Bruno 1988, *The Pasteurization of France,* trans. Alan Sheridan and John Law, Harvard University Press, Cambridge, MA and London, UK, pp. 5 – 7.

Latour Bruno Winter 2004, 'Why Has Critique Run Out of Steam? From Matters of Fact to Matters of Concern,' *Critical Inquiry - Special issue on the Future of Critique*, Vol 30 No 2, pp. 25-248.

Lavin, Sylvia 2004, *Form Follows Libido: Architecture and Richard Neutra in a Psychoanalytic Culture*, MIT Press, Cambridge, MA and London, England.

Wallenstein, Sven-Olov 2009, *Biopolitics and the Emergence of Modern Architecture*, Princeton Architectural Press, New York.

Wear, Andrew 2008, 'Place, Health, and Disease: The Airs, Waters, Places Tradition in Early Modern England and North America,' *Journal of Medieval and Early Modern Studies*, Vol 38, No 3, pp. 443-465.

Zenou, Yves; Boccard, Nicolas 2000. 'Racial Discrimination and Redlining in Cities,' *Journal of Urban Economics*, Vol 48, No. 2, September 2000, pp. 260-285.

When Public Health and Planning Closely Intersect
Five Moments, Five Strategies

Ann Forsyth

Trained in planning and architecture, Ann Forsyth is a professor of urban planning at the Harvard Graduate School of Design. From 2007-2012 she was a professor of city and regional planning at Cornell. She taught previously at the University of Minnesota, directing the Metropolitan Design Center (2002-2007), Harvard (1999-2002), and the University of Massachusetts (1993-1999) where she was co-director of a small community design center, the Urban Places Project.

Professional public health and urban planning are practices with intertwined histories, intersecting and diverging at various points in the past century or so. Both fields developed in their contemporary form as responses to a set of conditions arising from industrialization, urbanization, and migration. They looked forward to cleaner, safer, healthier, and more supportive places and communities. Their histories demonstrate multiple specific interconnections from slum clearance and anti-sprawl advocacy to traffic safety and water supply protection.[1]

This chapter focuses on five key intersections that represent both a substantive interest and a methodological approach:

- Documenting and analyzing social conditions in neighborhoods, towns, and cities,
- Reforming the city with targeted social interventions in places,
- Regulating cities and regions for health outcomes,
- Building model communities, and
- Coordinating diverse actors to make places healthier.

These are important moments. However, they were not necessarily those seen as most important overall, particularly in the field of public health. When the Centers for Disease Control and Prevention in 1999 articulated ten great public health achievements of the 20th century, these included: immunizations, infectious disease control, workplace safety, healthier mothers and babies, family planning, fluoridation of water, tobacco seen as a health hazard, safer and healthier foods, work to decrease deaths from heart disease and strokes, and motor vehicle safety. While some of these overlapped with urban planning activities, planning was not the main actor. For example, motor vehicle safety, the area with perhaps the most obvious links, has increased due to changes in vehicle and highway design, laws (e.g. safety belts and anti-drunk driving), and secondarily the work of planners to protect pedestrians with mechanisms like traffic calming. This reflects the complexities of intervening in specific places, and the difficulties of population-wide solutions to the problems of specific localities.

1 Sloane 2006; Lopez 2012.

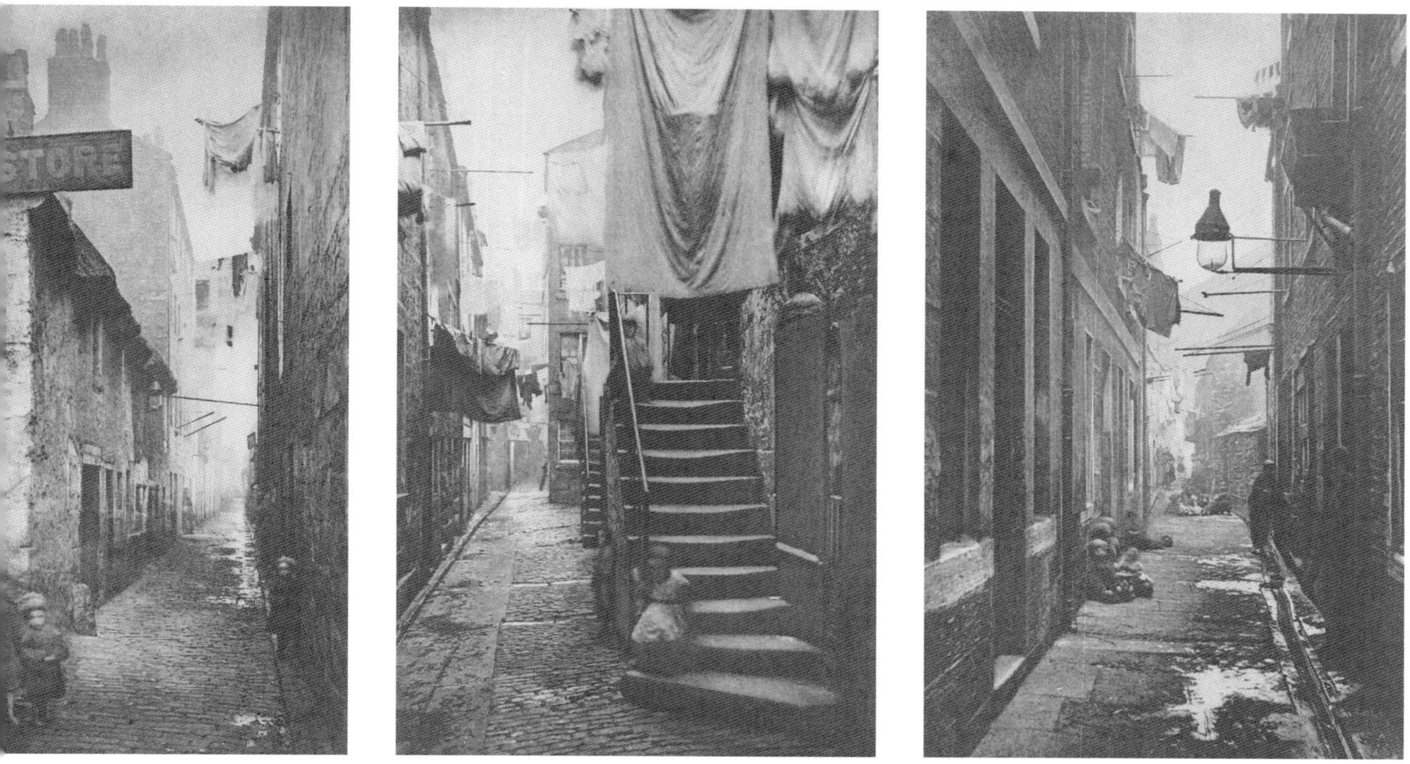

Figure 1-3 (Above) Thomas Annan's 1868 photos of Glasgow.

Documenting + Analyzing

In the nineteenth century Britain led the world in industrialization and urbanization. The relatively stable, if hierarchical and unequal, world of Jane Austen novels, set in the late 18th and very early 19th century, was transformed into the more chaotic and ruthless world of Charles Dickens some decades later. As industrial urbanization spread more globally, those documenting and analyzing the situation worked to systematically understand the resulting poverty, disease, and inequality. They communicated these problems to a set of opinion leaders and policy makers who had ignored or just not grasped their magnitude. This work in the middle and later part of the nineteenth century included:

- Written reports based on observations of living conditions—compellingly Engel's Condition of the Working Class in England in 1844.[2]
- Mapping of disease—most famously the early 1850s maps by Snow of the Broad Street pump cholera outbreak in London.
- Photography of living conditions—Annan's early photography of Glasgow taken in between 1866 and 1871, but also Riis's (1890) work on How the Other Half Lives in New York.[3]
- Surveying and mapping of poverty and in equality—exemplified by Booth's poverty maps of London and DuBois' work on race in Philadelphia in the 1980s.

Showing the interplay between crowded conditions, poverty, and unhealthy housing and work places, the earliest of these analyses and exposés predate both the public health and planning fields, at least in their

2 Engels 1943.

3 Annan 1900; Riis 1890.

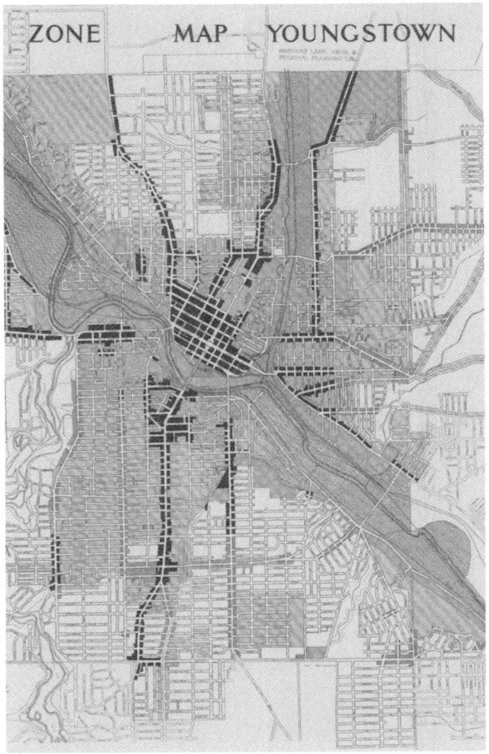

Figure 4 (Right) Youngstown, OH zoning map.

professional form. Public health organized earliest on a large scale, with the British Public Health Act passed in 1848 and the American Public Health Association founded in 1872.[4] Urban planning, though founded later, also sees these kinds of social analyses and critiques as part of its heritage.

4 British Library 2015.

Reforming

People did not stop at analysis but set about cleaning up the city: installing sewers, collecting wastes, and building public parks. Over time, however, a relatively new way of reforming the city emerged that involved setting community programs within neighborhoods and interacting directly to improve the lives of those who had migrated to urban areas. The iconic form of the settlement house emerged in the period of the 1860s through the 1890s, first in Britain and then in the U.S.[5] Though taking different forms in different countries and even cities, the basic idea was for university-educated people to settle in a poor community and bring educational, training, and health programs to the community. The kinds of people working in these settings tended to be interested in other aspects of reform such as labor laws, maternal health, and housing.[6] Playgrounds—compact and child-centered parks—are another offshoot of this movement in the late 19th and early 20th centuries.[7] What makes them different to some other approaches is that the programs such as classes and play activities and not just the places are key. In the U.S. this was also the movement where women found a very substantial leadership role, although they were less welcome in early city planning.[8] The legacy can be seen in programmed open spaces and community centers.

5 Scheuer 1985.

6 Spain 2001.

7 Cranz 1982.

8 Spain 2001.

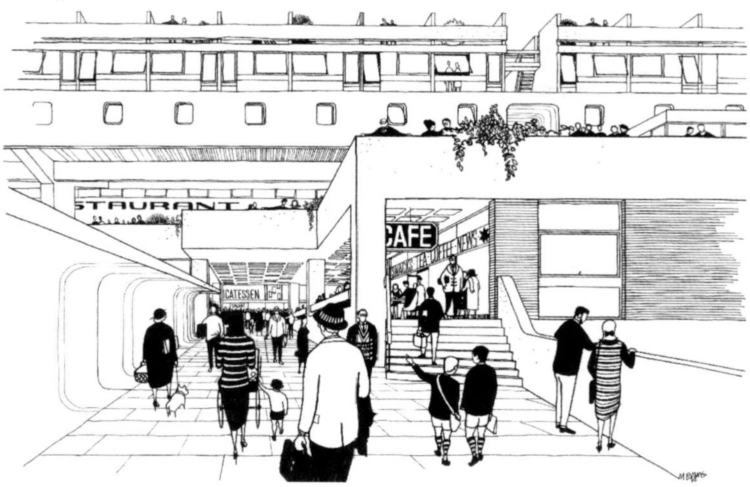

Figure 5 (Right) This drawing of Geoffrey Copcutt's design was prepared by Michael Evans c.1963. Cumbernald blends modernism and the garden city tradition. Its early road hierarchy with four levels and a Radburn-style layout completely separated pedestrians from cars and resulted in a reduction of accidents in the mid-1960s to 23% of national averages (Forsyth and Crewe 2009b; Sykes et al 1967, 9).

Regulating

Such methods of intervening could only help a limited number of people. To make a larger difference others moved to regulate aspects of the city related to health, from housing standards to factory locations. Such approaches needed many more workers to monitor and enforce, providing jobs for fledgling professions. While some regulations were specific to each field—such as food safety to public health—there have been many areas where both fields have been involved:

- Improving natural lighting, ventilation, and sanitation in housing, a key concern of the nineteenth century.
- Reducing industrial hazardous emissions and moving polluting industries further from residences saw a burst of activity in the nineteenth and early twentieth century to create early ordinances including zoning.
- Comprehensively planning neighborhoods, cities, and regions, starting in the early twentieth century but only really coming of age in the second half
- Limiting the kinds of activities in places through regulations like zoning.
- Making air and water cleaner from industrial pollutants, which reached a peak of activity in the 1970s.
- Working to reduce, mitigate, and manage climate change.

Such regulations, while sparking controversy from time to time, now seem part of the landscape of life. They are not all the same. Some are clearly linked to human health—for example regulating industrial emissions—while others such as zoning may take health as an excuse for regulations based on other values.[9]

9 Lopez 2012

Building

Intervening in the existing city obviously has limitations because it is very hard to undo the patterns of the past. Building model homes, neighborhoods, districts, and towns has great appeal as one can start from scratch to test innovations without the burden of the past.

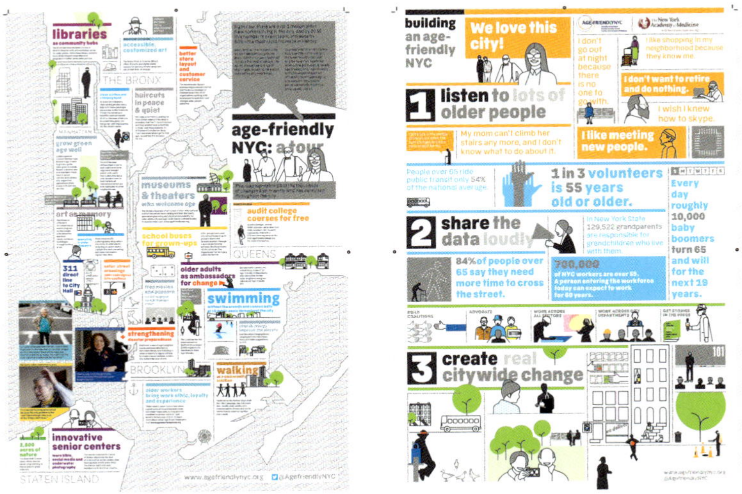

Figure 6 (Left) Age-Friendly NY overview.

- In the nineteenth century model company towns and some colonial settlements led the way at the neighborhood scale and above.
- The idea took off with the movement based on the garden city idea of new, compact, and decentralized towns set in a productive landscape.
- However, a modernist trajectory of towers in the park is also part of this movement to bring people closer to light and air, provide some level of collective services, and generally rethink the industrial city.
- Programs of new towns, or large-scale self-contained cities, spread after the Second World War.
- While very large scale developments are difficult to pull off—they take a lot of time and resources—model neighborhoods still remain in vogue from New Urbanism to Net Zero Energy Neighborhoods.

Such physical innovations can be tremendously inspiring and there are many classic examples of models developments that created livable, and arguably healthier places. This is the tradition of this book—of prototypical models and inspirations. But the models did not fit well everywhere, sometimes due to their physical form and other times because of the cultural and organizational context those forms needed to be part of. High-rise public housing does better in Singapore than in St. Louis, for example.[10]

10 Forsyth and Crewe 2009a.

Coordinating

Finally, in the last part of the twentieth century it was obvious that there was a great deal of activity in health policy and programming in areas related to health, but this didn't always add up to a healthier environment. Coordinating diverse actors involved in various social, economic, and environmental policy areas, as well as engaging community members, could solve some of those problems. The poster child for this type of activity is the WHO Healthy Cities program that has a well-honed process aimed at obtaining high level political support, creating a shared vision, and developing new organizational structures for coordination. It has gone through several phases, most recently focusing on topics such as healthy urban planning, health impact assessment, healthy aging, health equity, and health in all policies.[11] The WHO's Age-Friendly Communities program has

11 Tsouros and Green 2010.

many similarities. Obviously these activities are at the intersection of health and planning but also of a great many other fields and professions from social work to business and education.

Reflections

Documenting, analyzing, reforming, regulating, and coordinating have been and still are key strategies for understanding and intervening for healthier environments. Planners and environmental designers often have high hopes that their activities will solve pressing human problems and they certainly can. However, health outcomes have many causes from biology to the broader culture. The environment, from the building to the neighborhood, is only one of these. If created in a way that is coordinated with other programs and policies, from early childhood education to services for the frail and aged, such environments can of course do much more. This is the story of the best of the health and place interventions. They use multiple strategies which is perhaps why coordination has emerged as a major approach in recent decades. It is likely to remain important in the future.

Figure Credits

Figure 1-3, Annan, Thomas 1900, photos earlier, *The Old Closes and Streets of Glasgow. Glasgow,* Collection of the British Library. Accessed 4 August 2015, http://www.bl.uk/collection-items/the-old-closes-and-streets-of-glasgow.

Figure 4, Medicus, Fred C 1937, *Building zone map Youngstown, Ohio,* map. Youngstown, OH : City Planning Commission. Harvard Library Collection. Accessed 4 August 2015, http://id.lib.harvard.edu/aleph/013610057/catalog.

Figure 5, Michael Evans, 1963, *Drawing of Cumbernauld Town Centre,* © Royal Incorporation of Architects in Scotland, Accessed 12 January 2016, http://canmore.org.uk/site/70557/cumbernauld-cumbernauld-town-centre-general.

Figure 6, *Age Friendly NY*, PDF, Accessed 12 January 2015, http://www.nyam.org/agefriendlynyc/docs/agefriendlynyc_fullsize_11am_071713.pdf.

References

Annan, Thomas 1900, photos earlier, *The Old Closes and Streets of Glasgow. Glasgow,* Collection of the British Library. Accessed 4 August 2015, http://www.bl.uk/collection-items/the-old-closes-and-streets-of-glasgow.

British Library 2015, Public Health timeline. http://www.bl.uk/learning/histcitizen/21cc/publichealth/background/timeline/publichealthtimeline.html.

Center for Disease Control 1999, Achievements in Public Health 1900-1999, *Morbidity and Mortality Weekly Report.* Accessed 4 August 2015, http://www.cdc.gov/about/history/tengpha.htm.

Cranz, Galen 1982, *The Politics of Park Design,* MIT Press, Cambridge, MA.

Engels, Friedrich 1943, orig 1845, *The Condition of the Working-Class in England in 1844,* Trans. F.K. Wischnewetzky, George Allen and Unwin, London. Accessed 4 August 2015, http://www.gutenberg.org/files/17306/17306-h/17306-h.htm.

Forsyth, Ann and Crewe, Katherine 2009a, 'A Typology of Comprehensive Designed Communities Since the Second World War', *Landscape Journal 28,* 1: 56-78.

Forsyth, Ann and Crewe, Katherine 2009b, 'New Visions for Suburbia: Reassessing Aesthetics and Place-making in Modernism, Imageability, and New Urbanism', *Journal of Urban Design 14, 4*: 415-438.

Greenwich House 2015, History. Accessed 4 August 2015, http://www.greenwichhouse.org/about/history.

Lopez, Russell P 2012, *The Built Environment and Public Health.* Jossey-Bass, San Francisco.

Riis, Jacob 1890, *How the Other Half Lives: Studies Among the Tenements of New York*, Charles Scribners and Sons, New York.

Spain, Daphne 2001, *How Women Saved the City*, University of Minnesota Press, Minneapolis.

Tsouros, Agis and Green, Geoff 2010, 'Healthy Cities: Lessons Learned' in *Urban Health, Global Perspectives.* Vlahov, David; Boufford, Jo Ivy; Pearson, Clarence E.; and Norris, Laurie (eds), Jossey-Bass, San Francisco.

Scheuer, Jeffrey 1985, *Legacy of Light: University Settlement's first century,* University Settlement Society of New York, New York. Accessed 4 August 2015, http://www.socialwelfarehistory.com/organizations/origins-of-the-settlement-house-movement/.

Sykes, Andrew; Livingstone, J.M.; and Green, Maurice 1969, Cumbernauld 67: A Household Survey and Report Occasional Paper Number 1, University of Strathclyde, Department of Sociology.

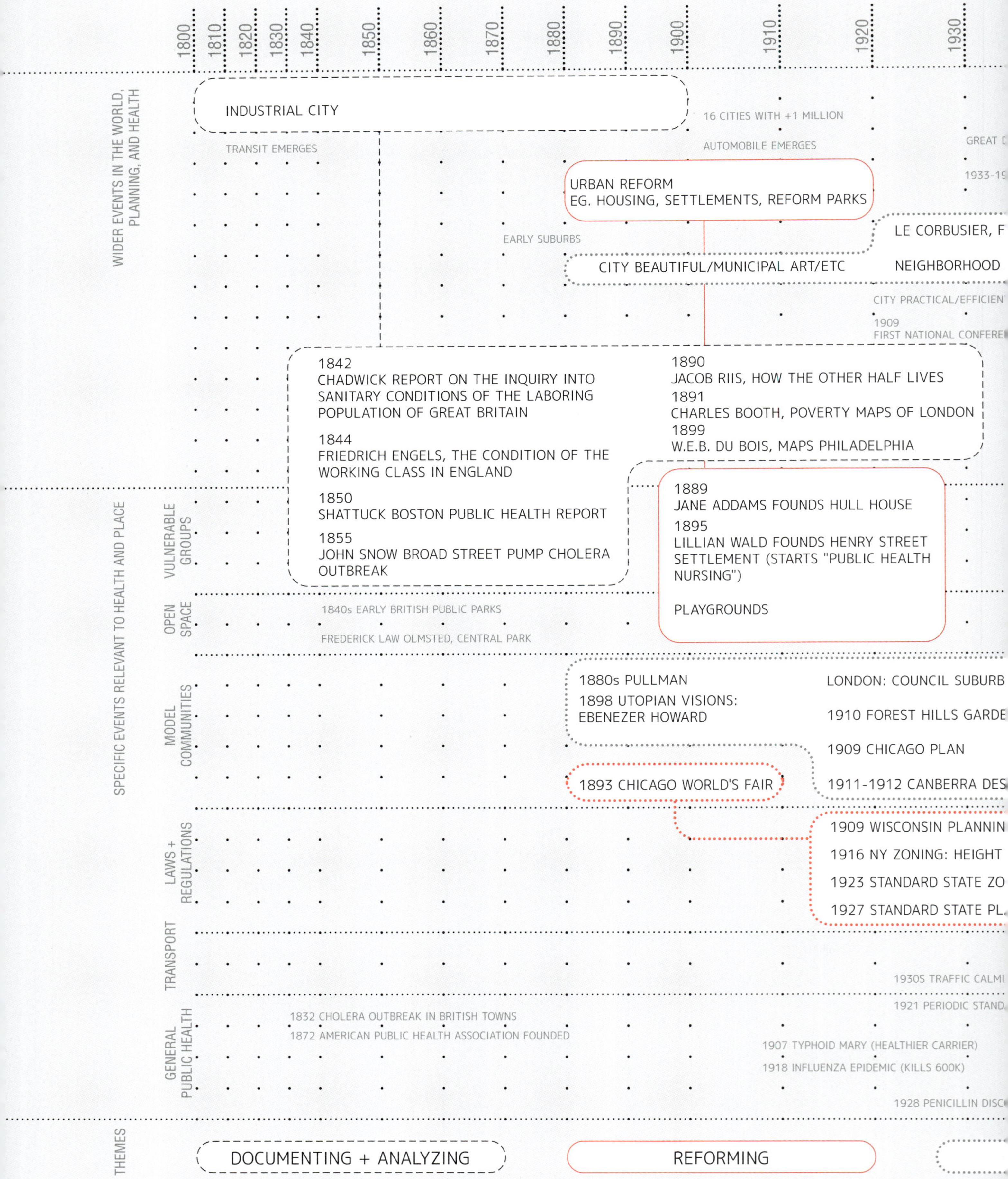
1800
1810
1820
1830
1840
1850
1860
1870
1880
1890
1900
1910
1920
1930
WIDER EVENTS IN THE WORLD, PLANNING, AND HEALTH
INDUSTRIAL CITY
16 CITIES WITH +1 MILLION
TRANSIT EMERGES
AUTOMOBILE EMERGES
GREAT D
1933-19
URBAN REFORM
EG. HOUSING, SETTLEMENTS, REFORM PARKS
EARLY SUBURBS
LE CORBUSIER, F
CITY BEAUTIFUL/MUNICIPAL ART/ETC
NEIGHBORHOOD
CITY PRACTICAL/EFFICIEN
1909
FIRST NATIONAL CONFERE
1842
CHADWICK REPORT ON THE INQUIRY INTO SANITARY CONDITIONS OF THE LABORING POPULATION OF GREAT BRITAIN
1844
FRIEDRICH ENGELS, THE CONDITION OF THE WORKING CLASS IN ENGLAND
1850
SHATTUCK BOSTON PUBLIC HEALTH REPORT
1855
JOHN SNOW BROAD STREET PUMP CHOLERA OUTBREAK
1890
JACOB RIIS, HOW THE OTHER HALF LIVES
1891
CHARLES BOOTH, POVERTY MAPS OF LONDON
1899
W.E.B. DU BOIS, MAPS PHILADELPHIA
SPECIFIC EVENTS RELEVANT TO HEALTH AND PLACE
VULNERABLE GROUPS
1889
JANE ADDAMS FOUNDS HULL HOUSE
1895
LILLIAN WALD FOUNDS HENRY STREET SETTLEMENT (STARTS "PUBLIC HEALTH NURSING")
PLAYGROUNDS
OPEN SPACE
1840s EARLY BRITISH PUBLIC PARKS
FREDERICK LAW OLMSTED, CENTRAL PARK
MODEL COMMUNITIES
1880s PULLMAN
1898 UTOPIAN VISIONS:
EBENEZER HOWARD
LONDON: COUNCIL SUBURB
1910 FOREST HILLS GARDE
1909 CHICAGO PLAN
1893 CHICAGO WORLD'S FAIR
1911-1912 CANBERRA DES
LAWS + REGULATIONS
1909 WISCONSIN PLANNIN
1916 NY ZONING: HEIGHT
1923 STANDARD STATE ZO
1927 STANDARD STATE PL
TRANSPORT
1930S TRAFFIC CALMI
1921 PERIODIC STAND
GENERAL PUBLIC HEALTH
1832 CHOLERA OUTBREAK IN BRITISH TOWNS
1872 AMERICAN PUBLIC HEALTH ASSOCIATION FOUNDED
1907 TYPHOID MARY (HEALTHIER CARRIER)
1918 INFLUENZA EPIDEMIC (KILLS 600K)
1928 PENICILLIN DISC
THEMES
DOCUMENTING + ANALYZING
REFORMING

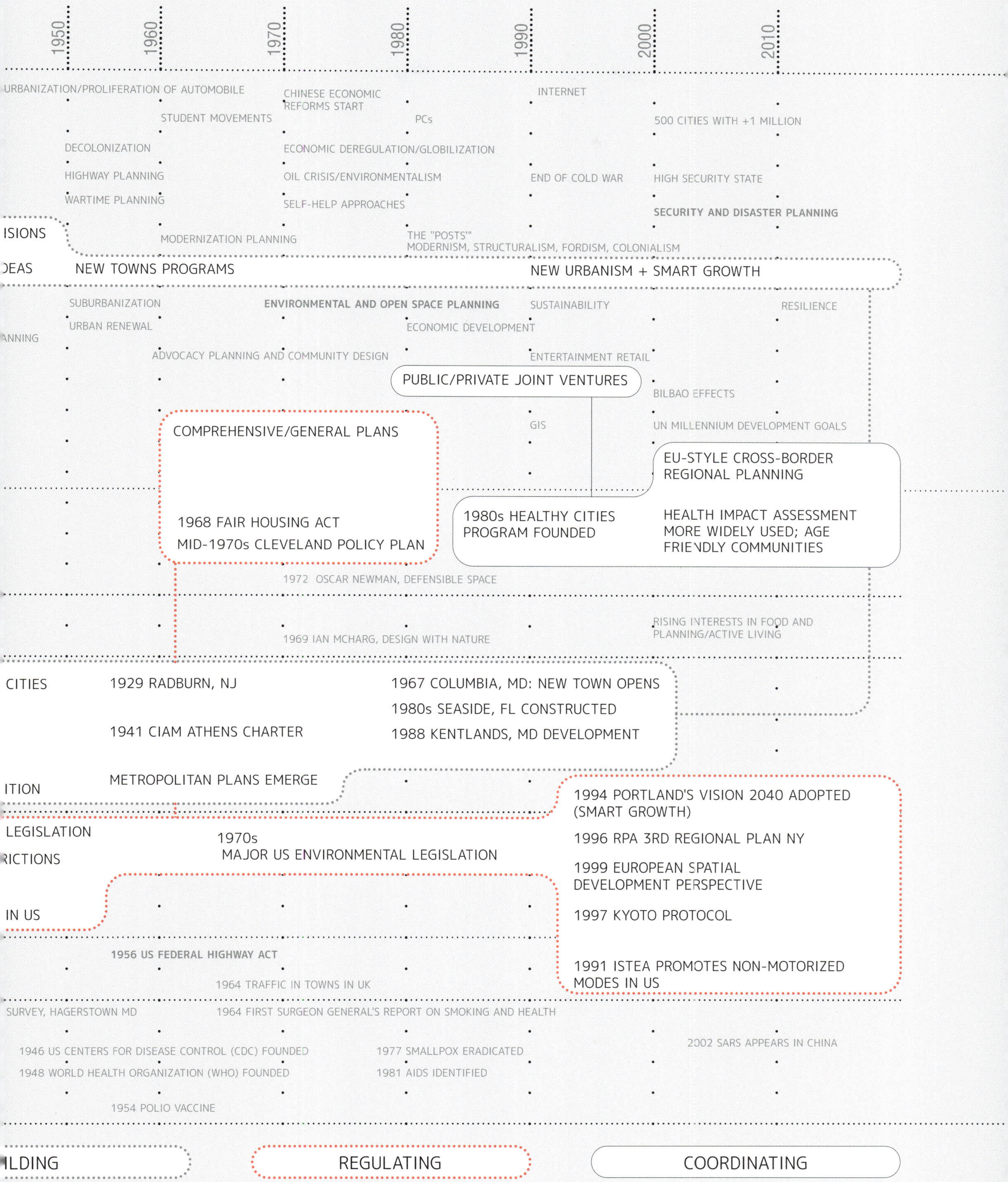
1950
1960
1970
1980
1990
2000
2010
URBANIZATION/PROLIFERATION OF AUTOMOBILE
CHINESE ECONOMIC REFORMS START
INTERNET
STUDENT MOVEMENTS
PCs
500 CITIES WITH +1 MILLION
DECOLONIZATION
ECONOMIC DEREGULATION/GLOBILIZATION
HIGHWAY PLANNING
OIL CRISIS/ENVIRONMENTALISM
END OF COLD WAR
HIGH SECURITY STATE
WARTIME PLANNING
SELF-HELP APPROACHES
SECURITY AND DISASTER PLANNING
ISIONS
MODERNIZATION PLANNING
THE "POSTS"
MODERNISM, STRUCTURALISM, FORDISM, COLONIALISM
DEAS
NEW TOWNS PROGRAMS
NEW URBANISM + SMART GROWTH
SUBURBANIZATION
ENVIRONMENTAL AND OPEN SPACE PLANNING
SUSTAINABILITY
RESILIENCE
URBAN RENEWAL
ECONOMIC DEVELOPMENT
ANNING
ADVOCACY PLANNING AND COMMUNITY DESIGN
ENTERTAINMENT RETAIL
PUBLIC/PRIVATE JOINT VENTURES
BILBAO EFFECTS
COMPREHENSIVE/GENERAL PLANS
GIS
UN MILLENNIUM DEVELOPMENT GOALS
EU-STYLE CROSS-BORDER REGIONAL PLANNING
1968 FAIR HOUSING ACT
MID-1970s CLEVELAND POLICY PLAN
1980s HEALTHY CITIES PROGRAM FOUNDED
HEALTH IMPACT ASSESSMENT MORE WIDELY USED; AGE FRIENDLY COMMUNITIES
1972 OSCAR NEWMAN, DEFENSIBLE SPACE
RISING INTERESTS IN FOOD AND PLANNING/ACTIVE LIVING
1969 IAN MCHARG, DESIGN WITH NATURE
CITIES
1929 RADBURN, NJ
1967 COLUMBIA, MD: NEW TOWN OPENS
1980s SEASIDE, FL CONSTRUCTED
1941 CIAM ATHENS CHARTER
1988 KENTLANDS, MD DEVELOPMENT
METROPOLITAN PLANS EMERGE
ITION
1994 PORTLAND'S VISION 2040 ADOPTED (SMART GROWTH)
LEGISLATION
1970s
MAJOR US ENVIRONMENTAL LEGISLATION
1996 RPA 3RD REGIONAL PLAN NY
RICTIONS
1999 EUROPEAN SPATIAL DEVELOPMENT PERSPECTIVE
IN US
1997 KYOTO PROTOCOL
1956 US FEDERAL HIGHWAY ACT
1964 TRAFFIC IN TOWNS IN UK
1991 ISTEA PROMOTES NON-MOTORIZED MODES IN US
SURVEY, HAGERSTOWN MD
1964 FIRST SURGEON GENERAL'S REPORT ON SMOKING AND HEALTH
1946 US CENTERS FOR DISEASE CONTROL (CDC) FOUNDED
1977 SMALLPOX ERADICATED
2002 SARS APPEARS IN CHINA
1948 WORLD HEALTH ORGANIZATION (WHO) FOUNDED
1981 AIDS IDENTIFIED
1954 POLIO VACCINE
ILDING
REGULATING
COORDINATING

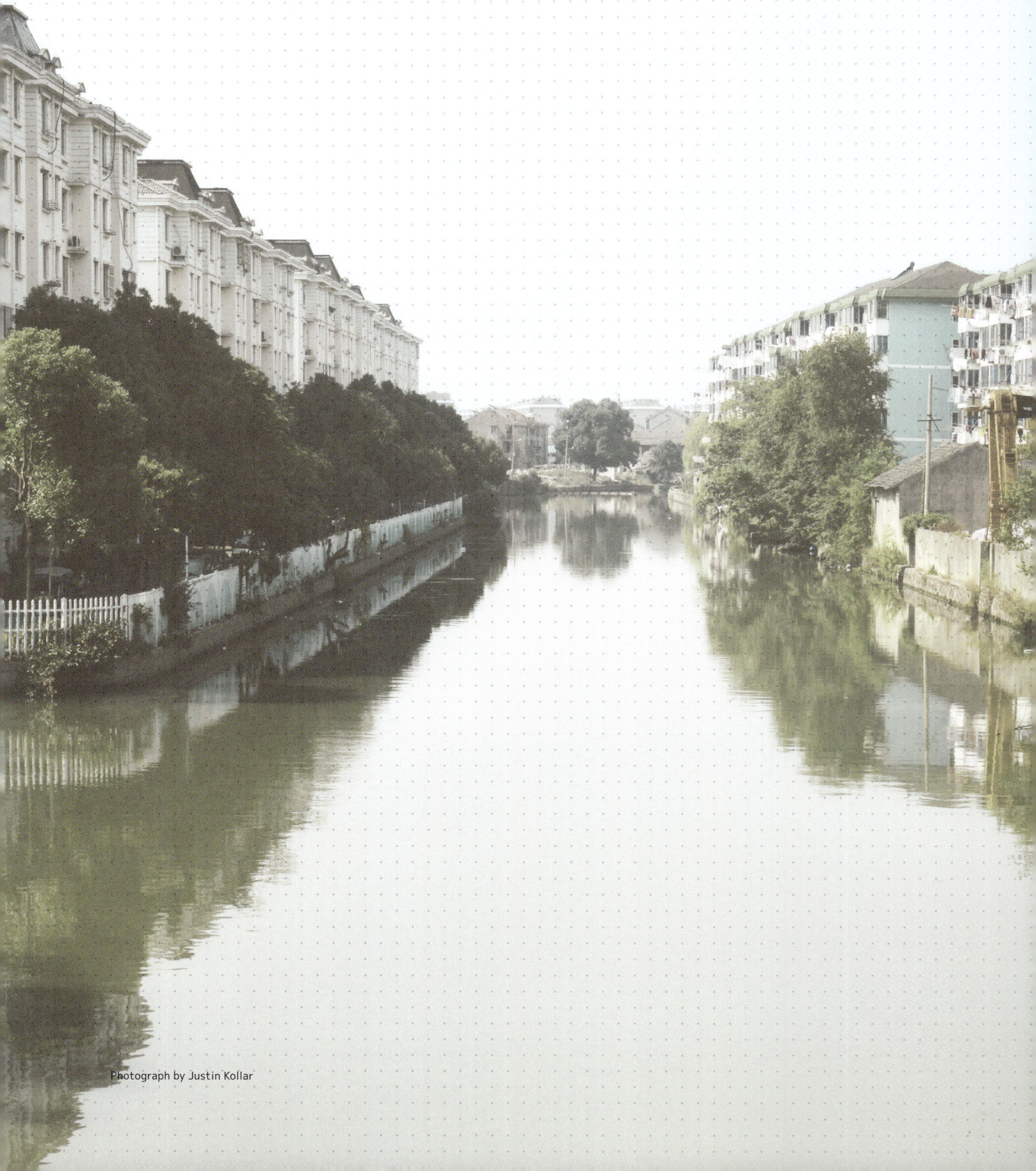

Photograph by Justin Kollar

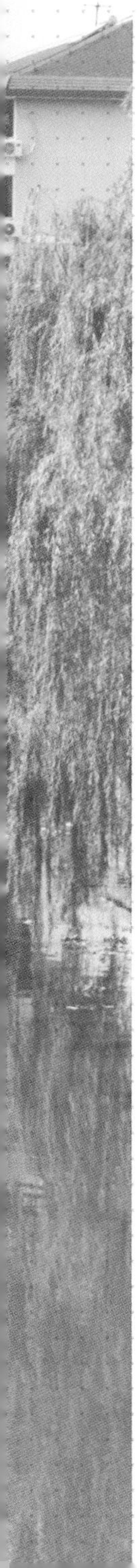

Chapter 2

The Social Determinants of Health

An Interview with Dr. Ichiro Kawachi, Leire Asensio Villoria + David Mah, 3rd March 2015

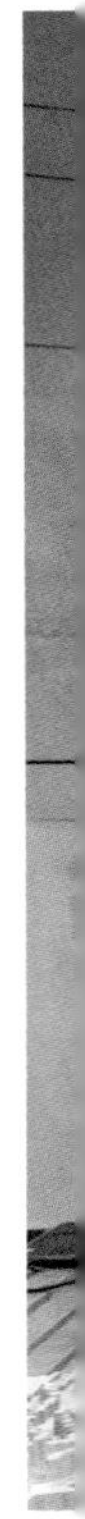

Ichiro Kawachi, MB.ChB., Ph.D., is the John L. Loeb and Frances Lehman Loeb Professor of Social Epidemiology, and Chair of the Department of Social and Behavioral Sciences at the Harvard School of Public Health. Dr Kawachi received both his medical degree and Ph.D. (in epidemiology) from the University of Otago, New Zealand. He has taught at the Harvard School of Public Health since 1992.

Kawachi is the co-editor (with Lisa Berkman) of the first textbook on Social Epidemiology, published by Oxford University Press in 2000 (new & revised edition published in 2014, with Lisa Berkman & Maria Glymour). His other books include *Neighborhoods and Health* with Lisa Berkman (Oxford University Press, 2003), *Globalization and Health* with Sara Wamala (Oxford University Press, 2006), *Social Capital and Health* with S.V. Subramanian & Daniel Kim (Springer, 2008), the *Oxford Handbook of Public Health Practice* with Charles Guest, Walter Ricciardi & Iain Laing (Oxford University Press, 2013), *Global Perspectives on Social Capital and Health* (Springer, 2013) with Soshi Takao & S.V. Subramanian, and *Behavioral Economics and Public Health* with Christina Roberto (Oxford University Press, forthcoming). His current NIH-funded R01 project is focused on the longitudinal impacts of community social cohesion/social capital on functional recovery after the March 11, 2011 Great Eastern Japan earthquake and tsunami.

Dr, Kawachi is the Co-editor in Chief (with S.V. Subramanian) of the international journal Social Science & Medicine. He is an elected member of the Institute of Medicine of the US National Academy of Sciences.

Using the World Health Organization's broad definition of health, encompassing physical, psychological, and social wellbeing, the book is organized in a manner that allows a range of issues associated with these different areas of health to be introduced to a design audience. Dr Ichiro Kawachi is a leading scholar and researcher in the field of social epidemiology.

His work on the social determinants of health is significant for designers because of its acknowledgment of the contextual as well as the compositional approaches to studying public health. His focus on the relationship between health and neighborhoods offers the design field a bridge to a potential dialogue with the public health field and a window into the ways in which the physical environment may have a role to play in affecting public health and particularly; the social determinants of health.

We spoke with Dr. Kawachi on the 3rd of March, 2015.

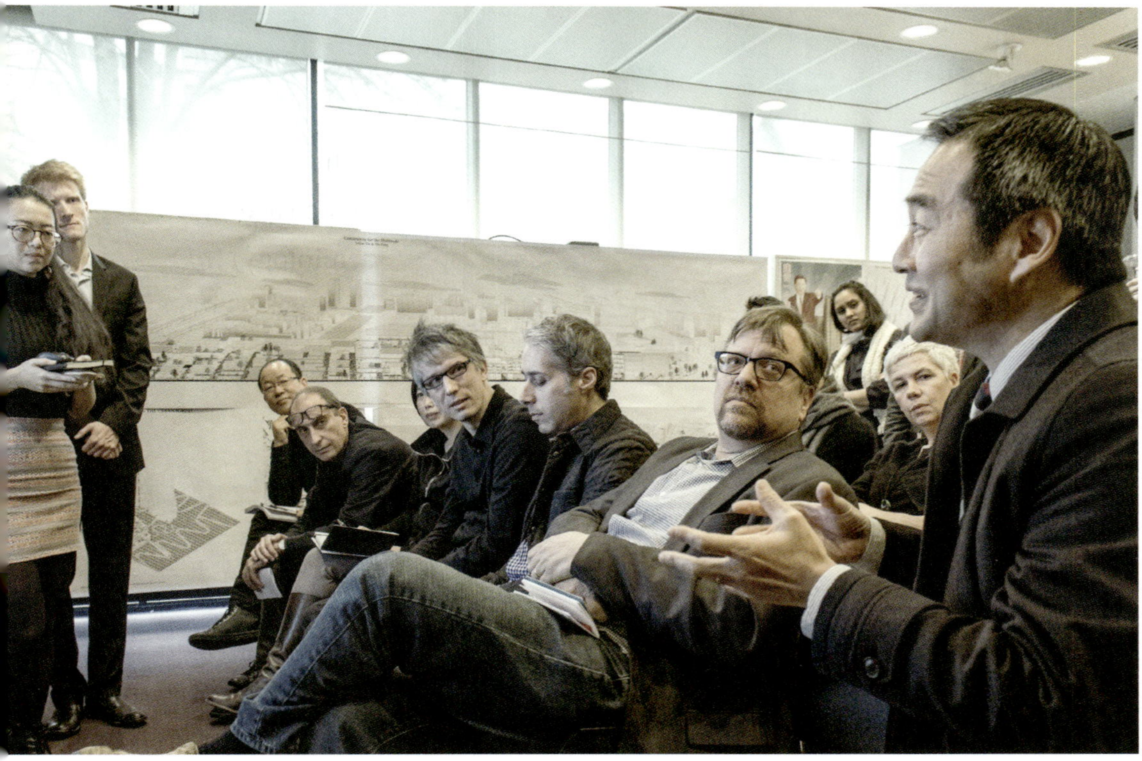

Figure 1 (Left) Dr. Ichiro Kawachi speaks to Harvard Graduate School of Design students.

HAPI As an introduction, we wonder if you could offer some definition or description of a number of terms for a lay design audience.

The first is social epidemiology.

IK It might be best to start with the World Health Organization. The WHO defines the social determinants of health as the conditions under which people are born, they learn, they grow up, they work, they age etc.[1] So all of these things, when we pause to think about it, affect health because we now know that your parent's wealth affects your health in later adulthood, your quality of schooling, the kind of work that you do and your job security, and naturally among all these factors, the residential environment where you live matters for health. So social epidemiology is simply the study of social determinants of health using what we call epidemiologic methods, which is really just the application of statistics, in order to understand medicine.

HAPI Social capital.

IK Social capital is one of the factors that we think drives people's health. Social capital is defined as the resources that are available to people through their social connections and social networking. Some people call it social network capital. If you are an economist, capital means any stock of resource that is accumulated over time. There are many types of capital ranging from financial to human capital. Social capital is the recognition that when we are connected to other people, those relationships have inherent value because we are able to call upon our social connections to obtain valuable resources such as information, emotional support, and social reinforcement. Social capital is just a buzzword to describe all these things. From a social determinants perspective, we think it is interesting because social capital can be described as existing not only within social relationships but relationships that are embedded within places such as neighborhoods.

1 World Health Organization. Closing the gap in a generation: health equity through action on the social determinants of health. Report from the Commission on Social Determinants of Health. Geneva: WHO; 2008. Also available from: URL:http://www.who.int/social_determinants/thecommission/finalreport/en/index.html [cited 2009 Jan 8].
"The social determinants of health are the conditions in which people are born, grow, live, work and age."

We can think of neighborhoods as being high or low in stocks of social capital. I always give the example, if you live in a neighborhood where your neighbors are constantly looking out for each other such as my neighborhood for example, when our children were growing up, if we had forgotten to pick them up from the school bus stop, our neighbors, without our asking, would bring them home with their own children and we would do the same for them. If our snow blower broke down, we could always go to our neighbors and borrow one. This type of resource that we are able to access from social relations that are embedded within a neighborhood is what we would call neighborhood social capital.

HAPI And finally, behavioral economics, which has a resonance and importance for the work that you have been pursuing.

IK Behavioral economics is a branch of economics and behavioral science, using novel and emerging insights in psychology and neuroscience aimed at trying to change people's behavior. There are a few interesting connections between behavioral economics and social determinants of health. One of them is that behavioral economics recognizes the importance of nudges.[2] These are what Richard Thaler would call the default options in the environment which steer people towards behaving in healthy ways or behaving in ways that are in their long-term interest. And so there are many kinds of things that are in the environment that are nudges, if I pause to think about it, the features of the built environment can be nudges. If you were to encourage people to socialize in a particular street, you may have to build wider footpaths. That is an example of an environmental nudge. You could connect some of these ideas all the way back to Jane Jacobs.

The other intersection between behavioral economics and my field is that behavioral economists recognize the importance of social norms and social influence. They recognize human behavior is not simply dictated by the rational agent who calculates the costs and benefits of doing something. We are often influenced to do something just because someone else in our environment is doing it, which has connections to the ideas associated with social capital.

2 A term developed by Richard Thaler and Cass Sunstein in their book *Nudge, Improving Decisions About Health, Wealth and Happiness.* (Thaler, Richard and Sunstein, Cass 2009, *Nudge, Improving Decisions About Health, Wealth and Happiness,* Penguin Books, New York.)

HAPI It is clear that in your own work, you have a strong interest in the relationship between health (and in particular social health) with neighborhoods or places. You appear to be interested in both the compositional and the contextual.

Part of that context is the physical environment. Why has there been a growing interest from the public health field in looking again at the physical environment?

IK I believe one of the stimuli to the resurging interest in the built environment within the public health field was the obesity epidemic. The obesity epidemic came upon us rather suddenly over the last twenty years, generally across the world many places have been experiencing a similar phenomenon. Initially it was all put down to individual factors like personal dietary habits and exercise patterns. However, we came to realize that it was not sufficient to explain the epidemic by resorting to individual explanations because when you look at a city like Boston, there is an enormous variation in obesity rates. Even when you take into account compositional characteristics such as whether a neighborhood is composed of people of a

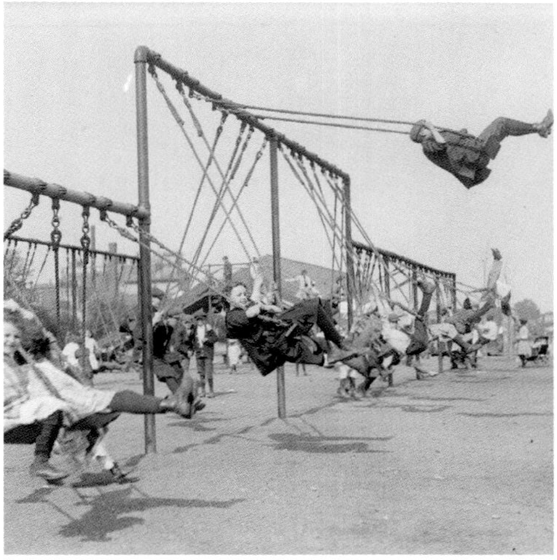

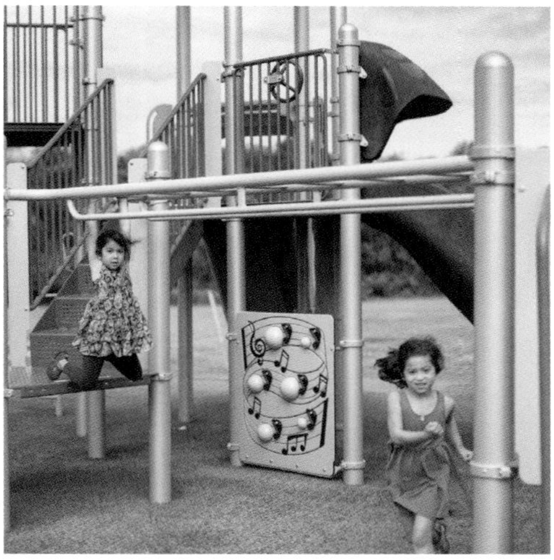

Figure 2 (Adjacent, Left) Boston playgrounds, ca. 1934.

Figure 3 (Adjacent, Right) Boston playgrounds, ca. 2012.

certain socioeconomic class or race and ethnic groups, you still see variation, which we attribute to differences in the environment. That is what turned many of us in the public health field towards the contextual influences on health outcomes such as obesity. Once you recognize this, it opens us up the possibility that you may be able to tackle an epidemic like obesity not just by counseling individuals but by improving the environment.

HAPI Have you been able to find certain patterns or reach any conclusions on the contextual importance for public health?

IK I think we have. The environmental research on obesity has concentrated on the physical activity environment and the food environment. Both are characteristics of the neighborhood environment, if you will. On the physical activity environment side we have found walkability is important for encouraging people to walk to work. Another example is one we found in Boston neighborhoods, where one of our former graduate students conducted a citywide audit of the safety of all parks and playgrounds around the city and she discovered that according to the level of wealth of the Boston neighborhoods, there is a clear gradient in the safety of playground equipment. That's an important environmental barrier to getting parents to take their children out to get some physical activity. On the food environment side, there are a lot of studies that show that neighborhoods that have higher levels of obesity also tend to be the neighborhoods that have worse access to food amenities. These neighborhoods tend to have access to fewer grocery stores and the grocery stores that they do have, tend to stock less reduced fat and reduced salt products. These same neighborhoods are more often targeted by fast food companies. So the overall environment does not encourage healthy eating habits. That is an important "nudge." We think that if you have a fast food outlet near your neighborhood, all other things being equal, you would be more tempted to go there.

HAPI While all places vary based on their specific circumstances and the effects on health are compounds of many different influences, are there any notable examples that you have encountered in your work that illustrate the efficacy of space or place in fostering or affecting public health and more specifically; social health? One example we came across in your books was the David Barker study of Burnley and Colne[3] where the back-to-back house

3 This example is discussed by Sally Macintyre and Anne Ellaway in *Neighbourhoods and Health: An Overview.* (Kawachi, Ichiro and Berkman, Lisa (eds.) 2003, *Neighbourhoods and Health: An Overview*, Oxford University Press, New York, p.29).

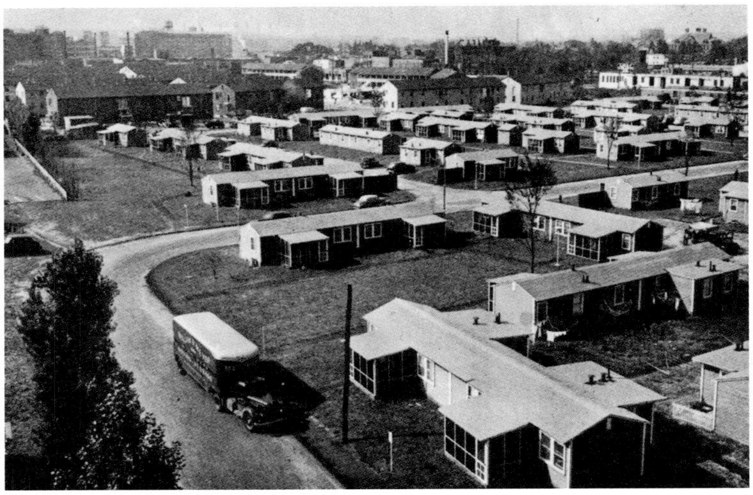

Figure 4 (Left) Westgate housing, MIT campus.

typologies having no cross ventilation and refrigeration facilities affected the adult health of its population through its impact on their early childhood development. That's obviously a case where a housing typology had a negative effect on the health of its residents.

IK I think that we are really just at the beginnings of these kinds of collaborations to find out whether design can influence the social determinants. Housing is a very important issue for public health. Clearly there is a lot of research into housing and health done by my colleagues. There are many things that we can conclude from these kinds of studies such as the recommendation to retrofit houses with insulation, so that you may reduce the incidences of colds and asthma, the importance of having appropriate air-conditioning and heating and so on. However in relation to the broader issues such as housing and social interaction, I think that we are just at the beginning of our understanding.

I have seen examples such as retirement homes built in Finland where there was the provision of a common space at the intersection of the two wings of the center where the residents could congregate in between the two wings. Having this space is very important for encouraging social interaction.

I believe a lot of this goes back to Leon Festinger's research from the 1950s on college dormitories,[4] where you had a kind of natural experiment, where students would be randomized to different buildings in this brand new housing complex for college students. He discovered over time as he went back to interview the college students, that the students located at the end units ended up getting to know fewer people from the complex, where as those towards the center who had more opportunity for casual interaction with people within the complex ended up having many more social ties.

The way that Jane Jacobs describes that the presence and width of sidewalks can help to determine whether people may be likely to linger and talk with their neighbors or if they simply speed by is another example. The fact that the height of apartment buildings can affect the possibility for parents to look over their children on the ground floor is another example of the built environment potentially having an effect on social practices. These are among a range of examples that we think should, in theory, matter for health outcomes but I believe that we are very much at the beginning because

4 Festinger, Leon; Schachter, Stanley and Back, Kurt 1950, *Social Pressures in Informal Groups; a Study of Human Factors in Housing*, Stanford University Press, Stanford, CA.

we just have not collaborated enough with designers or architects to be able to put a lot of these ideas into practice.

HAPI There are a lot of these environmental conditions that designers also intuitively believe have an effect on the social and general health of residents. Typically designers can test them by developing designs that address these issues and if lucky enough also build iterations of these ideas. But there have been many instances where certain typologies that have been applied in a particular context fail to meet social and health ambitions and in other contexts, the very same typologies are considered a success. An example is the type of public housing that was associated in many parts of the west as exemplifying the failure of High Modernism in delivering social and health reforms. However in parts of South East Asia, you could argue that these same housing types operate just fine.

IK I think that's right. Context is very important. I think this gets back to what we were just saying before which is that health is determined by multi-level influences and it is not sufficient to work on just one level and hope that the built environment will fix everything. Because people's lives are contextualized in the sense that the living environment matters but so does what they are doing the rest of the time. Do they have a job? How long do they take to commute and many other issues.

HAPI An interesting example is a town that you have talked about in Pennsylvania called Roseto.[5] What we found interesting about this was the description of the rising affluence of that community reflected in the increasingly private nature of their neighborhoods. While they may have previously socialized on their front porches, the community slowly removed these features of their houses as they enjoyed greater prosperity. It was interesting that this also coincided with a significant increase in the incidence of deaths through heart disease, upsetting what was a remarkably low rate of heart disease compared to the national average.*

5 Roseto is a town located in Pennsylvania. It became the focus of public health officials in the 1961 because of the considerably low rate of heart disease amongst its immigrant Italian community. Public health studies confounded researchers when individual behaviours were studied. The community had adopted personal dietary and lifestyle habits that were seen to be unhealthy. Cooking with lard, widespread smoking, and alcoholic consumption was typical. Yet the rate of heart disease and crime were considerably lower than the national average. This was subsequently seen to be an effect of the social cohesion and capital that the community enjoyed. Interestingly, these statistics readjusted to match national averages in the subsequent generations of the community where many of the social practices and ties were abandoned by the younger generations of Roseto residents for more mainstream American practices.

IK It was an Italian immigrant community, so if you go to many small towns in Italy, they still do that don't they? There are two communal habits. One is that people take their stroll after dinner. That is the time when the towns' people walk and meet their neighbors. Then the other is for when they don't want to walk, they sit on their front steps and converse with their neighbors across the road. I guess they brought that kind of culture to Roseto until they got sucked in by the American dream of having the gigantic front lawn that sets the house back.

HAPI As designers our main currency is the definition of space and organization of material. Even when we are dealing with more temporal conditions like programming, we typically address them through the articulation of spaces and material organizations. How do you think that the public health field may benefit from a dialogue or exchange with designers of the built environment?

IK I think it would make the things that we have been theorizing about in our field very real. Public health interventions tend to be in the public health arena. So we typically intervene through education, changing incentives (like taxes and so forth), or through direct regulation where we can pass public health legislation to prevent smoking indoors for instance. But when we talk about social determinants of health, a lot of the actions are in areas that are outside the realm of public health. The area of housing is one such case. That's where we really have to rely upon the people in those other fields to understand the public health consequences of what they do. I think that's the connection that has to be made.

For example, in American neighborhoods, when there is a discussion within a school district to decide where to locate the school, there is a process for doing that. There is typically a planning board where people come to give testimony and advice for where the appropriate location of the school would be. Typically within these processes, there is representation from the education officials, transport officials, and there may even be some local business interests but public health is rarely there. We are very seldom represented at the table in order to provide our input on what would happen if you located a school in a particular place with respect to patterns of walking to school versus driving and so forth. That's where I think we have been a little bit naive and haven't been able to take that next leap.

HAPI This leads to the next part of the question which is what do you think are the best ways to facilitate a dialogue or exchange between professionals within the design and public health field?

IK I think it has to happen first through the exchange at the level of academia in order to break down these disciplinary silos in order to understand where each field is coming from. You then have to do some demonstration projects and interventions to show to policy makers that these ideas actually work and then from there you would scale up in the real world. This is the kind of sequence by which I think ideas end up being put into practice in some way. This dialogue we are having now I think is the first step and it's often the step that takes the longest.

HAPI Yes, we think we are also jumping into the deep end with regards to what you do within your field as well.

IK I have been at the Harvard School of Public Health for twenty three years now and the Harvard Graduate School of Design has been there the whole time. The first doctoral student at the GSD whose committee I served on only happened about five years ago. Then just recently we started to interact with Ann Forsyth's group and yours and what astonished me when I came to sit on the review of your studio was that they were talking about social capital and essentially these are public health concepts or at least they have health consequences. There is a lot of research that indicates that social interaction and social capital can enhance or have an adverse impact on health. I thought it was really astonishing.

HAPI The relationship between public health and the physical environment can make the design field optimistic, and at the same time; extremely uneasy. This uneasiness comes from a number of historic episodes in their convergence. There have been key moments that have been appropriated by many in our field as pointed lessons as to why architecture should be, at the very least ambivalent, and at most; dismissive of the efficacy of architecture to deliver on its social ambitions.

One of these moments can be seen in the social and public health

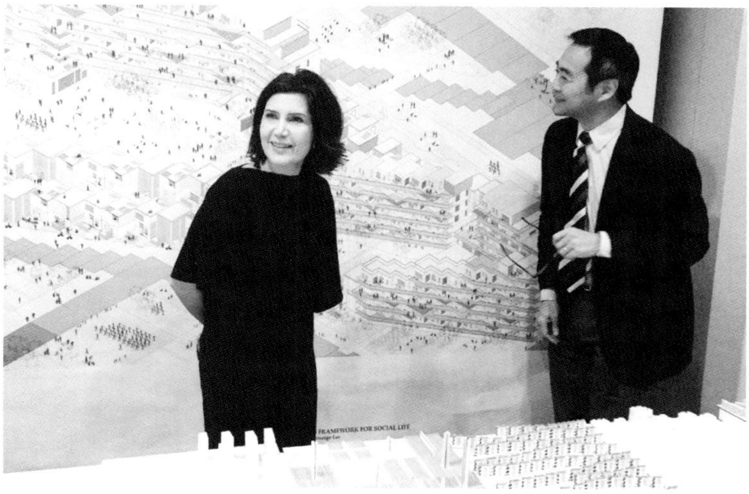

Figure 5 (Left) Dr. Ichiro Kawachi with Farshid Moussavi at Harvard Graduate School of Design studio reviews. (Image courtesy Harvard Graduate School of Design).

reformers of Victorian England. The impetus for slum and rookery clearance then was the pairing between physical and moral health. This was reflected in the physical fabric of the rookeries, the aggregation of abandoned mansions and hovels. Their spatial intricacy and density of bodies, their lack of hierarchy between private and public spaces, and the ambiguous nature of these spaces were seen to be cradles of physical and moral ills.

This led to the development of proposals that broadened the attention for social and health reform from the design of institutional buildings to the reform of domestic environments. A notable result was the model house developed by Henry Roberts under the influence of the social and health reformer; Sir Edwin Chadwick.

This model proposed a clear separation of circulation and private spaces as well as a clear organization of the interior of family units that prioritized the private nature of domesticity in reaction to what reformers saw as the pathological ambiguity of the spaces that the urban poor were living in.

This raises an interesting issue which is this highly private idea of domesticity, which became a standard for future domestic projects.

In China, you can see this as something that is also happening again, where prior to the housing reform and the opening up of housing to a market system, the *Danwei* operated as the unit that would accommodate both the private and public lives of its members. In fact many of what would have been considered private functions were communal activities such as cooking, dining and even ablutions.

With the rising prosperity in China, the tendency has been to adopt more and more, the private, modern sensibility of domesticity. There is a gradual erosion of the intricate nature of private and public spaces in domestic life. Within the new *Xiaoqu* developments, this complexity or intricacy is reduced to the very abrupt divisions between private and public spaces.

What are your observations of this issue of an increasingly private sensibility towards our living environments and its effect on the wider city in relation to your work on social health?

IK I think in a way it is inevitable isn't it? I think it's very difficult to reverse those kinds of trends and maybe it's not even desirable to stand in the way of it. One of the criticisms of the work of social capitalists is that we get accused of trying to turn the clock back in some ways. I think the question is not about trying to preserve ways of interaction that people no longer want to engage in. We have to think about how we can recreate these kinds of interactions within the conditions that are set by these new trends. And that may be by trying to encourage social interactions in workplaces where people are spending an increasing amount of their time as opposed to in their private homes. Or if you are going to build new types of built environments, it would be good to consider what is possible, without going to the extent of making people use a shared bathroom or communal kitchens. I think that is really homework for the urban designers to a certain extent isn't it. I think you need to think of designs that enable people to do that.

In my own research experience, it is extremely important that when you design new living arrangements, you should set aside space that enables people to socialize and interact. My current research that is funded by the NIH (National Institutes of Health) is based upon social capital and the recovery of older people after the March 11 earthquake and tsunami in Japan. In that disaster, a whole lot of people lost their homes and so they had to be moved to temporary houses built by the municipal authorities in the affected areas.

And that is like a natural experiment where people could design the houses in all sorts of ways. The most important thing that we discovered in relation to assisting older people in their recovery is that whatever arrangement you put the container housing into, you should provide a public space. You need to leave a space for communal meeting where people can come together and maintain their social links that existed prior to the disaster. We are finding now, especially amongst the elderly that if they don't have that opportunity then they rapidly start to lose function. They end up getting stuck at home, they have no reason to go out and that is one of the most distressing things that can happen if you are over the age of seventy. There are some lessons like that we can usefully apply in design principles.

HAPI It does seem that elderly care in Japan is quite well known for being advanced relative to many other practices in the world. What lessons can we take away from your work with seniors there?

IK Yes, but what is interesting is that while it is very advanced, there is tremendous variability as well. We are trying to explain that variability by patterns of social capital. There are enormous differences in how people are doing after the disaster. Some people are rapidly losing function and becoming disabled and others are able to maintain their vitality. More often than not, we are finding that this is done through social interaction. Every day they get dressed, if they are elderly ladies they would apply makeup and they would go out and visit their neighbors. This is very important. We underestimate that element. The technological notion is that the maintenance of functioning in old age is dependent on having correct medications and care from the geriatrician. But it isn't. What you do outside of interaction with medicine and health care, what you do during your day is extremely important as well.

HAPI It is being suggested that issues of chronic disease or lifestyle diseases are an area where the physical environment can have an effect on offering or encouraging life practices that foster better physical, social, and psychological health.

What do you think about this? Can design of the built environment foster or encourage healthier behavior or lifestyle practices? Or is it just a matter of, at the very least, not constraining it, where Foucault has said that there are no liberating architectures per se, but only constraining architectures. Earlier, you used the concept of the nudge, do you think that the built environment has a role to play in enticing certain behaviors?

IK Absolutely, there are all sorts of architectural things that are nudges aren't there? The classic nudge that Thaler describes is when you design a new building, where you place the stairs vis a vis the elevator has a very important impact. For instance, when you came into the Kresge building today (the building of the Harvard School of Public Health), did you notice the stairs? Most of the time, the staircase is typically shoved into a darkly lit corner of the building, making it very unattractive to find, to locate and to use. Whereas the elevators are typically given prime space. That's a nudge. Thaler calls it choice architecture. It's not always referring literally to architecture but we are in a way becoming architects of people's choices and that also applies to the way that buildings are designed it seems to me. I think there are a lot of things that potentially could be done. And by the way, that is not within the public health realm but that's in the realm of design.

I am convinced that these small, unconscious decisions add a tremendous amount to people's daily habits. Most people's daily habits with regard to exercise and diet are formed by hundreds of unconscious decisions that would frankly be a hassle if you were forced to think about it every time. So we typically take the default options presented to us every time. I think design can really help to nudge people in their long-term self-interested direction. I think that is true not only of building design but of environmental design too isn't it? Sometimes it also happens by accident too. I think of, for instance again, Japan where people seem to be extremely

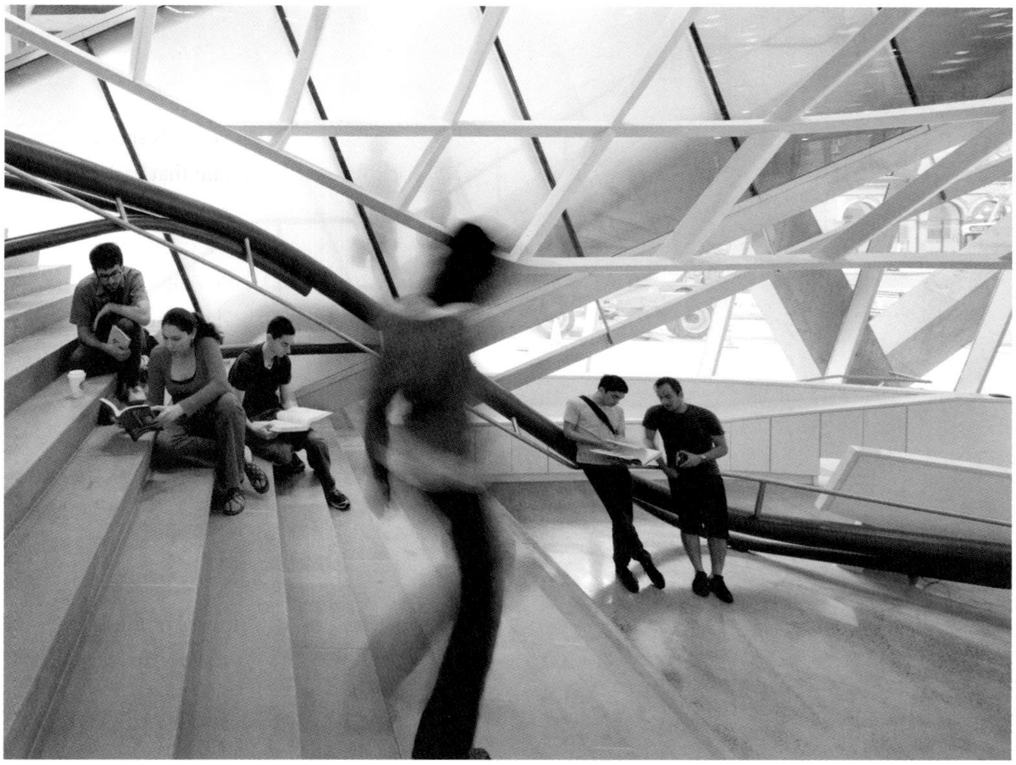

Figure 6 (Left) Cooper Union school of architecture, designed by Morphosis Architects, Inc.

mobile and physically active. The elderly in Japan are very "genki" (as we say in Japanese); full of vitality. I think part of the reason is that the environment is arranged in such a way that it encourages unconscious physical activity. If you have ever travelled to Tokyo, in a lot of the train stations, they do not have escalators. So it forces people to take the stairs up and down including my eighty-year-old mother. It's just extraordinary that people do this without complaining just because that is the environmental default.

HAPI That's true, and in Japan the general population seems to have a high longevity.

IK Absolutely, it's the highest longevity in the world and that longevity partly is because people don't become disabled. I once, just out of curiosity, when I was taking a vacation in Japan, wore a pedometer to see how many steps I'd end up taking just by doing casual stuff around Tokyo and I could easily reach seven or eight thousand steps just by traipsing up and down the train station steps to get from one platform to another. It was quiet an interesting lesson for me.

HAPI Interestingly, a little study we did in the research group was to look at the physical environment of these so-called "Blue Zones."[6] We found that in many (although not all) of these places such as the villages in Sardinia and Icaria, the natural environment could be quite challenging to mobility. The natural topography in those places is quite steep and if you consider what the residents there have to negotiate physically every day in relation to universal design standards, it certainly isn't compliant with what is considered comfortable.

6 Blue zones are geographic and demographic areas in the world where a particular population has been identified to live considerably longer and healthier lives. The work on identifying these zones was initiated by by Gianni Pes and Michel Poulain as well as Dan Buettner who brought it to the attention of the general public in a series of articles in National Geographic magazine.

IK I think that's all connected actually. With all these Blue Zone people, they all latch onto personal habits like diet and what they're doing in terms of smoking and drinking etc. But I think you have to see the broader

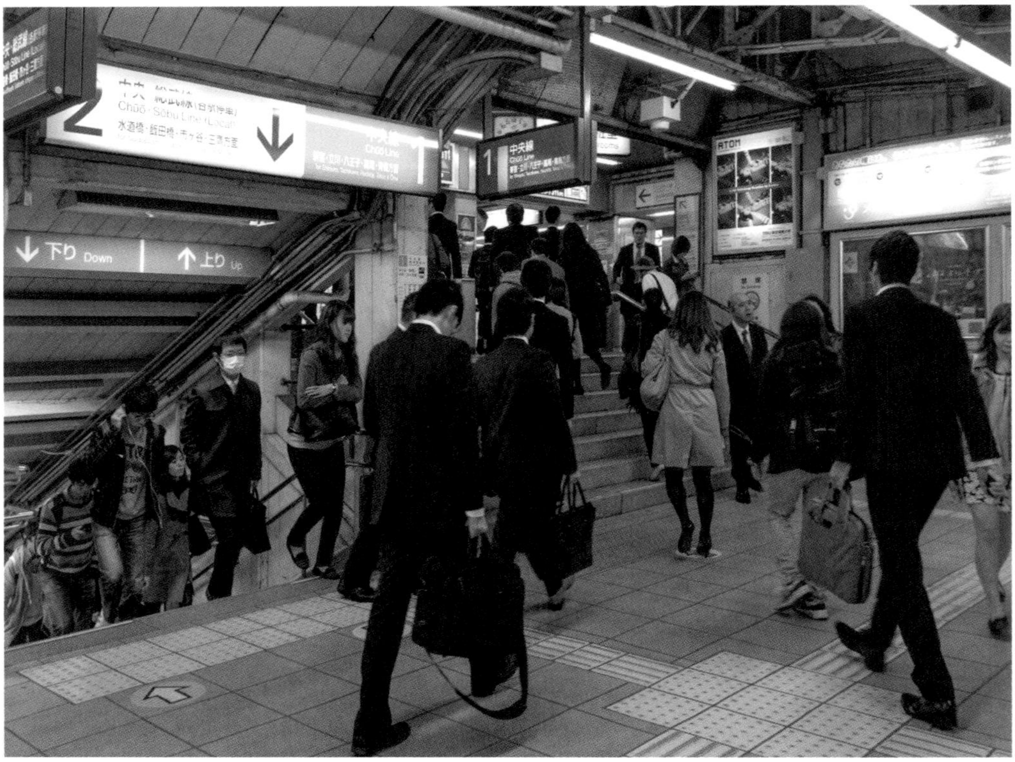

Figure 7 (Left) Commuters take the stairs at a Tokyo metro station.

picture, step back beyond the individual. What does their environment look like? And I do suspect that the built environment is a big part of it. Of course you could also step back even further than that and say that they also reflect infrastructure investments by governments and local authorities and that is very important too.

HAPI For your field, is there any value in the, let's call it aesthetic, communicative, or expressive capacities of the built environment? Is there any potential value you can see in the qualitative aspects of space beyond the functional or programmatic but also let's say the capacity for the design of spaces and places to captivate or engage the public?

IK Yes, absolutely. I do. I think we underestimate it but only because in public health we are rather bad at quantifying it. I always say, we fall under the trap of the "build it and they will come" illusion. That if we provide exercise facilities, people will naturally come or if we build meeting amenities, people will gather but I think the aesthetic features are extremely important. Plus you need whatever it is that the context provides in terms of encouraging people to come forwards and participate. I don't think we have done a good job of unlocking that. When you refer to expressive qualities are you referring to aesthetics?

HAPI There are some designers who believe that the built environment can be communicative or expressive. That it can communicate or express certain ideas or that it can even be made to affect certain sensations.

IK Yes, I see. How do you quantify that? That seems to me to be the 'je ne sais quoi' of design doesn't it? I agree with that. No doubt there could be some science developed that helps to clarify how people respond to the environment. But we have not been able to quantify that very much. Actually, last month I was in Edinburgh meeting with a group of architects. They have an interdisciplinary project called mood, mobility, and place at the University of Edinburgh which is a collaboration of public health geographers and architects. One of the things I found interesting that they were doing was they were trialing new sensory equipment that people wear like a helmet fitted out with EEG (electroencephalography) sensors. They then make people walk through a neighborhood and try to figure out how these people respond affectively to what they see. I thought it was very interesting; they were trying to get real-time objective data in the real environment of how these people experienced features of neighborhoods emotionally, as pleasurable or anxiety-causing. Maybe if we could use some objective information like that we might be able to begin to tease out what it is that to us seems like fairly similar scenarios to ones that are going to encourage people to get out to ones that people are going to avoid. Maybe it's too pie in the sky but it seems like an interesting approach.

HAPI Certainly we know it has an effect. How we measure or evaluate it is something we need to figure out and agree on.

IK So far we have relied on building it and waiting and seeing if people will come and use it in the way that you intend. It's a very time consuming and expensive process. It would be ideal to have a better idea about what it is in the environment that people are responding to before we build it. I think the problem is that as people in public health, we haven't really emphasized the aesthetic aspects, so that is a missing element that designers can bring to some extent. So that the consideration is not only about functionality but also beauty or how pleasing it is.

HAPI Perhaps we can ask you about social isolation, where the problems of segregation include inhibiting the possibility for multistranded and weak ties or the capacity to build networks that offer information dissemination such as employment opportunities. To build upon the strength of local connections, balanced with the need to construct bridges with other communities, appears to be one of the ambitions for people invested in the social determinants of health.

I wonder if you could elaborate on this idea of social bridges or links and the role that the physical environment or physical artifacts may play in facilitating or even operating as these links.

IK I do think that the physical environment can encourage and discourage social interaction as we said. The flip side is social interactions can still exist and even be very powerful within deteriorated conditions. I think that is the kind of mistake that we have made in the past. When we do slum clearance for the residents' "own good" for example, we may end up improving their housing conditions but on the other hand, inadvertently destroy existing social connections. That's a lesson we have learned a few times over the history of public health and I think you really have to think about what it is exactly that you are providing and what are you doing to preserve the strengths that are there and to be able to recognize these assets even in conditions where the physical side of it may be quite deteriorated. I don't know if that answers the question but you need to understand that the flip side of the environment being able to encourage social interaction is not the same as saying that bad environments have bad social relations. This is not necessarily true. Often in the worst slums, you have the strongest social bonds and social capital which can get destroyed when you force people to relocate to brand new houses.

HAPI We were struck by something that you made clear in the book you edited with Lisa Berkman, *Neighborhoods and Health*, that neighborhoods which are seen to have a very strong social bond can often also be seen to experience incredible tensions when you scale up. The conflicts between the tightly knit Catholic and Protestant communities in Northern Ireland are an example you cited. It is an interesting point for us, as we are becoming more and more aware that we cannot address a problem by looking at it from one scale or through a single disciplinary lens alone. We are becoming aware again that we benefit from looking across the many scales of concern that are addressed by the different design disciplines, from architecture and landscape to urban planning.

IK When you say scale I think that relates somewhat to the multi-level concept.

HAPI Yes, for us it may often be spatial. For you it encompasses many other aspects as well.

IK Spatial scale is also a form of multi-level, but multi-level can also apply to the way we conceptualize what happens at the individual level, within families, the community, and the wider society.

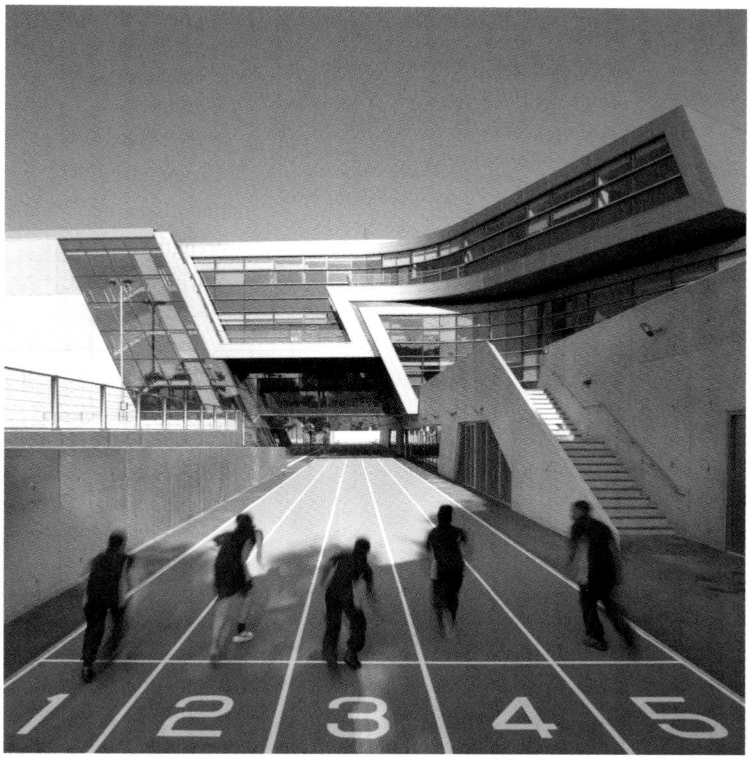

Figure 8 (Left) Evelyn Grace Academy designed by Zaha Hadid Architects.

HAPI Yes, multi-levels for you can be more challenging in that sense. (laughter).

Finally, given the complex issues of the increasing segregation of our cities and neighborhoods along socioeconomic lines and what you have called a withdrawal from civic engagement and responsibility by those who can afford to do so, what are the ways that you think, may allow us to address the delivery of better public health in a more equitable manner?

IK I don't believe there is a magic bullet. Or at least if there is one, we haven't found it. I think we must not be naive that fixing one thing will cure these ills, because increasing social isolation is part of a pattern of larger forces such as the rising income inequality and the fact that families are having to work longer hours at work and having to work further from homes which increases commuting times and reduces the amount of time available for investing in social relations in their neighborhoods and in their families etc. By fixing one thing, we can't hope to reverse some of these trends. You need solutions at multiple levels as we just discussed. Having said that I think you have to intervene wherever you can because maybe it is that neighborhood design elements may be the key to unlock some of these processes. But I cannot offer a definitive answer.

HAPI This is also something that we constantly have to consider for our field. How can we be effective and affect change or improve people's lives?

We recently attended an interesting lecture[7] discussing the book *Capital in the Twenty-First Century* by Thomas Pikkety.[8] At one point, a graph by Pikkety charting gains in labor and gains in capital was discussed. If you remember, the chart described how throughout history, gains in capital are typically far higher than gains in labor. Only at a particular point during the twentieth century can we see gains in labor and gains in capital…

7 Reiner de Graf, The Risk of Realism a lecture presented at the Architectural Association School of Architecture, London on November 25th 2014

8 Pikketty, Thomas 2014, *Capital In The Twenty First Century*, trans. Arthur Goldhammer, Belknap Press, Cambridge.

Graph 1 (Right) Thomas Pikkety's chart of gains in labor in relation to gains in capital. (Source: Thomas Pikkety 2014. Redrawn).

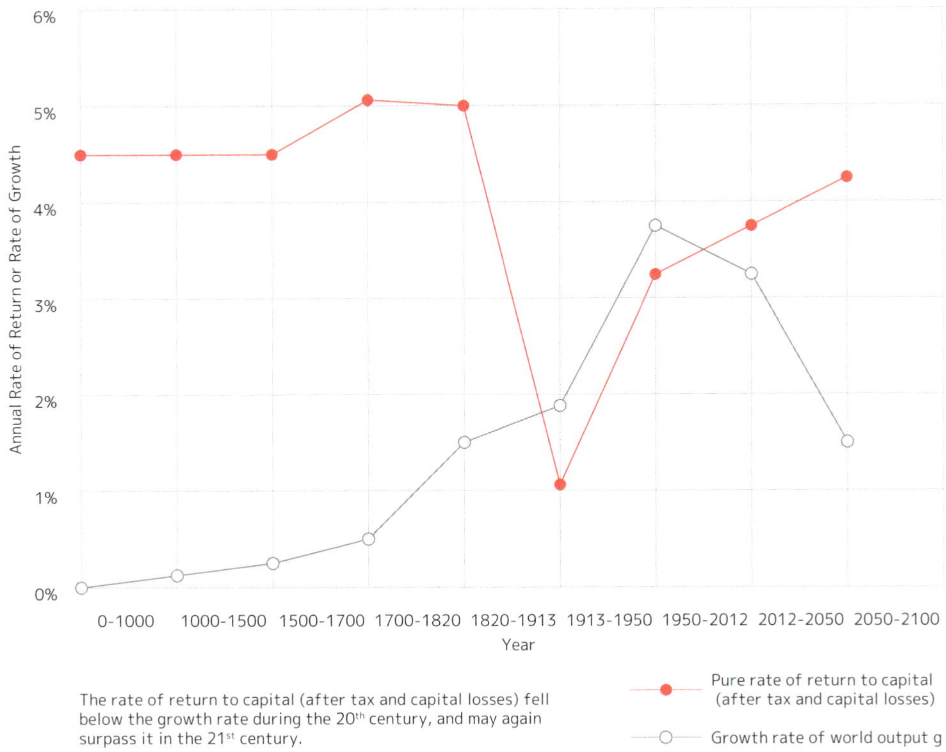

IK Yes, there was a compression. You know, he says that's a historical accident. We had this massive war where a lot of the capital got destroyed.

HAPI One interesting thing in that lecture was the decision to compare this period to the moment when architecture was most actively optimistic in generating theories and mainfestos for architecture and the city. It listed many of the seminal books on the city by architects and what it found was that nearly all of them were produced in this period.

IK Oh that's interesting. So, because a lot of the cities were destroyed, this posed a huge opportunity for architects and planners? They had the opportunity to start from zero?

HAPI The argument is also that a lot of this was related to the fact that there was a stronger state and a tax base. For instance, in the west, public housing was an important issue and was actually being implemented at a very large scale.

IK Yes, it was a moment of social cohesion. People had sacrificed so much up and down the social hierarchy. JFK served alongside a boiler maker's son for instance. So it was easier for governments to say, "We need to be all in this together." Food rationing was just the tip of the iceberg. That was when they rolled out these massive social protections. In was in the aftermath of world war two that the British introduced the NHS (National Health Service) for example. It was a certainly a window of opportunity. Having said that, no one is going to advocate world war (laughter). But there must be some lessons that we can extract from what worked.

I never thought that this massive wholesale destruction is mirrored in what was happening the field of architecture and design. That's very interesting. It's fascinating.

But you know, another thing that Pikkety says is that no society tolerates the level of wealth inequality that we have been approaching. History tells us that this often leads to an explosive cascade which leads to reforms again. I kind of suspect that we may be reaching another one of these periods where people will say, "enough!"

HAPI Interestingly, during the Victorian reform, that was a period where a lot of these social and health reforms such as slum clearance and public housing were driven by philanthropy. Where many of the wealthy members of society recognized that if they didn't do anything…

IK …it would bounce back on them. Yes, the massive cholera epidemics were things that could not only affect the workforce if you were a capital owner but actually literally affect your own health through a carry over or spillover effect on you.

I think that some of the inequality we are seeing now has some of these characteristics as well. When we think about Ebola or many of these issues that capture the public imagination, they usually involve some spillover from lack of investment in one part of the world that can affect people who would otherwise be quite comfortable leading their lives.

Figure Credits

Figure 1, Harvard Graduate School of Design 2014, *Dr. Ichiro Kawachi speaks to Harvard Graduate School of Design students*, photograph. In possession of: Harvard Graduate School of Design.

Figure 2, *Boston playgrounds*, 1934, Boston Public Library, Leslie Jones Collection.

Figure 3, Lin, Soe 2013, photograph. Creative Commons Attribution 2.0 Generic license; Desaturated. Accessed 4 August 2015, https://www.flickr.com/photos/soelin/9272217192/in/album-72157634613776864/.

Figure 4, Festinger et al. 1963, *Social Pressures in Informal Groups: A Study of Human Factors in Housing*, Stanford, California: Stanford University Press, 1963, p. 2

Figure 5, Harvard Graduate School of Design 2014, *Dr. Ichiro Kawachi with Farshid Moussavi*, photograph. In possession of: Harvard Graduate School of Design.

Figure 6, Baan, Iwan, *Cooper Union School of Architecture*, photograph. Morphosis Architects. © Iwan Baan Accessed 4 August 2015, http://morphopedia.com/.

Figure 7, LotsaSmiles Photography 2015, *IMG_6711*, photograph. Creative Commons Attribution-ShareAlike 2.0 Generic license; Desaturated. Accessed 4 August 2015, https://www.flickr.com/photos/lotsasmilesphoto/23138830689/.

Figure 8, Hayes, Luke 2010, *Evelyn Grace Academy*, photograph. Zaha Hadid Architects. © Luke Hayes Accessed 4 August 2015, http://www.zaha-hadid.com/architecture/evelyn-grace-academy/.

The Built Environment and Mental Well-being

An Interview with Dr. Gary Evans, Leire Asensio Villoria + David Mah, 12 July 2015

Dr. Gary Evans is the Elizabeth Lee Vincent professor at the College of Human Ecology at Cornell University in Ithaca, New York. He is an environmental and developmental psychologist interested in how the physical environment affects human health and well-being among children. Evans' specific areas of expertise include children's environments, the environment of childhood poverty, cumulative risk and child development, environmental stressors, and the development of children's environmental attitudes and behaviors.

Professor Evans received an Honorary Doctorate from Stockholm University in Sweden in 2006 and is a former member of the MacArthur Foundation Network on Socioeconomic Status and Health and currently serves on the Board of Children, Youth, and Families for the National Academy of Sciences. He is the 1997 recipient of the EDRA Career Award and Past-President of the Division of Environmental Psychology of the International Association of Applied Psychology. Evans has received a Senior National Research Service Award from the National Institute of Child Health and Human Development. He has a Ph.D. in environmental psychology with post-doctoral training in psychoneuroendocrinology and in human development. Professor Evans has given several hundred lectures and invited talks in over thirty-five different countries. He is also the recipient of numerous teaching awards.

HAPI The investment in studying relationships between physical health and the environment has a long-standing history. However, it did seem that public health shifted more towards medicine and the compositional (the characteristics of individuals) factors of health once the hygiene movement was seen to have "done its job." However, now it seems that contextual factors are being studied again and this time also in relation to mental and social health. What do you think are the reasons for this return to the study of the physical environment?

GE I believe a couple of reasons are responsible for this. One is the fact of people recognizing that when you focus just on the individual, there are still inherent limitations in that. The idea that all of health is down to personal choices and personal decisions and genes and all these individual factors, well, people just realized that, yes, those are important but just as there were limitations in the hygiene and public health movement, the flip side of that is that there are also limitations on focusing only on individual factors. I think the other reason, coming a lot from the public health side, is the cost effectiveness of some of these larger macro changes. It's much more efficient, it's easier. B.F. Skinner, the behavioral psychologist, said that it's easier to change the environment than it is to change behavior.

HAPI You have focused your work on the relationships between the built environment and mental health. Could you explain the idea of direct and indirect effects of the built environment on mental health?

GE The basic idea of a direct effect of the built environment, or the social environment for that matter, is when the relationship or the impact it has on human health is not mediated. It doesn't go through or is not filtered through any other factor or any other process. An example is, if it gets hot enough, you're going to sweat. So that's a direct effect of the physical environment and in terms of mental health, or more broadly human behavior, if it's loud enough it's difficult to hear.

An indirect effect is really talking about this idea of a mediated effect. The idea that some of these effects are not direct but are related with things like, for example, how the person is experiencing it or how they're perceiving it. Fear of crime is a nice example of that. So you could have the same objective physical situation, and there are in fact some correlations between design and crime. However the way that person perceives that or how they judge that situation in terms of risk, for example, can also influence both how they react to it and the reality of how the environment influences crime. So that can be an example of an indirect effect.

Figure 1, 2 (Below) Under-utilized and under-valued spaces in Philadelphia, PA and Cumbernauld, Scotland. (Source: Flicker. Images by Ann Forsyth/Design for Health).

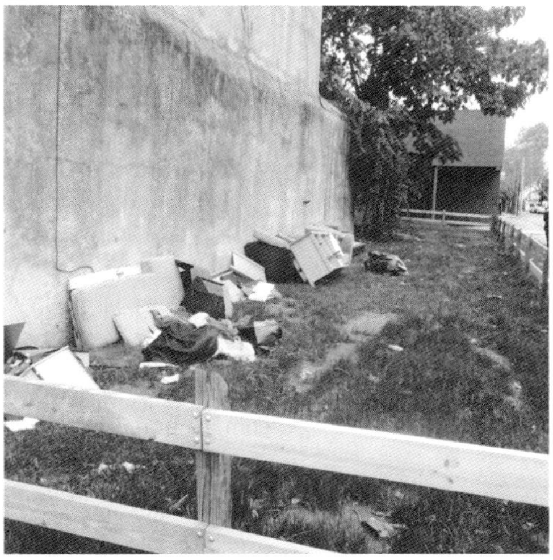

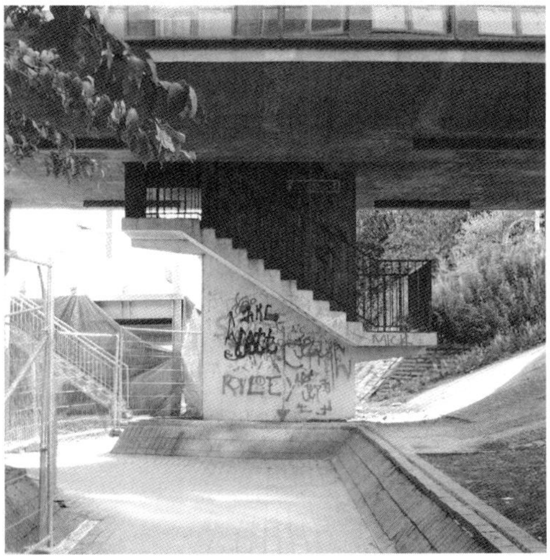

HAPI It is clear from a number of examples you cite in your work, that the ways in which the built environment is configured can greatly affect the ways in which we can live out our lives and hence impact our social and mental health. It appears that the organizational aspects of architecture or urban design can greatly limit the opportunities for social interaction, which can lead to isolation that could trigger many mental health issues. Could you say something about this? The idea that the organizational aspects of the built environment can limit the lifestyles of its occupants.

GE A concept that I like to use, which kind of ties into indirect effects, is a concept called affordances. And what I or other people mean by that is; opportunities or constraints. Or in other words, you have a lot of choice, a lot of latitude but the environment at any scale including the neighborhood scale can make it easier or harder to do certain things. Probably the classic example would be an ecological behavior example, where you have a person whose values and attitudes all line up to be committed to wanting to reduce their use of the car and they would like to use mass transit, but if it is very difficult to access mass transit, if the schedules are not appropriate or the geographic proximity is not there, you're not going to be able to use mass transit. So I think that's a nice example of thinking about this idea of how an organizational factor can affect choices. So in this case, it is the way in which the scheduling, the location, and the proximity affect the ease in which you can use something.

Another way to think about the organizational is at the institutional level. So institutions in themselves also have all kinds of rules, cultures, and rituals. Those can have a big influence. For example, a school may have available resources but perhaps because of rules or concerns about legal issues, people don't have access to those or there are ways that access is restricted in the ways that you could use it.

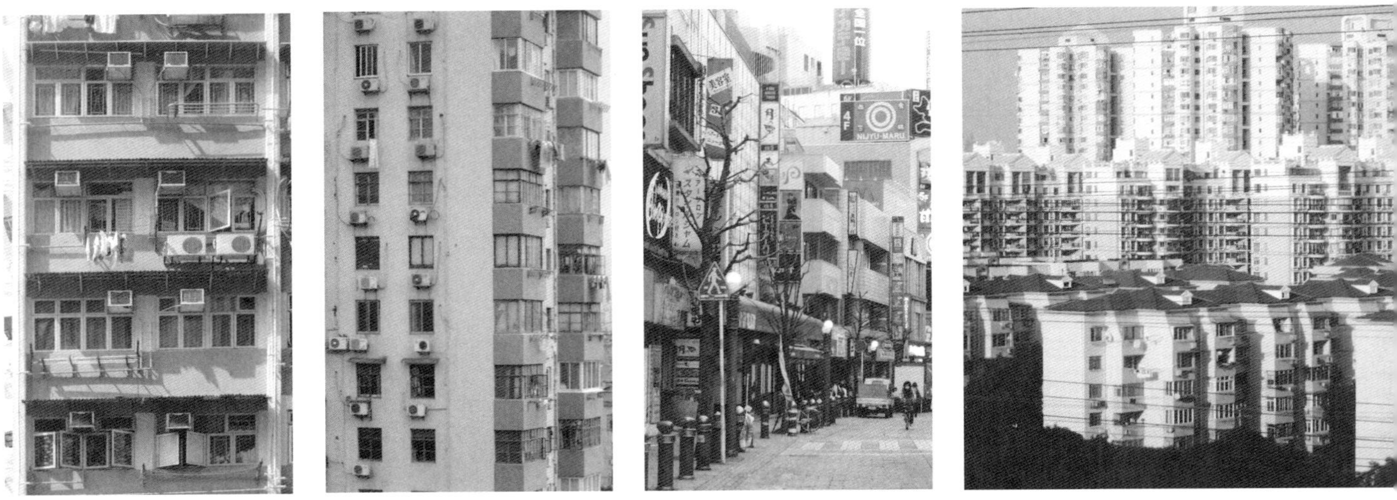

Figure 3-8 (Above) Highrises from (left to right) Hong Kong, China; Souzhou, China; Chiba, Japan; Souzhou, China; Mexico City, Mexico; and Hong Kong, China. (Source: Flicker. Images by Ann Forsyth/Design for Health).

HAPI We were very interested in your findings on high-rises and the effects that these building types can have on mental well-being. What was interesting about the notion that high-rises were potentially harmful, was that it was due to the social isolation that comes with a building type that typically doesn't embed more social spaces within them. It seems that if we are going to persist with building high-rises, and it doesn't look like they will be going away anytime soon, we would be forced to reconsider that building type as something that threads different types and scales of social spaces throughout the building. If this were something that is done, is there hope for the high-rise? Is the high-rise a write off?

GE - No, I don't think it's an inherently negative solution. You've touched right away one of the really critical issues, which is a very functional use of privacy. That is the idea of privacy as a regulation of social interaction rather than solitude. Think of privacy as your ability to regulate social interaction. One of the problems with high-rises—and this particularly interrelates to the social environment—if we take as an example, low-income mothers who are a particularly vulnerable sub-group for high-rises. They have difficulties regulating social interaction partly because of social and economic reasons but also because of the physical environment.[1] So I don't think that it's an inherently negative building type or a failure. I don't think that this type of environment inherently can't work. I think it could work but I think the key is thinking about the role of regulating social interaction. So if you want to be by yourself and you need to be with your family, you can do that. But if you need a break or you want to develop friendships and social capital and all of those kinds of important things, you need to have a physical environment that facilitates that rather than that makes it impossible.

HAPI We were also similarly struck by your findings with buildings that have deck access. It seems here that shared spaces with no sense of ownership, or which in some sense; cannot be controlled by residents, add to anxiety. It seems that part of a more intelligent design practice would include the careful organization of a range of different scales and types of social spaces that may be associated with different types of sociability. From

1 See Evans, Gary 2003 December, 'The Built Environment and Mental Health', *The Journal of Urban Health* 80 (4), pp. 536-555.

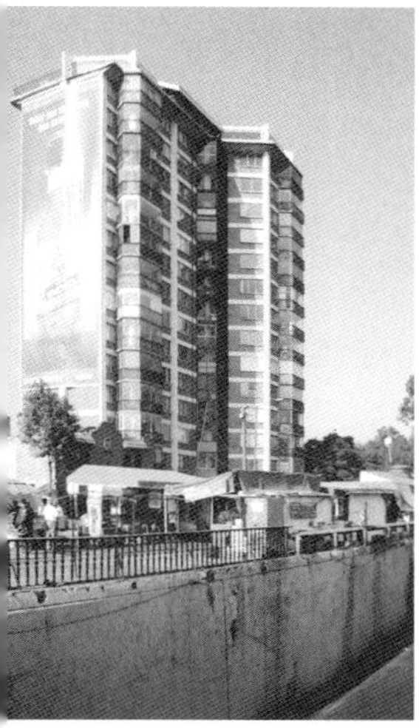

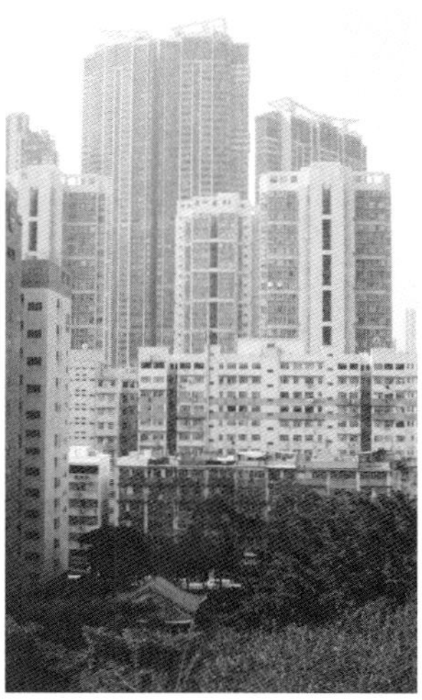

large public spaces to more intimate social spaces and even social spaces that allow us to be alone. Can you say something about this?

GE Well if we go back to the idea of privacy as regulating social interaction, I think one of the key features that affords that, or facilitates that, is a hierarchy of space. Going from very public to very private you have to have access to be able to do that. And of course this relates to the idea of power and efficacy. Yes, so I think having a gradient is very critical. A really interesting group to think about this is adolescents. If you think about adolescents and what make spaces work well for them, one of the things [is that] adults have this feeling that adolescents have to be constantly monitored and supervised. Of course that's the last thing an adolescent wants. This is an example where social control and organizational factors come in. So if you don't figure out a way to allow the adolescents to at least have the perception, if not the reality, of a space where they can just be with their friends and not feel like they are being monitored constantly, they're going to find a way to do that which you're probably not going to be happy with. So it's better to try and figure a way to do it where it's semi-regulated or semi-safe because it's going to happen anyway. So do you want it to happen in the subway for instance or do you want to let them have a safe space for themselves.

HAPI It was also interesting for us to see your findings that Alzheimer's patients or other institutional settings for the mentally challenged benefit greatly from adopting a more domestic atmosphere and organization.[2] It suggests to break the scale down and allow for a more intimate surrounding (rather than large wards that house many patients). Suites and corridors were seen to assist the quality of life for these patients. It has a very interesting parallel with the work of William Tuke at the York retreat[3] that adopted a domestic layout and atmosphere. Also the notion of a more social arrangement of furniture to facilitate a more social atmosphere is interesting to us as designers. Here the issue seems to be about the functional arrangement of spaces but it also seems to be about establishing settings with particular atmospheres and moods. As designers, many of us believe that what we do affects people in more ways than simply accommodating functions but can also affect people's moods and sensations.

The examples of the domestic atmosphere of institutional buildings, and the effect that green spaces can have on people's well-being,[4] both address the role that the built environment plays, which is not just about the way it enables or hinders certain life practices, but about how it affects people through the way that a particular space can make you feel or what kind of mood it puts you in. Do you think there is some value for research in this area? Do you think architecture's affective capacity is a significant component of the ways the built environment impacts mental health?

GE Sure, that kind of relates to the indirect effects. If the less tangible qualities of the built environment wind up making people feel alienated or unsafe or they feel that they can't own or they can't control it, then that's going to get in the way of an awful lot of things. So, yes, I think it's a legitimate area of research. One thing to be careful of in the research is the correlation between perception and health. If I'm measuring meaning, affect, emotional qualities, social qualities, and the social climate of the space and you ask the

2 Ibid.

3 The York Retreat, is an institution in England for the treatment of people with mental health needs, started by William Tuke, a Quaker, in 1796.

4 For instance, see Ulrich, R.S. 1984, 'View through a window may influence recovery from surgery', *Science* 224, pp. 420–421.

same person about their mental health or their physical health, there's a high probability of some tautological findings there. Because I'm using the same reporter to talk about, say, "what's the ambiance of this room like?" and then I ask the same person, "how much do you like it?" Well those are going to be highly correlated partly because of this tautological problem. So I think the way around that is to get some measure of that in the aggregate. So you ask twenty-five people about the space and then you measure a different twenty-five people's mental or physical health. , So there is a way to get out of that problem since the only way you can get at things like meaning, symbolism, sense of neighborhood, and sense of ownership is to ask people.

I don't think that's appreciated enough in the public health and design fields, where people who care about the environment and try to understand what role it plays in health and behavior. But because they're available, they'll ask people about the environment and then they'll ask the same people about their health and then they'll show that they're related. I would be very careful about that. The other thing about that work that is important, that resonates for designers, is that with too much of that kind of social science research in particular, you don't help the designer or the planner because you haven't said what the connection is between the physical environment and the perception or the physical environment and the ambient qualities. You have to get back to that in some way.

HAPI In your article, "The Built Environment and Health," you state that higher residential densities interfere with social support and this can subsequently increase psychological distress. This would seem to be a fair statement from intuition. There has even recently been a study that diverse neighborhoods in the United States can actually have lower rates of trust as well as political and civic engagement.[5] Some studies also point towards the notion that a high proportion of rentals in a neighborhood can also affect civic engagement in a neighborhood. While none of these are by default characteristics of all high-density urban neighborhoods, it would be fair to say that many high-density neighborhoods are composed of one of the two scenarios (or a combination of both). Is there a lesson in this for how we should urbanize? It seems there is an implicit lesson here that seems to favor mid- or low-density. Is it more complex than this?

5 See Putnam, Robert 2007, 'E Pluribus Unum: Diversity and Community in the Twenty First Century, The 2006 Johan Skytte Prize Lecture', *Scandinavian Political Studies* 30(2), pp. 137 - 174.

GE One thing that's very important is to be careful about what kind of density we are talking about. Because this is an area where I think there has been quite a bit of confusion and miscommunication. It looks like the really critical issue is people per room. So when you're talking about density and you're talking about urbanization, you're talking about number of people per census tract or square mile, there's some evidence that there's some real benefits from high-density. It turns out that people walk more and so you get some of the physical activity effects, you get the Jane Jacobs eyes on the streets, so you get some of those benefits. It comes back to the privacy issue. If you can't regulate your social interaction and particularly in a space that you expect to be able to do that it could be a problem. I don't expect to be able to regulate our social interaction here in a busy café, it may still be a problem. But if this was my house and I can't do that then it's a much bigger

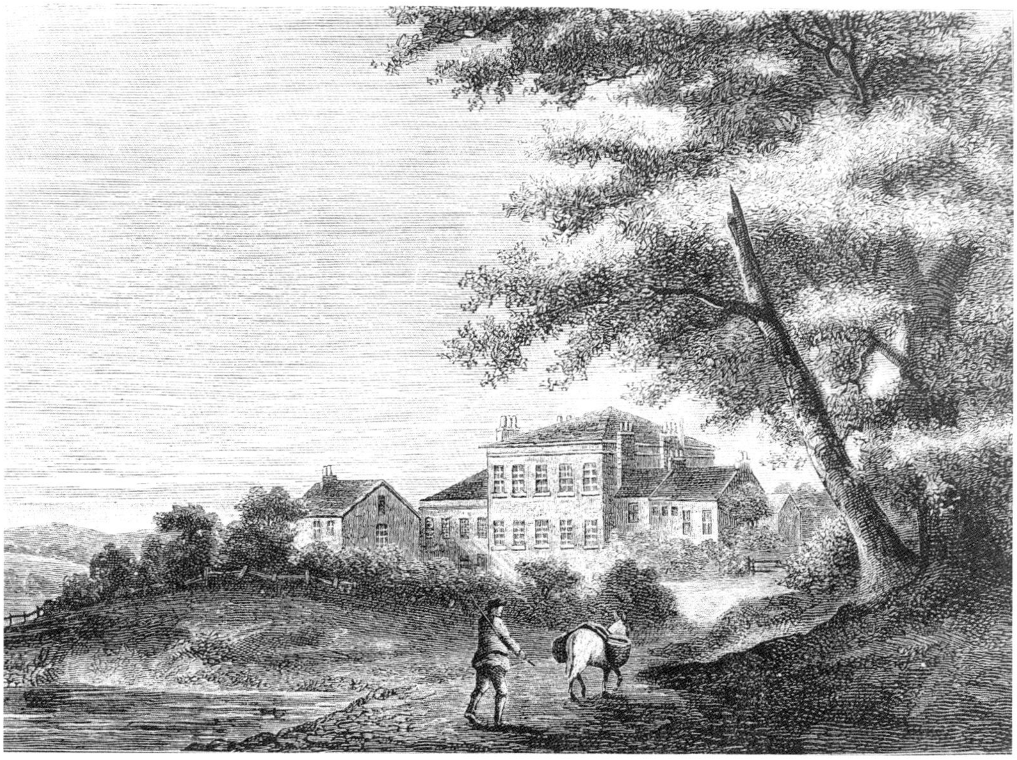

Figure 9 (Above) Engraving of the original building of The York Retreat by Cooper after Cave, ca 1796.

problem. I think that the density lesson is that the issue is more related to if you are having trouble regulating your social interaction. I think there is a lot designers can do even at the micro-scale to make that work better. So a concrete example is if you have a given amount of space, (a kind of spatial syntax issue), I think having more depth, having more places that you can separate yourself from others even though the total square footage is the same. Changing the people per room, I think can really make a big difference.

HAPI That's a good point because there is always a danger of taking that information about density and correlating it with the assumption that low-density urbanization is better for health.

GE I think that there is actually some evidence that low-density is worse, particularly at the areal level.

HAPI There is the idea presented in your work that the study of single environmental exposures was not sufficient to understand the whole context. For example, adults living in crowded domestic settings within high-density neighborhoods exhibited more mental stress than those who lived in crowded domestic settings in low-density neighborhoods. It would seem understanding the multiple scales of the context would be important.

GE We don't know a lot about that by the way. That's a really ripe area of work. Analogously, we know very little about housing quality and neighborhood quality. Good-quality housing in a bad neighborhood or vice versa. We don't know a lot about that.

HAPI It would seem from all this that there is a great argument for providing well-considered spaces for the general population. There seems to be some need for designers and public health people to have a dialogue, especially if the built environment can possibly affect mental health in so many ways.

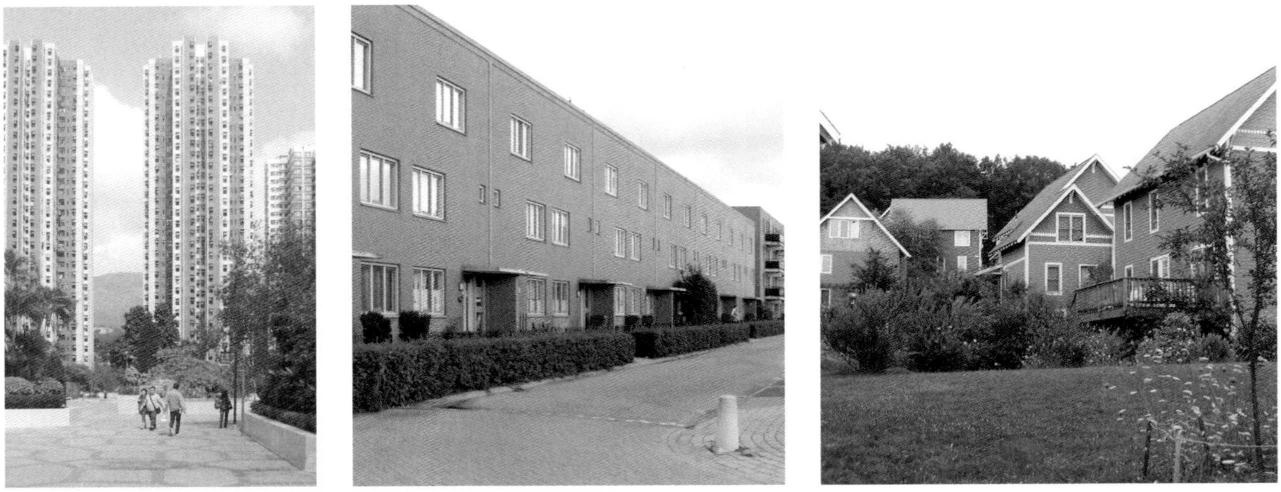

Figure 10-12 (Above) Varying community densities from (left to right) Hong Kong, China; Almere, Netherlands; and Amherst, MA. (Source: Flicker. Images by Ann Forsyth/Design for Health).

GE Absolutely.

HAPI What do you think is the best way that both fields can work on this issue?

GE I think one of the best ways is to bring people together who have similar interests and different backgrounds. So finding planners and designers and people from public health field who are most interested in the role of design environment or the planned environment in human health and well-being, and then working on a problem together. It should also ideally be a real problem, I think. In some ways I think it's the same as with the best teaching. Some of the best education you can get, I think, is when you are working with a group of people and they're not all trained like you, there's some diversity there, including your background, and then you've got a problem you're trying to solve. Ideally I think that's the way that it would work best.

HAPI So some sort of a multi-disciplinary....

GE Absolutely and again, ideally with a real problem too so that you have to try and apply your collective knowledge and intelligence to real issues. For example, now I have these theories, I have this knowledge, let's try to work with redesigning the ninth ward of New Orleans after Katrina. Do you simply rebuild it the same way that it was? Well, that doesn't seem like a good idea. So what should we do?

And China is a really good example. In some ways, that situation is a case of where there is the opportunity to work on these problems. One of the things that comes up a lot and I am sure that you've heard this yourself is that, "well, you can't prove it," "you don't know..." the causality issue, right? Well those decisions on how to build or rebuild large numbers of neighborhoods are going to get made anyway, whether you weigh in or not. So, I think that what your job is as a scholar, whether as a scientist or a designer is to say, "Here's what we know with confidence and here's what we think. We can't prove its true but this is what we think." And then the decision makers have that input when making their judgments.

HAPI At least they're informed...

GE Yes, and I think part of your job is to let people know your best guess at the quality of the evidence. So for example, the evidence is that if you where you live is high-density, you will socially withdraw, which is ironic because what this means is that if you live closer to people and you have less social support. Well that evidence is actually really solid. The evidence that high-density exterior environments lead to physical activity, I'd say that evidence is moderate. I'm not saying there's no evidence but it's not nearly as good as the other evidence. So I think that letting people know this when we are advising them is part of our job.

HAPI Can social and cultural contexts affect what the thresholds are for acceptable densities? Does what is acceptable or tolerable as high-density differ according to context? If you can excuse me I'll approach the question anecdotally. When I was an undergraduate student in Australia, the university I was attending, had a large number of overseas students, mainly from Asia. I clearly remember my surprise when many of my classmates would complain about how difficult it was for them to sleep in the quiet of the Australian suburbs. Many of them had come from living in major Asian cities, where they had grown accustomed to constant noise. In order to sleep they would need to keep the television on. Do you think there is a cultural or contextual difference between what is considered acceptable for high-density or what may be considered as acceptable for crowdedness?

GE Well people very clearly adapt and they can learn to cope with these sorts of situations. Human beings, for good or for bad, are very adaptable and usually those adaptations and copings have some real benefits. On the other hand they will often have some side effects that are not anticipated. A nice example of that, which I use when I teach, is that a really common way in which people would be able to cope or hide levels of noise or acoustical interference is that they will learn to ignore sound. So they just learn to tune it out. The problem is, when you learn to do that as a child, you tune out speech and then it interferes with your ability to read because reading is a language-based phenomena. So that's an example where, yes, it is sort of adaptive if you live in a high-rise that's over a freeway and it's really noisy, you just learn to tune it out. It is true that people learn to be adaptive but there are

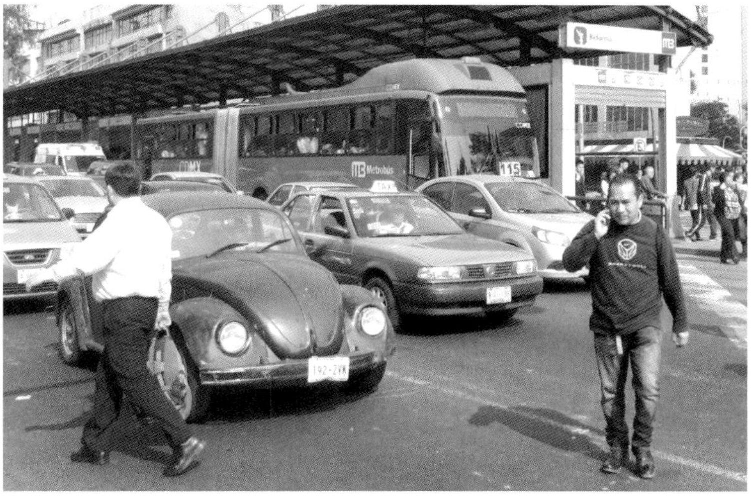

Figure 13 (Left) Mexico City, Mexico: Adapting to noise of heavy traffic. (Images courtesy Ann Forsyth/Design for Health Flickr).

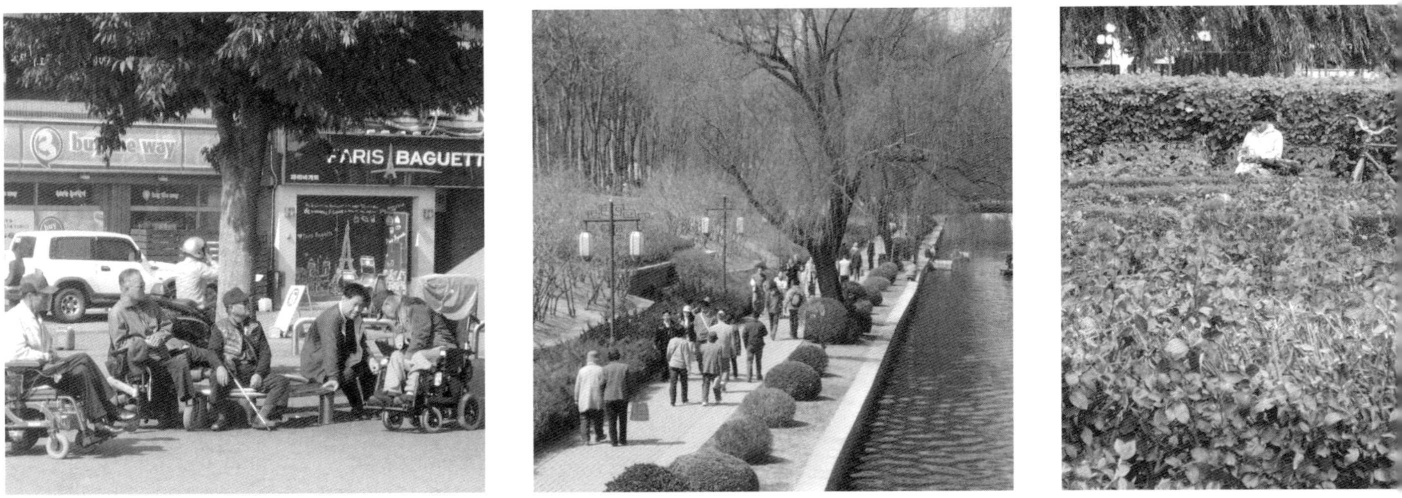

Figure 14-17 (Left) Built environments and different levels of social engagement as seen in (clockwise from top left) Daejeon, South Korea; Stockholm, Sweden; Boston, MA; and Beijing, China.

side effects to this. One of the things that means is we should pursue multi-methods in our studies. So for example, people who work in open offices, over time learn to habituate to that noise which comes with open plans. But then if you take some measures of things like, how cognitively fatigued they are for say executive functioning, you see a negative effect. So, the same exact person who, on a self-report, is saying the level of noise disturbance is five on a ten point scale, because they've gotten used to it, well they may have gotten used to it but they pay a price.

HAPI Actually it's a very good point, because there was a period when designers were promoting open plan offices for productivity reasons but there seems to be studies coming through that show that this form of working environment can actually compromise productivity.

GE And it also depends on what kind of productivity. That's where context comes in, so if you want to establish a team-based interactive exercise, if you need spontaneous, unplanned meetings and communication, there's some value in those kinds of spaces. But as we were talking about before in relation to a hierarchy of spaces, that person also needs a private space where they can shut the door.

HAPI In many ways it all seems to be pointing towards the value of providing a diverse series of spatial experiences.

GE And I think the job for designers is to try to locate what the relevant dimensions of that continuum are.

HAPI Finally, where do you think the valuable research areas are for design and public health in relation to the links between mental health and the built environment?

GE One big one is the measurement problem. I don't think we have a very good handle on how to measure the quality of the physical environment particularly at the more macro scales. I'll give you an example of what I mean, if you do a web search on neighborhood quality and you look at all the articles that come up, ninety-five percent or more are using socioeconomic status as the ways in which they define neighborhood quality. So they're not defining it in physical terms. So looking into what are the relevant dimensions

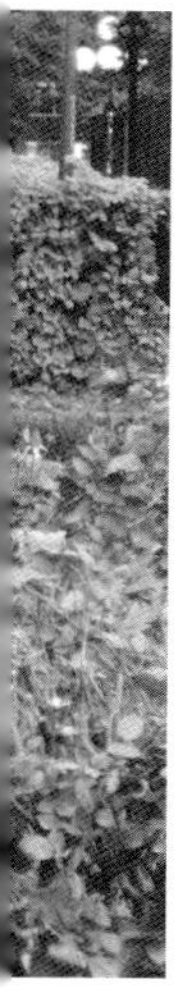

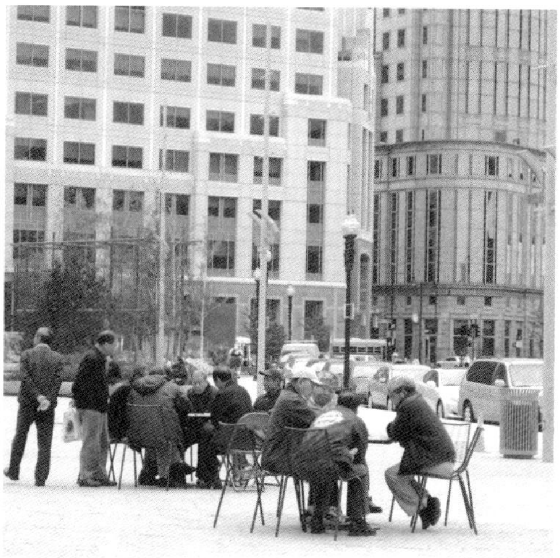

and characteristics of the environments that are potentially salient and figuring out how to measure them well is a big research opportunity.

I think another big line of research that I am particularly interested in is the interrelationship between social class and environmental experiences. I was reading something recently, it was a historical analysis, and it turns out that there is some evidence that our lives are even more segregated now by class than they have been historically. And so there are many people who have no contact, other than through the media, of someone of a different social class and particularly wealthy people. So I think that the whole role of class and ethnicity and income poverty is very important.

The final thing is there are some very fascinating things that are happening now in biology, particularly epigenetics. Epigenetics essentially puts forward that phenotypes are influenced by experience. Genes do not change, so for example, poverty does not affect genes, the environment does not affect genes, (other than in really early in utero), but what it does affect is the switching on and off of the genes. And there are biological mechanisms that explain this which are relatively well worked out. So for example, take inflammation. We are finding some evidence that a lot of diseases are turning out to be inflammatory. Obesity for instance is partly an inflammatory disease, cardiovascular disease is an inflammatory disease. The phenotype for sensitivity for reacting to the environment in terms of an inflammation is influenced by early experience. So I think that some of these developments in biology that are going beyond nature and nurture and looking into locating some of the mechanisms that explain how this happens are going to be a really important area of research in the long term.

HAPI To realize what the different triggers are....

GE Yes, and another one which is obvious is social media. I have a graduate student who is doing a Ph.D. (she's an architect by training) on the role of the settings in which people are using social media, which has not been looked at very much... the physical settings. We know that there's some benefits and costs of all of this attention to your social media. But are those moderated by certain settings? Are certain settings more likely to increase or decrease that kind of behavior? I think that's fascinating.

Figure Credits

Figure 1-8, 10-17, Forsyth, Ann 2011-2015, *Design for Health Collection*, photograph collection, Accessed 4 August 2015, https://www.flickr.com/photos/designforhealth/.

Figure 9, Cooper after Cave, *ca 1796, Original building of The Retreat, York, Instituted 1792.* Wellcome Library, London, Creative Commons Attribution 4.0 International.

Promoting Physical Activity for All Ages

Laura Smead

Laura Smead is a research associate in urban planning for the Health and Places Initiative at Harvard's Graduate School of Design. With master's degrees in both urban planning and psychology, Ms. Smead has specialized knowledge on health, aging, climate change, and sustainable urban planning. Her contributions to the Health and Places Initiative include being the primary author of research briefs on health and place, contributing to the development of a new suite of health impact assessment tools for planners, and co-authoring a guidelines book on creating healthy neighborhoods.

Introduction

Overview

The built environment can facilitate or create barriers for physical activity, and this effect varies by persons' age. To show this, the findings of twenty-four reviews (2002-2015) on the topic were analyzed and categorized by age group: children and adolescents (< 18 years), adults (18+ years, ideally aged 18-64), and older adults (aged 60+ on average). The reviews demonstrate that different age groups, especially young children, have their physical activity enabled or constrained by distinctive aspects of the built environment. These features were sometimes quiet environments that support adults walking or cycling for transportation. This chapter argues that more attention should be paid to the wide variety of people who walk, cycle, and play in urban areas.

Background

Physical activity is a well-known and critical factor for overall health: reducing the risk of chronic diseases as well as increasing longevity, well-being, and weight control.[1] The World Health Organization's (2010) Global Recommendations on Physical Activity for Health recommended accumulating at least 60 minutes of moderate-to vigorous-intensity physical activity daily for children and young adults (420 minutes weekly), and at least 150 minutes of moderate-intensity physical activity weekly for adults and older adults. According to the WHO (2010), "physical inactivity levels are rising in many countries with major implications for the prevalence of noncommunicable diseases (NCDs) and the general health of the population worldwide."[2]

1 WHO 2014.

2 WHO 2010, 7.

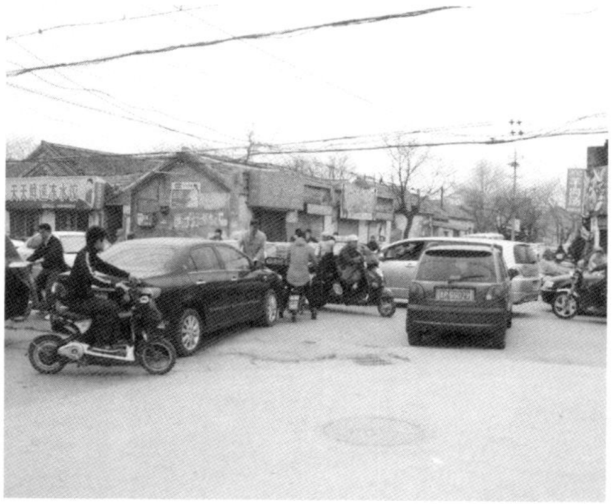

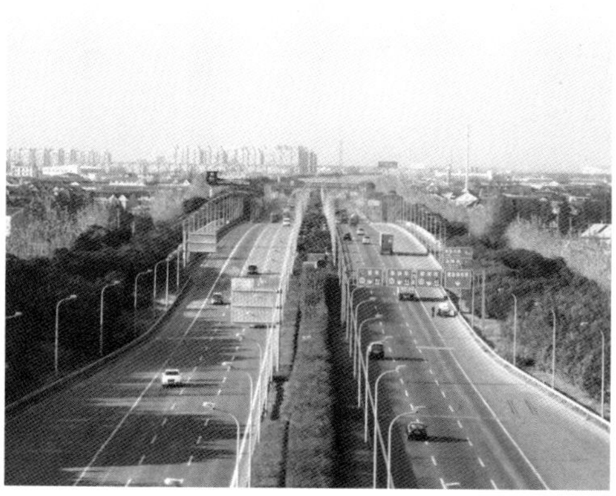

Figures 1, 2 (Left) Traffic density and speed, and a lack of sidewalks can be barriers to physical activity for children.

The built environment includes all spaces that people create or modify: such as buildings, street patterns, land use, green spaces, and transportation. There are four main settings for physical activity: at work (e.g. physical labor), at home (e.g. household chores, gardening), for recreation or exercise (e.g. hiking, sports, playing), and for transportation (e.g. walking or cycling to a destination). This review focuses on recreational physical activity (or exercise) and transportation-related physical activity as those are the settings that neighborhood built environments are most likely to affect.

Physical activity in the built environment can be convenient and attractive, but too often the environment is unpleasant, difficult to navigate, or inaccessible—especially for the very young or older adults who may face more mobility difficulties. For example, the figures above show that barriers can include poorly maintained and dirty surroundings, a lack of pedestrian infrastructure or traffic safety, or large, or fast moving roads with no way for pedestrians or cyclists to cross.

What We Know About Physical Activity in the Built Environment

- Walking and cycling for transportation: A large proportion of the research on physical activity in the built environment focuses on adults walking or cycling for transportation. This category also shows some of the strongest connections in the literature; that a strategically designed, compact, connected, mixed-use community is correlated with walking or cycling to destinations (for transportation).[3]
- Recreational activity or exercise: There is less consistent evidence connecting adults and recreational activity or exercise in the built environment; rather, other factors ranging from cost to personal preferences may be more important (Bauman et al. 2011; Lovasi et al. 2009; HAPI 2014 Physical Activity research brief). However, access to recreational facilities such as well-maintained playgrounds or parks seem to play a larger role for children or older adults.[4]
- Pedestrian amenities[5] and aesthetics:[6] While pedestrian amenities and aesthetics create an enjoyable and pleasing environment, the weight of the evidence suggests they are not strongly related to physical activity. In this analysis, pedestrian amenities had the weakest connection to physical activity across all age groups, although aesthetics were slightly more related to older adults general physical activity or adult's recreational physical activity (see Tables 2 and 3). However,

3 Bauman et al. 2012; Durand et al. 2011; Ewing and Cervero 2010; Fraser et al. 2010; Frost et al. 2010; Krizek et al. 2009; McCormack and Shiell 2011; Saelens et al. 2003; Sugiyama et al. 2012; van Holle et al. 2012.

4 Ding et al. 2011; Rosso et al. 2011; van Cauwenberg et al. 2011; Trost et al. 2002; Wendel-Vos 2007, 425.

5 Pedestrian amenities refer to features like seating, lighting, well-maintained sidewalks, and public toilets.

6 Aesthetics refer to features like overall greenness, and perceptions of a pleasing environment.

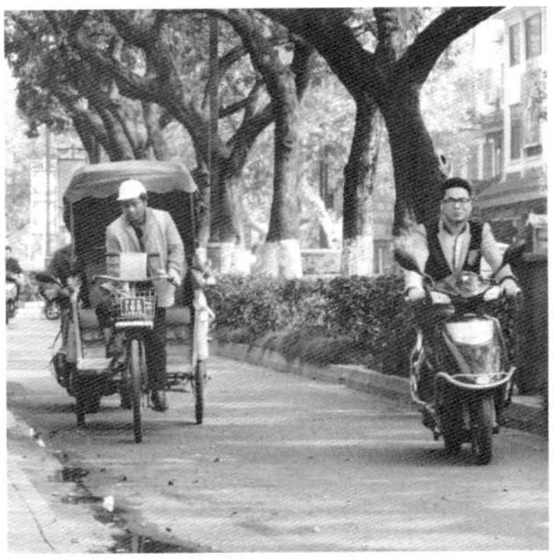
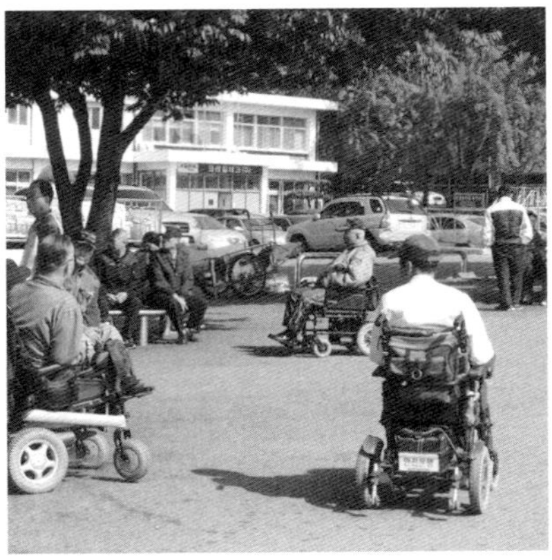
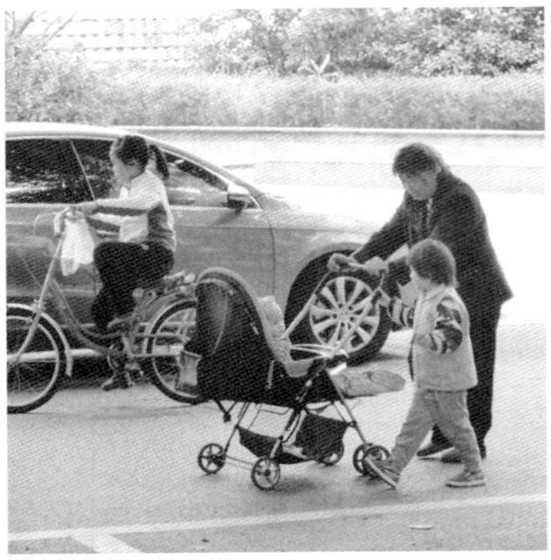

Figures 3-5 (Above) The illustrations show a range of different types of people who are active in the built environment: able-bodied adults, those dependent on wheelchairs, older adults, and young children.

high-quality pedestrian amenities are still important for older adults and children, who are more likely to need places to rest, and for whom narrow sidewalks, high curbs, and poorly maintained sidewalks can be a barrier to walking.[7] Aesthetics also have other important health promoting features, such as street tree canopies for cooling and urban comfort, views of green for mental health, and perceptions of safety and neighborhood quality (social capital).[8] So these features are still useful for other reasons.

7 Skiba and Zuger 2009, 23-24; Van Cauwenberg et al. 2011, 467; WHO 2007.

8 APA 2011; Barton and Pretty 2010; Bjornstrom and Ralston 2014; Bowler et al. 2010a; Bowler et al. 2010b; Coon et al. 2011; de Nazelle et al. 2011, 775; French et al. 2014; Wood 2008, 15; Lee and Maheswaran 2010; Maller et al. 2005.

How the Analysis Was Conducted

Data Inclusion

Articles were selected from English-language research on physical activity and the built environment for each of three age groups: children and adolescents (ages < 18 years), adults (aged 18+, ideally aged 18-64), and older adults (average age 60+). Priority for inclusion in the analysis followed this order: systematic review or meta-analysis[9] published after 2009, comprehensive or other review published after 2009, systematic review or meta-analyses published after 2000, comprehensive or other reviews published after 2000, and lastly, a large-scale survey study. Overall, 24 studies were included: of which, 12 were systematic reviews or meta-analyses, 11 were comprehensive literature reviews, and 1 was a large qualitative study. The adult age group had both the most available research and the strongest research quality. The research on children was the most limited. However, each age category analysis includes at least one systematic review published after 2009. Since almost all of the work on this topic has taken place in only a handful of countries—particularly the United States, Australia, and the U.K.—one large-scale international study (N= 11,541 individuals surveyed with 11 countries represented) was included.

9 Systematic reviews conduct a comprehensive search of the literature using a detailed plan and search strategy, to avoid bias in the evidence they select. They synthesize large bodies of evidence and can include a meta-analysis component, which uses statistics to combine data from many studies into one summary effect size (Petticrew and Roberts 2008; Uman 2011).

Data Coding

For each article, built environmental characteristics were categorized (adapted from Bauman 2012, Ding et al. 2011, and McCormack 2011), and the strength of connection between these features and physical activity was assessed categorically (i.e. high, medium, uncertain or mixed, no connection, or not assessed) based upon the findings of the article. For

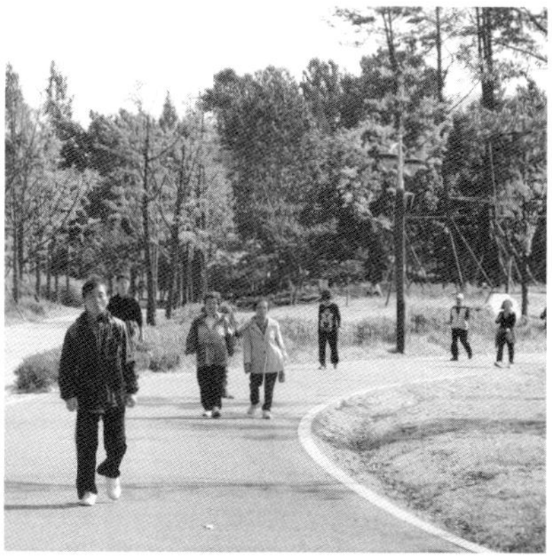

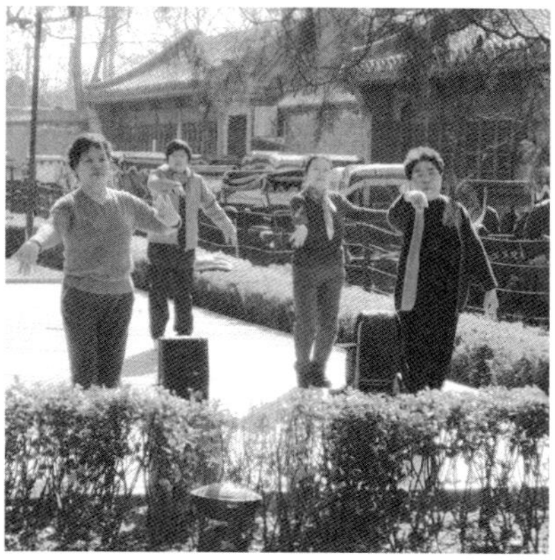

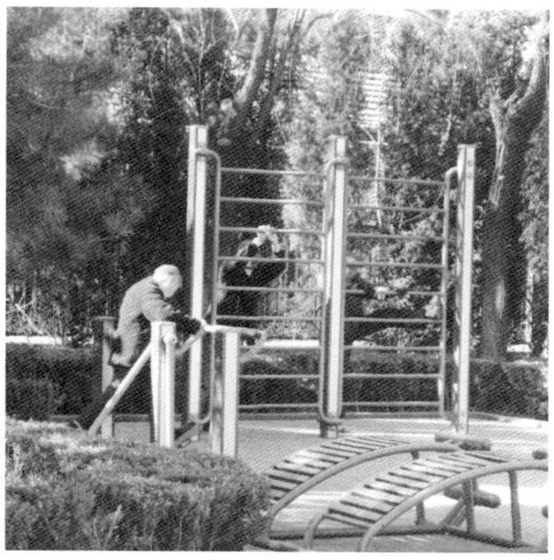

Figures 6-8 (Above) Greenspaces and recreational facilities in urban places may include parks, playgrounds, beaches, pools, off-road trails, community centers, recreation centers, picnic areas, sports fields, or exercise equipment, for instance.

example, an article may have found a characteristic (e.g. land use mix) to be "significantly"[10] or "strongly" related to physical activity, therefore it was given a score of "high," Or an article might describe a characteristic as being "somewhat related" or "weakly related" to physical activity, and therefore it was given a score of "medium," Where results were described as mixed, uncertain, or varied across context or groups, items were coded as "uncertain or mixed," A couple of studies found a built environmental characteristic was related to decreased physical activity, in which case the results were coded "negative," Environmental characteristics not found to have any relationship to physical activity for a particular age group were coded "No connection,"[11] Finally, if a built environmental category was not included in a particular study, that item was coded "not assessed."

Data Ranking

Built environment characteristics were then roughly ordered by the strength of their connection to physical activity within each age category, and summarized from highest connection to least connection. Environmental characteristics with mostly "high" degrees of evidence were categorized as "essential" features to promote physical activity in the built environment. Characteristics with mostly "medium" connections were categorized as "highly recommended." Characteristics with more "uncertain" evidence or "no connection" were categorized as "Good-to-do."

Data Summarizing

Finally, results were summarized to compare the most useful built environmental characteristics for promoting physical activity overall, and to compare each age category with each other. As before, more weight was given to "high" degrees of evidence, and less weight to "uncertain or mixed" findings. For each environmental characteristic, articles where it was not assessed were excluded from the summary. For example, if pedestrian amenities were assessed in 16 out of 24 total articles—only those 16 articles would be used to summarize the degree of evidence.

10 Please note that while a built environment characteristic may be related to physical activity significantly in a statistical sense, the magnitude of the effect is quite small.

11 It is important to note that researchers and journal editors tend to prefer to publish studies that find a positive (or statistically significant) effect to studies that find a negative effect or no effect. This can lead to publication bias toward studies that find positive effect in the available literature.

Table 1 Built environmental features promoting physical activity (recreational and transportation) for children and adolescents (ages < 18 years).

Legend: Strength of Evidence	+++ High	+ Medium	+- Uncertain or mixed evidence	o Low or no connection	x Not assessed
Study Characteristics	**Ding et. al. 2011**	**Davison and Lawson 2006**	**Giles-Corti et al. 2009**	**McGrath et al. 2015**	**Sallis and Glanz 2006**
Ages	ages 3-18	ages 3-18	Unspecified, <18	8-17 years	Unspecified, <18
Publication period of studies included	1993-2009	1989-2006	1985-2009	2000-2013	1990-2005
Number of studies included	103	33	113 articles cited	23 (of which 14 for metanalysis)	82
Report type	Review	Review	Narrative Literature review	Systematic review and metaanalysis	Review
Built environment characteristics					
Land use mix[12] (residential, commercial)/ or destinations (shops/ services/jobs)	+++	+ Destinations within walking distance	+ Destinations within walking distance, older children	+ Destinations, adolescents	+
Residential or population density (population per unit area)	+++	+-	+ Older children	+-	+
Street connectivity (density of connections, intersections per area, etc.)	+	+-	+ More for older than younger children	+-	+-
Walkability[13]	+++	x	+ More for older than younger children	+	+++
Transit proximity/access	x	+	x	x	+
Parks (access/density/proximity)	+-	+	+	+ For adolescents, not children	+
Recreation facilities (access/ density/proximity)	+++	+++	+ Especially sports centers	+ Play facilities, playgrounds - for adolescents not children	+++
Low traffic speed/volume	+++ <13 years only	+++	+	+	+++
Walking / biking facilities (sidewalks, bike lanes, trails)	+-	+ Sidewalks, not bike lanes	+ Sidewalks	+ Sidewalks, walking tracks	+
Pedestrian safety structures (crosswalks, traffic lights)	+++ <13 years only	+++	+ Primary school children	x	+
Safety (from neighborhood disorder or crime)	+ <13 years only	+ Objective crime rates and deprivation, not perceived safety	+ Perceptions of safety and objective crime, especially girls	+ Perceptions of safety of parents of younger children	+-
Aesthetics (variety/diversity/ vegetation)	+-	+-	+- Limited evidence	x	x
Pedestrian amenities (benches, toilets, lighting)	o	x	+- Lighting, younger children	+- Limited	x

12 Defined as co-locations of different land uses within walking distance: such as residential, commercial, or non-profit/institutional. May or may not include mixed-use buildings. Conventionally, ideal walkable distances between residential and other uses range from ¼-1/2 mile (400-800 meters).

13 Walkability is a composite score, which may be perceived walkability (e.g. the Neighborhood Environment Walkability Scale (NEWS)) or an objective walkability index (e.g. scores the presence and distance of neighborhood attributes based on physical observation or GIS analysis). Walkability scores include features such as residential and commercial density, land use mix, street connectivity, access to recreational facilities and transportation, safety (traffic/crime) and aesthetic elements.

Research Findings

Findings for Different Age Groups

Children (< 18 years)

Recent literature finds proximity of recreational facilities, low traffic speeds and volumes, pedestrian safety infrastructure, overall walkability,[13] and destinations within walking distance to be the most important built environmental characteristics connected to physical activity among children and adolescents (see Table 1). Table 1 also shows that safety concerns (both traffic and crime) are more important for promoting physical activity among younger children (<13 years), while destinations (recreational, parks, shops, etc.) may be more important for older children (> 13 years) who have more independence from their parents.

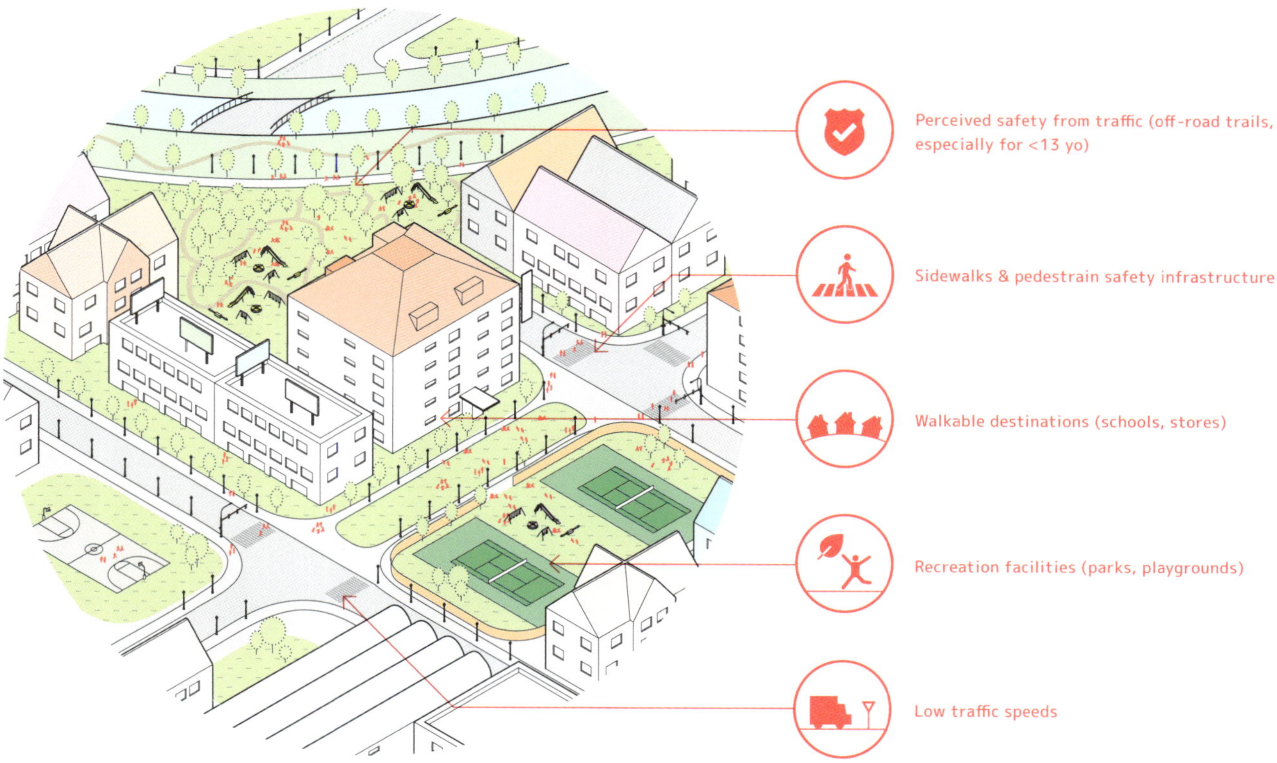

Figure 9 (Above) Diagram of ideal and recommended characteristics to employ for children.

Built environment characteristics to promote physical activity (recreational and transportation)[14] *For ages <18 years, based on evidence presented in Table 1.*

Essential:

- Access to recreational facilities (e.g. a neighborhood or school play area, or recreational equipment)
- Low traffic speeds and density (e.g. less than 30mph or 48kph)
- Overall walkability (may be a perceived or objective composite score, see sidenote 8)
- Pedestrian safety infrastructure (e.g. controlled intersections,[15] crosswalks, etc.)
- Residential proximity to walkable destinations[16] (e.g. distance from home to school, parks, stores)

Highly recommended:

- Parks (access/density/proximity)
- Transit proximity and access
- Walking/biking facilities (e.g. sidewalks, bike paths)
- Residential or population density (e.g. dwelling unit/acre, population/unit area—children are more likely to be close to neighbors, destinations or services)
- Safety from neighborhood disorder or crime (e.g. might be perceptions of safety or an objective measure such as violent crime rates)

Good-to-do

- Pedestrian amenities (e.g. benches, public toilets, water fountains)
- Aesthetics (e.g. street trees, landscaping, green roofs, green walls)
- Street connectivity (which prioritizes pedestrians and cyclists over cars)

14 This is inclusive of both physical activity for transportation or recreation. For the purposes of this study I don't distinguish between the two since the goal is simply to promote physical activity generally. Physical activity in most studies refers to walking, however, cycling and other recreation (jogging, playing etc.) were included in some articles—especially for children.

15 Controlled intersections have traffic lights, stop signs, or yield signs

16 Conventionally around ¼ - ½ mile walking distance or 400-800 meters

Table 2 Built environmental features promoting physical activity (recreational and transportation) for adults (ages 18-64).[17]

Legend: Strength of Evidence +++ High + Medium +- Uncertain or mixed evidence o Low or no connection x Not assessed

Study Characteristics	Bauman et al. 2012	Casagrande et al. 2009	Duncan et al. 2005	Forsyth and Krizek 2010	Frost et al. 2010	Humpel et al. 2002
Ages	18+	18+	Unspecified, <18	8-17 years	18+	18+
Publication period of studies included	2002-2011	2000-2005	1989-2005	1977-2008	2000-2008	1989-2001
Number of studies included	9	10	16	300+	20	19
Report type	Review of systematic reviews	Systematic review	Meta-analysis	International literature review, (active transp)	Systematic review	Review
Built environment characteristics						
Land use mix (residential, commercial)/ or destinations (shops/services/jobs)	+-	o (destinations within walking distance)	+ Shops and services within walking distance	+++	+-	+ Shops, non-residential
Residential or population density (population per unit area)	+-	x	x	+++	x	x
Street connectivity (density of connections, intersections per area, etc.)	+-	x	x	+	x	x
Walkability[18]	+-	x	x	+	x	x
Transit proximity/access	+	x	x	+	+-	x
Parks (access/density/proximity)	x	x	x	x	+-	+
Recreation facilities	+	o	+	x	+++	+
Low traffic speed/volume	x	+	+	+	+++	+- Yes perceived, no objective
Walking / biking facilities (sidewalks, bike lanes, trails)	x	+ Sidewalks	+ Sidewalks and footpaths, cycle lanes not assessed	+ Bike infrastructure, sidewalks inconclusive for adults, important for children	+ Sidewalks, Trails	+ Cycle path access, no connection for sidewalks
Pedestrian safety structures (crosswalks, traffic lights)	x	o	x	+ Children	x	x
Safety (from neighborhood disorder or crime)	x	+	o (High crime)	x	+++ Perceived	o
Aesthetics (variety/diversity/ vegetation)	+-	o	x	x	+	+
Pedestrian amenities (benches, toilets, lighting)	o	o (Lighting)	o (Lighting)	+- Lighting	+- Lighting	o (Lighting)

17 This is inclusive of both physical activity for transportation or recreation. For the purposes of this study I don't distinguish between the two since the goal is simply to promote physical activity generally. Physical activity in most studies refers to walking, however, cycling and other recreation (jogging, playing etc.) were included in some articles—especially for children.

18 Walkability is a composite score, which may be perceived walkability (e.g. the Neighborhood Environment Walkability Scale (NEWS)) or an objective walkability index (e.g. scores the presence and distance of neighborhood attributes based on physical observation or GIS analysis). Walkability scores include features such as residential and commercial density, land use mix, street connectivity, access to recreational facilities and transportation, safety (traffic/crime) and aesthetic elements.

(Table 2 continued.)

McCormack and Shiell 2011	Owen 2004	Saelens and Handy 2008	Sallis et al. 2009	Sugiyama et al. 2012	Trost et al. 2002	Van Holle et al. 2012	Wendel-Vos 2007
18+	18+	All	18-65	18+	18+	18-65	18+
1996-2010	1997-2004	2002-2006, mostly 2005-2006	Data collection 2002-2003	1997-2011	1998-2000	2000-2011	1980-2004
33	18	42	N=11,541 adults, 11 countries	46	38	70	47
Systematic review	Review	Review	Qualitative study	Systematic Review	Systematic Review	Systematic Review	Systematic Review
+++	+	+++	+ Many shops nearby	+++ Destinations within walking distance	x	+ Destinations within walking distance	x
+	+	+++	o (single family homes not significant)	x	- Urban location is negative	+-	x
+	x	+	o	+	x	+-	x
+++	o	x	x	x	x	+++	x
+	+	x	+	+		o	x
+-	+	+	x	+	x	x	x
+-	+	o	+ Low-cost	+	+	--	+
o	+- Yes, transport.; no for other PA	o	x	o	o	x	o
+- More important for cycling; trails more important for recreation than transportation	+ Sidewalks	+- More for recreation, not for transportation	+ Sidewalk and bicycle facilities	+ Sidewalks	o Sidewalks	+	+
x	+-	x	x	o	x	o	o
x	o	+-	o (Perceived crime)	o	+ "Neighborhood safety" but not high crime rates	c	o
o	+ Yes for recreation, not for transportation	o	x	+ Recreational, not utilitarian	+	o	+-
+-	o (Lighting)	x	x	x	o (Lighting)	x	x

Able-bodied Adults (18-65 years)

Evidence suggests that strategies to promote active transportation are most effective for able-bodied adults (see Table 2). Land use mix, overall walkability, street connectivity, walking and biking infrastructure, and access to transit are among the most consistent and influential strategies. There is less consistent evidence connecting built environmental features with recreational physical activity, although access to parks and were found to be important for this type of physical activity.

Built environment characteristics to promote physical activity (recreational and transportation)[19] *For ages 18-65 years, based on evidence presented in Table 2.*

Essential:

- Land-use mix/ residential proximity to walkable destinations[20] (e.g. distance from home to work, parks, stores)
- Overall walkability (may be perceived or objective composite score)
- Walking and biking facilities (e.g. sidewalks, bike paths)
- Street connectivity (which prioritizes pedestrians and cyclists over cars)

19 This is inclusive of both physical activity for transportation or recreation. For the purposes of this study I don't distinguish between the two since the goal is simply to promote physical activity generally. Physical activity in most studies refers to walking, however, cycling and other recreation (jogging, playing etc.) were included in some articles – especially for children.

20 Conventionally around ¼ - ½ mile walking distance or 400-800 meters

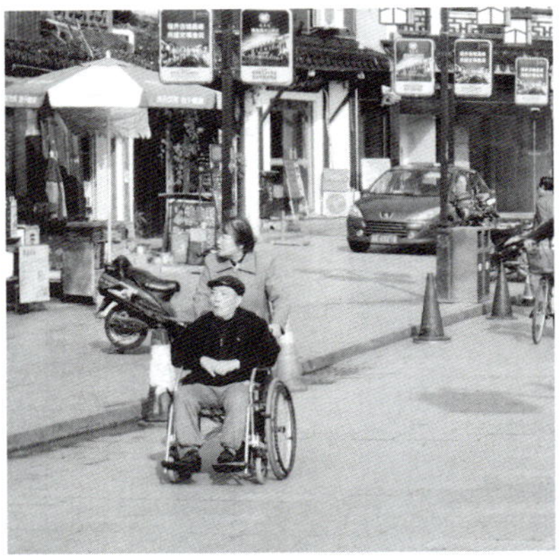

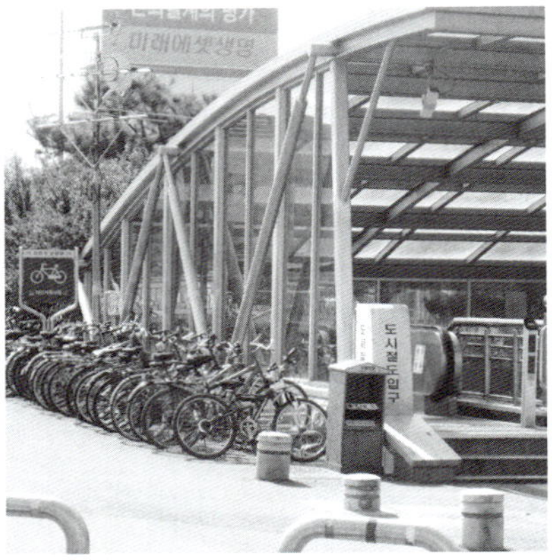

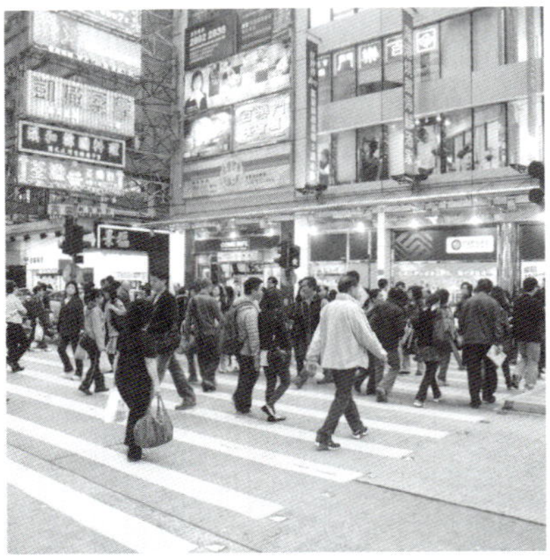

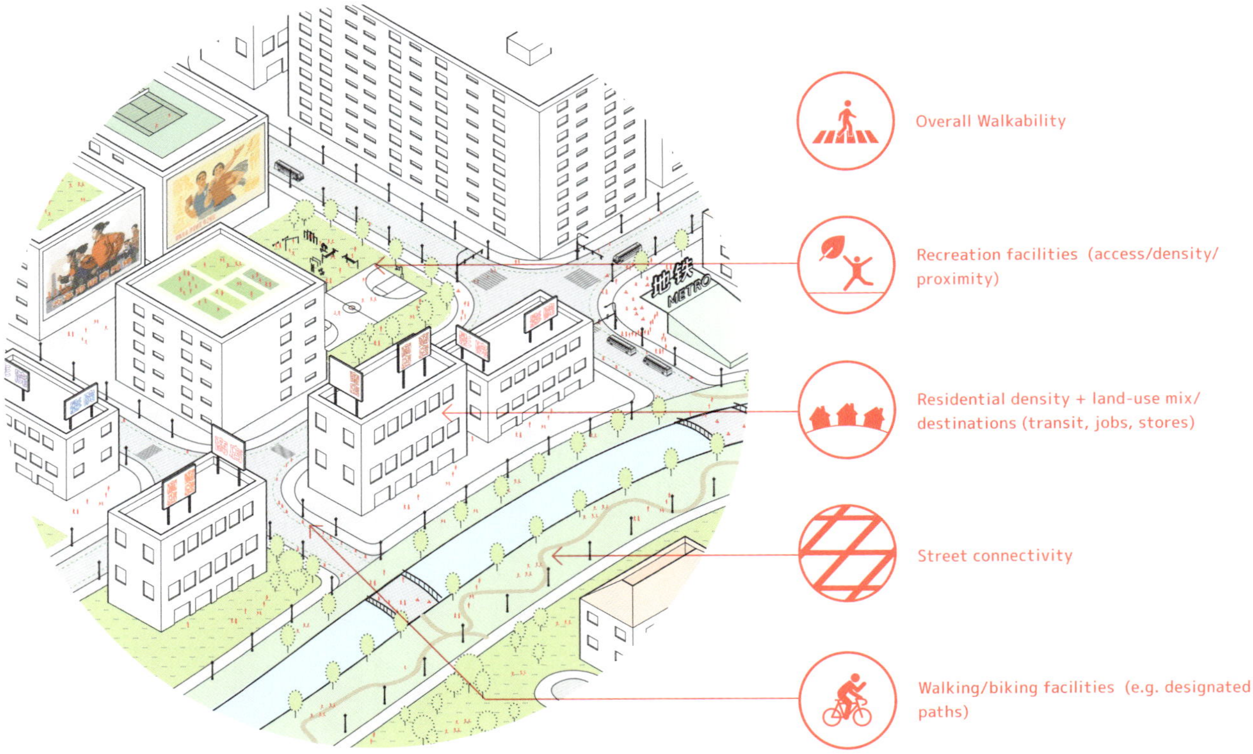

Figure 10-12 (Top) Photographs of recommended characteristics for able-bodied adults.

Figure 13 (Middle) Diagram of ideal and recommended characteristics to employ.

Figure 14 (Right Page, Full Bleed) Photograph of a poor physical environment that can make healthier life practices challenging.

- Parks (access/density/proximity)
- Transit proximity and access

Highly Recommended:

- Access to recreational facilities (access/density/proximity) (e.g. such as a neighborhood gym, pool, green space, or recreational equipment)
- Residential or population density (more likely to be close to neighbors, destinations, or services)
- Aesthetics (e.g. street trees, landscaping, green roofs, green walls)
- Low traffic speed/volume (e.g. less than 30mph or 48kph)

Good-to-do:

- Safety from neighborhood disorder or crime (might be perceptions of safety or an objective measure such as violent crime rates)
- Pedestrian safety structures (e.g. controlled intersections,[21] crosswalks, etc.)
- Pedestrian amenities (e.g. benches, public toilets, water fountains)

21 Controlled intersections have traffic lights, stop signs, or yield signs.

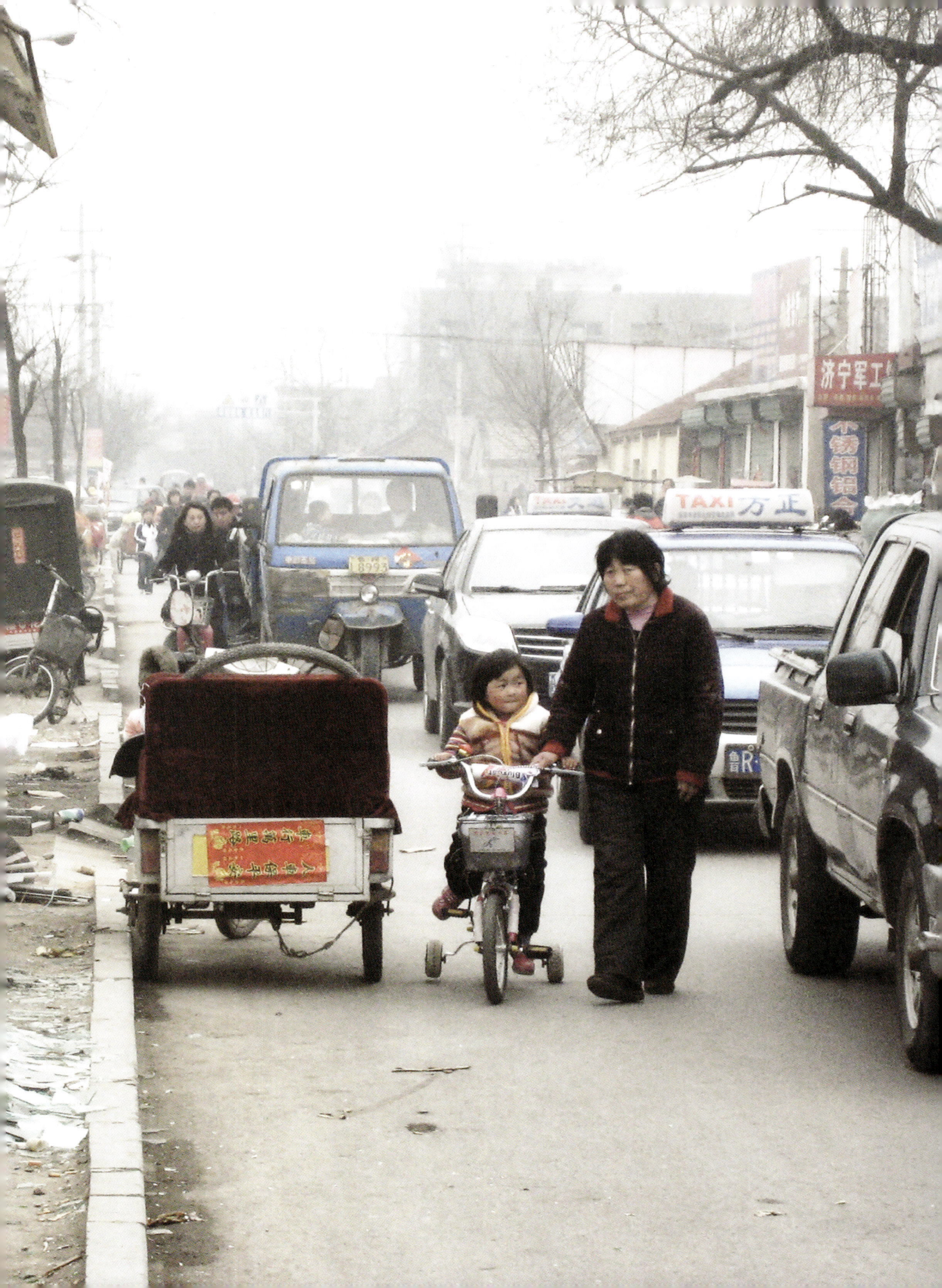
济宁军工
TAXI 万正

Table 3 Built environmental features promoting physical activity (recreational or transportation) for older adults.[22]

Legend: Strength of Evidence	+++ High	+ Medium	+- Uncertain or mixed evidence	o Low or no connection	x Not assessed
Study Characteristics	**Cunningham and Michael 2004**	**Moran et al. 2014**	**Rosso et al. 2011**	**Van Cauwenberg et al. 2011**	**Van Stralen et al. 2009**
Ages	All, but highlights studies specific to seniors	65+	60+	Average age 65+	Average >50 years, minimum 40 years
Publication period of studies included	1966-2002	1996-2012	1990-2010	2000-2010	1990-2008
Number of studies included	27 (6 specific to seniors, results below)	31	17	31	59
Report type	Comprehensive review	Systematic review, qualitative literature	Comprehensive review	Systematic review	Review
Built environment characteristics					
Land use mix (residential, commercial)/ or destinations (shops/services/jobs)	+- Destinations within walking distance	+ Access to daily destinations	+	+	+-
Residential or population density (population per unit area)	x	x	+	+-	x
Street connectivity (density of connections, intersections per area, etc.)	x	x	+	+-	o
Walkability	x	x	+	o	x
Transit proximity/access	o	+ Sheltered bus stops, senior services	o	o	x
Parks (access/density/proximity)	x	+ Green open space, age appropriate	+-	x	x
Recreation facilities (access/ density/proximity)	+-	+ Indoor gyms, indoor pools, buildings for older adults, low-cost	+-	+	+-
Low traffic speed/volume	o	x	o	o	+-
Walking / biking facilities (sidewalks, bike lanes, trails)	+- Sidewalk	+ Sidewalks, connectivity, and maintenance important; separation between walking and cycle paths	+-	o	o
Pedestrian safety structures (crosswalks, traffic lights)	x	- Zebra-crossing, inadequate signal timings	+	+-	x
Safety (from neighborhood disorder or crime)	+	+ Related to street lighting and maintenance	x	+-	+
Aesthetics (variety/diversity/ vegetation)	+	+	x	o	+-
Pedestrian amenities (benches, toilets, lighting)	o (Lighting)	+ Rest areas, street lights, public restrooms	o	o	o (Lighting)

22 This is inclusive of both physical activity for transportation or recreation. For the purposes of this study I don't distinguish between the two since the goal is simply to promote physical activity generally. Physical activity in most studies refers to walking, however, cycling and other recreation (jogging, playing etc.) were included in some articles—especially for children.

Older Adults (65+ years)

Modifying the built environment to support increased physical activity and mobility, and to facilitate independence is necessary for older adults' quality of life as they age. Safety from neighborhood disorder or crime, land use mix, and access to recreational facilities was found to be important for promoting physical activity (both for transportation and recreation) in older adults. Residential or population density, access to parks, and aesthetics were also found to have some connection. However, physical activity was found to be less associated with the built environment for older adults than other age groups. Older adults tend to have higher rates of chronic diseases and mobility challenges,[23] and those with mobility challenges have lower levels of physical activities (at least in the United States).[24] It could be that mobility challenges and other individual factors make it difficult for an enabling built environment to have an effect on older adults' physical activity. Rather, older adults may prefer to get physical activity in other ways (e.g. at home, in the garden, driving to a gym, etc.).

23 Timiras 2007, 33.

24 CDC 2009.

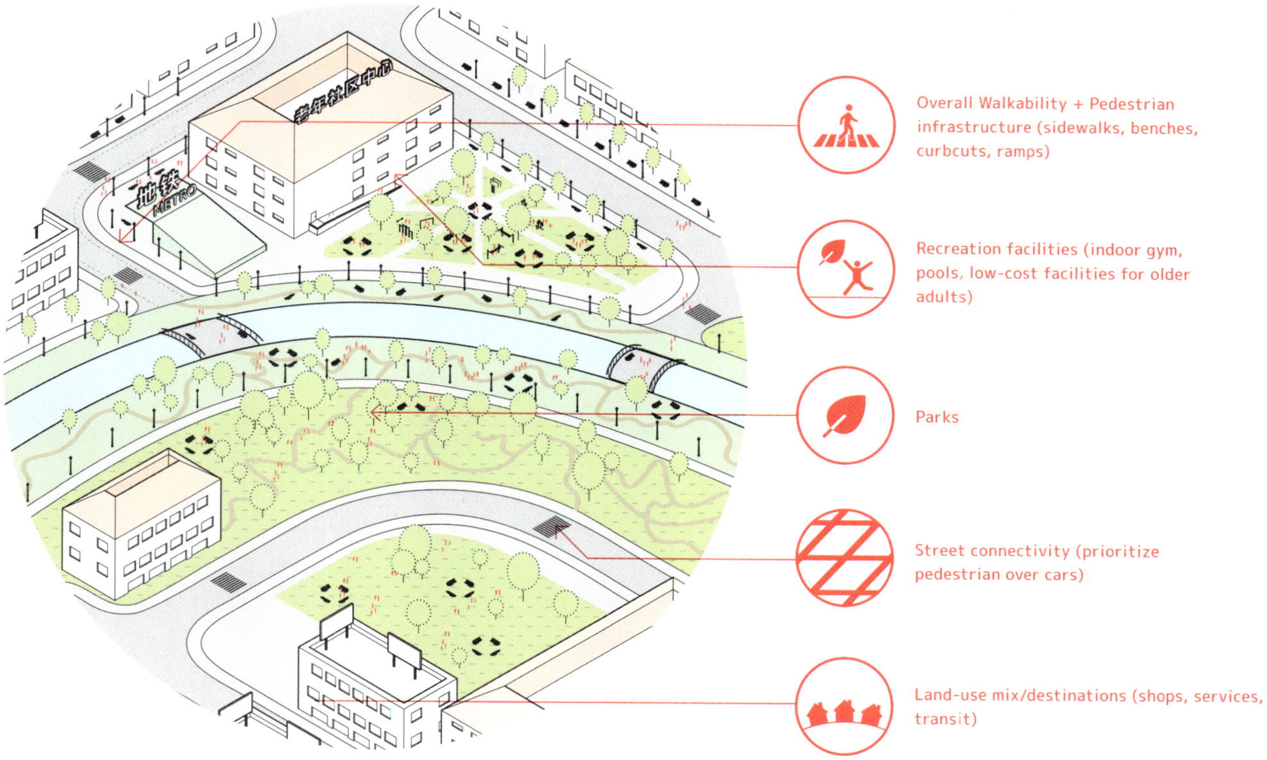

Figure 15 (Above) Diagram of ideal and recommended characteristics to employ for older adults.

Built environment characteristics to promote physical activity (recreational and transportation)[25] *For ages 65+ years, based on evidence presented in Table 3.*

Essential

- Safety from neighborhood disorder or crime (e.g. might be perceptions of safety or an objective measure such as violent crime rates)
- Land-use mix/ residential proximity to walkable destinations[26] (e.g. distance from home to school, parks, stores)

Highly Recommended

- Residential or population density (e.g. dwelling unit/acre, population/unit area—more likely to be close to neighbors, destinations or services)
- Parks (access/density/proximity)
- Recreational facilities (access/density/proximity) (e.g. such as a neighborhood gym, pool, green space, or recreational equipment)
- Aesthetics (variety/diversity/vegetation) (e.g. street trees, landscaping, green roofs, green walls)

Good-to-do

- Street connectivity (which prioritizes pedestrians and cyclists over cars)
- Overall walkability (may be a perceived or objective composite score)
- Walking and biking infrastructure (e.g. sidewalks, bike paths)
- Pedestrian safety infrastructure (e.g. controlled intersections,[27] crosswalks, etc.)
- Transit proximity/access
- Pedestrian amenities (e.g. benches, public toilets, water fountains)

25 This is inclusive of both physical activity for transportation or recreation. For the purposes of this study I don't distinguish between the two since the goal is simply to promote physical activity generally. Physical activity in most studies refers to walking, however, cycling and other recreation (jogging, playing etc.) were included in some articles—especially for children.

26 Conventionally around ¼ - ½ mile walking distance or 400-800 meters

27 Controlled intersections have traffic lights, stop signs, or yield signs

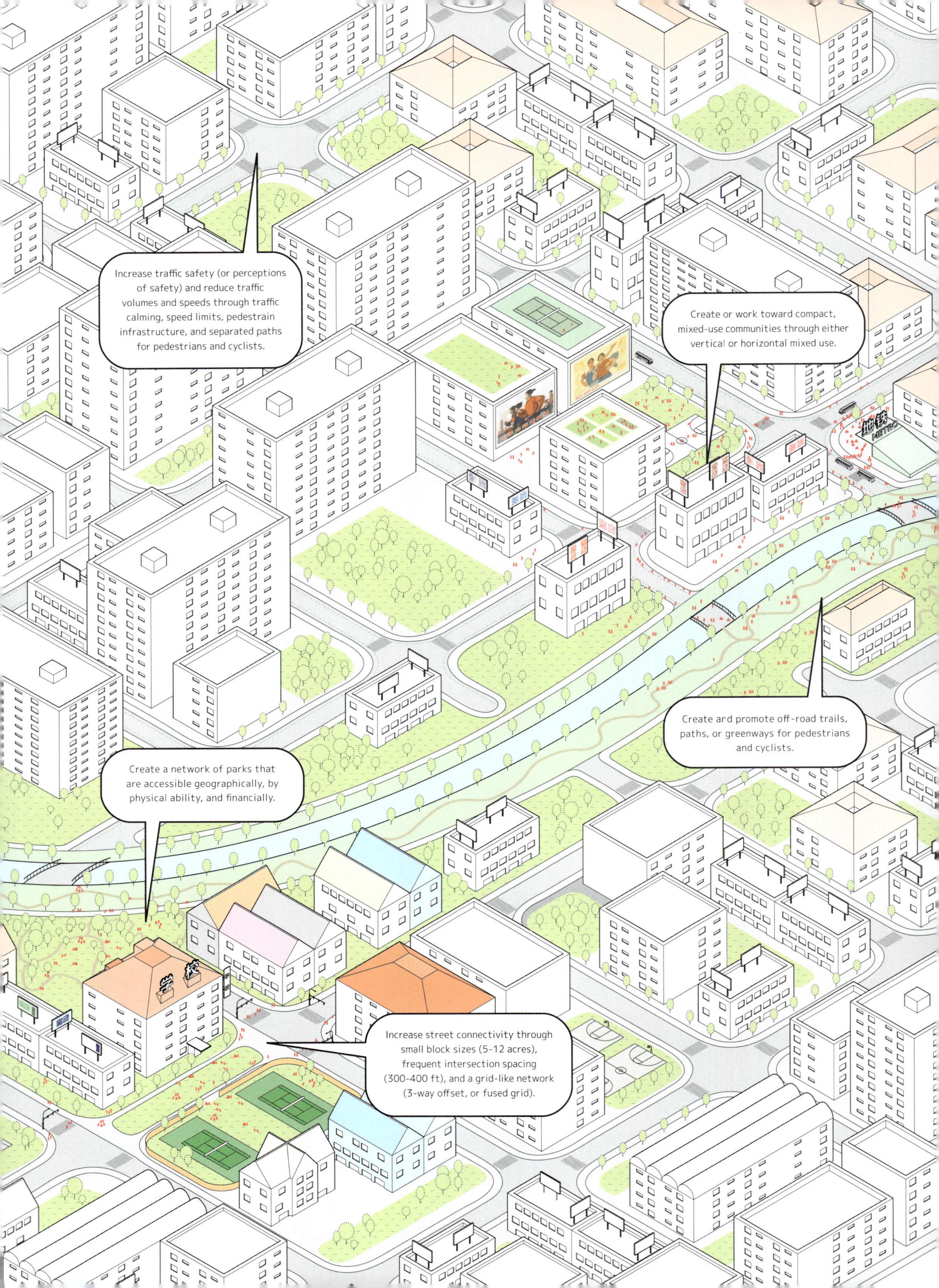
Increase traffic safety (or perceptions of safety) and reduce traffic volumes and speeds through traffic calming, speed limits, pedestrain infrastructure, and separated paths for pedestrians and cyclists.
Create or work toward compact, mixed-use communities through either vertical or horizontal mixed use.
地铁 METRO
Create and promote off-road trails, paths, or greenways for pedestrians and cyclists.
Create a network of parks that are accessible geographically, by physical ability, and financially.
学 校
Increase street connectivity through small block sizes (5-12 acres), frequent intersection spacing (300-400 ft), and a grid-like network (3-way offset, or fused grid).

Table 4 Summary table of built environmental features promoting physical activity by age.[28 29]

Legend: Strength of Evidence	+++ High	+ Medium	+- Uncertain or mixed evidence	o Low or no connection
Built environment characteristics	**All Ages**	**Children**	**Adults**	**Older adults**
Land use mix (residential, commercial)/ or destinations (shops/services/jobs)	+++	+++	+++	+
Residential or population density (population per unit area)	+	+++	+	+
Street connectivity (density of connections, intersections per area, etc.)	+	+	+	+-
Walkability	+++	+++	+++	+-
Transit proximity/access	+	+++	+	o
Parks (access/density/proximity)	+	+++	+	+
Recreation facilities (access/density/ proximity)	+++	+++	+	+
Low traffic speed/volume	+	+++	+-	o
Walking / biking facilities (sidewalks, bike lanes, trails)	+	+++	+	+-
Pedestrian safety structures (crosswalks, traffic lights)	+-	+++	o	o
Safety (from neighborhood disorder or crime)	+-	+++	o	+
Aesthetics (variety/diversity/ vegetation)	+-	+-	+-	+
Pedestrian amenities (benches, toilets, lighting)	o	o	o	o

28 Source: Modified and updated from Health and Places Initiative. 2014. Physical Activity, Health, and Place. A Research Brief. Version 1.0. http://research.gsd.harvard.edu/hapi/.

29 This is inclusive of both physical activity for transportation or recreation. For the purposes of this study I don't distinguish between the two since the goal is simply to promote physical activity generally. Physical activity in most studies refers to walking, however, cycling and other recreation (jogging, playing etc.) were included in some articles—especially for children.

Figure 16 (Opposite page, Left) Overall diagram of recommended characteristics

Key Strategies for All Ages

The following table summarizes the strength of connection between neighborhood characteristics and physical activity (either for transportation or recreation), by age. The three strategies found most consistently to promote physical activity across all age groups were land use mix (or destinations), overall walkability, and access to recreational facilities.

Built environment characteristics to promote physical activity (recreational or transportation)[29] across all years, and comparing year-groups with each other based on evidence presented in Table 4.

Essential:

- Land-use mix/ residential proximity to walkable destinations (e.g. distance from home to school, parks, stores)
- Overall walkability (may be a perceived or objective composite score)
- Access to recreation facilities (e.g. such as a neighborhood or school play area, gym, pool, or recreational equipment)

Highly Recommended:

- Parks (access/ proximity)
- Residential or population density (e.g. dwelling unit/acre, population/ unit area—more likely to be close to neighbors, destinations or services)
- Walking/biking infrastructure (e.g. sidewalks, bike lanes, trails)
- Street connectivity (which prioritizes pedestrians and cyclists over cars)
- Transit proximity/access
- Low traffic speed/volume (e.g. less than 30mph or 48kph)

Good-to-do:

- Safety from neighborhood disorder or crime (e.g. might be perceptions of safety or an objective measure such as violent crime rates)
- Pedestrian safety infrastructure (e.g. controlled intersections , crosswalks, etc.)
- Aesthetics (e.g. street trees, landscaping, green roofs, green walls)
- Pedestrian amenities (benches, toilets, lighting)

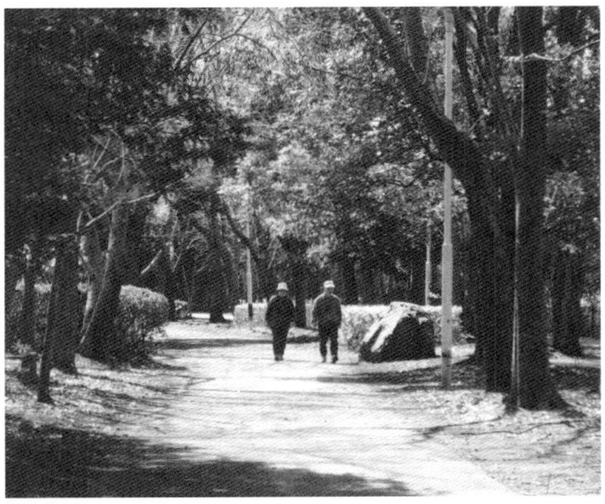

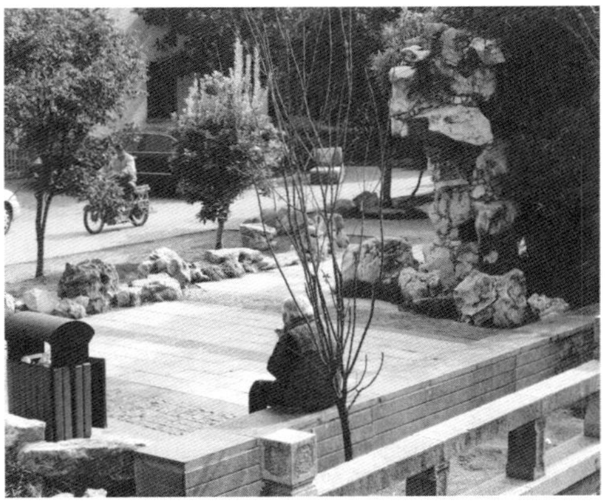

Figures 17-18 (Above) Street tree canopies can provide cooling and urban comfort, while benches can provide places to rest for children and older adults.

What We Don't Know: Research Limitations

Planning and design can make a difference, but we should be modest about how big a difference

Planning and urban design can generate opportunities for physical activity for all ages by creating a more walkable and accessible environment with plenty of recreational resources and green spaces. However, it is important to keep in mind that there are many determinants of physical activity besides the built environment—and these likely have a greater effect. They include:

- Individual characteristics (psychological, biological, intrapersonal)—demographics and individual characteristics play a large role in physical activity levels, such as mobility impairments, gender, income-level, car-ownership, or confidence.[30] For example, those with low incomes may be more affected by the built environment's effect on recreational physical activity (and have less time for leisure activities), but they are also more likely to be physically active during work or commute than those with higher incomes.[31]
- Interpersonal, national policy, and global determinants—these factors include social support, cultural norms, the larger-scale urban planning and transport sectors, and national physical activity and health policies.[32] For example, the Netherlands is known for its national cycling-friendly norms, policies, and planning interventions which have steadily increased its proportion of the population going to destinations on foot or bicycle (active transportation) over the years.[33]
- Natural environment—factors like topography, climate, and weather further enable or create barriers for physical activity outdoors.[34] For example, hilly landscapes might be a barrier to walking for some, but an opportunity for hiking for others.

These findings emphasize the importance of local context, individual factors, and community factors. There is no "one size fits all" when it comes to promoting physical activity through urban design. *So the key is to provide options for physical activity for diverse types of people, especially those who may have different needs than able-bodied adults—the very young, the elderly, and the mobility impaired.*

30 Abraham et al. 2010; Bauman et al. 2012; Casagrande et al. 2009; Trost et al. 2002; Van Der Horst et al. 2007.

31 Bauman et al. 2011; Lovasi et al. 2009.

32 Bauman et al. 2012, 259; Trost et al. 2002; Van Der Horst et al. 2007.

33 Pucher and Buehler 2008.

34 Bauman et al. 2012, 259.

Directions of correlation and self-selection issues.

Are active people more likely to seek out environments where they can walk or cycle for transportation? Or does the environment cause people to be more active? Does physical activity for transportation lower body-mass-index or are leaner people more likely to do active transportation? While there is growing evidence that environmental factors promote (or inhibit) physical activity, research in this area is still very limited and inconsistent in evaluating confounding variables, and therefore unable to clearly determine causality and direction of association.[35] Additionally, most studies are cross-sectional (conducted at one point in time), which cannot show before and after effects which the built environmental changes (e.g. changes in physical activity after a new trail is added, for example). The link to obesity is even weaker.[36] For example, there is growing evidence that urban sprawl may not significantly effect obesity for disadvantaged groups. Rather, other factors like the food environment, places to exercise, or neighborhood safety are more important.[37]

35 Wanner et al. 2012, 499, Yang et al. 2010, 7.

36 Faulkner et al. 2009, 3; Sallis and Glanz 2006.

37 Lovasi et al. 2009, 7, 15; McCormick and Shiell 2011, 8.

What comes next?

Children were more likely to have "high" degree of connection between the built environment and physical activity, while older adults have the least and most uncertain degree of connection. While this may be due to the smaller number and more qualitative studies for these age groups, it is worth looking into in future research. It could also be that strategies to promote physical activity in the built environment for children are actually more effective than other age groups. Fortunately, this is an area where research has been growing rapidly. Unfortunately, much of it comes from only a few countries—the U.S. and Australia being prominent—though recently there has been more international work in a variety of environments.

Comprehensive approaches to promote physical activity address more than just places alone—they deal with people, policies and place together. Health et al.'s (2012) systematic review evaluated the usefulness of recent (2000-2011) evidence-based interventions in physical activity. They "recommended environmental and policy approaches [to] include creation and improvement of access to places for physical activity with informational outreach activities, community-scale and street-scale urban design and land use, active transport policy and practices, and community-wide policies and planning. Thus, many approaches lead to acceptable increases in physical activity among people of various ages, and from different social groups, countries, and communities."[38] Therefore, to affect behavior in the greatest way, urban designers must partner with other private and public groups to do many different kinds of interventions, all in the same direction.

38 Heath et al. 2012, 272

Figure Credits

Figures 1-8, 10-14, 17, 18, Smead, Laura 2014, photographs. In possession of: The author: Smead.

References

Abraham, Andrea; Sommerhalder, Kathrin; and Abel, Thomas 2010, 'Landscape and well-being: a scoping study on the health-promoting impact of outdoor environments,' *International Journal of Public Health 55*, pp. 59–69.

American Planning Association 2011, 'Policy Guide on Planning and Climate Change,' *American Planning Association*. https://www.planning.org/policy/guides/pdf/climatechange.pdf.

Barton, Jo and Pretty, Jules 2010, 'What is the Best Dose of Nature and Green Exercise for Improving Mental Health? A Multi-Study Analysis,' *Environmental Science and Technology 44(10)*, pp. 3947–55. doi: 10.1021/es903183r.

Bauman, Adrian; Guansheng Ma; Cuevas, Frances; Omar, Zainal; Waqanivalu, Temo; Phongsavan, Philayrath; Keke, Kieren; Bhushan, Anjana; for the Equity and Non-communicable Disease Risk Factors Project Collaborative Group. 2011, 'Cross-national comparisons of socioeconomic differences in the prevalence of leisure-time and occupational physical activity, and active commuting in six Asia-Pacific countries,' *Journal of Epidemiology and Community Health 65*, pp. 35–43.

Bauman, Adrian E; Reis, Rodrigo S; Sallis, James F; Wells, Jonathan C; Loos, Ruth JF; and Martin, Brian W 2012, 'Correlates of physical activity: why are some people physically active and others not?' *Lancet 380*, pp. 258–271.

Bjornstrom, Eileen ES and Ralston, Margaret L 2014, 'Neighborhood built environment, perceived danger, and perceived social cohesion,' *Environment and Behavior* 46(6), pp. 718–744.

Bowler, Diana E; Buyung-Ali, Lisette; Knight, Teri M and Pullin, Andrew S 2010, 'Urban Greening to Cool Towns and Cities: A Systematic Review of the Empirical Evidence,' *Landscape and Urban Planning* 97, pp. 147– 155. Accessed November 16, 2013. doi:10.1016/j.landurbplan.2010.05.006.

Bowler, Diana E; Buyung-Ali, Lisette; Knight, Teri M and Pullin, Andrew S 2010, "A systematic review of evidence for the added benefits to health of exposure to natural environments", *BMC Public Health* 10(1), p. 456.

Casagrande, Sarah Stark; Whitt-Glover, Melicia C; Lancaster, Kristie J; Odoms-Young, Angela M; Gary, Tiffany L 2009, 'Built Environment and Health Behaviors among African Americans: A Systematic Review", *American Journal of Preventative Medicine* 36(2), pp. 174–181.

Coon, J. Thompson; Boddy, K; Stein, K; Whear, R; Barton,J and Depledge, MH 2011, 'Does Participating in Physical Activity in Outdoor Natural Environments Have a Greater Effect on Physical and Mental Wellbeing than Physical Activity Indoors? A Systematic Review,' *Environmental Science and Technology* 45, pp. 1761-1772. Accessed February 20, 2014. doi:10.1021/es102947t.

Centers for Disease Control and Prevention 2009a, 'Physical Inactivity and People with Disabilities,' *CDC*, Atlanta, GA. http://www.cdc.gov/ncbddd/documents/ physical-inactivity-tip-sheet-_phpa_1.pdf.

Cunningham, Grazia O. and Michael, Yvonne L 2004, 'Concepts guiding the study of the impact of the built environment on physical activity for older adults: a review of the literature,' *American Journal of Health Promotion* 18(6), pp. 435-443.

Davison, Kirsten K and Lawson, Catherine T 2006, 'Do attributes in the physical environment influence children's physical activity? A review of the literature,' *International Journal of Behavioral Nutrition and Physical Activity* 3(1), pp. 19.

de Nazelle, Audrey; Nieuwenhuijsen, Mark J; Antó, Josep M; Brauer, Michael; Briggs, David; Braun-Fahrlander, Charlotte; Cavill, Nick et al. 2011, 'Improving health through policies that promote active travel: A review of evidence to support integrated health impact assessment,' *Environment International* 37(4), pp. 766–77.

Ding, Ding; Sallis, James F; Kerr, Jacqueline; Lee, Suzanna and Rosenberg, Dori 2011, 'Neighborhood Environment and Physical Activity Among Youth: A Review,' *American Journal of Preventative Medicine* 41(4), pp. 442–455.

Duncan, Mitch J; Spence, John C and Mummery, W Kerry 2005, 'Perceived environment and physical activity: a meta-analysis of selected environmental characteristics,' *International Journal of Behavioral Nutrition and Physical Activity* 2, pp. 11.

Durand, CP; Andalib, M; Dunton, GF; Wolch, J and Pentz, MA 2011, 'A systematic review of built environment factors related to physical activity and obesity risk: implications for smart growth urban planning,' *Obesity Reviews* 12, pp. 173–182.

Ewing, Reid, and Cervero, Robert 2010, 'Travel and the built environment: a meta-analysis,' *Journal of the American Planning Association* 76(3), pp. 265–294.

Faulkner, Guy EJ; Buliung, Ron N; Flora, Parminder K and Fusco, Caroline 2009, 'Active school transport, physical activity levels and body weight of children and youth: A systematic review,' *Preventive Medicine* 48, pp. 3–8.

Forsyth, Ann and Krizek, Kevin 2010, 'Promoting walking and bicycling: assessing the evidence to assist planners,' *Built Environment* 36(4), pp. 429–446.

Fraser, Simon DS and Lock, Karen 2010, 'Cycling for transport and public health: a systematic review of the effect of the environment on cycling,' *European Journal of Public Health* 21(6), pp. 738–743.

French, Sara; Wood, Lisa; Foster, Sarah Alexandra; Giles-Corti, Billie; Frank, Lawrence and Learnihan, Vincent 2014, 'Sense of community and its association with the neighborhood built environment,' *Environment and Behavior* xx(x), pp. 1–21.

Frost, Stephanie S, Turner Goins, R; Hunter, Rebecca H; Hooker, Steven P; Bryant, Lucinda L; Kruger, Judy and Pluto, Delores 2010, 'Effects of the Built Environment on Physical Activity of Adults Living in Rural Settings,' *American Journal of Health Promotion* 24(4), pp. 267–283.

Giles-Corti, Billie; Kelty, Sally F; Zubrick, Stephen R and Villanueva, Karen P 2009, "Encouraging walking for transport and physical activity in children and adolescents. How important is the built environment?' *Sports Medicine* 39(12), pp. 995-1009.

Health and Places Initiative 2014, Physical Activity, Health, and Place. A Research Brief. Version 1.0. http://research.gsd. harvard.edu/hapi/.

Heath, Gregory W; Parra, Diana C; Sarmiento, Olga L; Bo Anderson, Lars; Owen, Neville; Goenka, Shifalika; Montes, Felipe; Rownson, Ross C for the Lancet Physical Activity Series Working Group 2012, 'Evidence-based intervention in physical activity: lessons from around the world,' *Lancet 380*, pp.272–281.

Humpel, Nancy; Owen, Neville and Leslie, Eva 2002, 'Environmental factors associated with adults' participation in physical activity: a review. *American Journal of Preventative Medicine* 22(3), pp. 188-199.

Krizek, Kevin; Forsyth, Ann and Baum, Laura 2009, 'Walking and Cycling International Literature Review,' Melbourne: Department of Transport Walking and Cycling Branch.

Lee, ACK and Maheswaran, R 2010, 'The Health Benefits of Urban Green Space: A Review of the Evidence,' *Journal of Public Health* 33(2), pp. 212–222. Accessed February 21, 2014. doi, pp. 10.1093/pubmed/ fdq068.

Lovasi, Gina S; Hutson, Malo A; Guerra, Monica and Neckerman, Kathryn M 2009, 'Built Environments and Obesity in Disadvantaged Populations,' *Epidemiologic Reviews* 31, pp.7–20.

Maller, C; Townsend, M; Pryor, A; Brown, P and St. Leger, L 2005, 'Healthy nature healthy people: Contact with nature as an upstream health promotion intervention for populations,' *Health Promotion International* 21(1), pp. 45–54.

McCormack, Gavin R and Shiell, Alan 2011, 'In search of causality: a systematic review of the relationship between the built environment and physical activity among adults,' *International Journal of Behavioral Nutrition and Physical Activity* 8, pp. 125.

McGrath, Leslie J; Hopkins, Wil G and Hinckson, Erica A 2015, 'Associations of Objectively Measured Built-Environment Attributes with Youth Moderate–Vigorous Physical Activity: A Systematic Review and Meta-Analysis,' *Sports Medicine*, pp. 1-25.

Moran, Mika; Van Cauwenberg, Jelle; Hercky-Linnewiel, Rachel; Cerin, Ester; Deforche, Benedicte and Plaut, Pnina 2014, 'Understanding the relationships between the physical environment and physical activity in older adults: a systematic review of qualitative studies,' *International Journal of Behavioral Nutrition and Physical Activity* 11, pp. 79.

Owen, Neville; Humpel, Nancy; Leslie, Eva; Bauman, Adrian and Sallis, James F 2004, 'Understanding environmental influences on walking. Review and research agenda,' *American Journal of Preventive Medicine* 27(1), pp. 67-76.

Petticrew, Mark and Roberts, Helen 2008, *Systematic reviews in the social sciences: A practical guide.* John Wiley & Sons.

Pucher, John and Buehler, Ralph 2008, 'Making cycling irresistible: lessons from the Netherlands, Denmark and Germany,' *Transport Reviews* 28(4), pp. 495-528.

Rosso, Andrea L; Auchincloss, Amy H and Michael, Yvonne L 2011, 'The urban built environment and mobility in older adults: A comprehensive review,' *Journal of Aging Research* 1, pp. 1–10.

Saelens, Brian E and Handy, Susan L 2008, 'Built environment correlates of walking: a review,' *Medicine & Science in Sports & Exercise* 40, no. 7 Suppl, pp. S550.

Saelens, Brian E; Sallis, James F and Frank, Lawrence D 2003, 'Environmental Correlates of Walking and Cycling: Findings from the Transportation, Urban Design, and Planning Literatures,' *Annals of Behavioral Medicine* 25(2), pp. 80–91.

Sallis, James F and Glanz, Karen 2006, 'The role of built environments in physical activity, eating, and obesity in childhood,' *The Future of Children* 16(1), pp. 89-108.

Sallis, James F; Bowles, Heather R; Bauman, Adrian; Ainsworth, Barbara E; Bull, Fiona C; Craig, Cora L; Sjöströmm Michael et al. 2009, 'Neighborhood environments and physical activity among adults in 11 countries,' *American Journal of Preventive Medicine* 36(6), pp. 484-490.

Skiba, Isabella and Zuger, Rahel 2009, *Barrier-Free Planning*, Birkhauser, Basel.

Sugiyama, Takemi; Neuhaus, Maike; Cole, Rachel; Giles-Corti, Billie and Owen, Neville 2012, 'Destination and route attributes associated with adults' walking: a review,' *Medicine & Science in Sports & Exercise* 44 (7) (07), pp. 1275–86.

Timiras, Paola S 2007, *Physiological Basis of Aging and Geriatrics, Fourth Edition*, Informa Healthcare USA, Inc., New York, New York.

Trost, Stewart G; Owen, Neville; Bauman, Adrian E; Sallis, James F and Brown, Wendy 2002, 'Correlates of adults' participation in physical activity: review and update,' *Medicine & Science in Sports & Exercise.*

Uman, Lindsay S 2011, 'Systematic reviews and meta-analyses,' *Journal of the Canadian Academy of Child and Adolescent Psychiatry* 20(1), pp. 57.

van Cauwenberg, Jelle; De Bourdeaudhuij, Ilse; De Meester, Femke; Van Dyck, Delfien; Salmon, Jo; Clarys, Peter and Deforche, Benedicte 2011, 'Relationship between the physical environment and physical activity in older adults: a systematic review,' *Health & Place* 17(2), pp. 458–469.

Van der Horst, Klazine; Paw, MJ C A; Twisk, Jos WR and Van Mechelen, Willem 2007, 'A brief review on correlates of physical activity and sedentariness in youth,' *Medicine & Science in Sports & Exercise* 39(8), pp. 1241.

van Holle, Veerle; Deforche, Benedicte; Van Cauwenberg, Jelle; Goubert, Liesbet; Maes, Lea; Van de Weghe, Nico and De Bourdeaudhuij, Ilse 2012, 'Relationship between the physical environment and different domains of physical activity in European adults: a systematic review,' *BMC Public Health* 12(1), pp. 807.

van Stralen, Maartje M; De Vries, Hein; Mudde, Aart N; Bolman, Catherine and Lechner, Lilian 2009, 'Determinants of initiation and maintenance of physical activity among older adults: a literature review,' *Health Psychology Review* 3(2), pp. 147-207.

Wanner, Miriam; Götschi, Thomas; Martin-Diener, Eva; Kahlmeier, Sonja and Martin, Brian W 2012, 'Active transport, physical activity, and body weight in adults: a systematic review,' *American Journal of Preventive Medicine* 42(5), pp. 493–502.

Wendel-Vos, W; Droomers, M; Kremers, S; Brug, J and van Lenthe, F 2007, 'Potential environmental determinants of physical activity in adults: a systematic review,' *Obesity Reviews* 8, pp. 425–440.

World Health Organization (WHO) 2007. 'Global Age-Friendly Cities: A Guide,' *World Health Organization*, Geneva, Switzerland. http://whqlibdoc.who.int/publications/2007/9789241547307eng.pdf?ua=1.

World Health Organization 2014, 'Physical activity,' Fact sheet No 385. Geneva, Switzerland: World Health Organization. http://www.who.int/mediacentre/ factsheets/fs385/en/. Accessed June 25, 2014.

Wood, Lisa, Tya Shannon, Max Bulsara, Terri Pikora, Gavin McCormack, and Billie Giles-Corti. 2008, 'The anatomy of the safe and social suburb: An exploratory study of the built environment, social capital and residents' perceptions of safety,' *Health and Place* 4, pp. 15–31.

World Health Organization (2010) Global Recommendations on Physical Activity for Health

Yang, Lin, Shannon Sahlqvist, Alison McMinn, Simon J. Griffin, and David Ogilvie. 2010, 'Interventions to promote cycling: systematic review,' *BMJ, pp. British Medical Journal* 341.

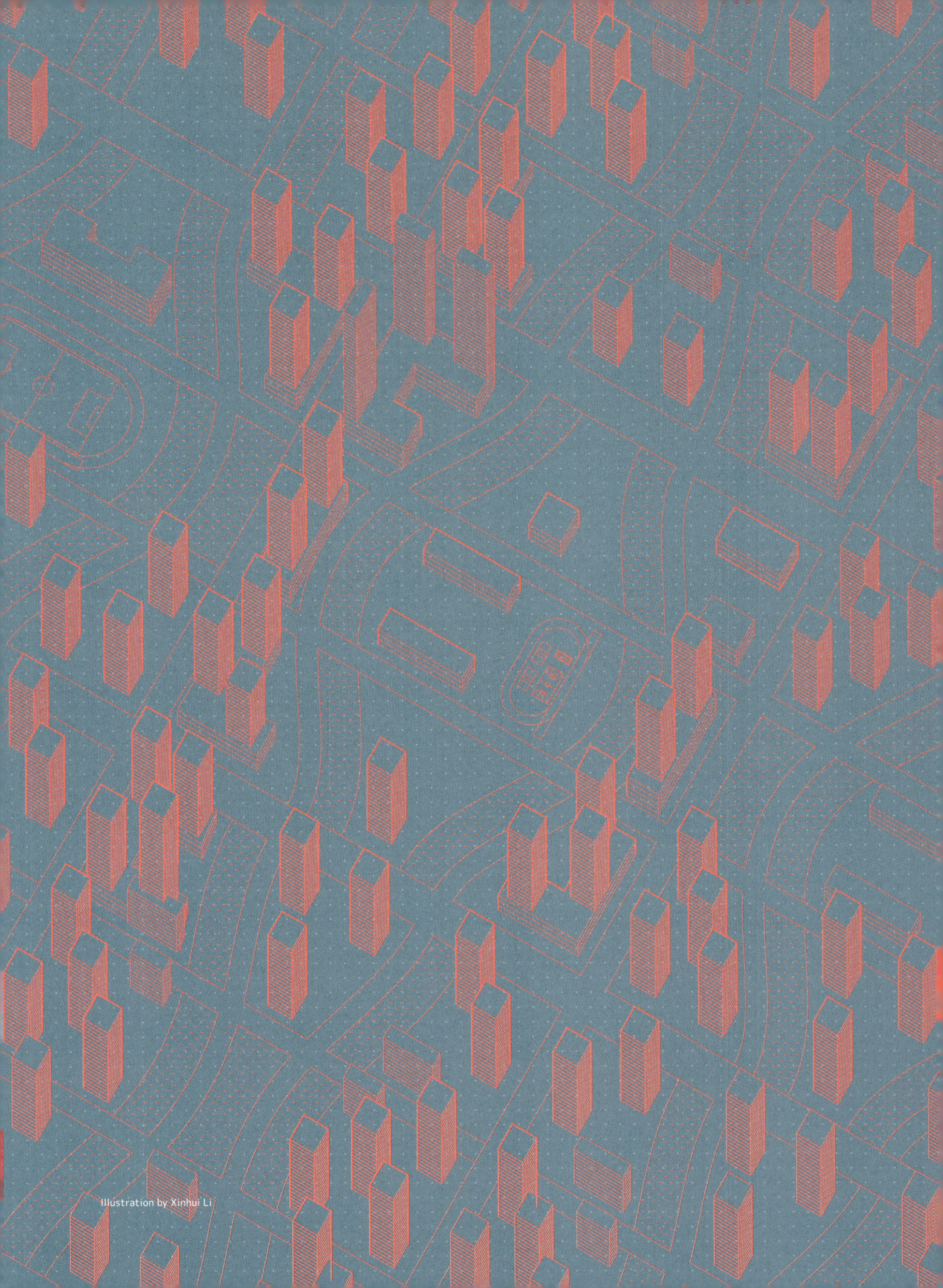

Illustration by Xinhui Li

The Chinese Superblock

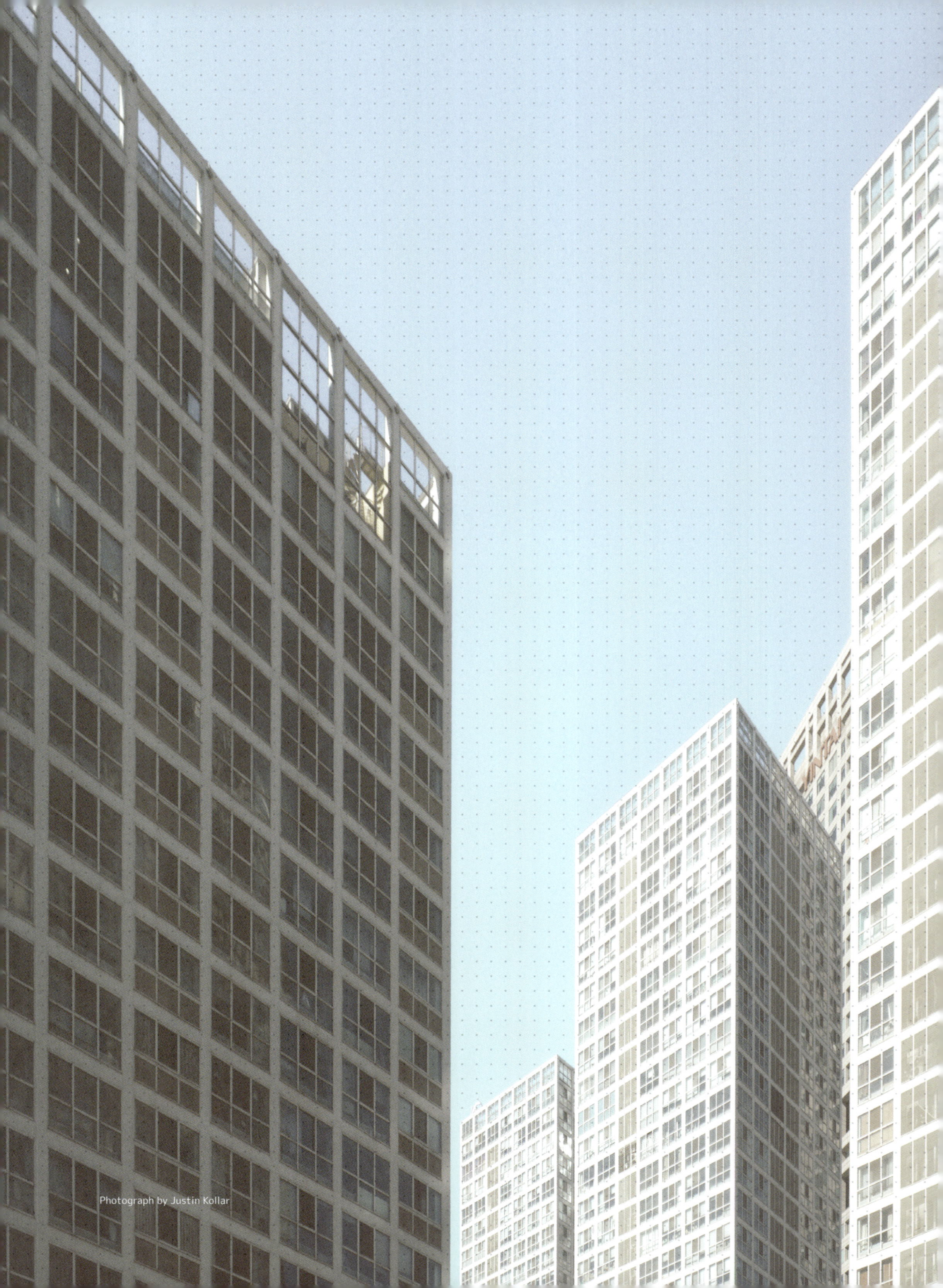

Photograph by Justin Kollar

Chapter 3

China's Modernist Superblocks

Peter G. Rowe + Har Ye Kan

Peter G. Rowe is the Raymond Garbe Professor of Architecture and Urban Design and a Harvard University Distinguished Service Professor at Harvard University where he has taught since 1985 and served as Dean of the Graduate School of Design between 1992 and 2004. He is an author or editor of numerous books, several of which deal with housing, including *Making a Middle Landscape, Modernity and Housing,* and *Modern Housing in China, 1840-2000.*

Har Ye Kan has been a Research Associate and Post-Doctoral Fellow at the Graduate School of Design, Harvard University, where she recently completed her doctoral degree. The author of several articles and book chapters dealing primarily with Chinese urbanism, she also served as an instructor with Peter Rowe in a graduate seminar on housing.

A defining feature of China's urban landscape is its modernist superblocks. Spreading out in a carpet-like fashion across the built-up fabric, these superblocks or megaplots typically occupy sites of some six hectares and above, and are bounded by wide arterial roads. They are commonly used as the basic configuration to structure Chinese neighborhoods with each block composed of a mixture of walk-up slabs and/or high-rise towers, supported by amenities such as community and retail services. Prosaic as they may seem, these large tracts have arguably been held as the standard template for urban expansion and adopted across most cities writ large since the beginning of the communist era. At the outset, under the *danwei* or 'work-unit' system, a rather full array of production facilities and community services were incorporated, before the privations of the Great Leap Forward and Cultural Revolution set about reducing the scope of building projects. Then again, in more contemporary projects, there have been noticeable shifts towards incorporating a greater diversity of programs and land uses once again, as well as attempts to resolve some of the problems arising from this mode of development. What follows is an analysis of how and why superblocks emerged as the prototype for urbanization in modern China, an evaluation of their efficacy, and commentary on recent design evolutions that seek to chart new pathways forward for their redevelopment.

Early Urban Blocks

The superblock, as defined by Alan Colquhoun, refers to a large tract of real estate which is financed and organized as a single entity.[1] The form of the superblock could be determined by the existing street pattern or it could be composed by a cluster of buildings or a single megastructure spanning an area across one or more adjacent blocks. More importantly, a superblock is distinguished by its 'total design' where it is generally conceived of as a whole. Blocks have been used for the organization of cities, including those in China, reaching far back into the early imperial times. The construction

1 Colquhoun 1981, 83-103. Also see Sarah Whiting, "The Invisible Superblock" in SOM, accessed September 30, 2013, https://www.som.com/publication/invisible-superblock.

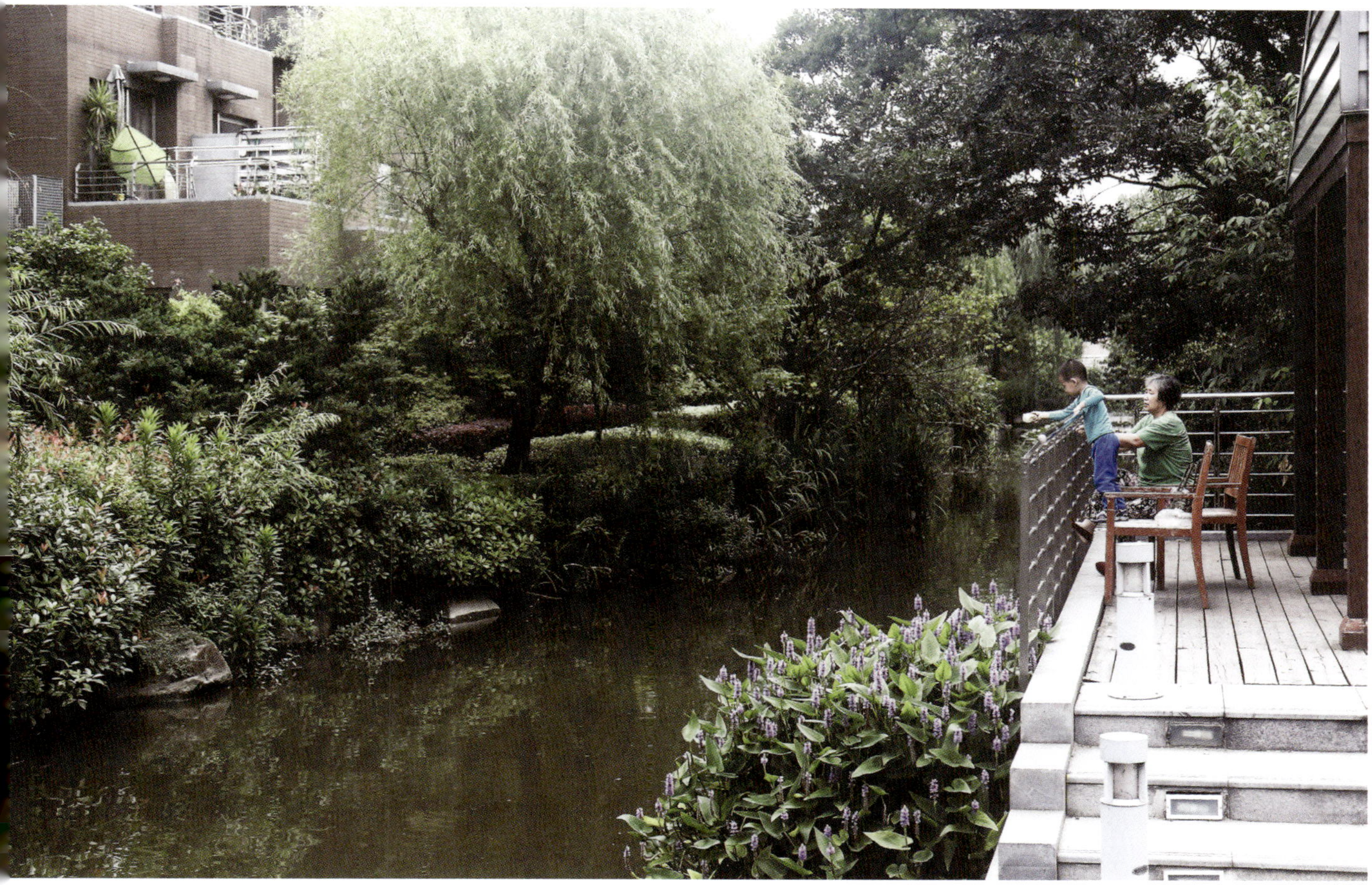

Figure 1 (Above) Inside Langrun Gardens by Vanke.

manual *Kaogongji (Record of Trades)* from the Book of *Zhou Li (Rites of Zhou)* compiled during the Spring and Autumn Period (771 to 476 B.C.) described the canonical form of the state capitals. In this idealized plan, the square-shaped cities measure nine *li* on side, with three gates on each side. Within the walled settlement are nine meridional and nine latitudinal streets, thereby giving rise to the grid iron pattern subdividing the city into blocks. Of the many Chinese capitals from the various eras, Chang'an from the Tang Dynasty is most renowned for its checkerboard block configuration. The street layout was formed by fourteen latitudinal and eleven longitudinal streets which divided the city into approximately 130 blocks, some of which were set aside for commercial, administrative, and religious purposes. 108 of these blocks were developed into walled residential wards of various sizes, ranging from roughly the equivalent of 27.5 hectares to 94.3 hectares in area.[2] Apart from other East Asian capitals such as Kyoto and Nara that were modeled after Chang'an, the imperial capitals from the Song, Yuan, and Qing dynasties adhered as much as possible to the gridded block pattern and the creation of residential wards.[3] In essence, Chinese cities have long maintained the practice of organizing residential spaces into walled, large-sized blocks.

While the block has long been a basic unit used in Chinese cities since the pre-modern era, the superblock is a modernist invention. The earliest adoption of the term refers to the German word *Siedlung* which largely refers to a human settlement and acquired a particular meaning in Vienna under the rule of the Austrian Socialist Party. Between 1919 and 1934, nearly a

2 The dimensions of the smallest wards in Chang'an ranged between 500–590 meters by 550-700 meters while the dimensions of the largest wards ranged between 660-838 meters by 1,020-1,125 meters.
See China Baike, "Sui Daxing Tang Chang'an Cheng Yizhi (Sui Daxing & Tang Chang'an Historic City Ruins)," accessed August 17, 2015, http://www.chinabaike.com/article/1/78/434/2007/20070520113556_2.html .

3 Steinhardt 1990.

dozen superblocks or the "people's palaces" were constructed as part of the goal to establish a Red Vienna. Combining housing units and communal facilities such as laundries, bathhouses, meeting rooms, cooperative stores, kindergartens, playgrounds, and clinics, these superblocks were meant to create new living environments that would socialize the workers and their families.[4] Around the same time, Le Corbusier's influential *Ville Radieuse* called for a "true geometrical lay-out" in which prefabricated towers in a park would be spread across a grid in large blocks, thereby allowing the city to function as a "living machine." Each tower or *Unité* would fully integrate similar sorts of amenities as in a Red Vienna superblock, thereby fostering a self-sustaining community.[5]

4 Levinson and Christensen 2003, 1241-1246.

5 Fishman 1977, 226-234.

Communist Clusters

A superblock concept that had the most profound impact on Chinese planning was the *mikrorayon* or microdistrict proposed by the 'urbanists' school in the Soviet Union during the 1930s under Stalin. Comprising planners and architects who argued for the creation of a compact socialist city or the Sotsgorod, the *mikrorayon* was based on four-sided *kvartal* blocks consisting of a cluster of four- to six-storey blocks of flats arranged around a quadrangle.[6] In fact, town planning in accordance to these four-sided *kvartal* blocks was elaborated by the 1935 Moscow Plan.[7] Each *kvartal* blocks had an average area of 6 hectares, enclosed by roads and built with facades facing the streets. As constituents of a *zhilkompleks* or a living region, the *kvartal* was to be supported by a crèche, kindergarten, club, and cafeteria; in comparison, the broader *zhikompleks* was to encompass shops, post offices, primary medical points, a savings bank, hairdresser, repair shops, sports facilities, and some internal open space with gardens and lawns.[8] This particular strategy was favored by Nikolai Kuzmin and the Vesnin brothers who sought to realize urban superblocks integrating communal housing and amenities in their plans. Aleksandr and Leonid Vesnin, for instance, drafted a plan for Novokuznetsk in 1930 that featured three residential districts with communal superblocks that had amenities connected to residential buildings by enclosed walkways.[9] While the *kvartal* became the predominant mode of urban organization or literal building block during the five-year-plans in the Soviet Union before the Second World War, they were often without the communal facilities originally intended to support the neighborhood. Hence, with the exception of the numerous *kvartaly* and a handful of experimental micro-districts that were constructed, most of the *zhikompleks* remained on the drawing board.

6 French 1995, 37.

7 Bater 1980, 27-30.

8 French 1995, 63 (cited from Novikov et al. 1934, 23).

9 Craft and Rowland 2003, 142-143.

In the late 1950s after the death of Stalin, the *zhikompleks* was revisited by Strumilin, and was recast as the *mikrorayon* or micro-district to serve as the basic unit of residential development.[10] The necessary daily or weekly services would be dispersed on the ground-floor levels of the apartment blocks. Ideologically, the *mikrorayon* exemplified the ideal communist residential neighborhood that lauded the family as the building block of a stable socialist society. In addition, the *mikrorayon* gained further currency with the introduction of large panel construction methods of building. The prefabricated units within the superblocks were intended to become completely integrated neighborhoods supported by social and commercial services that were readily accessible on foot to all residents. These blocks

10 French 1995, 81.

were envisioned to be a relatively self-sustaining, microcosmic, and amenable urban area where residents would live, work, and be educated in an environment that was protected from the grime and congestion of the industrial city outside. Planning and construction agencies in the Soviet Union embraced the superblocks because they could be easily built with industrialized housing and were compelling as exhibition models and mock-ups.[11] Known as *khruschevki*, the pre-fabricated residential buildings were typically five-storeys with separate one-, two- or three-room apartments with reduced ceiling heights between 2.2 and 2.5 meters. The *khrushchevki* and the *mikrorayon* were built quickly with minimum expenses to address the housing crisis after the Second World War, often resulting in similar-looking districts throughout the Soviet Union.[12]

With the founding of the People's Republic of China in 1949 following the Chinese Civil War, a growing housing shortage, particularly in cities, prompted an evaluation of the design of housing and planning. One of the earliest constructions of a planned residential district which began in 1951 was Caoyang Xincun (曹杨新村). Directly inspired by the Anglo-American neighborhood unit, the scheme was designed by Wang Dingzeng, who graduated from the University of Illinois at Urbana-Champaign. The residential area occupied a total area of 94.63 hectares with in which public buildings were erected in the center. Housing here was assigned by the work unit or the *danwei* on a meritocratic basis.[13] From 1951 to 1958, new residential districts based on the structure of the modified neighborhood unit were constructed in several parts of Shanghai, such as the East Shanghai Workers' Residential District (沪东工人住宅区). These new villages comprised several neighborhood clusters (街坊群), which are in turn constituted by a group of neighborhoods (街坊) or superblocks. The defining feature of this urban configuration was the use of arterial streets to enclose the neighborhood clusters, thereby forming an independent residential sub-district equipped with the services and amenities for daily living. Each self-contained neighborhood cluster was to occupy an area ranging from 50 to 100 square kilometers, and was intended to support a population of 30,000 to 40,000 persons. Free from any through traffic, the neighborhood cluster was to be furnished with a cultural and commercial center, located at the center of the site and with a service radius of 500 to 600 meters from the nearest public transportation stops.[14]

11 Ruble 1999, 269. See also Ruble 1993, 232-269.

12 Vihavainen 2009. See also Natalia Lebina, "Zhil'e: Kommunizm v otdel'noi kvartire" in Natalia Lebina and Aleksandr Christikov (eds.), Obyvatel'l reformy. Kartiny povsednevnoi zhizni gorozhan (Sankt-Peterburg: Neva/Letnii sad, 2003).

13 In February 1951 before construction began for Caoyang Xincun, the *danwei* was formalized by the central government as the basic tenet of social, economic, and urban organization. The *danwei* was not only the specific place of employment in which all workers were identified, but was also responsible for providing safety, welfare, health care, culture, education, and financial support to the workers. Each *danwei* thus constructed its own housing, child care, schools, clinics, shops, and services, governing the everyday life of the individual, and more importantly, became the means in which centrally determined policies and strategies were implemented. By 1957, a most 90% of the urban workforce belonged to either a state-owned or a collective-owned *danwei*.

14 Wang and Chen 1964, 8-9

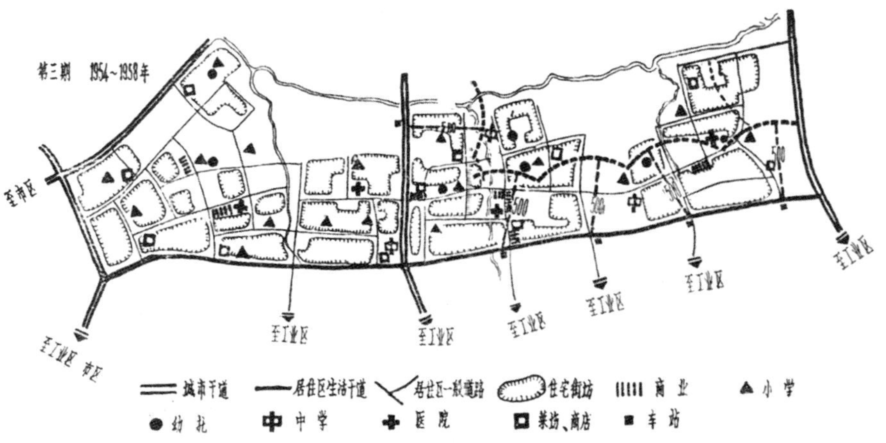

Figure 2 Site Plan of the East Shanghai workers' residential district showing the neighborhood clusters (Architecture Journal, 1964 Vol. 2, p. 9).

Although the planning of Caoyang was regarded as a success as it integrated the entire project within its surroundings, it was subsequently criticised for ideological reasons, following the introduction of the Soviet Union's ideas about residential area planning.[15] This is not surprising as assistance from Soviet architects and planners was significant during China's First Five-Year Plan from 1953 to 1958. In 1955, a group of Chinese architects led by Yang Tingbao (1901 – 1982), attended the 4th Congress of the International Union of Architects at The Hague.[16] Upon their return, they published a report in the 1955 edition of the 建筑学报(*Architectural Journal*), where Yang Tingbao highlighted the distinctions between the capitalist neighborhood units (邻里单位) and socialist *zhilkompleks* or "big neighborhoods" (大街坊) that were essentially superblocks.[17] According to Yang, the capitalist neighborhood unit referred to an area bounded by streets with major buildings situated in the neighborhood center. Commercial services and shops are typically clustered as a distinct complex, while secondary and low-rise residential buildings are located along the surrounding streets but are sometimes turned inwards. In comparison, the socialist *zhilkompleks* locate the major, large-scale buildings along the roads to shape the streetscape. Some social service amenities and green open space are situated within the *zhilkompleks*, and commercial shops are generally found at the ground-level of residential buildings facing the streets. In his perspective, the key divergence between the two typologies was the more holistic approach adopted by the socialist *zhilkompleks* as this was conceptualized as an integral component of the city whilst the relation between the capitalist neighborhood unit and the city remained unaddressed.[18]

15 Lu et al. 2001, 124.

16 Yang 1955, 69-82.

17 Ibid, 74.

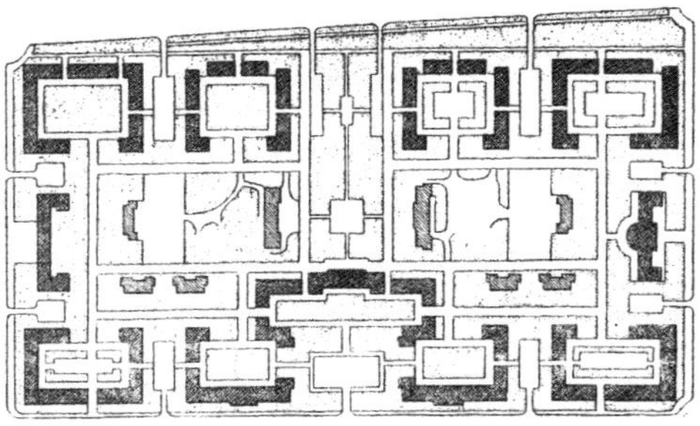

Figure 3 (Above) Typical Soviet Kvartal cited in Yang Tingbao's report.

18 Ibid, 74.

The growing friendship and political alliance between China and the Soviet Union led to the rapid promotion of socialist principles of design and planning, with the former closely following the trends of the latter. As such, the transformation of the *zhilkompleks* into the *mikrorayon* in 1956 correspondingly redefined the Chinese neighborhood cluster (街坊群) and residential area (居住区) into the micro-district (小区). This change was first formally introduced via a translation of M. Teweiersikeyi's article on "Housing, Neighborhood and Micro-district"(住宅街坊小区) in the journal *Urban Construction* "*城市建设译丛*" in 1956 and was quickly incorporated into the preliminary masterplan for Beijing in 1957.[19] As in the case of the neighborhood clusters in the pre-1958 hierarchy, the micro-districts were similarly encircled by arterial streets and constituted by several basic living units (基本生活单元) or residential clusters (住宅组) occupying superblocks. Unlike the neighborhood cluster scheme where the commercial and cultural services were congregated largely within a stand-alone complex, those in the post-1958 typology were combined with multi-storey residential buildings and occupied the ground floor of these blocks. Such an arrangement was first tested out in Minhang New Village in Shanghai (闵行新村) in 1958, with the objective of minimizing space requirements, improving the accessibility of these services and convenience extended to the residents, as well as enhancing the streetscape through the activity generated by these roadside shops.[20] Additionally, these shops either continually flanked one side of the street or were dispersed at two ends of each block. Not only was this layout notable for its adaptation of the

19 The micro-district was to replace the smaller "residential complex" of the 1953 plan, and to serve as the basic unit of residential districts, housing 10,000 to 20,000 persons within a 30 to 60 hectare site. This allowed the "small district" to be supplied with primary and secondary schools, kindergartens, shops, and other public services. (Sit 1985, 96-97).

20 Li and Xu 1964, 30-33.

traditional shophouse arrangement within these modern residential districts, but also for its resonance with the Soviet way of dispersing the amenities at the ground-floor of the residential blocks.[21]

21 Zhengzhou Engineering Institute Civil Engineering Department in 建筑学报 *(Architectural Journal)* 1973, 13-17.

More importantly, an article by Wang Shuoke published in the *Architecture Journal* in 1962 on "Planning and Design Explorations of Residential Districts" illustrated how the superblock was a basic unit in the planning and design of residential districts. Using examples in Shanghai, he highlighted how each neighborhood occupied and was organized as a superblock or a basic living unit. As shown in Figure 4, the enclosed superblocks were composed typically of parallel slabs, open space, a nursery, residents' dining hall, and some stores. Aggregates of these cellular units would then yield a neighborhood, or a microdistrict, and multiples of these would, in turn, form a residential district. As part of a nested hierarchy, the basic living unit in the form of a superblock became the foundation for urban development in communist China. Indeed, this popular spatial configuration was transplanted to various parts of China, including Zhengzhou, Wuhan, Changsha, Xiangtan and Guangzhou, and utilized in the construction of housing for work units and municipalities.[22]

22 Ibid, 13-17 & 43.

Post-Reform Templates

Although the superblock persisted through the depths of the Cultural Revolution even when architectural and urban planning practices were suspended, housing quality in general declined considerably. The official standards on living space issued by the Ministry of Building Industry was limited to no larger than four square meters per person and no larger than eighteen square meters per family by the late 1960s. It was only towards the end of the Cultural Revolution in 1973 that the State Construction Commission issued "Proposals for Revising the Building Standards of Apartments and Dormitories," stipulating that the floor space per family was to be 34-37 square meters and 36-38 square meters in extremely cold areas, and that multi-storey buildings should be the predominant type built for dormitories. Besides efforts to improve the living space per person, the post-reform era beginning around 1978 also saw the gradual dismantling of the *danwei* and shifts towards increasing densities as well as the commodification of housing. During this time, residential district development, however, continued to draw upon the housing typology, superblock arrangement, and inclusion of community services from the pre-reform era. Earlier on, in Shanghai, for instance, high-rise apartments ranging between 11 and 16 storeys were built beginning from 1972, arranged in parallel blocks. Notable projects there included the North Caoxi Road High-rises, Kangle Towers, and Huasheng Towers. Later, one of the earliest post-reform residential districts constructed was the Quyang Xincun residential district built on a 77.7 hectare-site in Hongkou District to house approximately 7,000 to 8,000 residents. Subdivided into six neighborhoods, the residential district was also equipped with a cultural-commercial center, a library, a large-scale department store, a book store, a sports stadium, a 200-bed government hospital, and other community service amenities.[23] Other major large-scale superblock developments in Shanghai during the 1980s and 90s included the 89-hectare Weifang Housing Estate in Pudong and the 137-hectare Gubei New District in Changning.

23 Shanghai Gazetteer, Hongkou District Gazetteer, "Quyang Xincun," accessed August 4, 2015, http://www.shtong.gov.cn/node2/node4/node2249/node4418/node20208/node21558/node62884/userobject1ai9095.html.

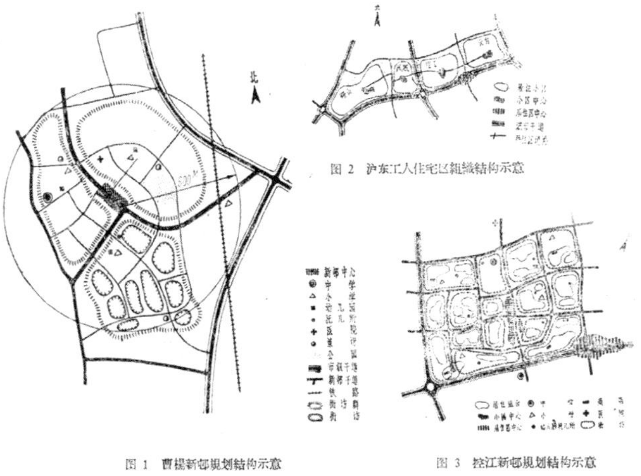

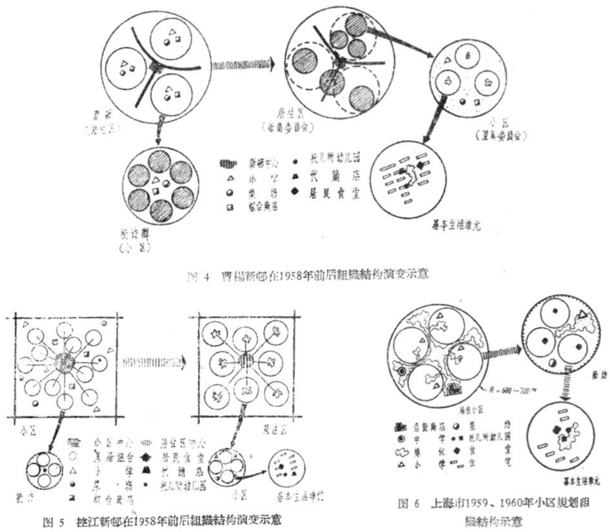

Figure 4 (Top, Left) Diagrammatic representation of the superblock forms of the neighborhood clusters and microdistricts in Caoyang Xincun, the East Shanghai Workers' residential districts, and the Kongjiang Xincun.

Figure 5 (Top, RIght) Diagrammatic nested hierarchy of the basic living unit within the microdistricts in Caoyang Xincun, the East Shanghai Workers' residential districts, and the Kongjiang Xincun.

Indeed, across the first two decades of the post-reform era, residential districts, or estates, have continued to be built within large-block configurations, incorporating ancillary levels of mixed use, and enclosed by broad and coarse-grained road networks. Regardless of the city that the residential districts were built in or the type of housing program that they were developed under, they all share the above similarities. Whether it is more up-scale market-rate, *anju* or 'comfortable housing' projects that are commercially built subsidized affordable housing, or 'economic and suitable housing' in the mega-residential districts on the urban periphery, the superblock has remained as the preferred mode of development. This is due in large part to the economies of scale reaped by having sizeable blocks of self-sustaining residential estates in the detailed control plans that can then be auctioned off to public or private property developers to realize as a whole. From an urban design perspective, China's superblocks reflect sustained adherence to modernist urban-architectural features, including the segregation of vehicular and pedestrian flows, mono-functional buildings that are separated from one another, and supposed efficiencies arising from the 'slabs in a park' configuration. Coincident with this widespread replication of enclave-like residential estates occupying large tracts of land is the emergence of the notion of a *shequ*—a community or collective. Intended to provide community services and to foster solidarity, the *shequ* was promulgated by the Ministry of Civil Affairs to fill the gaps in social and welfare provision with the waning of the *danwei* or work unit. Vanke, China's largest residential real estate developer, also exemplifies this social vision by seeking to create 'communities of happiness' based on a model of "security, participation, symbiotic relationships, and trust." To date, they have completed 405 of these communities, spanning from the conventional superblock mid- and high-rises to cultural villages.[24]

The constant rote application of this superblock template for much of urban residential construction in contemporary and emerging circumstances begs the question of whether this recipe is indeed appropriate or even all that effective. Since the economic reforms of 1978, much of the emphasis on housing has been placed on relatively basic provision of dwellings, infrastructural access, and community services. As income levels and living

24 Vanke Group, "Housing & Three Qualities That Make It Good," accessed August 4, 2015, http://www.vanke.com/en/service.aspx?type=26.

standards have improved over the past two decades with the country's ascendance as a global economic powerhouse, residential expectations have risen and diversified. Furthermore, against a backdrop of calls for greater environmental protection and remediation, as well as more compact development, this resource-consumptive mode of urban growth and accretion clearly entails larger ecological footprints. This is not to discount the fact that these residential enclaves offer serene, well-vegetated, pleasant living environs. Beyond the compounds, however, the coarse-grained network of megaplots and roads have not been able to keep up with the increasing private automobile ownership.[25] Traffic congestion has worsened in the past decade and pedestrian and bicycle circulation have been compromised due to the fuzziness in the intermediate rights of way.[26] Apart from associated environmental and social costs, wind analyses of China's predominantly north-south oriented superblocks show that the wide borders comprising roads or even canals tend to create wind tunnels and uncomfortable walking conditions, particularly during the winters.[27]

Another issue presented by the structure of superblocks is how their design as a 'whole,' limits the degree to which dynamic processes of local-level despecialization of use and other transformations can occur. The over-determined, functionally separated modernist approach to 'total design' constrains the possibility of allowing blocks to be restructured, retrofitted, and adapted to the changing needs and times of urban societies. In comparison, the finer-grained networks of blocks and streets in cities such as New York and Barcelona have facilitated the continual transformations and population growth of these places. While blocks in China measure some 400 meters by 300 meters on average, surrounded by streets around 30 to 50 meters, those in the Manhattan grid measure some 244 meters by 61 meters, separated by streets 18-meters in width, and avenues of only some 30-plus meters. In the Barcelona *Ensanché* grid, the blocks with chamfered corners, admitting light and air, are 113 meters by 113 meters, separated by roads of widths ranging between 20 and 30 meters. The blocks in Manhattan and Barcelona have also accommodated a mixture of uses from the outset, often within and across individual buildings in the same block. Scales of uses within each block can vary considerably, ranging from a modest corner convenience store on the ground level to high-rise commercial or institutional establishments occupying the entire block. In addition, some of the original buildings such as mid-rise industrial factories and apartments have been retrofitted, evolving successfully into private lofts, offices, boutique stores, and galleries in Manhattan's SoHo district. By contrast, the current Chinese practice where the land use, site coverage, floor area ratios, building heights, setbacks, green-space provision, parking requirements, service provisions, and road layouts are specified in the detailed control plans remains relatively inflexible, hindering potential despecialization of the blocks over time towards greater functional diversification. Encouraging appropriate levels of diversification with regard to land use, programs, and employment types would, in turn, also aid in curtailing excessively high levels of inter-district travel and traffic congestion, as evidenced by large-scale residential districts such as Huilongguan and Tiantongyuan north of Beijing that are further away from employment nodes in the city center.

25 Calthorpe, Peter 2012 August 13 'Weapons of Mass Urban Destruction,' Foreign Policy, accessed August 4, 2015, http://foreignpolicy.com/2012/08/13/weapons-of-mass-urban-destruction/.

26 "China's Soviet-Style Suburbia Heralds Environmental Pain," Bloomberg Business, November 7, 2013, accessed August 4, 2015, http://www.bloomberg.com/news/articles/2013-11-06/china-s-soviet-style-suburbia-heralds-environmental-pain . Also see Chris Busch, "Superblocks: Why China Must Embrace Mass Transit (Op-Ed)," LiveScience, June 7, 2013, accessed August 4, 2015, http://www.livescience.com/37293-chinese-superblock-streets.html.

27 Simulation of the wind conditions was conducted for some 25 neighborhoods in the cities of Beijing, Shanghai, Suzhou and Shenzhen as part of the Health and Places Initiative research project at the Graduate School of Design (2014-2015).

Figure 6 (Below) Photo of Huilongguan.

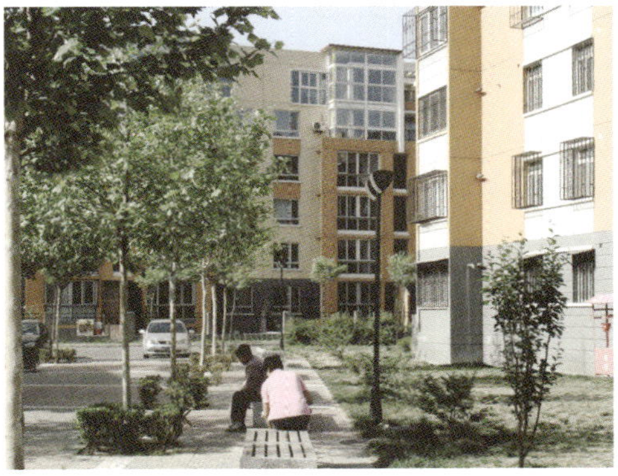

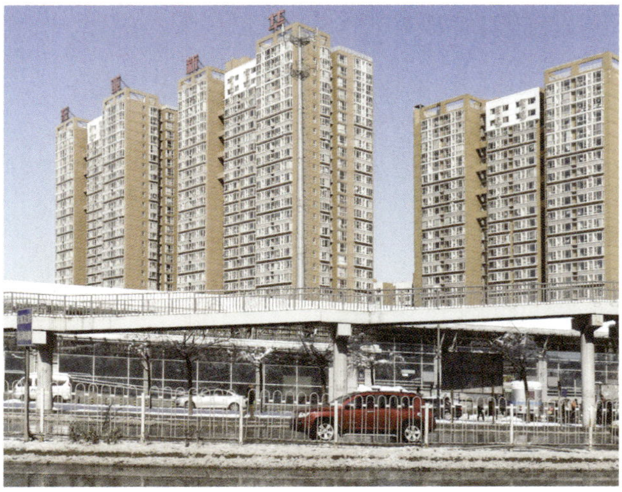

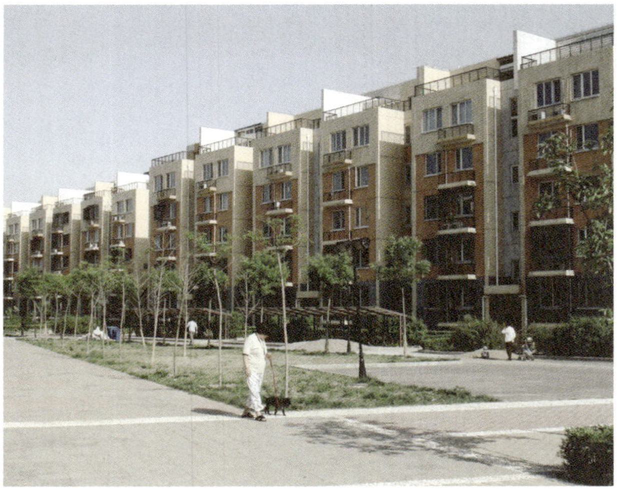

Figure 7 (Above, Left) Photo of Tiantongyuan.

Figure 8 (Above, Right) Photo of Huilongguan.

Opportunities & Recent Design Evolutions

Shortcomings of the superblock template have been recently acknowledged by some policy makers who have re-oriented urban planning towards more compact forms of development and improving diversity in urban environments.[28] At the same time, the large size and coverage of China's superblocks offer opportunities for design interventions that can enhance the estates' environmental performances, live-work circumstances, and infrastructural access. Vanke's Langrun Gardens, for instance, was developed to be the "first, green ecological residential district" in China. Occupying a 9.6-hectare site, the project incorporated a rainwater collection and recycling system into the neighborhood's themed landscape areas. Other environmental and ecological features include green roofs, vertical greening elements, the use of solar power and natural gas, double-glazed and high solar gain and low-E glass windows, as well as having a high green space coverage of 40%.[29] In this case and in many other ecological residential estates that were developed thereafter, the 'total design' nature of the superblocks lends itself well to undertaking interventions that would enhance the sustainability of these communities. Attempts at introducing a finer-grain of road and transit network with smaller blocks of mixed use activities have also been initiated by a collaboration between Calthorpe Associates, The China Sustainable Energy Program, and the ClimateWorks Foundation. The aim is to create active, vibrant urban communities that will be more sustainable, resilient, and energy efficient by designing these around the pedestrian, bicyclists, and transit. These ideas are currently being tested out in the planning and construction of Chenggong New Town in Kunming, and in Yuelai Eco-City in Chongqing.[30]

A project that effectively redeveloped what was originally a *danwei* superblock configuration is Jian Wai SOHO in central Beijing. The 34-hectare superblock was subdivided into nine smaller parcels by re-introducing a denser network of roads, effectively reducing the size of a typical block to around 300 meters by 200 meters. Within this expansive site, the entire Jian Wai SOHO development took up just 16.9 hectares spread across four and a half parcels.[31] The uses in each block were also varied to incorporate conventional office and retail spaces, as well as different types of home-office apartments which offered a higher degree of programmatic adaptability. To enhance the spatial

28 Qiu 2007.

29 Li Ju, "Shanghai Vanke Langrun Gardens, Vanke City Gardens Case Studies," accessed August 4, 2015, http://wenku.baidu.com/view/44bdc66b1eb91a37f0115c02.html.

30 "Low Carbon Cities: Principles and Practices for China's Next Generation of Growth," accessed August 4, 2015, http://www.calthorpe.com/files/China%20Design%20Manual%20Pamphlet.pdf.

31 "Jian Wai SOHO," SOHO China, accessed October 20, 2013, http://jianwaisoho.sohochina.com/en.

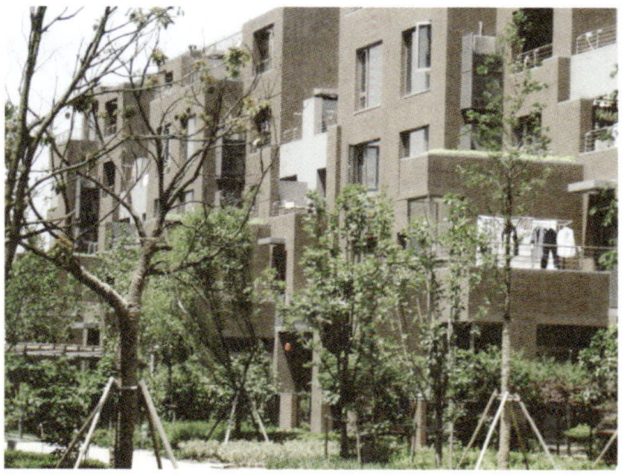

Figure 9 (Above) Photo of Vanke's Langrun Gardens.

32 Enlazado 2008, 226-241.

experience, the architect Riken Yamamoto explored what might be termed a 'field operation' to 'thicken' the ground plane. In the first few phases of the project, the checkerboard layout of nine slender towers and the four low-rise villas were combined with a plinth of underground parking and common living spaces together with a horizontal ground plane above for public open space. Sunken courtyards marked the common living spaces, crisscrossed by pedestrian pathways allowing residents and visitors to explore different aspects of the place in a maze-like manner.

Another contemporary project of note is Steven Holl's Linked Hybrid located in the northeast corner of Beijing beyond the Second Ring Road. Here, the focus was on introducing greater porosity to challenge the enclave-like condition of most superblock housing estates in China. To create a connected "city of spaces," passages lined with shops and public functions on the ground floor were designed to be open to be street.[32] Within the site, seven individual buildings were joined together by a C-shaped loop comprising a multitude of amenities servicing the residents, including a pool, a gym, cafes and stores, galleries, lounges, and viewing decks. In six out of the seven buildings, residential space was combined with commercial, recreational, and sometimes educational uses. Besides the effort to foster greater interactions with the broader urban fabric, the Linked Hybrid also installed some 600 geothermal wells under the reflecting pool encircled by the buildings to provide cooling in the summer and heating in the winter. Such a feature clearly leveraged the superblock's nature and the size of the site to be able to put in place such a large-scale system. In Shanghai, similar strategies of opening the estate to through pedestrian traffic and creating an artificial lake in the middle of an urban block to enhance the environmental amenity were used by the Canadian firm, B + H Architects, in their design for Top of the City I, a multi-tower residential development with podiums for retail and commercial space.

Figure 10 (Below) Jian Wai SOHO by Riken Yamamoto. Small open plaza with adjacent offices and residential complexes.

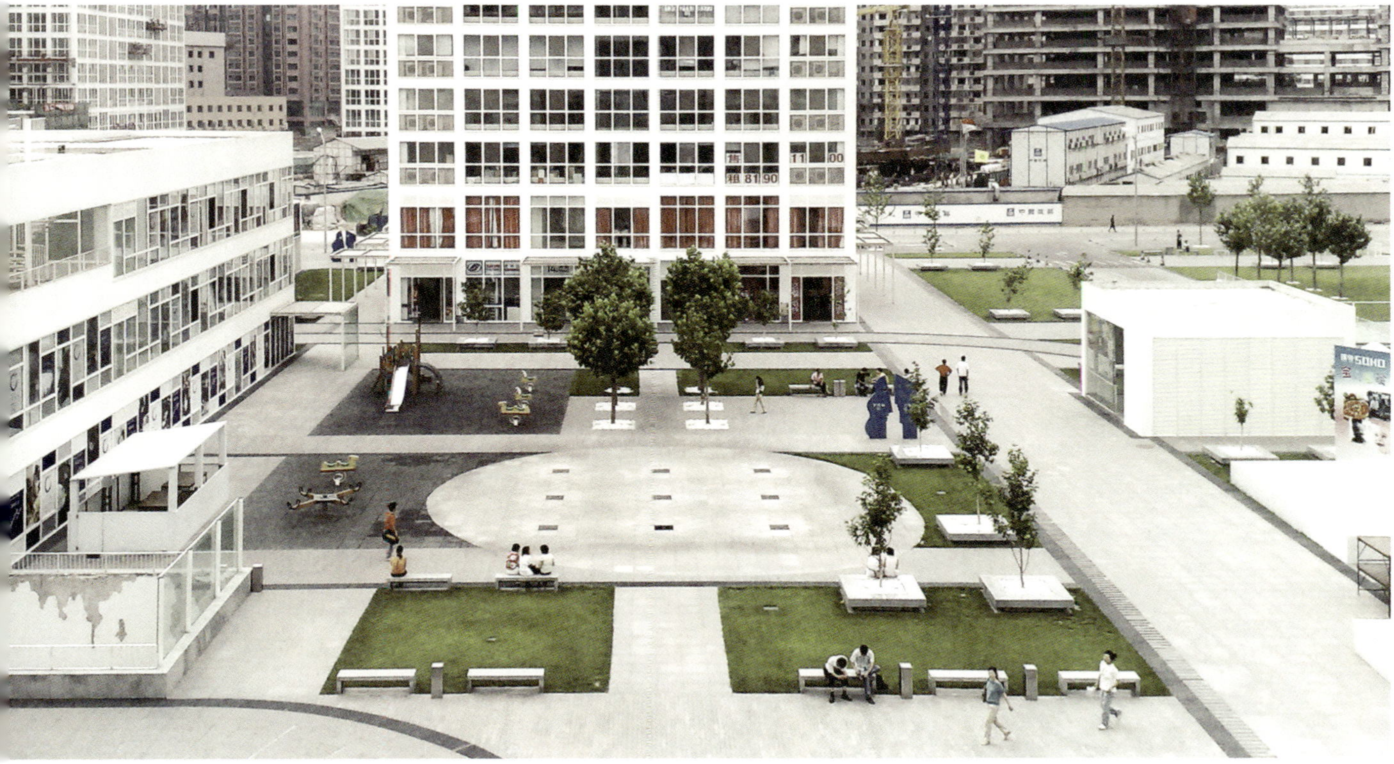

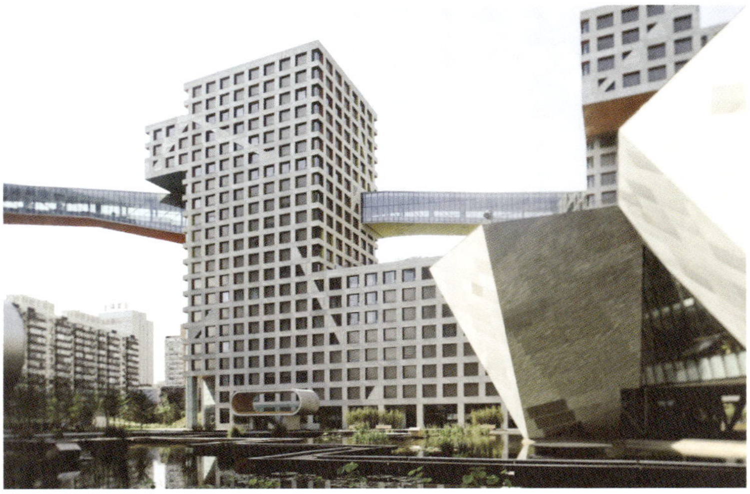

Figure 11 (Left) Photograph of linked hybrid by Steven Holl.

In conclusion, the gated 'slabs or towers in a park' style modernist superblock surrounded by wide thoroughfares has long been the template of urban development across China. While there have been tendencies towards the use of large block and wide grids even in imperial times, it was only since the Communist era under the initial Soviet influence that the superblock was applied extensively. The convenience of the 'total design' and the serene, typically tree-lined, and secured enclaves afforded by such a mode of development is to be recognized. However, as discussed, the modernist superblock also has its share of limitations, as well as the opportunities provided by these functional limitations. To be able to pursue the laudable goals of compactness and greater functional diversity in addition to improvements in environmental performance, there is a need to give pause for thought to current planning and design practices. Clearly, the first step would be to move away from overly-determined megaplot zoning in the master plans and detailed control plans to more refined, flexible reformulations at an urban district-, or block-level. For new developments, and for areas slated for redevelopment, this should entail proposing plans with smaller blocks and a denser network of streets and transit. Buildings within each block could also be designed to accommodate a variety of uses and programs in ways that can be repartitioned and remodeled over time. For existing blocks, there are opportunities for in-situ installation of public access networks, and the incorporation of environmental features such as water harvesting and renewable energy production systems, along with retrofitting of the buildings. Recent endeavors by foreign planners and architects in collaboration with Chinese developers have demonstrated alternatives to the superblock status quo and possibilities to harness environmental benefits by leveraging the scale of the block itself. The challenge is not insurmountable, and with sufficient will and receptiveness to change, China's cities and neighborhoods can be more human-scaled, diverse, and resilient.

Figure Credits

Figure 1, Rowe, Peter 2015, *Inside Langrun Gardens*, photo. In possession of: The author: Rowe.

Figure 2, *Site Plan of the East Shanghai Workers' Residential District*, Architecture Journal, 1964 Vol. 2. p. 9.

Figure 3, Tingbao, Yang, *Typical Soviet Kvartal*, Architecture Journal, 1955 Vol. 2, p. 75.

Figure 4, *Superblock Forms of the Neighborhood Clusters and Microdistricts in Caoyang Xincun, the East Shanghai Workers' Residential districts, and the Kongjiang Xincun*, Architecture Journal, 1962 Vol. 1, pp. 8-9.

Figure 5, *Nested Hierarchy of the Basic Living Unit, Caoyang Xincun, the East Shanghai Workers' Residential districts, and the Kongjiang Xincun*, Architecture Journal, 1962 Vol. 1, pp. 8-9.

Figure 6, Rowe, Peter 2015, *Huilongguan 1*, photo. In possession of: The author: Rowe.

Figure 7, Rowe, Peter 2015, *Tiantongyuan*, photo. In possession of: The author: Rowe.

Figure 8, Rowe, Peter 2015, *Huilongguan 2*, photo. In possession of: The author: Rowe.

Figure 9, Rowe, Peter 2015, *Langrun Gardens*, photo. In possession of: The author: Rowe.

Figure 10, Wiechers, S 2007, Jian Wai SOHO by Riken Yamamoto, photograph, Accessed 4 August 2015, https://www.flickr.com/photos/whoisstan/587837261/in/photostream/. Creative Commons Attribution-ShareAlike 2.0 Generic license; Desaturated.

Figure 11, Deutscher, R 2013, MOMA_Beijing - internal courtyard view, photograph, Accessed 4 August 2015, https://www.flickr.com/photos/bobarc/11448450033/in/photostream/. Creative Commons Attribution 2.0 Generic license; Desaturated.

References

Bater, James H. 1980, *The Soviet City: Ideal and Reality.* Hodder Arnold, p.27-30.

Busch, Chris 2013, 'Superblocks: Why China Must Embrace Mass Transit (Op-Ed),' *LiveScience*, 7 June. Accessed 4 August 2015, http://www.livescience.com/37293-chinese-superblock-streets.html.

Calthorpe Associates, *Low Carbon Cities: Principles and Practices for China's Next Generation of Growth.* Accessed 4 August 2015, http://www.calthorpe.com/files/China%20Design%20Manual%20Pamphlet.pdf.

Calthorpe, Peter 2012, 'Weapons of Mass Urban Destruction,' *Foreign Policy*, 13 August. Accessed 4 August 2015, http://foreignpolicy.com/2012/08/13/weapons-of-mass-urban-destruction/.

China Baike, 'Sui Daxing Tang Chang'an Cheng Yizhi (Sui Daxing & Tang Chang'an Historic City Ruins),' Accessed 4 August 2015, http://www.chinabaike.com/article/1/78/434/2007/20070520113556_2.html.

Colquhoun, Alan 1981, *Essays in Architectural Criticism: Modern Architecture and Historical Change*, MIT Press, Cambridge, MA, pp. 83-103.

Craft, James and Rowland, Daniel Bruce 2003, *Architectures of Russian Identity: 1500 to the Present*, Cornell University Press, Ithaca, pp.142-143.

Enlazado, Híbrido 2008, 'Linked Hybrid,' *El Croquis 141*, pp. 226-241.

Fishman, Robert 1977, *Urban Utopias in the Twentieth Century: Ebenezer Howard, Frank Lloyd Wright, and Le Corbusier*, Basic Books, New York, pp. 226-234.

French, R Antony 1995, *Plans, Pragmatism & People: The Legacy of Soviet Planning for Today's Cities*, UCL Press, London, p. 37.

French, R Antony 1995. *Plans, Fragmatism & People: The Legacy of Soviet Planning for Today's Cities*, UCL Press, London p.63, cited from Novikov et al. (1934:23).

French, R Antony 1995, *Plans, Pragmatism & People: The Legacy of Soviet Planning for Today's Cities*, UCL Press, London p. 81.

Lebina, Natalia 2003, 'Zhil'e: Kommunizm v otdel'noi kvartire,' *Obyvatel'I reformy. Kartiny povsednevnoi zhizni gorozhan*, eds Natalia Lebina and Aleksandr Christikov, Neva/Letnii sad, Sankt-Peterburg.

Levinson, David and Christensen, Karen (eds) 2003, 'Siedlung,' *Encyclopedia of Community: From the Village to the Virtual World Volume 2*, Sage Publications, Thousand Oaks, California, pp.1241-1246.

Li Ju, 'Shanghai Vanke Langrun Gardens,' *Vanke City Gardens Case Studies.* Accessed 4 August 2015, http://wenku.baidu.com/view/44bdc66b1eb91a37f0115c02.html

Li Yingzhe and Xu Hanhui 1964, 'Design of Ground-Floor Commercial Shops in Roadside Residential Buildings,' *Architectural Journal* Vol.1, ('沿街住宅的底层商店设计.' 建筑学报), pp. 30-33.

Lü Junhua, Rowe, Peter G. and Zhang Jie (eds) 2001, *Modern Urban Housing in China: 1840-2000*, Prestel, Munich, p. 124.

Panckhurst, Paul (ed) 2013, 'China's Soviet-Style Suburbia Heralds Environmental Pain,' *Bloomberg Business*, 7 November. Accessed 4 August 2015, http://www.bloomberg.com/news/articles/2013-11-06/china-s-soviet-style-suburbia-heralds-environmental-pain.

Qiu Baoxing 2007, *Harmony and Innovation: Problems, Dangers, and Solutions in Dealing with Rapid Urbanisation in China*, L'Arca, Milan.

Ruble, Blair A 1999, 'Housing the Citizens in Soviet Russia, 1955-90: The Tyranny of Technology,' *The European Cities and Technology Reader: Industrial to Post-Industrial City*, ed David C. Goodman, Routledge, London, pp.269.

Ruble, Blair A 1993, 'From Khrushcheby to Korobki,' *Russian Housing in the Modern Age*, eds William Craft Brumfield and Blair A. Ruble, Woodrow Wilson Center Press, New York, pp.232-269.

Shanghai Gazetteer, *Hongkou District Gazetteer*, 'Quyang Xincun.' Accessed 4 August 2015, http://www.shtong.gov.cn/node2/node4/node2249/node4418/node20208/node21558/node62884/userobject1ai9095.html.

Sit, Victor F.S. 1985, *Beijing: The Nature and Planning of a Chinese Capital*, pp. 96-97.

Jian Wai SOHO, SOHO China. Accessed 20 October 2013, http://jianwaisoho.sohochina.com/en.

Steinhardt, Nancy S 1990, *Chinese Imperial City Planning*, University of Hawai'I Press, Honolulu.

Vanke Group, *Housing & Three Qualities That Make It Good.* Accessed 4 August 2015, http://www.vanke.com/en/service.aspx?type=26

Vihavainen, Rosa 2009, *Homeowners' Associations in Russia after the 2005 Housing Reform.* Accessed 4 August 2015, http://www.iut.nu/members/Russia/HomeownerAssociations_Russia_2009.pdf

Wang Hua and Chen Qingzhuang 1964, 'Discussion of Several Issues in the Planning of Residential Districts in Shanghai,' *Architectural Journal* Vol. 2 ('上海居住区规划设计中几个问题的探讨.' 建筑学报), pp. 8-9.

Whiting, Sarah, 'The invisible Superblock,' SOM. Accessed 4 September 2013, https://www.som.com/publication/invisible-superblock

Yang Tingbao 1955, 'Report on the Proceedings of the 4th Congress of the International Union of Architects,' *Architectural Journal*, Vol 2, ('国际建筑师协会第四届大会情况报道.' 建筑学报), pp. 69-82.

Zhengzhou Engineering Institute Civil Engineering Department 1973, 'Investigation of Ground-Floor Commercial Shops in Residential Buildings,' Architectural Journal Vol. 2, ('住宅底层的商店建筑调查.' 建筑学报), pp. 13-17 & 43.

Spatial Foundation of the 'Aging in Place' Community, Shanghai

Yu Yifan

居家养老条件下的居住空间基础研究

——以上海为例

于一凡

Yu Yifan, Ph.D (EHESS, France, 2003), has been a professor at the Urban Planning Department of Tongji University since 1996. She has been a research fellow at the Harvard University Graduate School of Design and at Sorbonne University in Paris. She also serves as Vice President of the Shanghai Urban Planning Association, Deputy Secretary General of the China Real Estate Research Association, and Deputy President of the Sino-francophone Scholars Association (SORSA). Yu's practice and research focus on urban housing and city renovation, and she has published more than forty articles and has authored three books: *Urban Habitation Morphology*, *Urban Design Project* and *Atlas de Shanghai* (with UNESCO).

The community environment and senior service facilities play an important role in senior citizens' later years, both in psychological and physiological terms. It is, therefore, an essential foundation for the elderly who are 'aging in place.' Based on a series of surveys of current senior living conditions and related facilities in Shanghai, we found that the existing residential area's spatial organization is, as a whole, weak. There is also a lack of appropriate policy and technical guidance for new developments to include perspectives from the aging population. This essay concludes that a legislation system urgently needs to be established, and basic research together with targeted initiatives need to be implemented to meet the rapidly growing demands of an aging population in China.

China is the only country in the world that has an elderly population of over 200,000,000, and the elderly lifestyles of the aging population are becoming a significant part of the general social life in the country. As a consequence of the cultural tradition of aging in families, the "4-2-1" transformation of the family structure, and the current phenomenon of "getting old before getting rich" (未富先老), the government strongly promotes an "aging in place" strategy.

From the pilot projects of "aging in place" (居家养老) in Shanghai, Beijing, and Dalian during the early 2000s, to the national 12th five-year plan which lays out the specific measures of improving the living environment and constructing service facilities for seniors, "aging in place" is currently at an important stage of development. However, it is worth considering, what the current condition of the urban environment for "aging in place" is like. Are the spatial qualities of urban residential areas prepared for the transformation from "young populations" to "older populations"? What measures should be taken to prepare urban living environments for "aging in place"? This paper explores the elderly-adaptability of the spatial environment and its associated regulations in Shanghai's residential areas. The data used in this paper is from consecutive surveys on old-age suitability in Shanghai's common residential areas undertaken in 2010, 2011, and 2012 by the research team. The survey areas include nine neighborhoods and communities within the central city of Shanghai, and six new commercial housing and affordable housing residential areas. A total of 1,281 questionnaires were sent out, and 1,175 valid ones were received.

Translated by: Li Xinhui, Yang Han, Justin Kollar
Edited by: David Mah

The Central Universities Fundamental Research Funds for the project (0100219090); (Tongji) China Intelligent Urbanization Co-creation Center for High Density Region project (CIUC20140014)

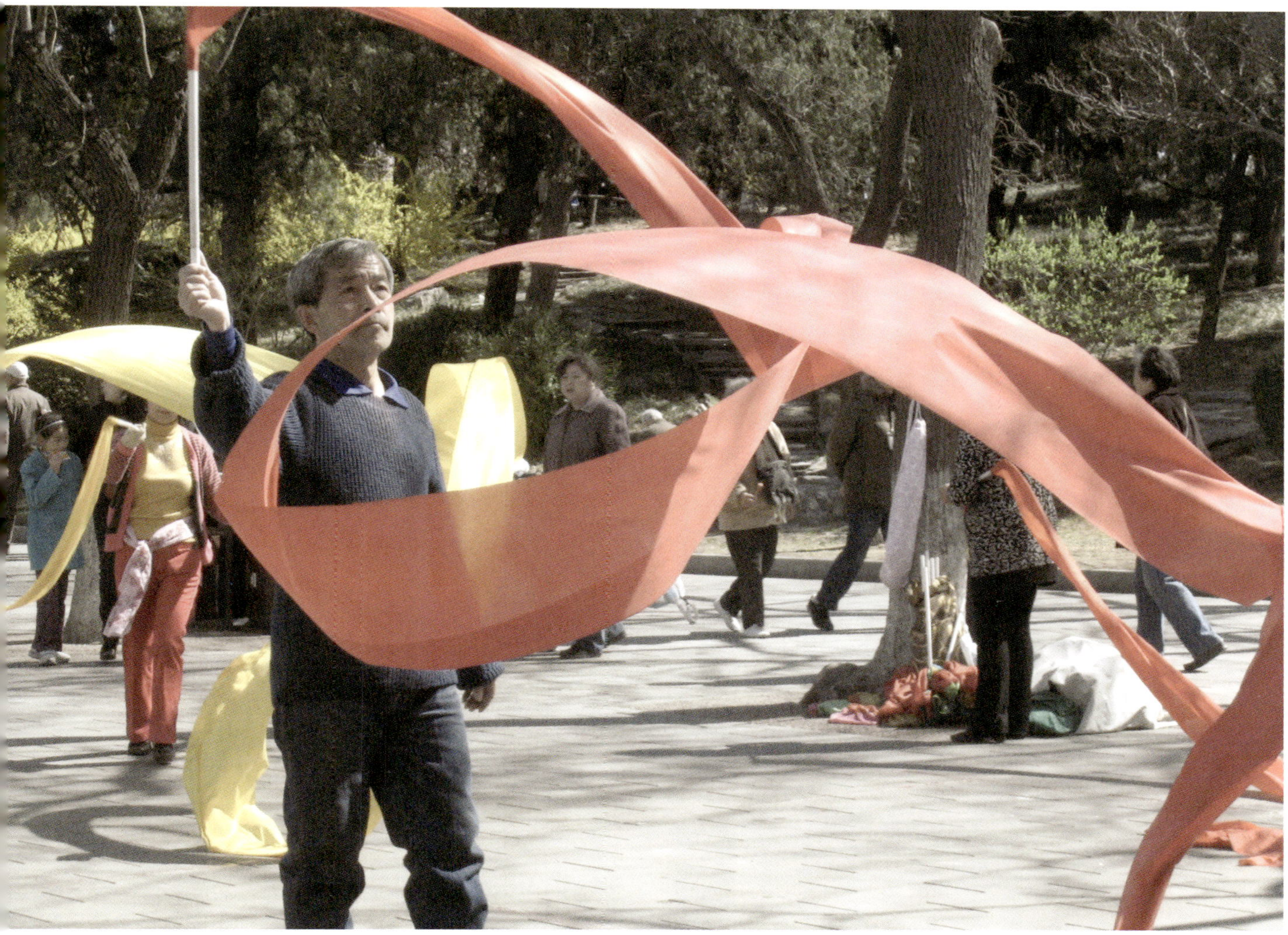

Figure 1 (Above) Many collective activities require the right context and ample space.

Physical Space for "Aging in Place"

Due to the degeneration of bodily functions, the elderly require smaller spaces for activity, but depend more on living spaces and service facilities. As an essential foundation for the "aging in place" strategy, the suitability of physical spaces and service facilities for old age largely determine the elderly's quality of life. The importance of this relationship also increases with age.

The physical space for "aging in place" consists of 3 parts: the interior living environment, the exterior living environment, and senior service facilities. Interior living environments refer to the space in a living unit, including the living room, bedroom, bathroom, kitchen, and balcony. It requires deliberate design and arrangement in terms of floor area, spatial arrangement, programs, circulation, as well as decoration and amenities. Exterior living environments refers to the residential area's outdoor environment, which is the primary space for the elderly's communication with the community and nature. It includes courtyards, gardens, and activity spaces, and requires consideration of spatial arrangement, size, roads and accessibility, outdoor facilities, and so on. Senior service facilities are service places providing assistance, day care, and entertainment for the elderly, and can be categorized according to three categories of functions: daily life care facilities, medical or health care facilities, and social activity as well as mental support facilities. (Figure 2)

Figure 2 Constitution of physical space for "aging in place."

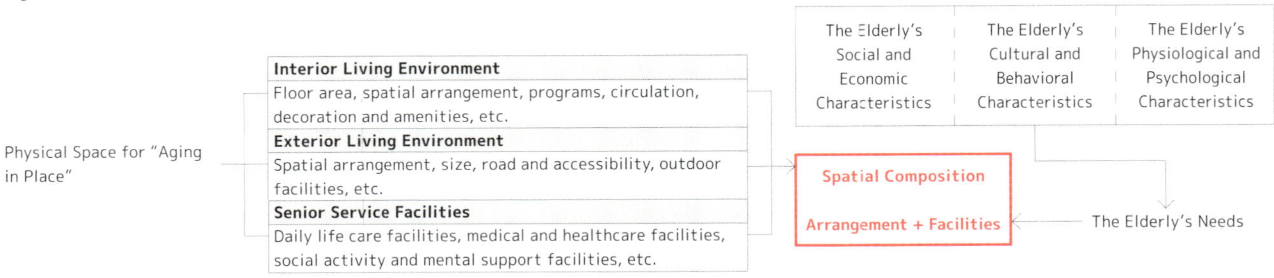

Providing adequate senior service facilities and living conditions that suit the physical and mental characteristics of the elderly is an important basis for both implementing the "aging in place" strategy and developing "spiritual civilization" (精神文明建设) in cities. However, due to the lack of attention to the aging population and design guidelines for the elderly in common living environments, the elderly-adaptability of interior and exterior environments and senior service facilities is generally far behind the rapidly developing needs of "aging in place."

Current Living Conditions

Interior Living Environment

China's aging urban population mostly live in collective housing units. Collective housing generally consists of historic residences, early pre-reform public housing, and new, commercial and affordable housing built since the 1990s. Housing that was built before the 90s generally has a low level of suitability for aging populations, and yet despite this, there is a high percentage of middle aged and elderly occupants. Common problems are small living areas, inadequate functions, and so on, resulting in safety hazards and to some extent inconvenience. In comparison, newly built housing usually has intact functions and improved sanitary conditions. However, these still lack specific design considerations for the elderly. The common problems are small bedroom spaces, narrow spaces in kitchens and bathrooms, absence of necessary handrails, signs for wayfinding, and so on.

In recent years, the emergence of commercial housing for the elderly on the real estate market has started to improve the suitability of housing for the elderly. However, most of them merely copy old age design models from Europe, the US, and Japan. Their systematic implementation and evaluations of suitability remain to be seen, and the lack of a cohesive technical system of standards makes it difficult to manage. Therefore, there are urgent needs for systematic and standardized regulations.

Exterior Living Environment

The suitability of exterior living environments for old age includes activity spaces and facilities, green space coverage, quality and design of water bodies, street environments, amenities, accessible facilities, and spatial qualities of exterior spaces. (Table 1) Due to technical and economic limitations, residential areas built earlier generally are not well adapted to elderly living. They usually

Table 1 Elements suitable for old age in exterior environment.

Elements suitable for old age in exterior environment	Items
Activity spaces and facilities	Public activity space and private activity spaces, exercise spaces, and supporting facilities
Green space coverage and water environment	Public green spaces, green spaces in between buildings, water bodies, and environmental cleanliness
Street environment	Street network, pedestrian network, parking lots
Amenities	Recreational facilities, shading and sheltering facilities, public restrooms, lighting facilities, sculptures, smart facilities and monitoring facilities
Accessible facilities	Signs, flatness and slip-resistance of plaza and paths, accessible ramps, handrails, paving color and material
Physical environment	Wind conditions, acoustic environment, light conditions

have limited space, conflicts in pedestrian and vehicular circulation, low green space coverage, and inadequate public activity spaces and accessible facilities. In comparison, new residential areas built in recent years have significantly improved the overall quality of the environment. However, as a result of insufficient attention to the elderly and the absence of relevant guidelines and regulations, newly built residential areas are not very suitable for aging either; for example, the prevalence of steps at entryways, safety hazards on paths, and alack of accessibly designed pedestrian pathways are very common, while plazas and exercise facilities, built without shading, are more formal than functional.

Summarizing the survey results, the main problems arising in the suitability for old age in different types of residential areas in Shanghai are as follows (1) public spaces and green spaces are not adequately functional or comfortable; (2) there are no adequate small spaces, benches or handrails suitable for the social behavior and habits of the elderly; (3) the safety, convenience, and identity of pedestrian networks needs improving; (4) the outdoor sign system, lighting system, resting and recreational facilities as well as landscape facilities need to be specifically designed for old-age; (5) physical

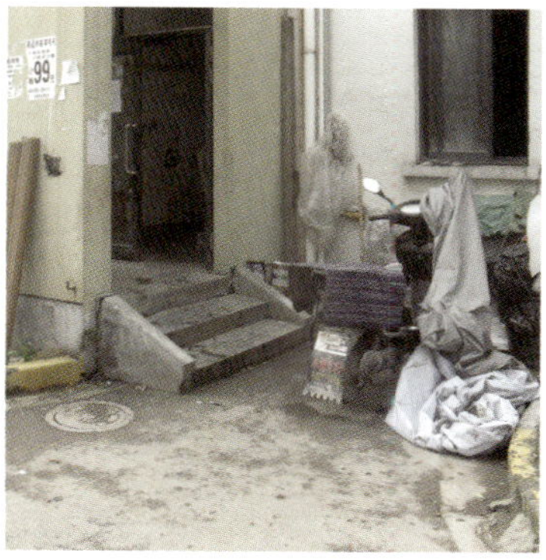

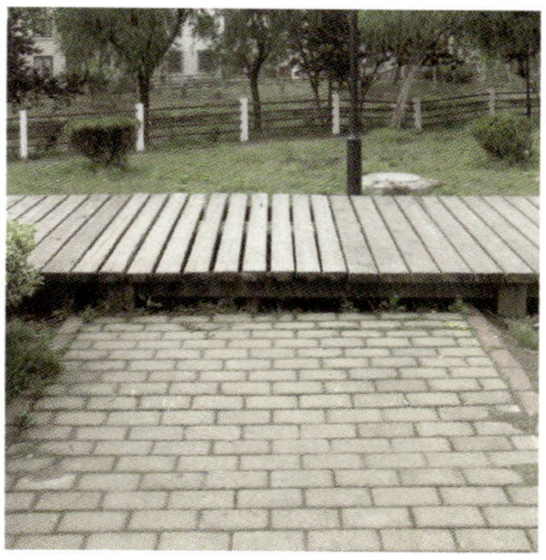

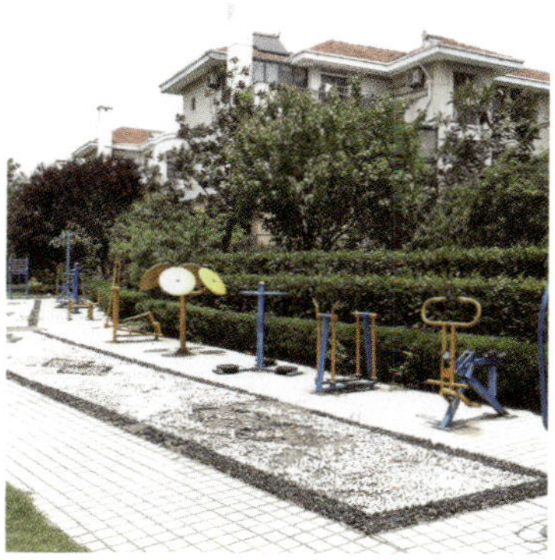

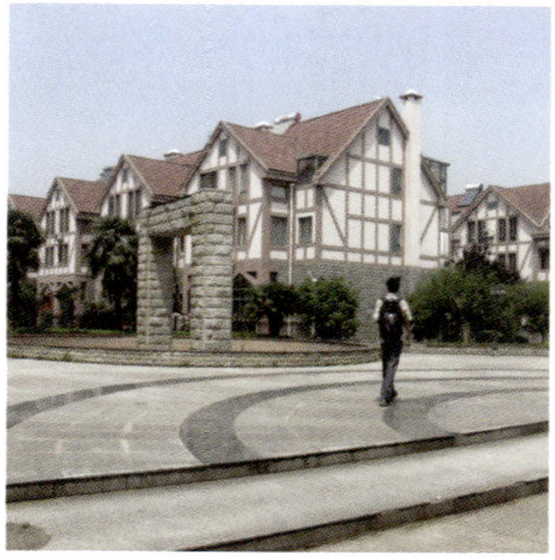

Figure 3 (Top Left) Building entrance in a new residential area in Shanghai.

Figure 4 (Top Right) Pedestrian path in a new residential area in Shanghai.

Figure 5 (Bottom Left) Exercise facilities in a new residential area in Shanghai.

Figure 6 (Bottom Right) Community plaza in a new residential area in Shanghai.

environments are not comfortable, for example, wind conditions, shading, and lighting are not properly considered in design. In addition, poor estate management and maintenance is also a major constraint on the suitability of residential areas for the elderly.

Current Conditions of the Senior Service Facilities

It is a common issue that China's urban residential areas have relatively low provision of services and facilities for "aging in place." In 2011, the result of our research group's study[1] regarding the existing residential areas in downtown Shanghai has found that clinics, activity rooms, and senior canteens are the top three needs of the elderly, among other possible senior service facilities in the city and the community. The survey has also found that the scope of daily activities of the urban elderly is within approximately 500 meters, but sentiments have reflected that there is a general lack of senior service facilities and venues within this radius. In 2012, our research group's study[2] on new residential areas in Shanghai's suburbs found similar results: medical help, meal assistance, and health care are the most needed services of the elderly. However, due to the fact that most of the respondents participating in the 2012 study were relocated to the suburbs from downtown they were generally dissatisfied by the developing suburban conditions. Besides adding community-level services and facilities, respondents feel that hospitals, colleges for the elderly, and public transportation also need improvement in the surrounding areas. (Figure 7)

1 The Study in 2011 on existing residential areas in downtown Shanghai selected six residential areas in three types – Linong, public housing, and new commercial real estate. A total of 420 questionnaires were sent out and 401 valid ones were retrieved.

2 The study on new residential areas in suburbs of Shanghai selected three of the first (2008) large residential areas in Baoshan, Jiading, and Songjiang, as well as three commercial real estate residential areas in the three districts. A total of 448 questionnaires were sent out and 437 valid ones were retrieved.

Figure 7 The most needed services for the elderly in downtown and suburban Shanghai.

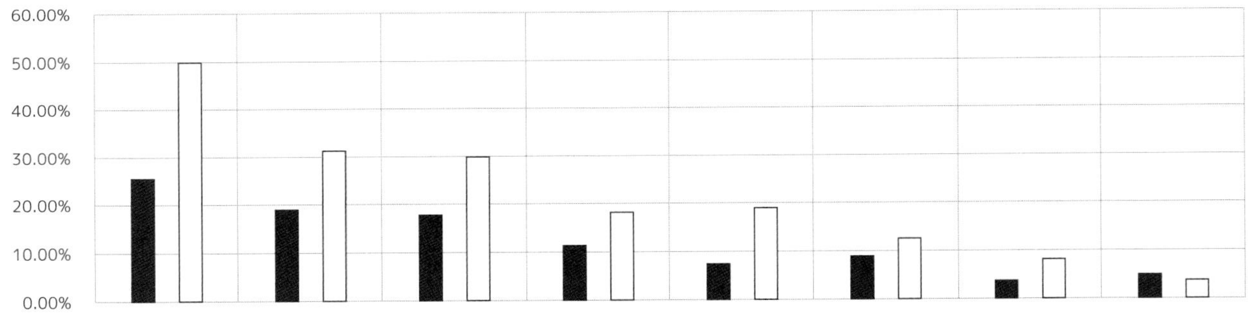

	Medical Help	Cooking Assistance	Health Care	Cleaning Service	Urgency	Spiritual Solace	Transport	Bathing
Downtown ■	26.40%	19.70%	18.50%	12.70%	7.70%	9.50%	4.00%	5.20%
Suburbs □	49.90%	32.30%	30.00%	19.20%	19.70%	13.50%	8.70%	4.10%

Source: the research group's studies in 2011 and 2012

The study has also found that low standards and design flaws in the provision of facilities are the main reasons that some existing senior facilities have been performing poorly. For example, in 2010, the study regarding Siping Rd Neighborhood (Yangpu District), Jiangning Rd Neighborhood (Jing'an District), and Dongming Rd Neighborhood (Pudong District) showed that all three neighborhoods had day-care centers that were significantly smaller than was adequate. Comparisons with ordinary Japanese day-care centers demonstrated that both the area per capita and the staffing were considerably less in the Shanghai cases. (Table 2)

Table 2 Day-care center comparision.

Neighborhood	Floor Area (m^2)	Area Per Capita (m^2/person)	Staffing (# persons)
Toyama City, Japan[3]	400	22	12
Chinese Standard[4]	750	x	x
Siping Rd (Yangpu)	370	12	6
Jiangning Rd (Jingan)	250	8	x
Dongming Rd (Pudong)	200	12	3

Source: the study conducted in 2010

3 Zhou 2011.

4 Codes for Community Senior Day-care Center (Jianbiao 143-2010), edited by the Ministry of Civil Affairs, approved by the Ministry of Housing and Urban-Rural Development and National Development and Reform Commission, implemented on March 1, 2011.

The data in the study further shows that the percentage and density of the elderly population varied significantly across neighborhoods and districts in downtown Shanghai – suggesting that by simply applying the same standards and quota, it would be difficult to meet the actual needs and situations of different neighborhoods. (Table 3).

Table 3 Distribution of the elderly in Shanghai neighborhoods

Neighborhood	Area (km^2)	Total Population	Population over 60	% of Pop. over 60	Elderly Pop. Density (1,000/km^2)
Siping Rd (Yangpu)	2.68	95,780	19,225	20.07	7.17
Jiangning Rd (Jingan)	1.84	85,267	22,841	26.79	12.41
Dongming Rd (Pudong)	5.95	100,000	21,756	21.76	3.66

Source: the study conducted in 2010

Moreover, the lack of systematic deployment and coordination also creates issues in the implementation of senior service facilities. "Code for Planning of City and Town Facilities for the Aged" (GB50437—2007), "Code for Construction of Community Senior Day-care Centers" (143-2010), and "Code for Residential District Planning & Design" (GB 50180-93[Ed. 2002]) have varying definitions and requirements regarding senior service facilities, and provide inadequate guidance towards composite uses of land and space.

Relevant Regulations and Policy Framework

It has been 15 years since the age structure of society in China has grown older,[5] and in major cities like Shanghai, significant aging of the population began as far back as in late 70s. However, the suitability of physical spaces and senior service facilities for the elderly in China is still at a low level, which is, to a great extent, a consequence of the lack of related laws, regulations, and the lagging development of technical standards.

5 China's population started aging since 1999.

Laws and Regulations

At the national level, the first law that addressed living spaces for the elderly was the "Law of the People's Republic of China on Protection of the Rights and Interests of the Elderly" (2012 Revision), which contains content related to building "livable environments" for the elderly. For the first time at the national level, this law defined the responsible parties and principles of building livable environments for the elderly, and brought up specific requirements for urban public service facilities, construction standards, accessible facilities, and livable senior communities.[6]

6 Law of the People's Republic of China on Protection of the Rights and Interests of the Elderly (2012 Revision).

In terms of the departmental regulations and design standards, the

Table 4 Relevant laws, regulations, and national standards.

Name	Year of Implementation	Government Body	Scope of Regulation
Constitution of People's Republic of China	1982	NPC	Basic social rights of senior citizens
Law of the People's Republic of China on Protection of the Rights and Interests of the Elderly	Issued in 1996 Revised in 2012	NPC Standing Committee	Public service facilities, construction standard system, accessible urban environment construction, livable community development for the elderly
Code for Design of Urban Roads and Buildings with Easy Access for Disabled Persons (JGJ 50-88)	1989	Ministry of Construction, Ministry of Civil Affairs, China Disabled Persons' Federation	Accessible facilities
Code for Design of Buildings for Elderly Persons (JGT 122-99)	1999	Ministry of Construction, Ministry of Civil Affairs	Housing for the elderly, nursing home, day-care center
Codes for Design on Accessibility of Urban Roads and Buildings (JGJ50-2001)	2001	Ministry of Construction	Accessibility construction
Code for Design of Residential Building for the Aged (GBT50340-2003)	2003	Ministry of Construction	Housing for the elderly, nursing home, day-care center
Basic Norms of Social Welfare Institutions for the Elderly (MZ008-2001)	2001	Ministry of Civil Affairs	Social welfare institutions providing nursing, rehabilitation, and day-care services for the elderly
Code for Planning of City and Town Facilities for the Aged (GB 50437—2007)	2008	Ministry of Construction	Residential buildings and public buildings for the elderly
Code for Planning of Urban Public Facilities (GB 50442-2008)	2008	Ministry of Construction	Urban public facilities, land use codes for senior facilities as a type of social welfare institutions
Guidance for Urban Elderly Comprehensive Welfare Institutions and Facilities (Trial)	2009	Ministry of Civil Affairs	Urban Elderly Comprehensive Welfare Institutions and Facilities
Guidance for Nursing Home Construction (Trial)	2009	Ministry of Civil Affairs	Nursing homes
Guidance for Construction of Honorable Military Persons Nursing Facilities (Trial)	2009	Ministry of Civil Affairs	Nursing facilities for honorable military persons
Codes for Community Senior Day-care Center (Jianbiao 143-2010)	2011	Ministry of Housing and Urban-Rural Development, National Development and Reform Commission	Service facilities for "Aging in place"
Codes for Construction of Senior Nursing Homes (Jianbiao 144-2010)	2011	Ministry of Housing and Urban-Rural Development, National Development and Reform Commission	Senior nursing homes
Code for Accessibility Design (GB50763-2012)	2012	Ministry of Housing and Urban-Rural Development	Accessible facilities
Basic Standard for Senior Care Organization (GB/T29353-2012)	2013	Ministry of Civil Affairs	Full-time senior care facilities, not including community day-care facilities
Design Code for Buildings of Elderly Facilities (GB50867-2013)	2014	Ministry of Housing and Urban-Rural Development	Nursing homes, senior care facilities, and senior day-care centers
Basic Standard for Clinics in Senior Care Institutions, Basic Standard for Nursing Stations in Senior Care Institutions (Trial)	2014	National Health and Family Planning Commission	Medical facilities in senior care institutions

Source: Compiled by the author.

rules regarding living spaces for the elderly started with the development of accessible urban streets and major public buildings in the 80s. As increasing attention was paid to the aging issue, a number of design regulations and standards regarding residential buildings and facilities for the elderly were also implemented since 1999, and the conditions of institutions for the elderly gradually improved. However, aside from technical regulations on design for accessibility and senior day-care centers, there are almost no national standards for residential area development suitable for the elderly. (Table 4)

In addition, there is a severe lack of content regarding old-age suitability in the technical standards guiding the development of general housing. In the "Code of Urban Residential Areas Planning & Design" (GB 50180-93[2002 Revision]), only five items mentioned regulations about the elderly, three of them are specific to site selection and sunshine rules for senior housing units, while the other two are general requirements that "opportunities of social activities should be provided for elderly and disabled persons." Similarly, the "Residential Building Code" (GB 50368-2005) does not include any specific requirements for meeting the needs of the elderly. These regulations can hardly provide adequate technical support for housing development and construction, nor can they effectively guide renovation in existing environments suitable for the elderly.

Local Policies and Actions

Since the 1990s, some cities with aging populations have started to implement policies and local codes to guide the development of senior care. Taking Shanghai as an example, the local codes and policies since 2000 include "Design Codes for Buildings of Facilities for the Elderly" (2000), "Regulations on Management of Senior Day Care Institutions in Shanghai" (2002), "Opinions on Strengthening the Management of Community Activity Rooms for the Elderly" (2005), "Notice of Shanghai Civil Affairs Bureau to Encourage Communities to Establish Food Service Stations for the Elderly" (2008), "Guidelines for Adding Elevators to Existing Multi-floor Residential Buildings in Shanghai" (2011), "The 12th Five-year Plan for Aging in Shanghai" (2012), "Guidelines for Developing Elderly-friendly City in Shanghai" (2014), "Guidelines for Promoting Pilot Projects of Livable Communities for the Elderly" (2014), "Guidelines for Planning and Management of Adding Elevators to Existing Residential Buildings in Shanghai (Trial)" (2014), and so on. Based on this, we can conclude that Shanghai is trying to address the provision of spaces for "aging in place."

Figure 8 (Below) A photo of a large group of elderly engaging in a healthy public space in the People's Park in Shanghai. (Image courtesy of Justin Kollar)

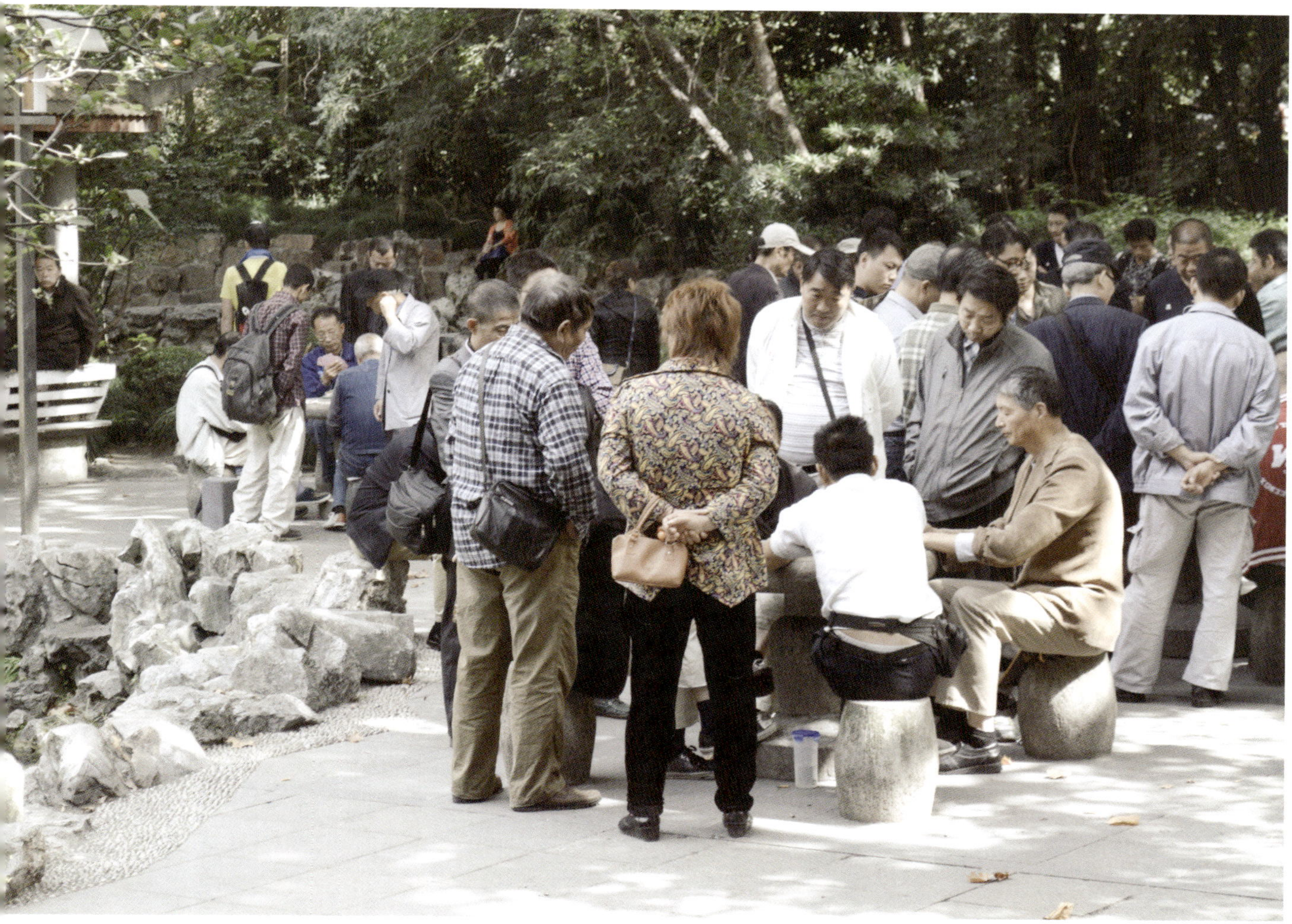

Since 2010, cities including Beijing, Shanghai, Guangzhou, Tianjin, Chengdu, and Hangzhou started to compile a "Special Plan for Layout of Urban Facilities for the Elderly." This is a helpful exploration for improving services for "aging in place" by promoting the collaboration among bureaus of civil affairs, public health, and planning management as well as by focusing on physical spaces for elderly service at the community level.

Ways to Optimize the Living Space for Rapidly Growing Demands of the Aging Population

Support from Regulations and Policies

The primary task of implementing "aging in place" is to establish and improve the regulatory and social security system. It requires not only comprehensive deployment across different levels, including housing, environment, and facilities, but also concerted action by multiple departments including the ones related to civil affairs, health, and planning. In order to prepare for the rapidly aging population, the state should promote the healthy development of the "aging in place" environment through legislation, while related departments should develop general residential standards for the aged. In addition, there should be a shift in the ideology of development; the arrangement of the physical environment and unbalanced distribution of senior service facilities should be less "priority based" and be more of a "universal benefit" for the entire elderly population. Such a transformation can be gradually achieved through the formulation and implementation of relevant policies. (Figure 9)

Figure 9 Regulation and policy system development of livable communities for the elderly.

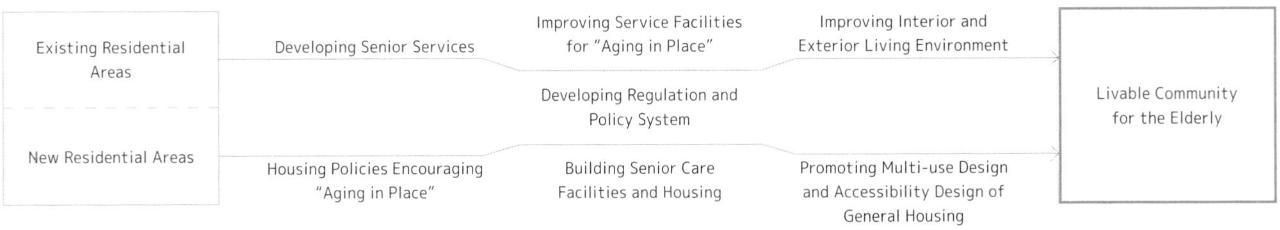
Existing Residential Areas
New Residential Areas
Developing Senior Services
Housing Policies Encouraging "Aging in Place"
Improving Service Facilities for "Aging in Place"
Developing Regulation and Policy System
Building Senior Care Facilities and Housing
Improving Interior and Exterior Living Environment
Promoting Multi-use Design and Accessibility Design of General Housing
Livable Community for the Elderly

Prevailing Scientific Research

The elderly share common demands toward space, yet also have personalized needs. Different spatial requirements reflect the diverse living habits across various lifestyles of the elderly, and directly affect the quality of living conditions and performance of public facilities. As an important foundation of knowledge, the research of urban space for an aging population urgently needs to be developed and expanded. Some scholars have made progress in this field, such as the research on living conditions based on the physiological and psychological characteristics of the elderly,[7] investigation and analysis regarding the existing problems of old-age suitability[8], research

7 Junmin Zhang 1998; Ping Huang 2003; Jiangping Wang 2009.

8 Renlu Hu 1995; Chunfa Zhou et al 2008; Peng Zhou 2009; Yishan Xu et al 2011; Guobin Kuai 2012; Yifan Yu and Jinping Chen 2014.

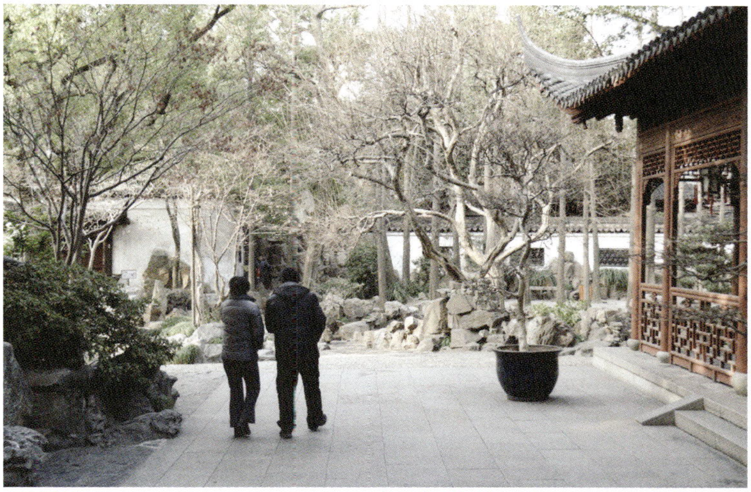

Figure 10 (Left) A photo of an elderly couple walking in a public garden. (Image courtesy of Justin Kollar)

on rehabilitating landscape design for the elderly,[9] research on planning and design methods for suitable environments for old age,[10] and research on behavioral characteristics and traveling patterns of the elderly.[11] Building adequate living spaces in response to the needs of "aging in place" is a long-term and systematic process, and therefore, related basic and applied research must be supported by the entire society.

9 Song Liu and Renzan Qian 2008.

10 Weihua Wang 1997; Jie Fu et al, 2004; Chunhua Yang 2009; Yanmin Zhou and Jingyi Lin 2012; Yunzhou Zhan, Fangfang Wu 2014.

11 Yanwei Chai 2005 and 2010; Jianzhong Huang and Meng Wu 2015.

Public Participation and Assessment of Implementation

As the primary user and benefit group, the elderly should actively participate in the development of suitable living conditions for old age. Moreover, the desires of the elderly are the major basis for taking proper measures in the rebuilding of the environment for old age. The survey results show that although there are common needs for modification of different aspects of the living environment to make them suitable for old age, the most urgent need of residents of Lilongs is the improvement of the interior of residential units. The most pressing need for elderly public housing residents is the addition of elevators to multi-floor residential buildings, while the primary need for the elderly residents in new residential areas is safety of travel.[12] It is clear that there are great disparities in knowledge of spatial needs regarding aging in various conditions. Only by fully understanding the desires of the elderly in earnest can satisfactory results be achieved.

12 Yu Yifan, Chen Jinping 2014.

To this end, it is necessary to establish an assessment system for evaluating the suitability of spatial conditions for old age based on public participation. This system would include procedures starting from planning and design, implementation, evaluating usage, assessment and feedback, to making appropriate modifications.

Development of Elderly-adaptability of Living Spaces

Residential units and areas are important spaces for the daily life of the elderly, where the spatial layout and amenities play a key role in physiological and psychological health. The primary concern of interior space is to ensure the safety, sanitation, and comfort for the elderly, as well as to provide necessary assistance facilities for advanced aged and disabled persons. Exterior living spaces directly affect the elderly's daily activities and willingness to go out, and thus should be built based on safety, accessibility, convenience, comfort, and according to the basic principles of developing a cohesive elderly-friendly city.[13] Specific measures should be taken for both the renovation of existing residential areas and, simultaneously, the planning and design of new residential areas in order to improve spatial and living conditions for the elderly step by step.

13 World Health Organization 2007.

Development of Senior Care Facility System

Supporting facilities for "aging in place" make up a part of the urban public service system. In consideration of the overall efficiency of the public service system, general urban facilities that also satisfy the needs of the elderly should share resources with elderly-specific facilities. Regarding the spatial layout and configuration of senior community service facilities, the "Special Plan for Layout of Urban Facilities for the Elderly in Shanghai" (2014) proposed three basic principles for planning: a balanced layout, differentiated configurations, and comprehensive provision of services. It also placed emphasis on modularity of programs and a multi-use implementation strategy.[14] In the future, the development of community service facilities for "aging in place" should be achieved primarily through the improved and researched configuration of senior care facilities in new residential environments. It also should make use of existing facilities and resources while developing new ones in existing towns,[15] and promote built-in senior care facilities within communities.

14 Zhan Yunzhou, Wu Fangfang 2014.

15 Wu Qingdong, Zhang Ling, Ran Lingfeng 2012.

Conclusions

Shanghai is one of the first megacities in China to have such a large aging population, hence, it has an early lead on research and practice regarding aging populations. Despite this, research shows that its living conditions are still poorly suited for old age, while also lacking relevant legislation and technical regulations. There is an urgent need to improve these conditions by deepening basic research, improving technical systems, and implementing appropriate planning and design initiatives.. It is predicted that the elderly population in China will reach 400 million, accounting for one-third of total population by 2050, whereby Chinese society will reach an advanced stage of aging (China's Fiscal Policy Report, 2011). Faced with the changes in the age-structure of the population, it is necessary to take appropriate measures to plan for old age.

Figure Credits

Figure 1, Forsyth, Ann 2011-2015, *Design for Health Collection*, photograph collection, Accessed 4 August 2015, https://www.flickr.com/photos/designforhealth/.

Figures 3-5, Yu, Yifan 2010, *New Residential Area in Shanghai*, photographs. In possession of: The author: Yu.

Figure 8, 10, Kollar, Justin 2014, *Shanghai*, photographs. In possession of: The author: Kollar.

References

Chai Yanwei 2010, *Urban elderly activity space in China* [中国城市老年人的活动空间], Science Press, Beijing, China.

Chai Yanwei, Li Changxia 2005, 'The spatial characteristics of shopping behavior of the Chinese urban elderly: A case study of Beijing, Shenzhen and Shanghai' [中国城市老年人日常购物行为的空间特征：以北京、深圳和上海为例]. *Acta Geographica Sinica*, 60(3), pp. 401-408.

Chen Jinping, Yu Yifan 2014, 'Senior Residents' wishes and demands in Elderly-adaptive Rehabilitation of Existing Resident Area in Shanghai' [上海既有住宅区适老化改造意愿和需求分析], *Shanghai Urban Planning Review* (5), pp. 98-101.

Chen Xiaowei, Fu Jie, Liu Qing 2004, 'How the Residential Area Planning should be Adapted to an Aging Population' [居住区规划应如何适应人口老龄化的要求], *Journal of Hebei Institute of Architecture* (2).

Hu Renlu 1994, 'A Preliminary Research on the Aged Urban Living Environment' [老龄化城市居住环境初探], *Architectural Journal* (10).

Huang Jianzhong, Wu Meng 2015, 'An Investigation and Analysis of Travel Characteristics and Related Factors of the Elderly Population in Megacities—The Case of the Central Area in Shanghai' [特大城市老年人出行特征及相关因素分析——以上海市中心城为例[J]. 城市规划学刊], *Urban Planning Forum* (2), pp. 93-101.

Kuai Guobin 2012, 'Neighourhood Planning for an Aging Society' [老龄社会的住区设计对策], *Shanghai Urban Planning* (3), pp. 127—131.

Lin Jingyi, Zhou Yanmin 2012, 'Analysis on the Development and Planning Principles of Senior Living Community' [我国养老社区的发展现状与规划原则探析], *Urban Planning* (1).

Liu Song, Qian Renzan 2008, 'A Preliminary Research on the Planning and Design of the Elder Complement Landscape' [老年人弥补性景观及其规划设计初探]. *Shanghai Urban Planning* (6).

Liu Wei 2010, 'Analyzing Elder Supported Home Mode in Sociological Perspective' [居家养老模式的社会学分析], *Forward Position* (9), pp. 122－125.

Wang Jiangping 2009, 'Planning and Design of the Elderly Living Environment' [老年人居住外环境规划与设计]. *China Electric Power Press*, p. 147.

Wang Weihua 1997, 'Imminent Needs for the Study of Characteristics and Measures regarding the Aged Urban Communities' [研究老年型城市社区规划特点及对策迫在眉睫]. *Urban Planning* (4), pp. 47—48.

World Health Organization 2007, 'Global age-friendly cities: a guide,' *WHO*.

Wu Fangfang, Yan Yunzhou 2014, 'Planning Strategies for Aging Megacities: A Case Study of Shanghai' [老龄化背景下特大城市养老设施规划策略探索——以上海市为例]. *Urban Planning Forum* (6).

Wu Qingdong, Zhang Ling, Ran Lingfeng 2012, 'Research on the Development Dilemma and Optimization Strategy of Public Service Facilities in Old Community' [冉凌风. 城市老社区公共服务设施发展困境与优化对策研究]. *Shanghai Urban Planning Review* (1), pp. 49-54.

Xu Yishan, Zhou Dian, Yu Zhenhui 2011, 'Study on the Outdoor Exercises of the Aged in Residential Area and Relevant Space Features: Case Investigation of Outdoor Exercises in Summer' [居住区老年人户外活动及其空间特征研究——夏季户外活动实态调查], *Architectural Journal* (2).

Yang Chunhua 2009, 'Dilemma and Solutions of 'Aging in Place' Urban Communities' [城市社区居家养老的困境和出路]. *Frontiers* (8), pp. 161—163.

Zhan Yunzhou, Wu Fangfang 2014, 'Planning Strategies for Aging Megacities: A Case Study of Shanghai' [吴芳芳. 老龄化背景下特大城市养老设施规划策略探索——以上海为例], *Urban Planning Forum* (62), pp. 38-45.

Zhang Junmin 1999, 'Planning Countermeasures for the Aged Communities' [面向老年人的居住区规划对策思考]. *Population Research*, 23 (3).

Zhou Chunfa, Zhu Hailong 2008, 'Housing for the Elderly: International Experience and China's Choice' [老年人住房政策:国际经验与中国选择], *Population & Economics*, 167 (2).

Zhou, Yan Min 2011, 'Architectural Design Elements for Elderly and Case Study 5: Japanese Daycare Center Funcional Configuration Analysis.' [老年建筑设计要点及案例分析系列五：日本日间照料中心的功能配置分析] [Blog] *Detailed Designs for Dwellings*. Accessed 4 August 2015, http://blog.sina.com.cn/s/blog_6218cf570100sbrj.html.

Zhou Peng 2009, 'A Survey on the Traditional Domesticity and Social Communication Styles of Shanghai Senior Citizens' [周芃:上海市乐龄者家居活动方式、社交活动方式调查研究], *Urban Planning Forum* (3).

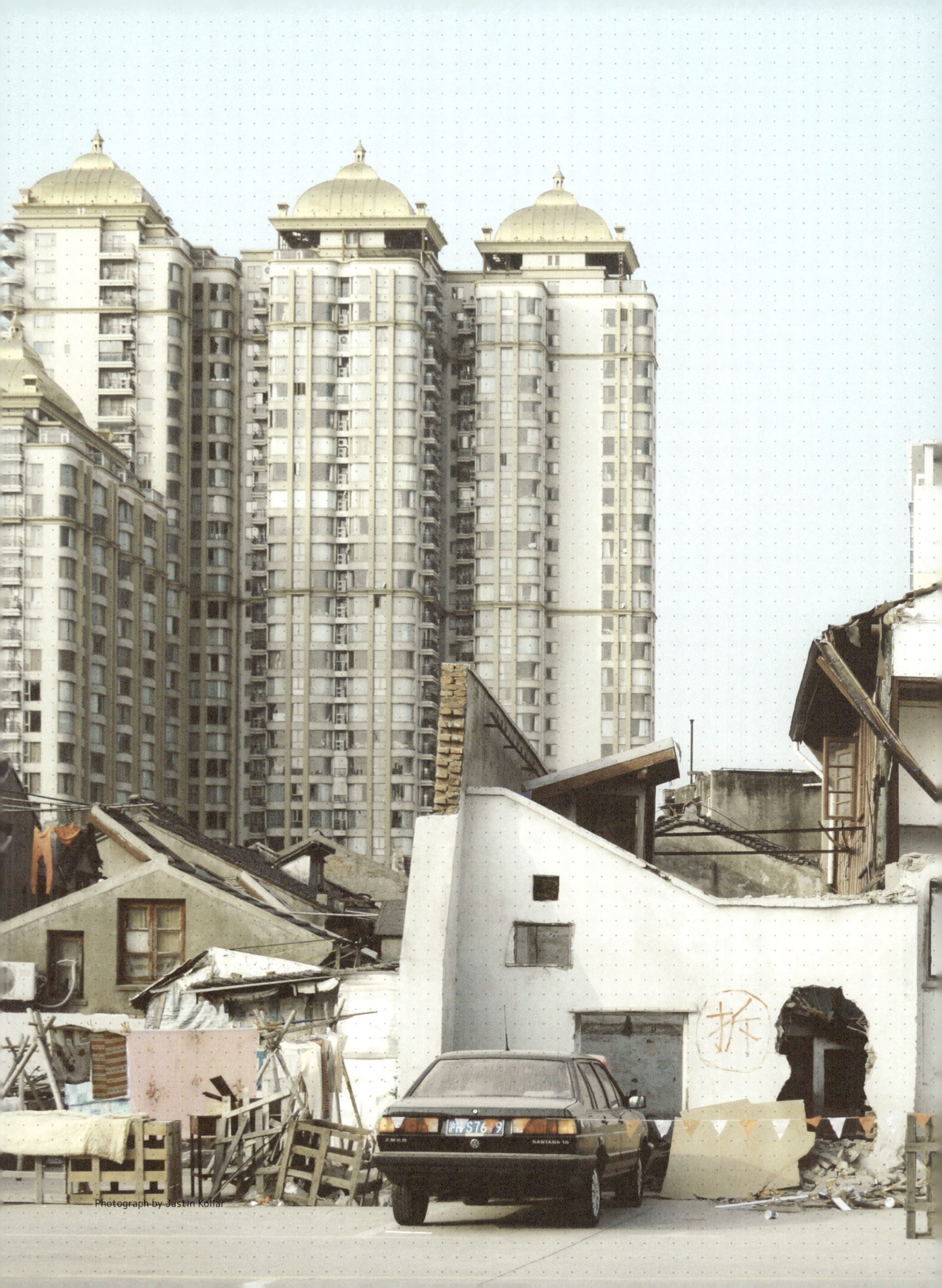

Photograph by Justin Kollar

Chapter 4

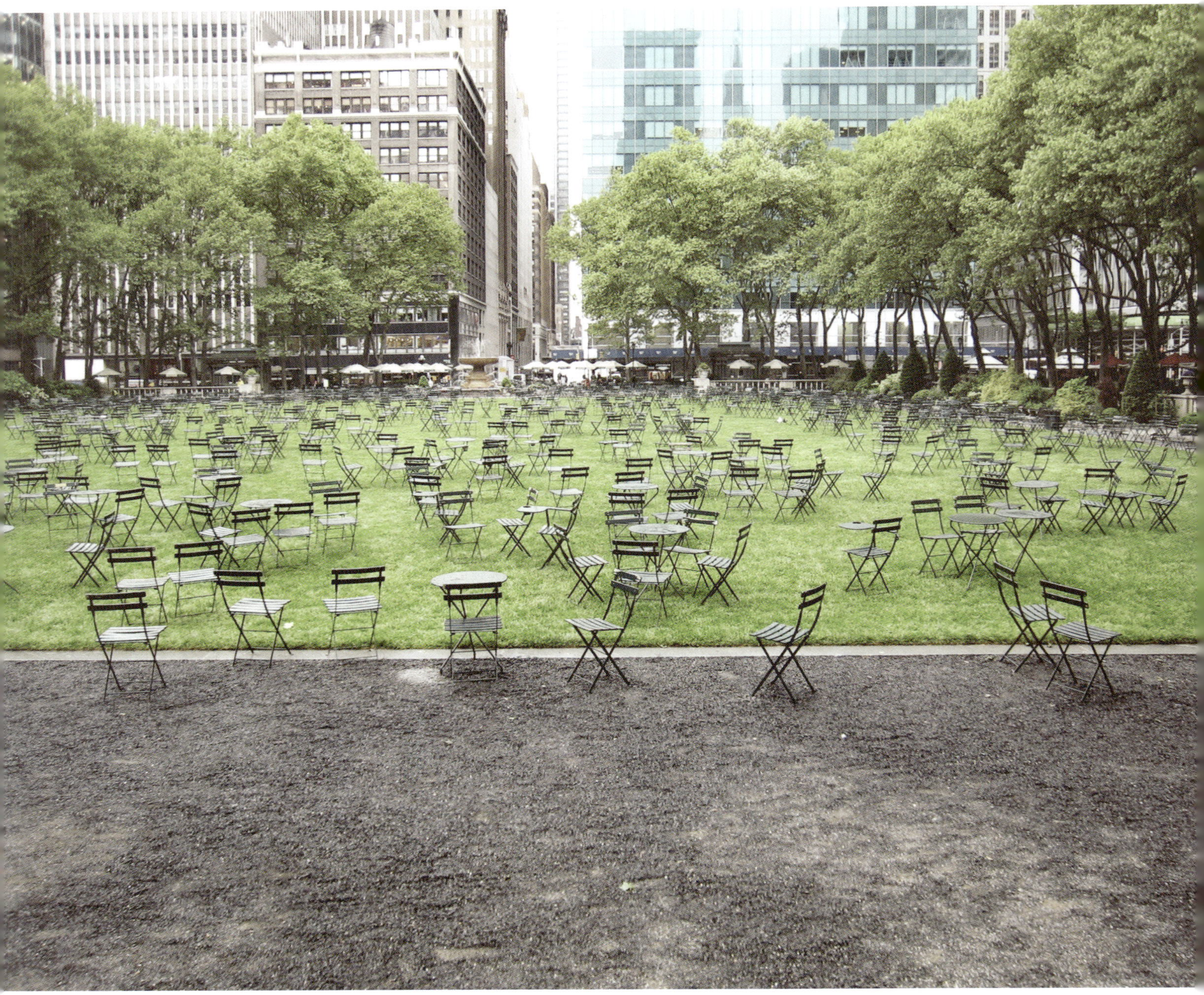

Photograph by Ann Forsyth

Research by Designers

Leire Asensio Villoria + David Mah

"The natural sciences are concerned with how things are...Design, on the other hand, is concerned with how things ought to be..."[1]

The established definitions for what constitute pure research on the one hand and design on the other, can typically put these two practices in opposition. In many ways pure or basic research is associated with making explicit or bringing to light what already exists. It has generated new theories, concepts, and knowledge of the world, while purporting to illuminate it. However, as a practice, it does not have the burden nor obligation for engaging directly with or transforming the world. Any of its transformative potential is typically contained to its capacity to augment or extend our understanding of what already exists. Design, on the other hand, is a projective act that is invested in acting on the world directly. It is, when materialized, by its very nature, always an interventional or transformational act.

As a result, design as a research activity is typically measured as a form of applied research, where the two practices share a primary goal in problem solving. Despite this shared goal, designers often refer to the practice of design as being distinct from the linear problem solving associated with scientific research process in an idealized form.[2] Design is often described as a recursive process, typically involving regular iteration and feedback between proposition and evaluation. This process, rather than assuming an unwavering deductive trajectory between a given problem or hypothesis and an optimized solution or conclusion, can, in some cases, even result in reframing the "problem." It can involve a critical reassessment of the enquiry presented at the start of the process, evaluating if indeed it is the appropriate issue to tackle when addressing a particular wider problem. But more typically, it involves negotiating a complex interplay of parameters and considerations that can make the idea of absolute optimization; elusive. It is, as described by some; both circular and conversational.[3]

The linear process of problem solving is of course conceivable for many "tame" design concerns that are framed by a narrow focus. For instance, a design research project that seeks to optimize structural solutions for certain material technologies can mirror a more linear method, if many of the constraints or parameters that often make demands of a building are either ignored or closely defined. However, if presented with more complex or multi-stranded problems with interdependent and occasionally conflicting parameters or influences, it becomes harder to fathom such a clearly defined path towards design resolution. "Wicked problems," a term originally used to describe confounding problems associated with social policy planning[4] is quite appropriate to describe many design problems facing contemporary designers, particularly those engaged with complex urban concerns.

In the case of the prototypes design research at HAPI, we were presented with a clear mandate to formulate propositions on how neighborhoods in China may be configured to enable healthier lifestyles and offer an improved quality of life. The nature of the research topic is in itself a "wicked problem" because of its starting point within a complex cultural, political and economic context[5] as well as the intricacy of the links between the many contextual factors that can affect health. Given the overall goal of the research initiative to offer templates for future urban development (and re-development or rehabilitation), the aim for the research project was less concerned with offering the absolute, best possible model but rather to elucidate a process for obtaining a wide range of good instantiations of neighborhood models. In order to address and manage the complexity of the task, the prototypes research project adopted a series of strategic approaches that included the adoption of, among others, a multidisciplinary approach and the leveraging of computational design processes.

1 Simon 1969, 114.

2 This assumption of a linear process associated with scientific research is in fact shown by Bruno Latour, amongst others, as an idealization.

3 "… design is characterized as a verb (rather than a noun), a way of acting carried out by a designer/actor, which is circular and conversational in form." Ranulph Glanville. The notion of conversation is elaborated in his keynote lecture at the 2005, Sint Lucas School of Architecture's Unthinkable Doctorate conference; "Design Propositions" where he refers to the cybernetician; Gordon Pask's description of architectural design as a conversation.

4 Rittel and Webber 1973, 153-169.

5 A succinct description of China's dynamism is perhaps well articulated by the architect, Rem Koolhaas' description of the attempts "to construct a coherent narrative about a landscape… [China] …that is changing by the minute" as being "seemingly impossible" quote from Work In Progress, Selections from Urban China Magazine, ed. McGetrick Brendan & Jun Jiang, 2009, Timezone 8 Limited, Hong Kong, China

Diverse Knowledge

To address the complexity of the topic, there were a number of strategies and approaches that were established. The first was to deliberately integrate a multidisciplinary understanding of the relationships between health and place, by engaging team members and advisors with expertise in a range of disciplines, (including architecture, planning, public health, real estate, and landscape architecture to name a few) to inform the project. Resonating with the notion put forward by Rittell and Weber[6] that collaborative approaches are an effective means to address "wicked" problems,[7] the research was deliberately structured to benefit from the combined intelligence of the diverse expertise of the teams.

6 Rittel and Webber 1973, 153-169.

7 Ibid.

Multiple Research Lines

Secondly, a series of parallel projects were also pursued by the GSD HAPI research teams. These included extensive systematic literature reviews on published health and place writings together with surveys and analysis of existing residential neighborhoods in China.[8] Together, these research projects generated a range of findings and conclusions that offer insights into the existing knowledge on health and place. In addition to these secondary research findings, data from fieldwork conducted in China provided important information on the current situation. While these exercises offer valuable "knowledge of"[9] the existing situation, the results of the research have also gone on to inform the development of a range of tools, including guidelines and health impact assessments that offer "knowledge for"[10] designers, policy makers, developers, government officials, and the wider public. In effect, these tools are intended as "knowledge for action" as much as they are effective as research that illuminates the prevailing conditions. The results, conclusions and data generated from these projects also guided the development of the prototypes design research project, which would subsequently also generate both "knowledge for and of."

Similarly, for the prototypes design research, we chose to approach the project through two different formats. One stream was conducted as a longer sustained research project developed within the core research group between 2014 and 2015 and the other through a semester long advanced level graduate design option studio course offered at the Harvard Graduate School of Design in the fall of 2014. The decision to pursue both lines of design inquiry was taken in order to leverage a range of strengths that each format allowed for cultivating different design approaches, addressing a wider range of issues and consequently generating a larger arsenal of proposals. On the one hand, the sustained research allowed for a detailed and systematic process that would elaborate on a longer focused project while the studio setting allowed for the more agile generation of an eclectic range of insights together with more visionary or speculative propositions for healthier neighborhoods.

8 These projects were led by Professors Ann Forsyth and Peter Rowe for the Harvard GSD's HAPI research project between 2013 to 2015.

9 "Although research in architecture has a long tradition, it uses, in the main, imported approaches that do not help architects do architecture. What is needed is a form of research coming out of architecture itself, producing knowledge that will help architects act. This is distinguished as "knowledge for" (action) in contrast to the academically more traditional "knowledge of" (what is)." From Ranulph Glanville's keynote lecture at the 2005, Sint-Lucas School of Architecture's Unthinkable Doctorate conference, "Design Propositions"

10 Ibid.

Managing Complexity

> "There once were two watchmakers, named Tempus and Hora, who manufactured very fine watches… The watches the men made consisted of about 1000 parts each. Tempus had so constructed his that if he put it down—to answer the phone, say—it immediately fell to pieces and had to be reassembled from the elements. The better the customers liked his watches, the more they phoned him and the more difficult it became for him to find enough uninterrupted time to finish a watch.
>
> The watches that Hora made were no less complex than those of Tempus. But he had designed them so that he could put together stable subassemblies of about ten elements each… Hence when Hora had to put down a partly assembled watch to answer the phone, he lost only a small part of his work, and he assembled his watches in only a fraction of the man-hours it took Tempus… (If) there is one chance in ten, that either watchmaker will be interrupted while adding one part to an assembly—then… it will take Tempus on average about four thousand times as long to make a watch as Hora."[11]

11 Simon 1962, 467-482.

The iterative (or more accurately, recursive)[12] nature of the design process, involving multiple increments of feedback between projection and reflection, was adopted for the prototypes core research group. The value of recursive processes includes the ability to address multifaceted problems by carefully focusing on smaller aspects of the wider concern in a considered sequence, gradually building up the complexity of the proposition with each subsequent iteration. This allows for the systematic management of the intricacy of the problem, where the various parameters and considerations can be identified and treated with the necessary focus as well as the more appropriate approach. The possibility of addressing various aspects of the project individually, by utilizing suitable methods and techniques for working on each subset of the problem, can also allow for the regulation of how the different types of knowledge and approaches from the diverse disciplinary team and parallel research projects may be best deployed.

12 Recursion is a term that is used in many different fields, however its specific meaning in computer science is related to the way in which a problem is resolved. In recursive processes, a larger problem is addressed by resolving smaller increments of the problem that gradually accumulate. Another aspect of this can be illuminated by defining recursive sequences as sequences where each item in the series is defined by its preceding items. When applied to the design process, this differs from a simple iterative process where in recursion, the results or conclusions from each iteration of the process informs subsequent steps in the process.

13 Steadman, 36-37.

Methods and Aims

> "The distinctive feature of the sciences of the artificial would be their effort to understand—where this is not consciously understood already—how artefacts are organized and how they function. The implication or hope would be that any understanding gained by the research could help designers to be more effective in their decision making. Architects would have a clearer picture of the range of strategic possibilities open to them, and the likely performance and properties of each alternative."[13]

The prototypes design research team was invested in a design research process aimed at, both generating and evaluating, a large range of possible Chinese neighborhood block organizations that perform well with respect to a number of identified health parameters. Informed by an understanding of the design process offered by Herbert Simon; as an "artificial science," the project focused on analyzing the existing and projected performance of the physical characteristics of the neighborhood superblocks. The performance criteria that were utilized as considerations were related specifically to contextual factors that are identified to be influences on the health and quality of life of its residents (through, among others, parallel HAPI research projects). The project adopted evidence-based design approaches that were informed by a range of quantifiable assessment criteria offered by the Health Impact Assessment, while also being guided by qualitative knowledge on the health impacts of place. Factors ranging from the walkability of the neighborhood together with access to opportunities for socializing were studied and included within the range of concerns integrated in the design of the blocks.

However, rather than remaining at the level of simply testing or applying recommendations and findings from the reviews, surveys, and health impact assessments, the prototypes research was also carried out to generate a range of findings and outcomes of its own. Through the use of computational design and evaluation techniques, patterns in the performance of a broad sample of both existing and

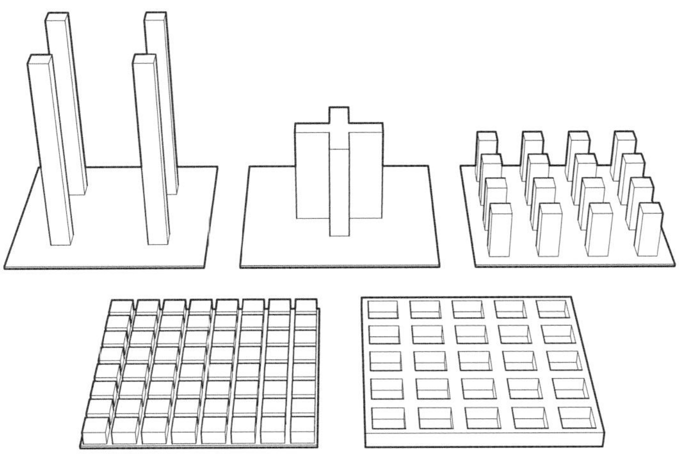

Figure 1 (Left) Illustrations based on Lionel March and Leslie Martin's land use and built form studies developed at Cambridge University in 1972.

projected neighborhood block design iterations could be produced and then studied both individually and comparatively. These findings on the relationship between different aspects of a block organization and its impact on health factors offer original knowledge that can be used to inform future design. The project sought to resonate with the aims of notable precedents of design research such as the land use and built form studies of Leslie Martin and Lionel March,[14] where it was pursued to uncover the performance or organizational benefits that may be achieved through specific design operations while also offering knowledge on the existing condition of urban neighborhood blocks in China.

14 See Lionel March and Leslie Martin's land use and built form studies developed at Cambridge University and published in *Urban Space and Structures.*

The research project also leveraged computational design tools and processes for their capacity to both generate and evaluate numerous design iterations, including already existing models. This opportunistic adoption of computational processes resonates with the origins of public health, where the nineteenth century English statistician; William Farr's utilized a calculating machine modeled on Charles Babbage's difference engine[15] to calculate life tables, an exercise that would come to define the origins of epidemiology. Furthermore, the collection of possible neighborhood block configurations that result from the process also present a range of design proposals that embed characteristics and performance ranges that satisfy many indicators and measurements for healthier places. Cumulatively, the design research prototypes project offers contributions to a knowledge for how we may practice urban design that better incorporates health concerns, while also identifying the actual effects that specific design operations may have on health related performances through the study of an extensive range of samples of existing and proposed organizations.

15 The difference engine was the earliest theoretical computing device, developed by the Englishman; Charles Babbage in 1882.

Generating Alternatives Versus Optimization

> "The subject of computational techniques need not be limited to optimization. Traditional engineering design methods make much more use of inequalities—specifications of satisfactory performance—than of maxima and minima… No one in his (or her) right mind will satisfice if he (or she) can equally well optimize; no one will settle for good or better if he (or she) can have best. But that is not the way the problem usually poses itself in actual design situations."[16]

16 Simon 1969, 119.

To paraphrase Herbert Simon, the process of optimization is intended to locate the best possible iteration of all the possible worlds, a process that he describes as "a purely empirical question, calling only for facts and ordinary declarative reasoning to answer for it."[17] In opposition to finding the best possible solution (which is often incomputable for many design problems[18]), Simon locates the "logic of design" as a practice of locating a range of satisfactory alternatives. This process is structured by what he terms as a bounded rationality that aims for solutions that "satisfice"[19] rather than optimize.

17 Ibid, 121.

18 Even, an example cited by Simon of a more abstract and bounded problem such as the traveling salesman problem, has proven to be computationally unfeasible for arriving at an optimal solution (looking for the most efficient itinerary for a salesman through even a moderate numbers of cities.)

19 'Satisfice' is a term coined by Herbert Simon which is a conflation between the words satisfy and suffice. It is a description for a decision making process that searches for solutions until an acceptable range of solutions are found rather than focusing on locating the optimal or best solution.

As described earlier, the HAPI design research process adopted the modularization of the larger complex problem of designing healthy neighborhood environments into smaller and more manageable components. This modularization also allowed the design team to either/both optimize for particular sub-problems (where applicable) and/or to locate a range of satisfactory solutions in other areas that do not have optimal solutions. What then became important in the subsequent process of defining the different iterations of design possibilities is the strategic selection of the factors to be addressed and the hierarchy in which these different sub-components are re-assembled.

The HAPI design research team was critical of the impulse to steer the research process towards an exercise in optimization, where the results of the project would be deemed as ideal, optimized models for healthy neighborhoods. This goal was problematic for the team due to two important reasons. The first is the idea of ideal universal models ignorant of context, the second is the notion of an optimized solution being one that is complete and fixed—an organic totalizing solution, both of which present a model of working that do not allow for the flexibility and variety needed for contemporary urban practice.

To illustrate an alternative position from a model of linear efficiency and optimization, designers can profit from revisiting an exemplar of urbanization that has become synonymous with a highly engineered generalized urban model, the Eixample by Idelfons Cerdà. Instead of the established narrative of Cerdà's

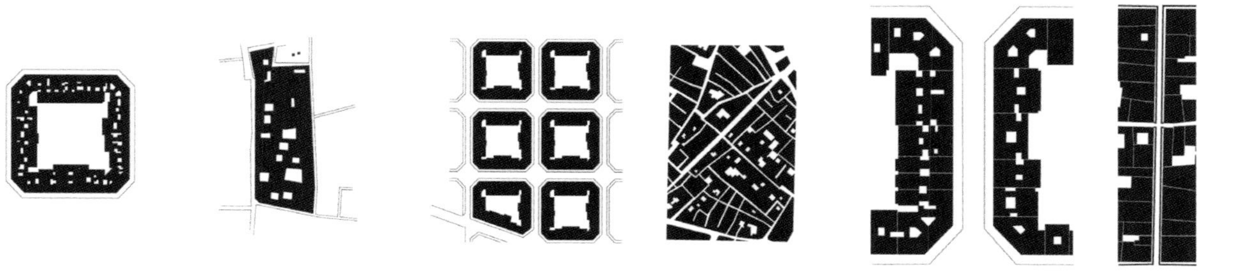

Figure 2 (Above) Scale comparison between Eixample and Barcelona's historic city center.

technical search for an optimized model for the city, the Eixample provides a way to reframe thinking about systemic and generalized modes of practice in urban design. Rather than focusing on Cerdà's original and revised plans for the Eixample, we may also solicit valuable lessons from looking at how this vital part of Barcelona has evolved over the last century and a half. Cerdà's plan, after its many years of evolution, ultimately offered a carefully managed yet differentiated urban fabric with an equally varied open space pattern, a system that was robust enough to accommodate subsequent generations of building types and open space patterns—and even changes to the grid itself. By reconsidering the nature of Cerdà's 'general theory,' we invoke a systemic model of urbanization that recognizes the possibility of ranges of distinction and differentiation.

Cerdà's techniques can just as easily be exploited for their capacities to generate diversity as they were for operating as searching mechanisms for perceived optimal solutions. The mathematical formulas Cerdá used to define the blocks' building and open space typologies may just as easily be interpreted for their capacity to locate alternative occupations for the block. Rather than relying on the accumulation of random expressions, these differences can be a consequence of coordinated systemic processes.

Generalized rules, like the ones developed by Cerdà, have the capacity to enable spatial, experiential, and organizational complexity, and to support a differentiated yet consistent and cultivated urban environment. When translated into bylaws and guidelines, these can be generational practices for elaborating urban landscape and urban fabric patterns. Rather than relying on willful and highly authored practices to yield desired urban qualities, designers can use this "bottom up" approach to develop urban spaces that offer flexibility within consistency. These designs may unfold over long timescales and evolve under the influence of different stakeholders, yet potentially retain the core strengths of a generalized model of urbanization.

The Evolution of Idelfons Cerdà's Eixample: From Organic Plan to Framework

> "A central premise of the sciences of the artificial is that artefacts—despite the fact that they are made by humans—can embody 'knowledge' or possess properties of which their makers and others are not aware."[20]

Cerdà's Eixample has often been compared with many of its contemporaneous urban plans and grouped into the general category of '19th-century metropolis.' Like many within this category, Cerdà's system for urban expansion assumed the form of the extensive isotropic grid. Cerdá elaborated his method for urbanization in several proposals written between 1855 and 1867, publishing *Teoría General de la Urbanización* in 1867.[21] The theory and plan as developed, while not implemented in their entirety, offered a highly comprehensive collection of rules for determining the morphology and layout

20 Steadman 2013, 36.

21 The first two volumes of this work, a conceptual presentation of urbanization and case study, were published as Teoría General de la Urbanización, Madrid: Instituto de Estudios Fiscale, 1867. The third (unpublished) volume held proposals that followed the theory. See Soria (1995) for a fuller explanation.

of infrastructure, urban blocks, property division, and open public spaces as well as the associations between these urban elements.

Cerdá's initial plan (1859) was a continuous grid of ~1,000 blocks, each 113.3 x 113.3m, extending over an area that occupied ten times the footprint of the old city.[22] This carefully regulated infrastructural system integrated transportation, public landscape spaces with over 30,000 cultivated trees, and a modern sewage system.[23] The characteristic chamfered corners of the *manzanas* (blocks) frame and articulate the corners of the urban environment, while improving flows of movement through its mesh-like system of streets. With the direct relationship between performance and morphology, with organization as a primary emphasis of the plan, Cerdá's work can be described as having been engineered rather than designed.[24] His plan reveals a method of optimization by which a number of parameters and variables are brought to an ideal level of performance, presented as archetypes, and organized into a set of patterns that could be generally proliferated. [25]

Probably as a result of Cerdá's clear systematization and elaboration into a general theory, the Eixample has been used to support arguments for the efficacy of universal implementation in design. Its systemic and repeated characteristics allow for unlimited and incremental urban development, while retaining an overall consistency. Certainly in comparison to other models of city planning prevalent at Cerdá's time, which relied more heavily on formal composition, the relative simplicity and repeatability of Cerdá's Eixample provided a manageable system for implementation.

However, the presumed determinism of the general theory that underpins the Eixample is in fact technically composed of a series of associations that allow for the possibility of generating differences and variations. We may extract alternative insights from the Eixample that are demonstrated both by the narrative of the plan's implementation and the evolution of its use, renovation, and transformation. The Eixample's persistence for over a century and a half as a vital site for Barcelona's urban life points towards its capacity for transformation and adaptation, facilitating changing urban practices, politics, economies, and lifestyles.

History and Challenges

Critiques of the Eixample have typically challenged the 'autonomous' nature of Cerdá's general theory of urbanization, suggesting it was motivated purely by technical reasoning. Attendant to this argument is the portrayal of the Eixample as a territorializing abstraction that lacks connection to context (social, historical, physical, or otherwise). It is true that the plan is biased towards optimization, suggesting the linear economies of efficiency associated with early engineering. The customary critical focus on hygiene and efficient mobility as performance drivers for Cerdá's plan further reinforce his association with engineering practices.

The Eixample has been appropriated as a cautionary tale of the failings of generalized and systemic

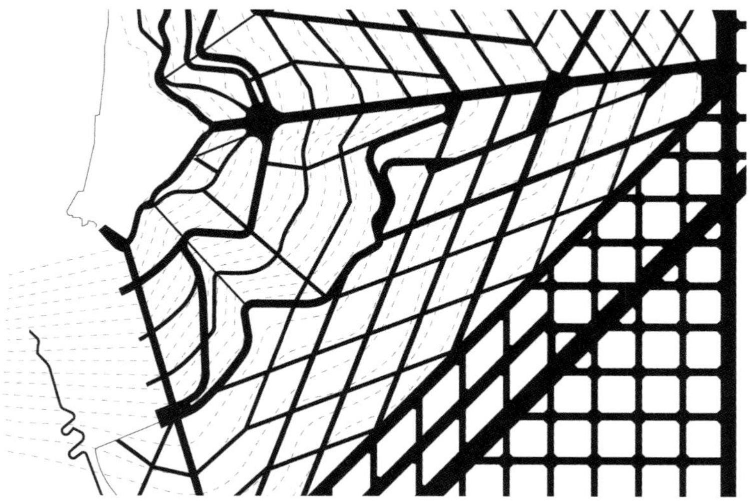

Figure 3 (Left) Proposed Eixample extension over Montjuic.

22 Aibar and Bijker, 24

23 In one plan iteration from 1855, 36.74% of the plan area is allocated for roads, 36.14 % for gardens and 27.12 % for buildings. (Soria y Puig, 23)

24 Cerda's professional affiliation as an Ingeniero de Caminos, Canales y Puertos (engineer of paths, channels and ports – much like today's civil engineer) is affirmed by the functional and performance ambitions that inform the Eixample.

25 Cerda presented the formula for the blocks as:

$$x=\frac{pv-2bd}{d} \pm \sqrt{\frac{pv}{d^2f}(pvf-4bdf-4b^2d)},$$

where x is the side of the block, 2b is the width of the street, f is the depth of the building site, d is the height of the facade, v is the number of inhabitants per house, and p is the number of surface square meters per person. Cerda took the values of the variables as 2b=20m, f=20m, d=20m, v=43, and p=40, obtaining 113.3 m, the length of the blocks in the Eixample. This equation was never discussed by Cerda, and it remains unclear whether the formula was generative of urban form, descriptive of the Eixample following its design, or some combination of the two. (Aibar and Bijker, 16)

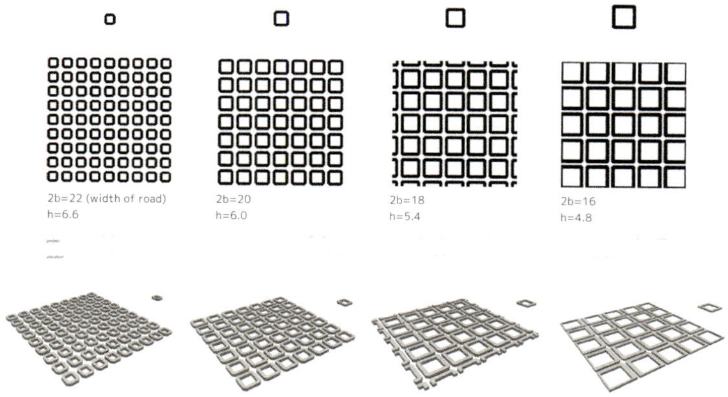

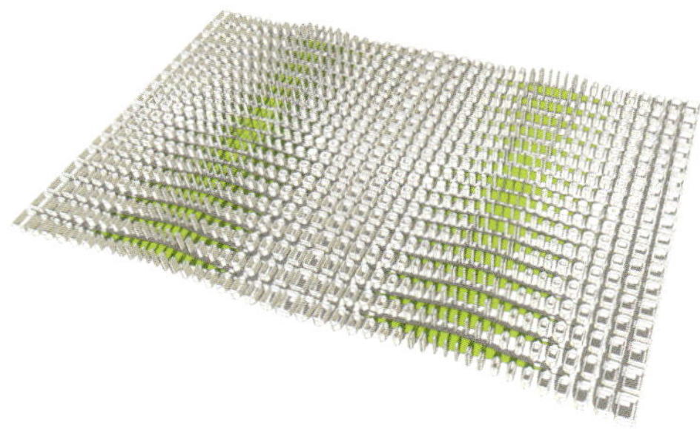

Figure 4 (Top, Left) Differentiation of Cerda's associative model for the Eixample.

Figure 5 (Top, Right) Hypothetical catalogue of different iterations of Cerda's rule.

models of urbanization to deliver urban environments with spatial and scalar diversity. It has also been celebrated as a precedent that supports the link between morphology and performance. Associative designers[26], in particular, pursue the claim of a tight causal relationship between expected performance and the plan's particular morphological and organizational characteristics. Their interest follows a characteristically faithful focus on Cerdà's plan as a model of an organic, "biologically formulated" system that reveals what Manuel de Sola Morales identified as the "abstract biological formulation of its principles."[27]

In principle, the "organic plan" works as a series of highly synchronized part-to-whole relationships (albeit with modest measures of wiggle room) and acquires value from this synchronicity between elements. The biologically formulated position is often coupled with a historical view of the frustrated implementation of Cerdà's full and authentic plan, which claims that the plan—in its absolute form—would have operated as a highly coordinated and nested series of associations across different scales of the urban environment. Under this conception, transformations and deviations from the original intentions of the plan compromise its efficacy.

Ironically, the biologically formulated interpretation of the Eixample may itself be characterized as teleological and deterministic. Cerdà's plan was not singularly motivated by the strict relationships between the organization and formalization of urban matter and its carefully engineered performance. Instead, his plan was a framework for transforming the urban environment. In place of a highly deterministic image for the city controlled by master plans, the landscape infrastructural grid in the Eixample offered an organizational structure that anticipated significant urban transformation and difference which can be seen in the numerous variations for defining the block developed and anticipated by Cerdà in two main iterations of his plan in 1859 and 1863. At the same time, the grid imparted a consistent overall organization and public character to the urban environment. Considered in this way, our understanding of the Eixample shifts: Cerdà's extension is not a definitive organic plan, but instead a looser framework for the evolution of the city.

The qualities of the plan considered as a framework are more easily discerned by considering the time-weathered version of the Eixample as the subject of study rather than the original plan and general theory alone. A study of the Eixample over time suggests a diversely scaled model for urbanization that locates and exploits the performance of different elements within the urban field, allowing for stochastic and localized practices to operate within its frame. A "framework" understanding of the plan reveals that processes of urbanization span multiple scales of the urban environment and are not bound in an organic totality. While loose affiliations occur across elements, they are not governed by strict part-to-whole relationships, and constituents may be defined (and redefined) independent of their context. The splitting of authority over the bylaws from the control of the grid, which occured during the implementation of the project, was a defining event: it may have altered the plan, but it enabled the Eixample to accommodate change. Ultimately, it transformed and distorted Barcelona's organic plan into a supple framework.

26 Associative design is a design practice that associates a number of performance parameters and variables with the development of geometric and organizational design models. The practice is invested in the use of multiple performance parameters and information as the main drivers of the design process.

27 de Sola Morales, 286.

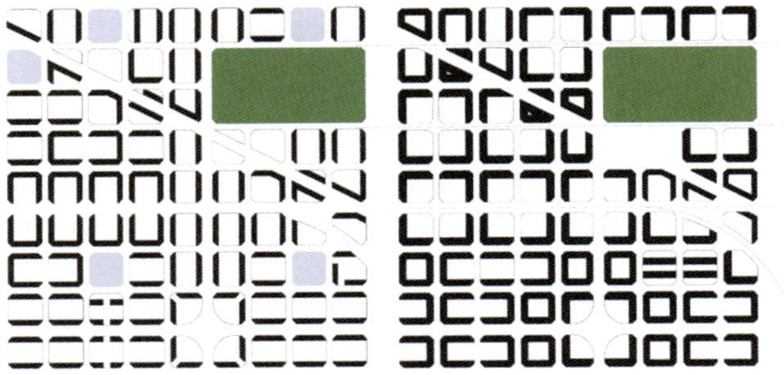

Figure 6 (Left) Comparison between proposed urban fabric in Cerda's 1859 and 1863 plans.

Difference and Adaptation

The Pla Cerdá gains value as a model for contemporary urbanization when our interpretation shifts from a focus on the design as an absolute metric definition of optimal urban organizations towards an understanding of the plan as a process that elaborates mutable associations. This suggests a shift from the geometrical definition of urban morphologies to the identification of their underlying topological relationships.

During the long course of its implementation, the grid of the Eixample—at first recognizable for its isotropism—has in fact absorbed and accumulated significant inflection and differentiation. Many of these changes index social and economic tendencies, such as the difference in perceived status (and consequently value) attached to different sides of the Eixample divided by the already distinguished Passeig de Gracia. Other changes reflect local watershed and climate patterns, such as the North-South ways that support a variety of landscape and planting patterns and treatments. The street meshwork itself has also evolved in a somewhat organic manner, as it adapts to the factors and variables that operate across a number of scales of influence.

One deliberate case can be seen in the speculative exercise developed by Cerdá for testing the possible propagation of the Eixample over Barcelona's Montjuïc hill, which showed the transformation from a regular to diagonal grid in response to the terrain. This exercise allows us to gain some insight into the latent possibilities embedded within the Pla Cerdá for difference and variation as a system in itself. The interface between a regulated urban grid and the particularities of a natural landform solicited an adjustment to the urbanizing grid itself. This perturbation to the urban form, influenced by the underlying landscape, is significant because it explicitly reveals the potential for a topological understanding of the Cerdá plan. Cerdá's decision to deform his system exposes the nature of his general theory as associative and topological rather than as absolute . Rather than using the regular grid as an archetype, the decision to deform and readjust its deployment suggests that Cerdà chose to view his grid as a system that could take on an adaptive function relative to different site conditions. This is significant when considered in light of many instances of the use of urban grids in Cerdà's time that would instead impose a regular archetypal grid optimized for flatness over terrain that would significantly compromise the performance of such a regular form.

Either as a deliberate reference to Cerdá's Montjuïc experiment or through serendipitous similitude, the Jardí Botànic de Barcelona (1999) adopts an analogous form of a differentiated grid modified to the topography of Montjuïc's slopes. A deformed lattice operates as the main structuring frame for the gardens, orienting the lines of the network into a series of switchbacks of circulation and, coincidentally, as the subdivision of the terrain into discrete garden plots. This interface between the grid and the strategically modulated topography of the site generates microclimates with differential exposure, shading, and humidity, and supports the careful cultivation of different geographic variations of the Mediterranean biome

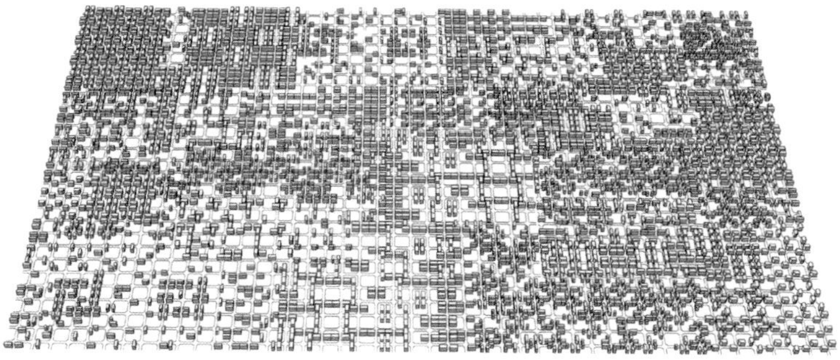

Figure 7 (Left) Hypothetical colonization of the Eixample with Cerda's different block types from the 1859 and 1863 plans.

Whether on varied terrain or in the flatter city center, Cerdá's incremental and recursive approach supported a design that could evolve over many generations, establishing a series of practices that may be carried out over a long timescale and by multiple participants. This approach reverberates with vernacular settlement practices – or in Christopher Alexander's terms, 'unselfconscious design.'[28] Further, it suggests a contemporary link to associative practices that establish generalized and systemic design methodologies, leveraging iteration and recursion within their creative processes. One strategy these practices have already extracted from the Eixample is an evolutionary design process that searches for an ideal end state. Alternatively, deployment of these processes could aim not towards a single anticipated goal, but rather towards a curated inventory of latent possibilities within a set of associations. This second approach promises to more radically re-appropriate the Pla Cerdá.

28 Alexander 1964.

Frameworks and Possibilities

"...the aim of design is not to find the truth, but to improve some characteristics of the world where people live"[29]

29 Rittel and Webber 1973, 153-169.

The design research project developed by the HAPI team sought to deliver a model of research that emerges from a design process. It engages with the specific issue of health and place by aiming to generate knowledge both for and of the organization of neighborhood blocks in China. However it, as with all design, it is a situated problem with many complex variables and factors.

What results is less of a singular optimized model and more a process for generating a range of neighborhood configurations. It identifies the specific design operations and some of their associated metric ranges that can be deployed to transform existing neighborhood block organizations and default design models into better performing spaces for healthier living. Beyond the scale of specific design operations, it also provides a large range of actual neighborhood configurations that may be referenced to guide both the design and renovation of neighborhood blocks. In effect, it presents, not just a model to emulate or repeat, but a design process that may be used to generate a wide range of possible solutions and to potentially integrate many different concerns as well as expertise by making the process suitable for collaborative work by making it accessible and manageable.

Following on from this goal, is the decision to structure the process so that the models that are offered by the research may allow for transformation and adaptability. Learning from the reading of the Eixample in Barcelona as an urban lesson, not just in relation to Idelfons Cerdá's organic plan but also in its evolution into a mutable framework, the project strategically adopted the rigor of Cerdá's original process with the acknowledgment of its value in locating a rich array of potential solutions. This was done by adopting two very specific lessons from this reinterpretation of Cerdà.

1) The urban grid, together with the open space pattern, is treated as a framework that may be inhabited by a wide array of possible block configurations. The nature of this framework is extended to the block itself, where a number of health-related performance criteria would restructure the superblock into a smaller grain through its subdivision into smaller sub-blocks. This is particularly valuable for the capacity to generate a range of different blocks through a simple series of different combinatorics and also allows us to implement new blocks or transform existing ones in a flexible and incremental manner.
2) The definition of the blocks and sub-blocks are inspired by Cerdà's use of associations between various elements of the block and numerous parameters to define a topological relationship that allows us to locate multiple organizations. Similar to his use of mathematical, relational formulas to link form or organization with performance, we developed associative models that ensure a certain range of performance while also allowing for the possibility of the generation of many different instantiations through the capacity embedded within these models to change variables.

The design and research strategy adopted here accepts the possibility and value of both showcasing and evaluating many different solutions to meet its dual obligations for providing templates for stakeholders to act with while simultaneously allowing us to study the qualities of neighborhood organizations in the aggregate. It acknowledges the value of studying the relationships between block organization and health factors while also recognizing and accounting for the possibility for transformations to the neighborhood configurations that may happen over time. This was adopted as a means to offer an approach that acknowledges the "wicked" nature of the relationships between health and place, the value of diversity and also the need for being mindful of the rigors demanded of design as a form of research.

Figure Credits

Figure 1, Illustration based on March, Lionel and Martin, Leslie (eds.) Built form studies in 1972

Figure 2, Kim, Jisoo 2015, *Scale comparison between Eixample and Barcelona historic city center*, drawing. In possession of: The author: Kim.

Figure 3, Kim, Jisoo 2015, *Proposed Eixample extension over Montjuic*, drawing. In possession of: The author: Kim.

Figures 4, 5, Suarez, Elizabeth; Freundt, Monica; Cho, Mijin 2013, Speculative Urbanizations Studio, drawings, Cornell University, studio led by Leire Asensio Villoria and David Mah.

Figures 6, 7, Raub, Martin; Zhang, Xiang; Peng, Chiayu 2013, Speculative Urbanizations Studio, drawings, Cornell University, studio led by Leire Asensio Villoria and David Mah.

References

Aibar, Eduardo and Bijker, Wiebe E. 1997, 'Constructing a City: The Cerda Plan for the Extension of Barcelona' in *Science, Technology, & Human Values*, Vol 22, No 1, Sage Publications, Inc. pp. 16, 24.

Alexander, Christopher A. 1964, *Notes on the Synthesis of Form*, Cambridge, MA: Harvard University Press.

De Sola Morales, Manuel 2008, *Ten Lessons on Barcelona*, Col-Legi D'Arquitectes de Catalunya. p. 286

Glanville, Ranulph 2005, 'Design Propositions', Keynote lecture at Sint-Lucas School of Architecture's Unthinkable Doctorate conference.

March, Lionel and Martin, Leslie (eds.) 1972, Urban Space and Structures, Cambridge University Press, Cambridge, UK.

McGetrick, Brendan (ed.) and Jiang Jun (aut.) 2009, Urban China Work In Progress. Selections from Urban China Magazine, Timezone 8 Limited, Hong Kong, China.

Rittel, Horst and Webber, Melvin 1973, 'Dilemmas in a General Theory of Planning', *Policy Sciences* 4, Elsevier Scientific Publishing Company, Amsterdam, pp. 153-169.

Simon, Herbert A. 1962, 'The Architecture of Complexity', Proceedings of the American Philosophical Society, Vol 106, No 6, pp. 467-482.

Simon, Herbert A. 1969, The Sciences of the Artificial, The MIT Press, Cambridge, MA, pp. 114, 119, 121.

Soria y Puig, Arturo 1995, 'Ildefonso Cerdà's General Theory of Urbanization', in *Town Planning Review* Vol 66 No 1, pp. 15-39.

Steadman, Phillip 2013, 'An 'Artificial Science' of Architecture', Design Research in Architecture: An Overview, Murray Fraser (ed.), Ashgate, pp. 36-37.

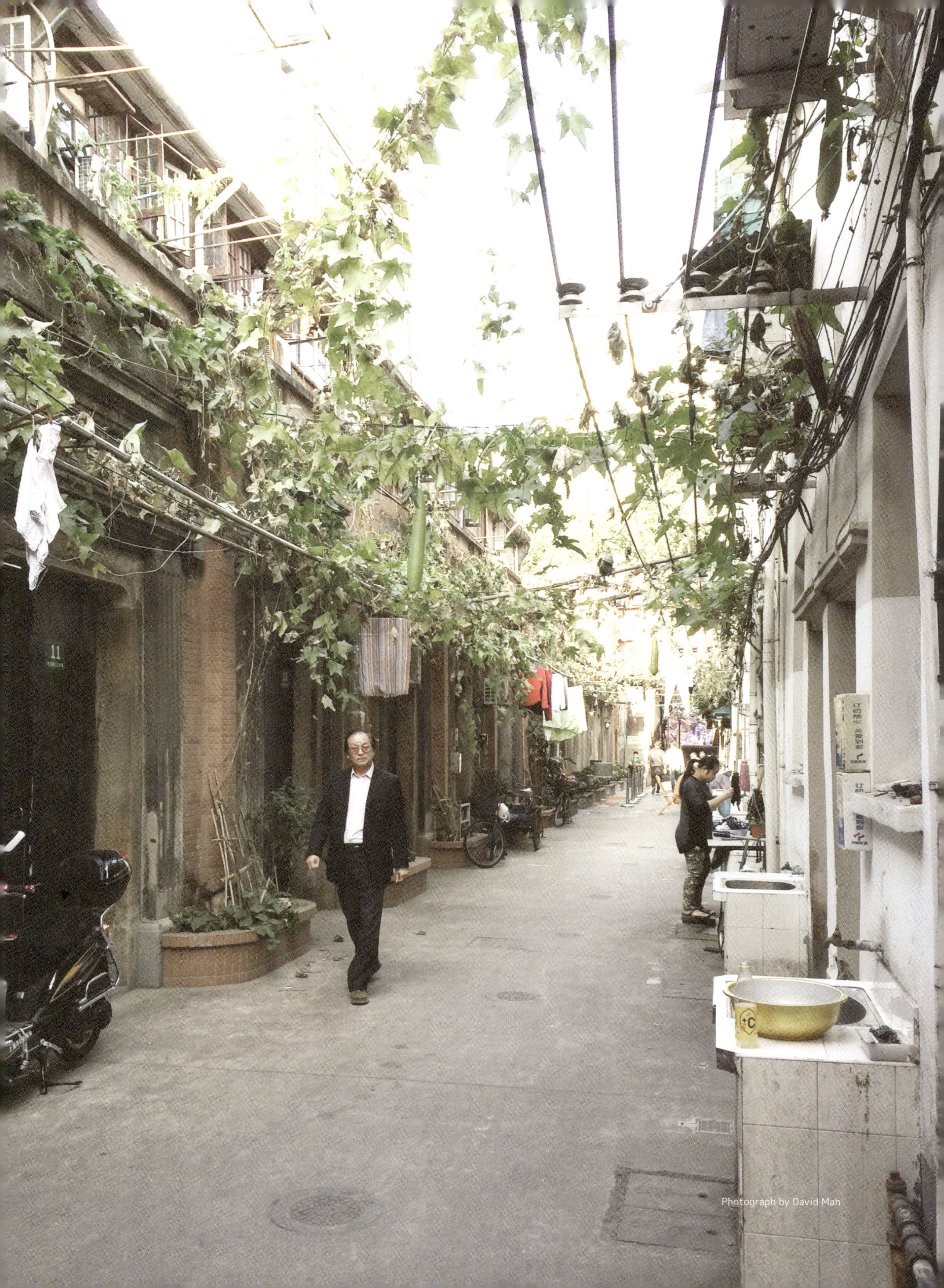

Photograph by David Mah

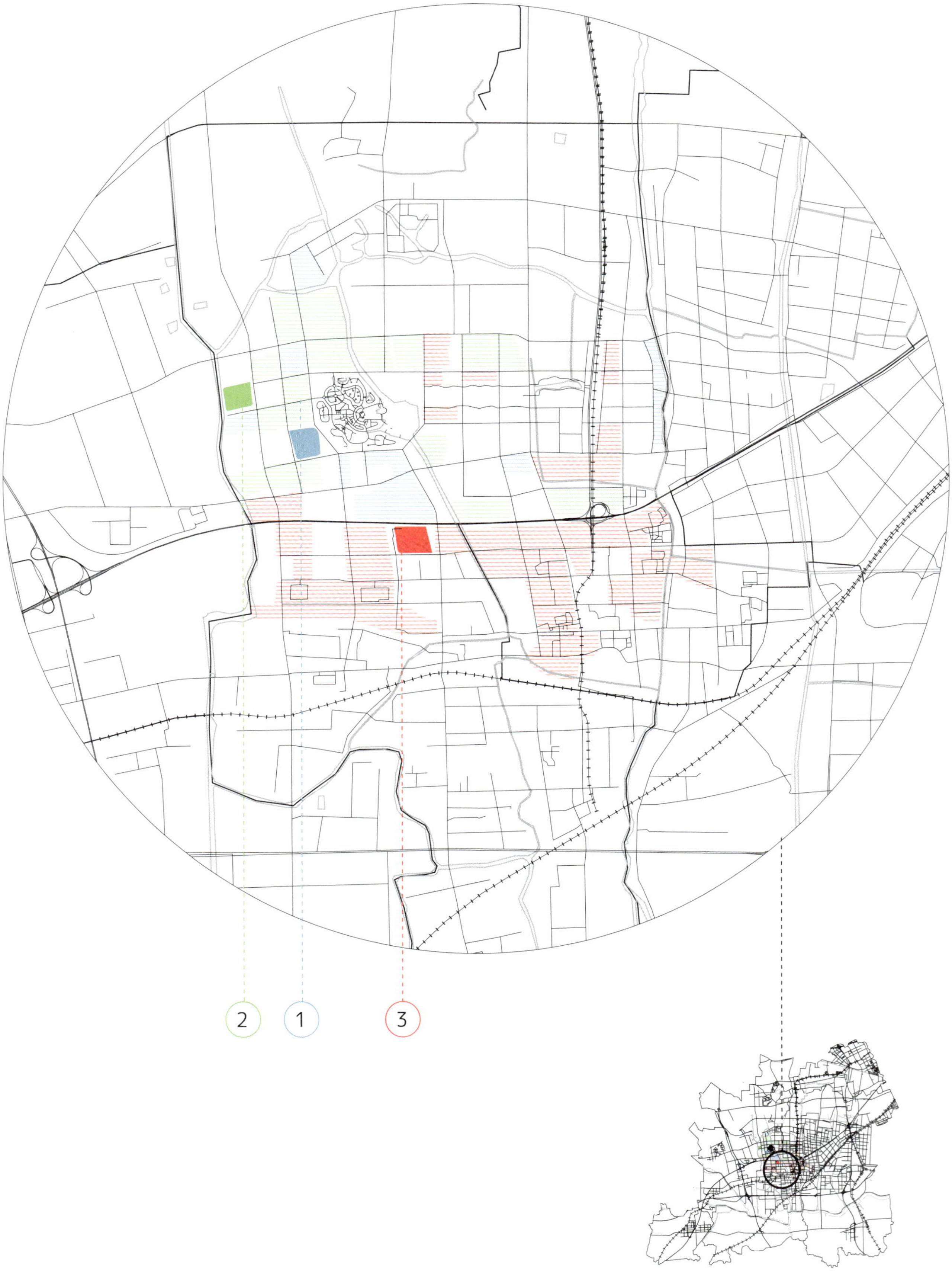
2
1
3

Design Research Process and Visualization

The prototype design research was predicated on a general aim to provide a series of guides, tools, and findings that may inform the design and renovation of newbuild as well as existing neighborhood blocks in China. The team identified a sample city, Songjiang, located on the periphery of Shanghai as a suitable model and proxy for cities in China. Its role as a secondary city to Shanghai provided an appropriate model for second- and third-tier cities, as well as towns, which are projected to be the areas of more significant growth and transformation in the future. By offering alternatives for how these cities may urbanize, we may also offer guidance on the future urbanization and reurbanization of the country.

We identified three main types of neighborhood block developments in new Songjiang city that were found to be the most repeated types. These constituted the main, normative development models for many of China's new towns and cities. The team chose to analyze and work from these models for three main reasons:

- Their configurations were standard and typical of many similar cities in China. The typical superblock configuration (around 400 meters by 400 meters) provided the appropriate scale in which the team believed it could focus in detail, yet still have the critical mass to consider it on the neighborhood scale (an area equivalent to eight Boston Back Bay blocks).
- By offering alternatives, or design transformations to these models, the team also recognized that it would provide guides on both newly built neighborhood blocks as well as ways in which existing blocks may be renovated and transformed to better perform in relation to a range of key health concerns.
- Finally, it was determined that the study and analysis of existing models and practices would also inform the implementability of the team's proposals as it would allow us to identify and integrate a range of existing practices and constraints (such as sunshine laws, fire regulations, and developmental standards) that would also help guide the project more specifically with regard to its capacity to be implemented within China's current development and construction culture.

Each type was analyzed and evaluated in relation to a number of important health indicators from the HAPI Health Impact Assessment in order to ascertain the existing strengths of the block configurations, as well as their shortcomings.

1 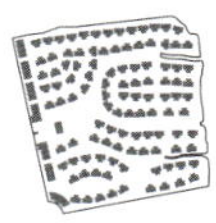

BLOCK TYPE 1: VILLA TYPE
Single family mix

2 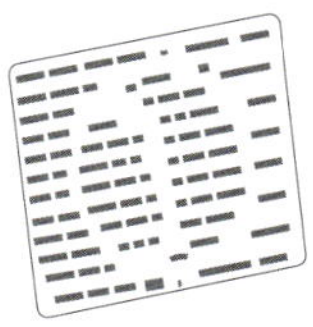

BLOCK TYPE 2: MIXED RESIDENTIAL A
Single family and apartment block mix

3 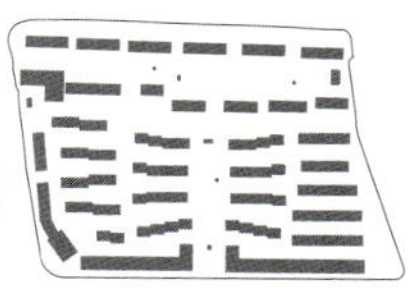

BLOCK TYPE 3: MIXED RESIDENTIAL B
Apartment block and high-rise mix

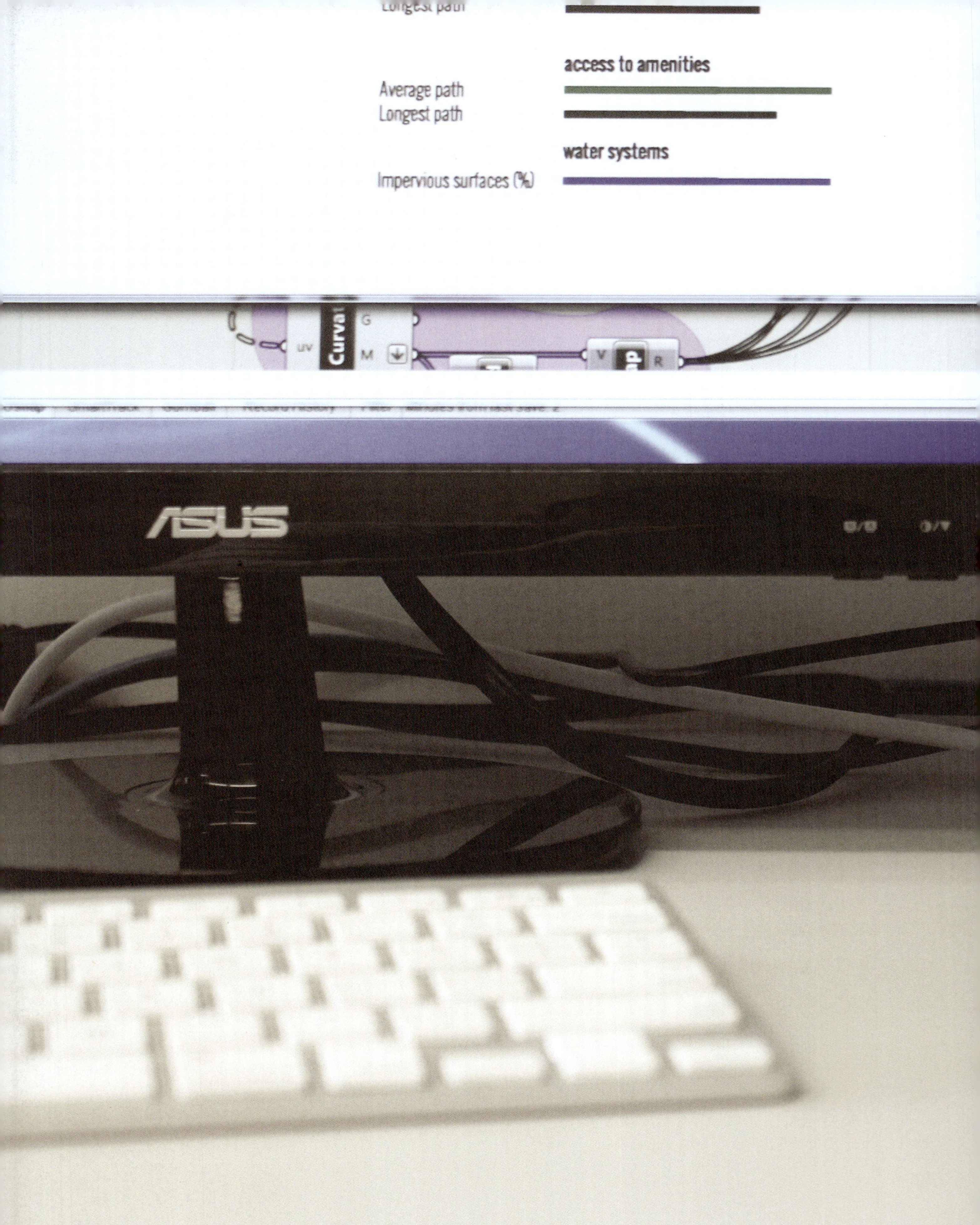

Photograph by Justin Kollar

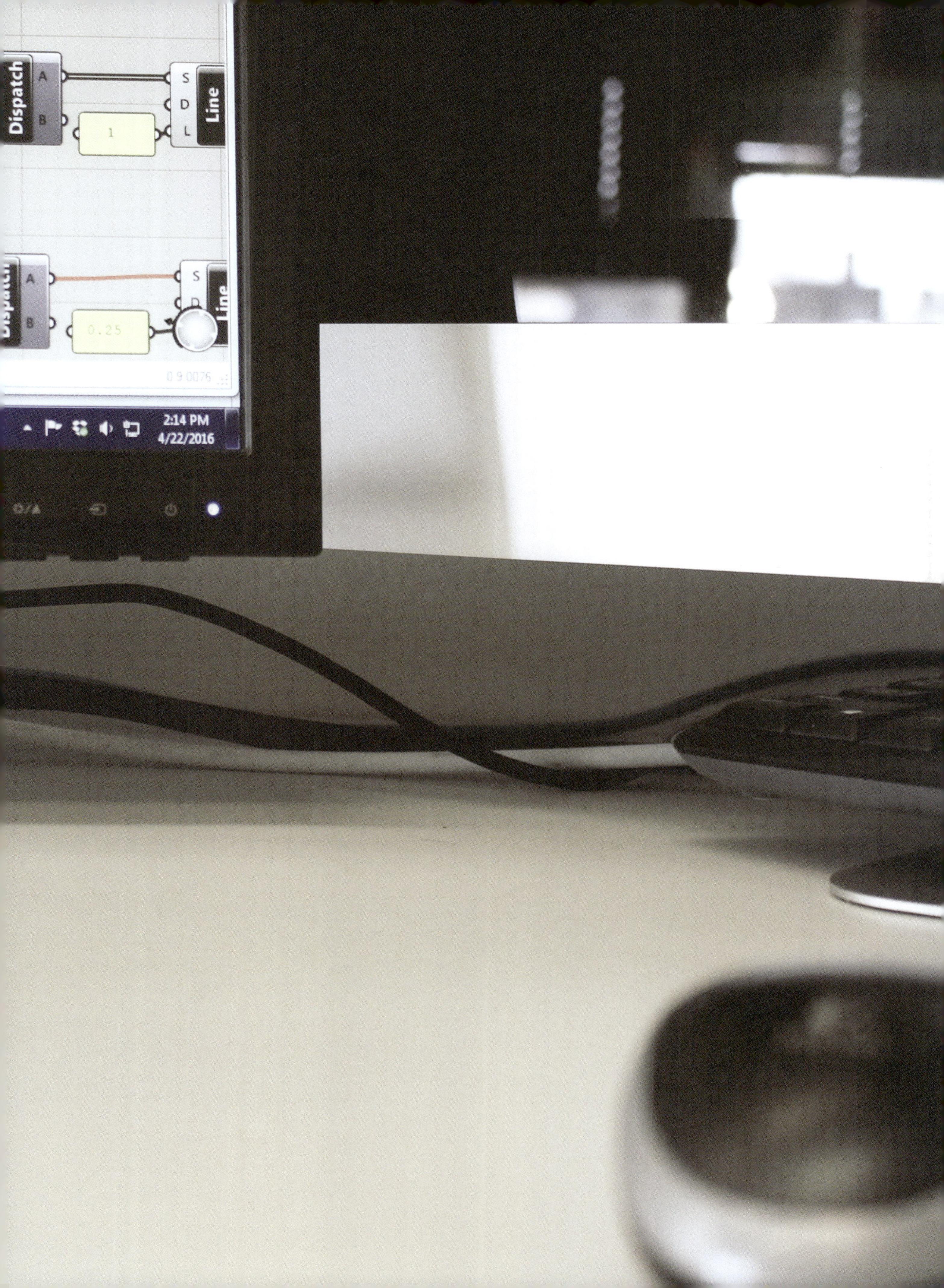
Dispatch
A
B
S
D
L
Line
1
0.25
2:14 PM
4/22/2016

Analysis: Songjiang Case Study

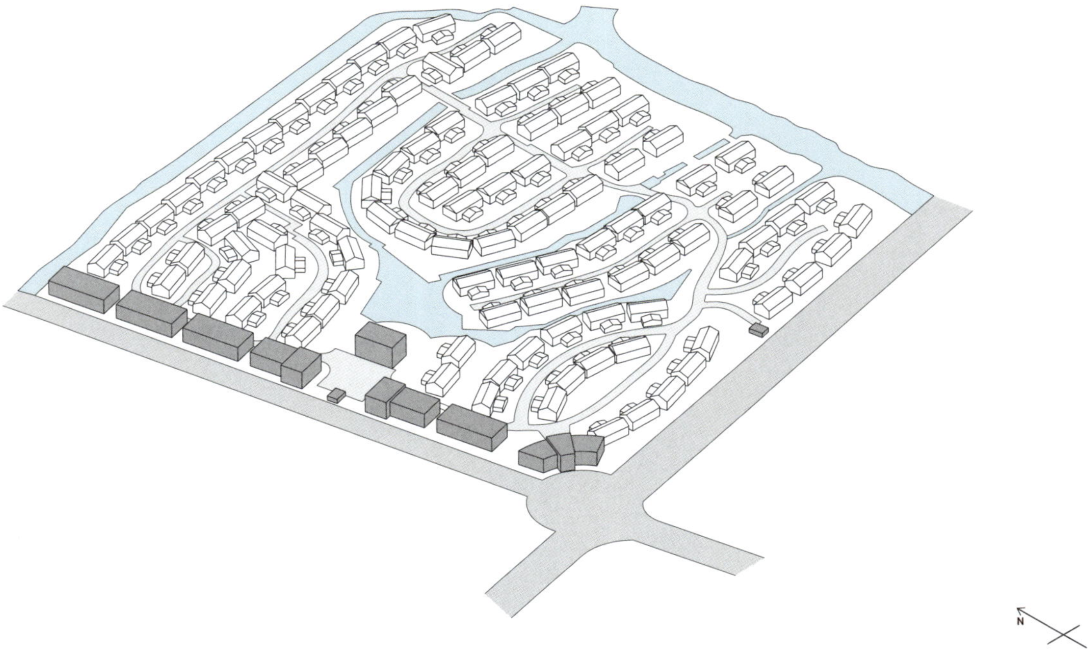

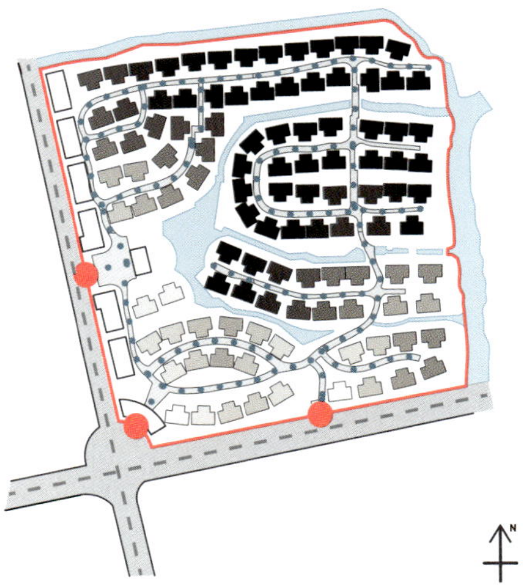

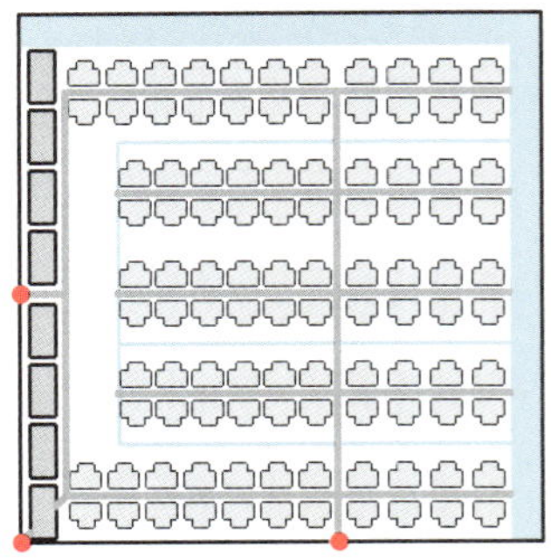

BLOCK TYPE **1**: VILLA TYPE

Site dimensions	400x400m
Site area	142,000 sq.m.
FAR	x
Population - estimate	~430*
Density	x
Total number of buildings	108
Built area	41,000 sq.m.

* assumption: average household size: 4

The villa neighborhood block utilizes detached single family or multi-family villas as the dominant building types. It is low density and approximates the suburban models found in many western countries. The typology has since come under scrutiny and has been largely abandoned or discouraged as a model of development. Though performing well in relation to open space provisions, overall it performs poorly in relation to walkability, access to amenities, and mixed uses among others. All block types were converted to a more normalized associative model. This allowed the team to generate a wide range of block organizations, that may act as normalized models, by adjusting variables of the organization structure.

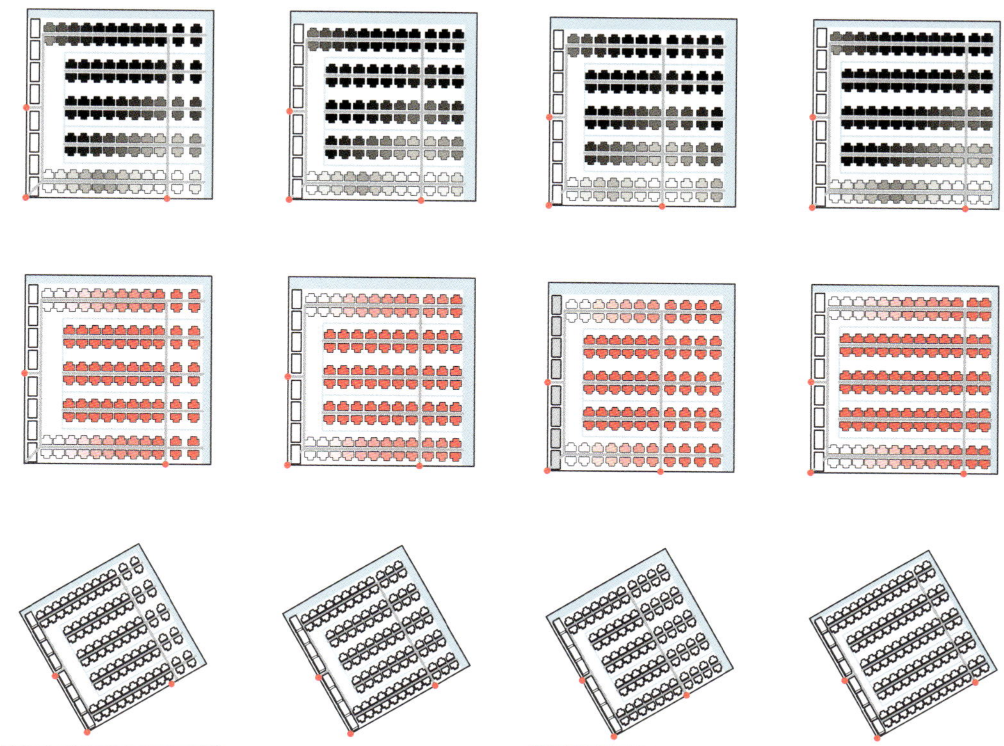

1B.00 **1B**.02 **1B**.04 **1B**.09

	1B.00	**1B**.02	**1B**.04	**1B**.09
Required Parking Lots	216	216	208	248
Ratio Lots/Units	2	2	2	2
steepness %				
street network length	2337	2309	2309	2424
intersections	10	10	10	10
direct path/detour %	67	68	68	65
long path-car (m)	1.2	1.1	1.1	1.3
long path-cycling (m)	1.8	1.7	1.7	2
long path-adult (m)	5.7	5.4	5.4	6.3
long path-older adult (m)	7.5	7.2	7.2	8.3
long path	476	457	456	526
avg path-car (m)	0.6	0.6	0.6	0.7
avg path-cycling (m)	1	0.9	0.9	1
avg path-adult (m)	3	2.9	2.9	3.2
avg path-older adult (m)	4	3.9	3.8	4.3
avg path	256	247	244	272
Units/Acre	2.73	2.73	2.63	3.14
OpenSpace/Person	67.21	63.24	66.06	58.01
Impervious Srfs %	34.96	34.85	34.03	38.57
Roads %	8.77	8.66	8.66	9.09
Open Spaces %	54.12	50.92	51.74	51.8
Amenities %	4	4	4	4
Mixed Use %				
Residential %	22.19	22.19	21.37	25.48
Population	1288	1288	1253	1429
No of Units	108	108	104	124
Coverage %	26.19	26.19	25.37	29.48
No of Buildings	116	116	112	132
FAR	0.6	0.6	0.59	0.67
Total GFA	96622	96622	93992	107144
Block area	160000	160000	160000	160000

1B.00 **1B**.02 **1B**.04 **1B**.09

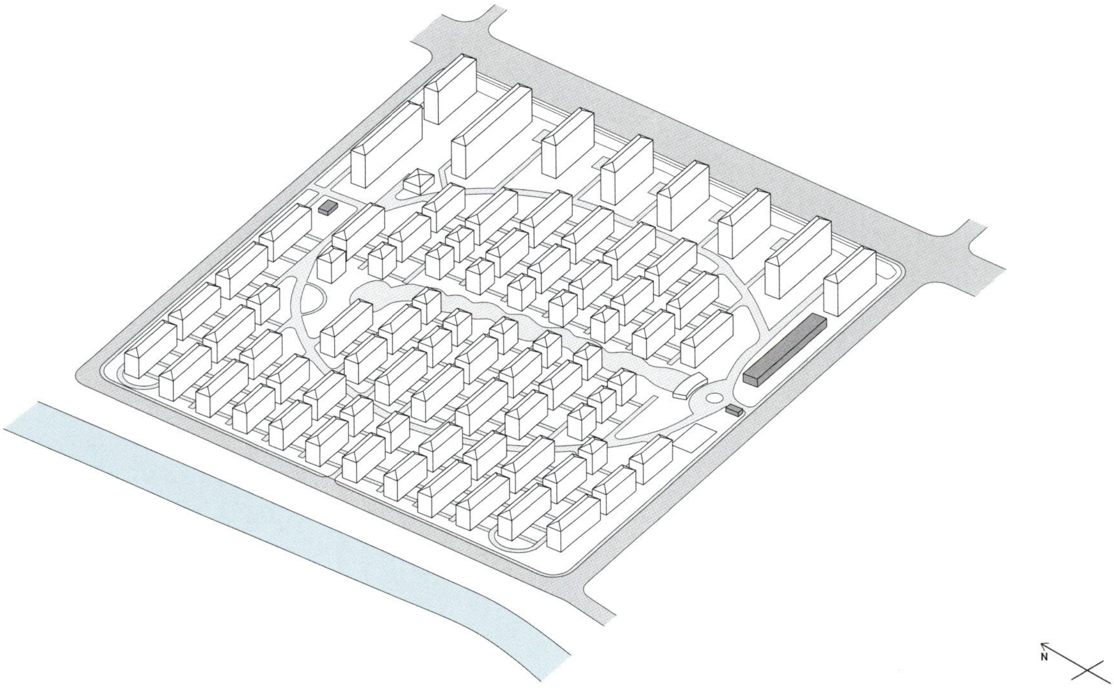

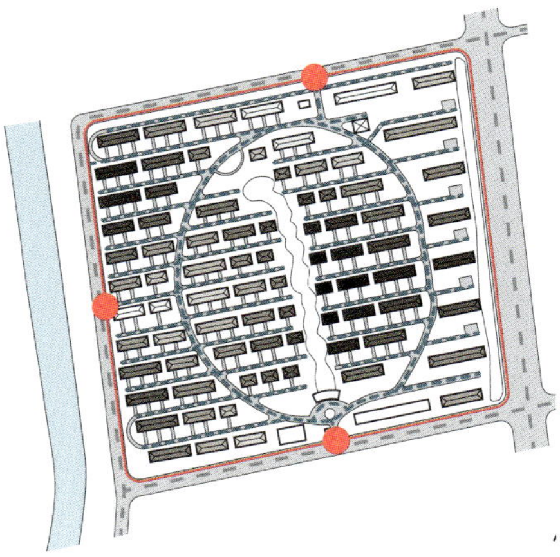

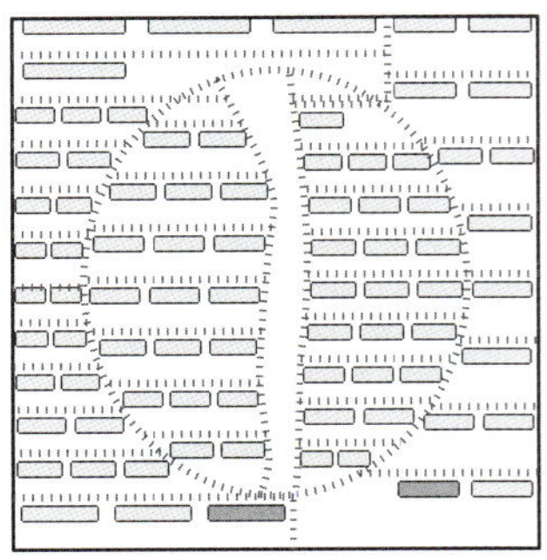

BLOCK TYPE **2**: MIXED RESIDENTIAL **A**

Site dimensions	355x390m
Site area	136,863 sq.m.
FAR	1.07
Population - estimate	~930*
Density	x
Total number of buidlings	82
Built area	27,970 sq.m.

* assumption: average household size: 4

Block type 2 is a mixed building type residential block with a range of slab buildings of varying heights. The slabs are arranged in a repetitive manner with a consistent East-West orientation, in accordance with an optimal arrangement for the Chinese "sunshine" law. There are slight variations in open space types based on the different building heights and their corresponding distances determined by the "sunshine" law. As with all the block types, these were normalized to a more "standard" configuration and converted in to an associative model that allowed for variations in their organizations to be generated and evaluated for their performance in relation to health associated parameters.

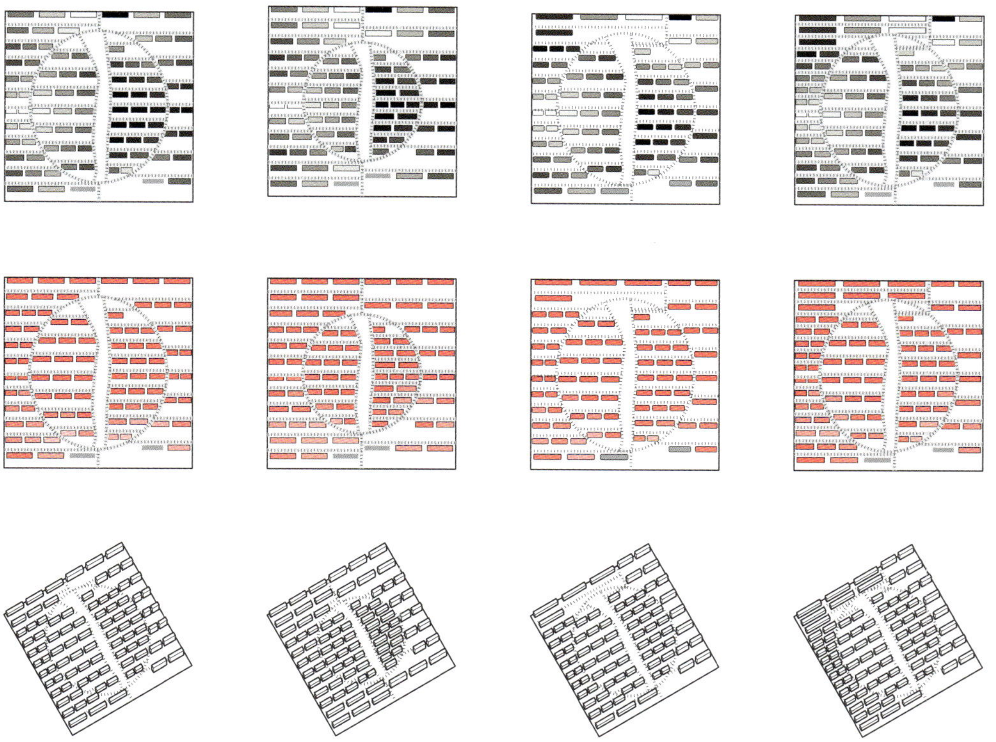

2B.00 **2B**.03 **2B**.05 **2B**.06

	2B.00	**2B**.03	**2B**.05	**2B**.06
Required Parking Lots	894	1002	866	963
Ratio Lots/Units	0.5	0.5	0.5	0.5
steepness %				
street network length	4551	4761	4787	5232
intersections	37	37	37	40
direct path/detour %	69	69	69	70
long path-car (m)	0.9	0.9	0.9	0.9
long path-cycling (m)	1.4	1.3	1.3	1.3
long path-adult (m)	4.5	4.2	4.1	4.1
long path-older adult (m)	5.9	5.5	5.4	5.4
long path	377	350	345	345
avg path-car (m)	0.5	0.5	0.5	0.5
avg path-cycling (m)	0.7	0.7	0.7	0.7
avg path-adult (m)	2.4	2.3	2.3	2.2
avg path-older adult (m)	3.1	3.1	3	2.9
avg path	199	197	190	185
Units/Acre	45.25	50.69	43.78	48.71
OpenSpace/Person	46.16	39.64	47.22	40.04
Impervious Srfs %	35.63	38.13	36.17	40.03
Roads %	17.07	17.85	17.95	19.62
Open Spaces %	64.37	61.87	63.83	59.97
Amenities %	0.62	0.67	0.63	0.63
Mixed Use %				
Residential %	17.94	19.61	17.59	19.78
Population	5033	5637	4869	5417
No of Units	1789	2004	1731	1926
Coverage %	18.56	20.28	18.22	20.41
No of Buildings	89	86	82	88
FAR	1.05	1.17	1.01	1.12
Total GFA	167333	187309	162203	179744
Block area	160000	160000	160000	160000

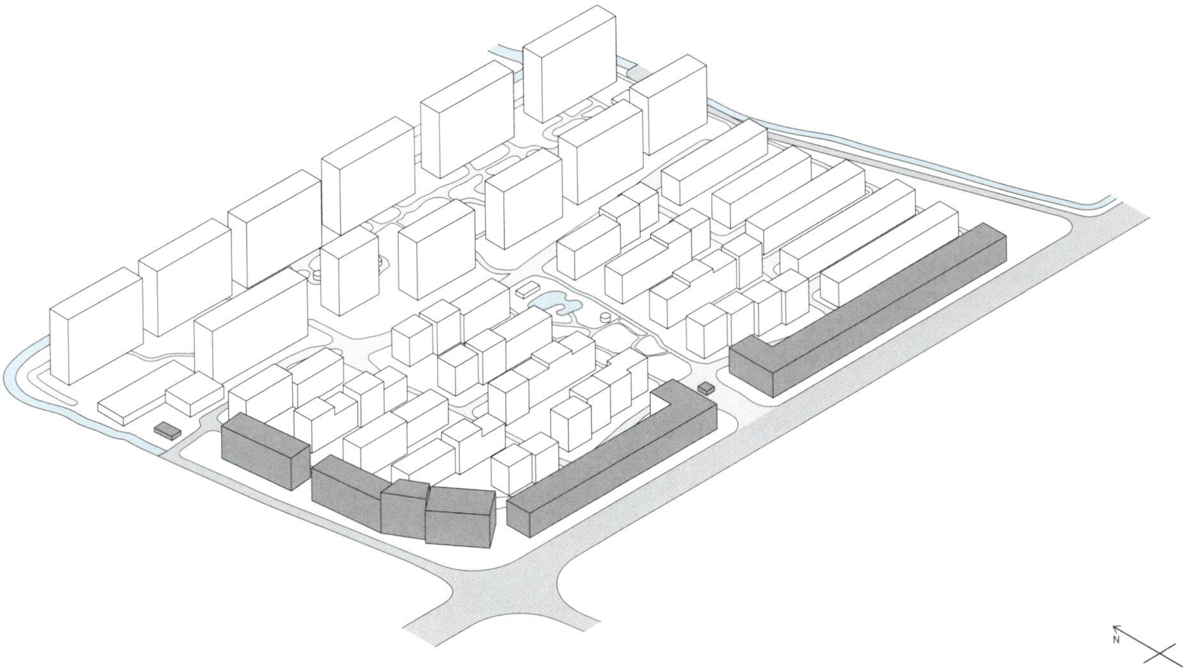

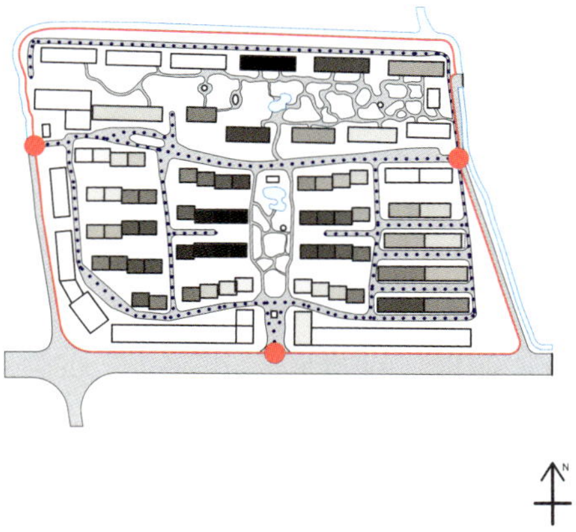

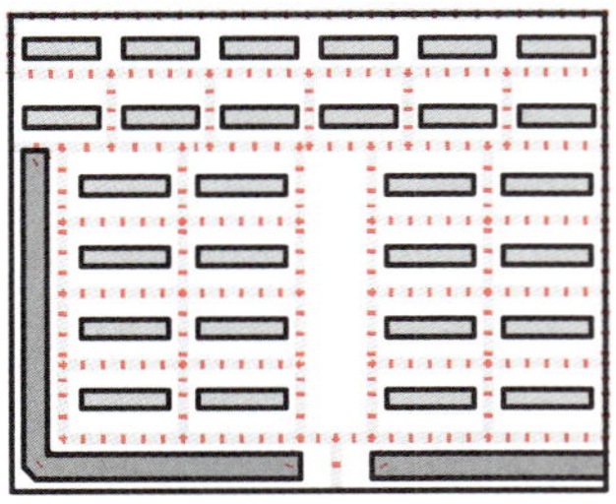

BLOCK TYPE **3**: MIXED RESIDENTIAL **B**

Site dimensions	460x365m
Site area	173,163 sq.m.
FAR	1.60
Population - estimate	~930*
Density	x
Total number of buidlings	82
Built area	27,970 sq.m.

* assumption: average household size: 4

This block type has a more varied range of building types. This resulted in a slightly more differentiated open space pattern and higher density than the other block types. A border of amenity and retail buildings are integrated within the block, adding a higher mix of uses than the other blocks. This was, as with all other block types, normalized in to an associative model and tested for health-based parameters. Out of all three blocks, this type offered the best range of performances.

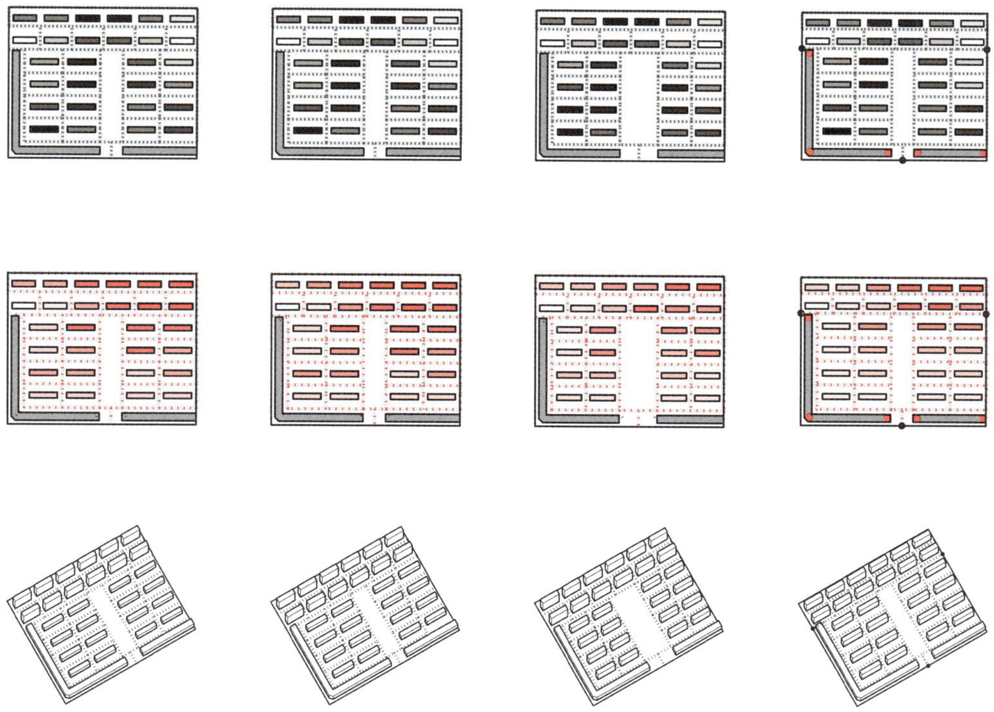

3B.00 | 3B.04 | 3B.09 | 3B.12

	3B.00	3B.04	3B.09	3B.12
Required Parking Lots	1591	1690	1885	1785
Ratio Lots/Units	0.5	0.5	0.5	0.5
steepness %				
street network length	5107	5107	4987	5129
intersections	40	40	40	40
direct path/detour %	80	80	79	80
long path-car (m)	0.7	0.7	0.7	0.7
long path-cycling (m)	1	1	1	1.1
long path-adult (m)	3.3	3.3	3.2	3.4
long path-older adult (m)	4.3	4.3	4.3	4.5
long path	275	275	270	285
avg path-car (m)	0.5	0.5	0.5	0.5
avg path-cycling (m)	0.7	0.7	0.7	0.7
avg path-adult (m)	2.2	2.2	2.3	2.2
avg path-older adult (m)	3	3	3	2.9
avg path	187	187	194	183
Units/Acre	65.20	69.24	77.25	73.15
OpenSpace/Person	33.73	31.7	29.2	30
Impervious Srfc %	34.7	34.7	33.1	34.7
Roads %	15.5	15.5	15.1	15.5
Open Spaces %	65.3	65.3	66.9	65.3
Amenities %	4.2	4.2	3.9	4.2
Mixed Use %				
Residential %	15	15	14.1	15
Population	8949	9503	10603	10041
No of Units	3182	3379	3770	3570
Coverage %	19.2	19.2	17.9	19.2
No of Buildings	30	30	30	30
FAR	1.86	1.95	2.1	2.04
Total GFA	367920	385650	416040	404520
Block area	197500	197500	197500	197500

3B.00 | 3B.04 | 3B.09 | 3B.12

	1B.00	1B.02	1B.04	1B.09	2B.00	2B.03	2B.05	2B.06	3B.00	3B.04	3B.09	3B.12
Required Parking Lots	216	216	208	248	894	1002	866	963	1591	1690	1885	1785
Ratio Lots/Units	2	2	2	2	0.5	0.5	0.5	0.5	0.5	0.5	0.5	0.5
steepness %												
street network length	2337	2309	2309	2424	4551	4761	4787	5232	5107	5107	4987	5129
intersections	10	10	10	10	37	37	37	40	40	40	40	40
direct path/detour %	67	68	68	65	69	69	69	70	80	80	79	80
long path-car (m)	1.2	1.1	1.1	1.3	0.9	0.9	0.9	0.9	0.7	0.7	0.7	0.7
long path-cycling (m)	1.8	1.7	1.7	2	1.4	1.3	1.3	1.3	1	1	1	1.1
long path-adult (m)	5.7	5.4	5.4	6.3	4.5	4.2	4.1	4.1	3.3	3.3	3.2	3.4
long path-older adult (m)	7.5	7.2	7.2	8.3	5.9	5.5	5.4	5.4	4.3	4.3	4.3	4.5
long path	476	457	456	526	377	350	345	345	275	275	270	285
avg path-car (m)	0.6	0.6	0.6	0.7	0.5	0.5	0.5	0.5	0.5	0.5	0.5	0.5
avg path-cycling (m)	1	0.9	0.9	1	0.7	0.7	0.7	0.7	0.7	0.7	0.7	0.7
avg path-adult (m)	3	2.9	2.9	3.2	2.4	2.3	2.3	2.2	2.2	2.2	2.3	2.2
avg path-older adult (m)	4	3.9	3.8	4.3	3.1	3.1	3	2.9	3	3	3	2.9
avg path	256	247	244	272	199	197	190	185	187	187	194	183
Units/Acre	2.73	2.73	2.63	3.14	45.25	50.69	43.78	48.71	65.20	69.24	77.25	73.15
OpenSpace/Person	67.21	63.24	66.06	58.01	46.16	39.64	47.22	40.04	33.73	31.7	29.2	30
Impervious Srfs %	34.96	34.85	34.03	38.57	35.63	38.13	36.17	40.03	34.7	34.7	33.1	34.7
Roads %	8.77	8.66	8.66	9.09	17.07	17.85	17.95	19.62	15.5	15.5	15.1	15.5
Open Spaces %	54.12	50.92	51.74	51.8	64.37	61.87	63.83	59.97	65.3	65.3	66.9	65.3
Amenities %	4	4	4	4	0.62	0.67	0.63	0.63	4.2	4.2	3.9	4.2
Mixed Use %												
Residential %	22.19	22.19	21.37	25.48	17.94	19.61	17.59	19.78	15	15	14.1	15
Population	1288	1288	1253	1429	5033	5637	4869	5417	8949	9503	10603	10041
No of Units	108	108	104	124	1789	2004	1731	1926	3182	3379	3770	3570
Coverage %	26.19	26.19	25.37	29.48	18.56	20.28	18.22	20.41	19.2	19.2	17.9	19.2
No of Buildings	116	116	112	132	89	86	82	88	30	30	30	30
FAR	0.6	0.6	0.59	0.67	1.05	1.17	1.01	1.12	1.86	1.95	2.1	2.04
Total GFA	96622	96622	93992	107144	167333	187309	162203	179744	367920	385650	416040	404520
Block area	160000	160000	160000	160000	160000	160000	160000	160000	197500	197500	197500	197500

(Left) A range of iterations of all three block types were generated and analyzed. These were subsequently evaluated according to a wide spectrum of health-related parameters. A comparative analysis was organized into an extensive matrix, of which a portion is represented here.

The three types identified as the dominant models of neighborhood superblock developments in Songjiang were studied in order to evaluate their relative performance in relation to health concerns (which were informed by a number of parallel research projects conducted within the Harvard GSD HAPI group. These included design briefs and Health Impact Assessments [HIA] developed by Professor Ann Forsyth's team, and the survey and study of Chinese neighborhoods conducted by Professor Peter Rowe's team). This study of existing models was conducted so that the prototypes research team could locate the qualities and organizational specifics of the existing block types which performed well, while also allowing for the identification of factors that were detrimental to healthy practices. It allowed the team to make informed judgments on the existing block type's suitability, resulting in the team choosing to focus its subsequent research on the mixed residential types, eliminating the villa block type for its poor function.

The comparative matrix visualized a larger consideration for the design research project, which was the acknowledgment of the wide array of factors that affect or contribute to health-related performance in places. While these initial evaluations were restricted to quantifiable indicators and parameters, it was already clear that, while it was easy to identify a range of block configurations that performed well or satisfactory across all criteria, it was not possible to locate an optimized iteration that was absolutely optimal for all criteria. In fact, it is unlikely that all categories had clear optimizable solutions. It is likely that many parameters had conflicting requirements, potentially canceling out the benefits of one criteria when optimizing for another.

So, while associative modeling allowed the team to rapidly generate a large sample of these blocks very quickly, it was not possible to find a totally optimized version overall. However, the benefit of the use of associative design techniques was the capacity to generate a wider range of blocks that provided a good and abundant study sample, as well as a rich collection of design options.

Following this initial assessment, the research team proceeded to analyze various aspects of the block organization in discrete steps, building complexity through an iterative and incremental process, with regular feedback and recursive steps.

Entrances + Accessibility

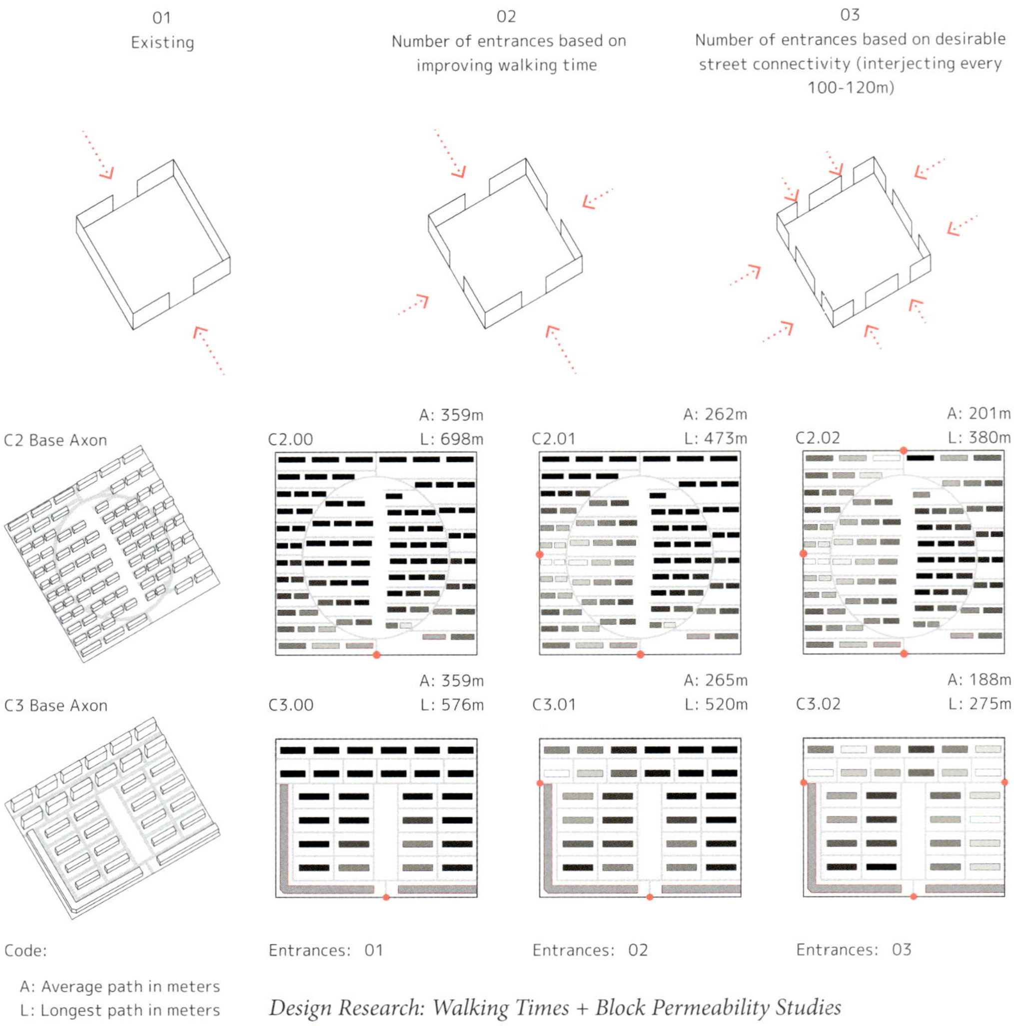

Design Research: Walking Times + Block Permeability Studies

One of the well-known criticisms of recent neighborhood block developments in China is the propensity to develop "superblocks" of roughly 400m x 400m dimensions with very low permeability. These often borrow from gated community models. Walled neighborhoods and domestic spaces also have a tradition in Chinese urbanization. This can be seen to discourage pedestrian activity as the distances people have to traverse on foot in order to move through and between the blocks can be significant enough to discourage people from walking. When studying the effects of increasing the permeability (or the number of entrances) of the perimeter of the typical neighborhood blocks, one of the aspects that we studied was the relationship between the number of entries and the average, as well as the longest distances between all the buildings in the block and the entrances.

Through the associative models, we were able to evaluate these values relative to a series of incremental scenarios that would involve a gradual insertion of entries in the block's perimeter. A color gradient was attached to the buildings in order to visualize the range of distances within the block, while the two distance variables were tracked and recorded as a graph for all the generated scenarios.

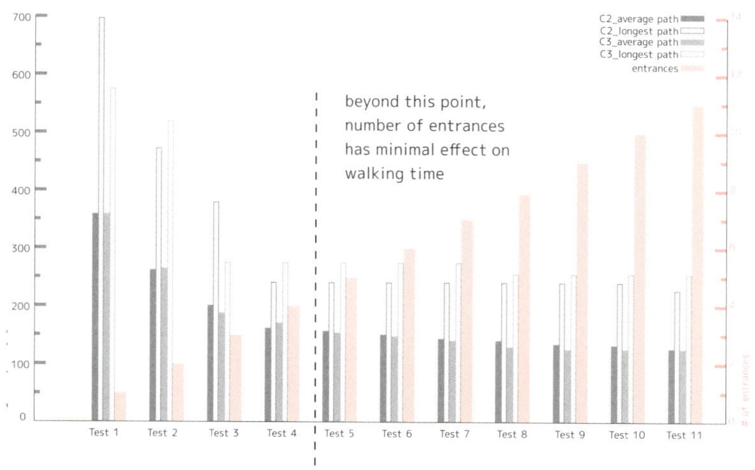

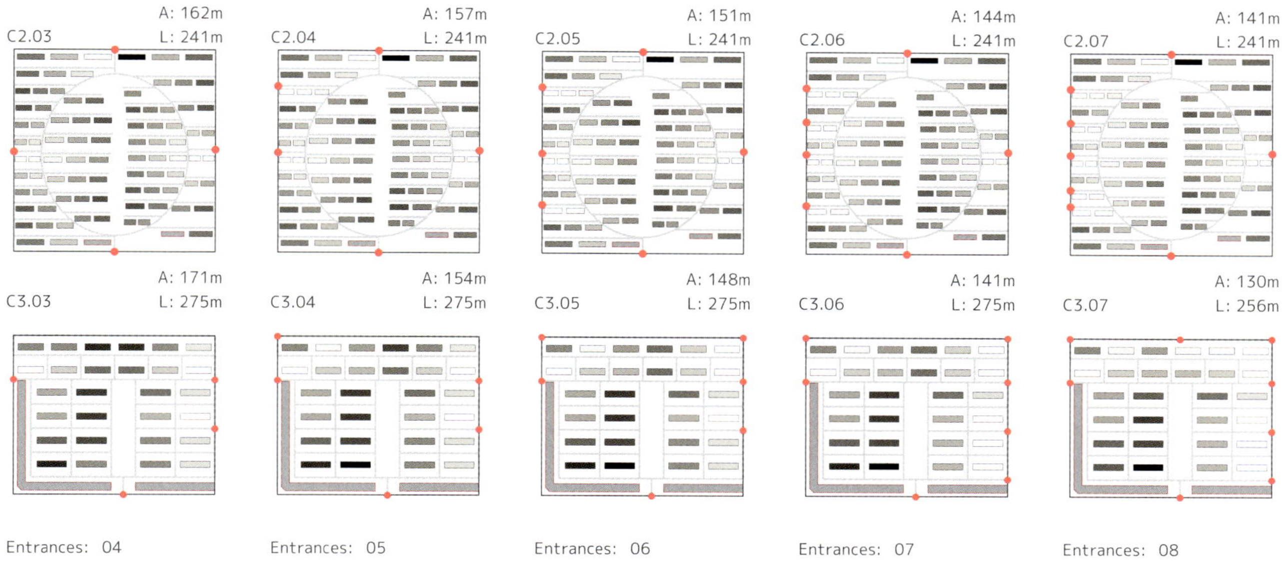

The resulting graph highlights a pattern in performance which can seem counterintuitive. Typically, it would be assumed that the higher the number of entries, the larger the reduction in walking distances. While this is generally true, we can see that most of the benefit in walking time reduction is achieved in the first four entrances. Beyond this, there are rapidly diminishing returns. While not an optimized solution, we can ascertain that four entrances, strategically placed, is more than sufficient to achieve good walking times, making the block more conducive to pedestrian use. This study offers specific knowledge of the performance of existing block types while also describing the effect that certain design operations (increasing the permeability of the block) may have on walking.

As described in the chapter on design research, the determination of organizational aspects of the block is often made by the evaluation of a number of different criteria. The final determination of an appropriate number of entrances (or a suitable degree of permeability) was not determined by this parameter alone, however, it was only made once an additional concern was considered. When taking into account the desirable street connectivity, a recommendation from extensive literature review and HIA's, it was found that eight entries, equally distributed around the block perimeter was appropriate, but not optimal. This allowed for street connectivity with intersections every 100-120m.

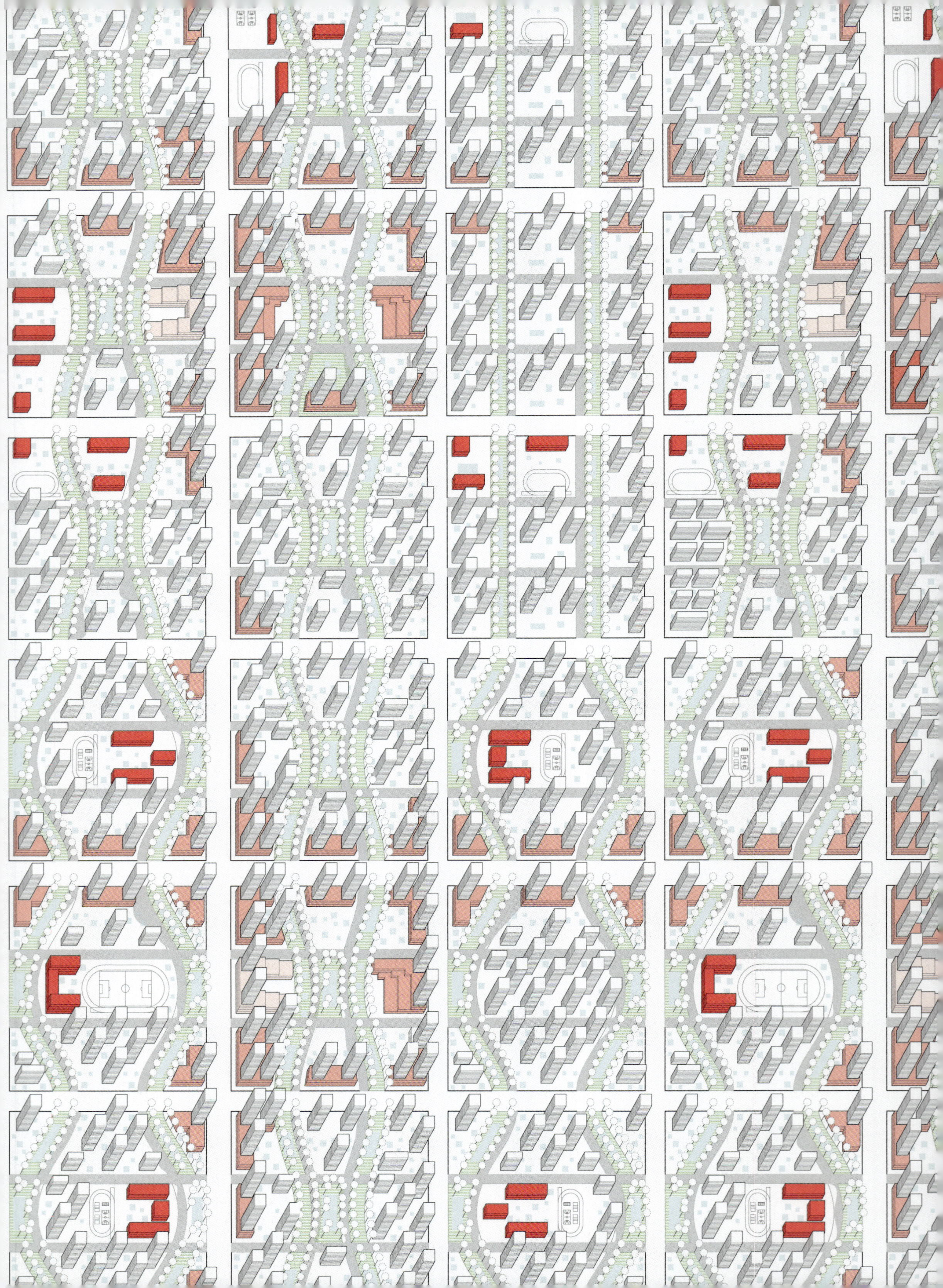

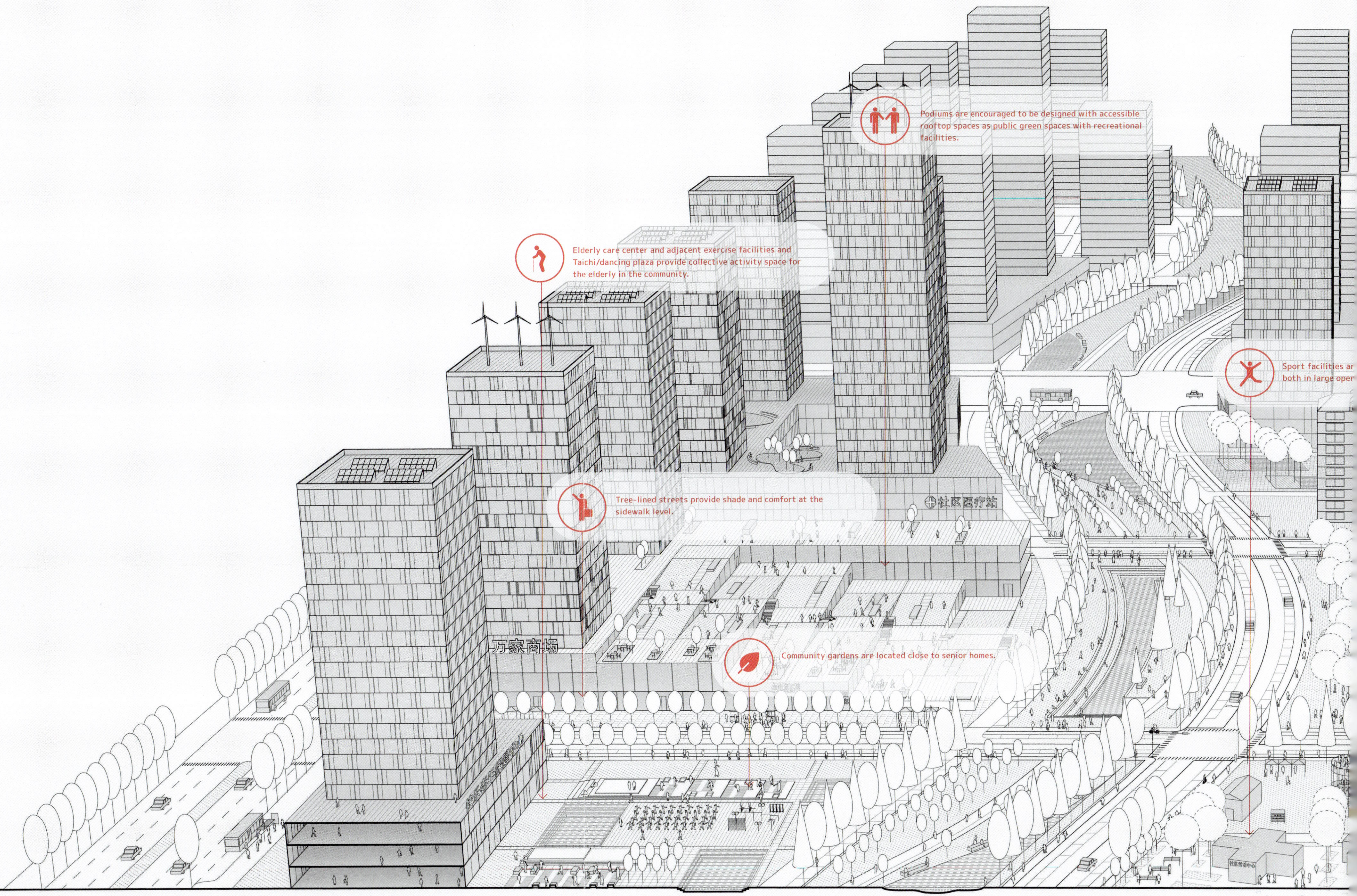
Podiums are encouraged to be designed with accessible rooftop spaces as public green spaces with recreational facilities.
Elderly care center and adjacent exercise facilities and Taichi/dancing plaza provide collective activity space for the elderly in the community.
Sport facilities ar
both in large oper
Tree-lined streets provide shade and comfort at the sidewalk level.
社区医疗站
万家商场
Community gardens are located close to senior homes.

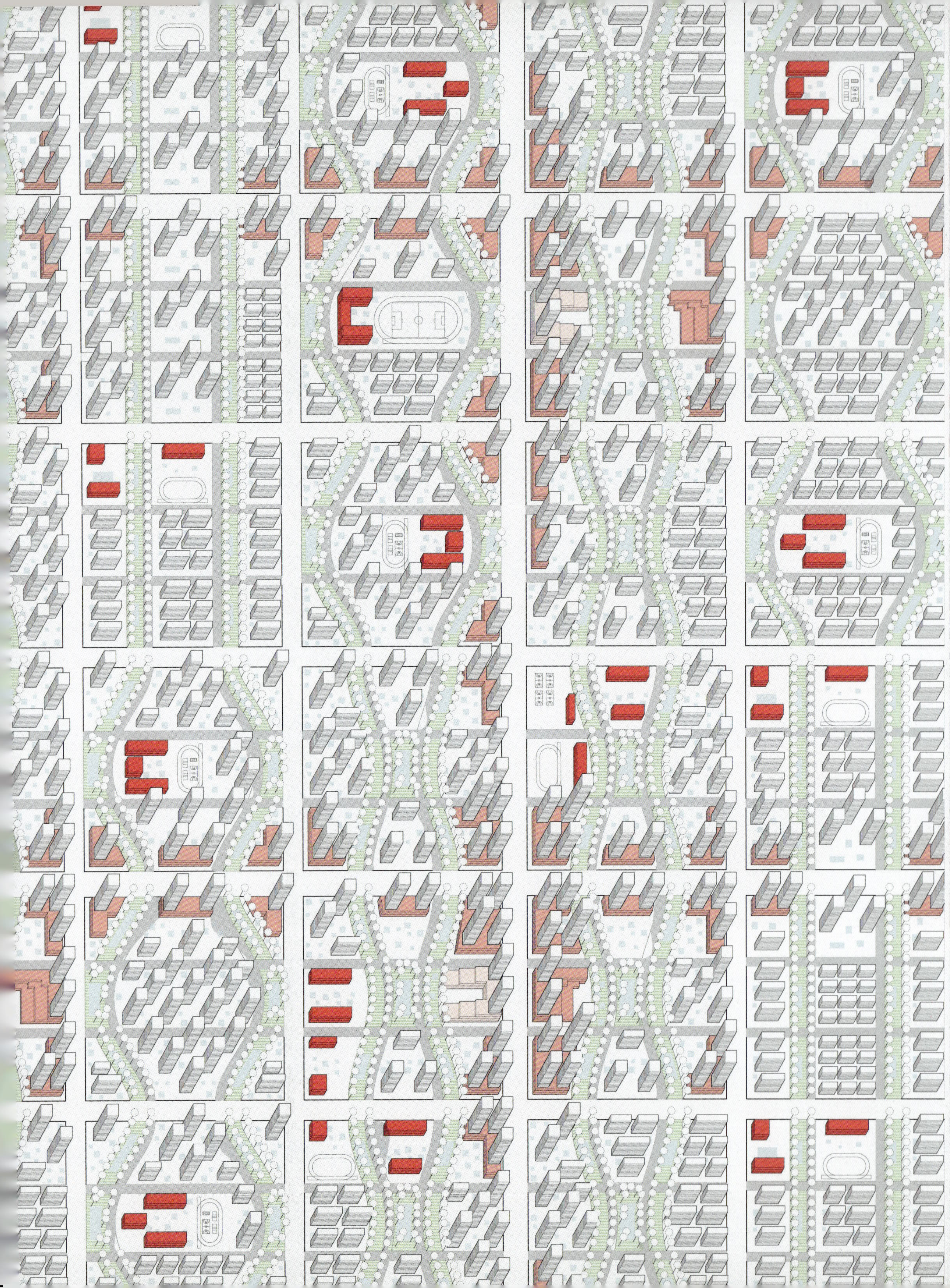

Scenario 1

High-rise, Podium, and Greenway Scenario

The scenario visualized here offers a version of the block that combines high-rise buildings with podium bases that allow for a series of ground conditions which accommodate different social spaces. Accessible podium roof levels allow for street activity to extend, offering a range of different views and experiences for residents and workers. Podiums may adopt courtyard or terrace formatting and help to frame smaller squares and community spaces at the ground level. A large greenway zone provides a significant public space with its own range of microclimates; produced by a careful arrangement of green and blue spaces.

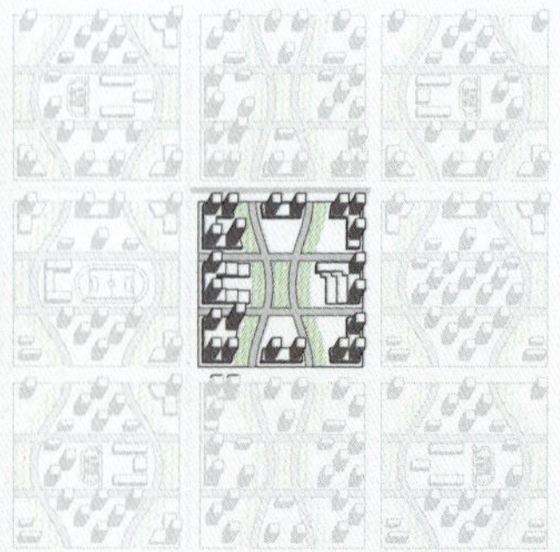

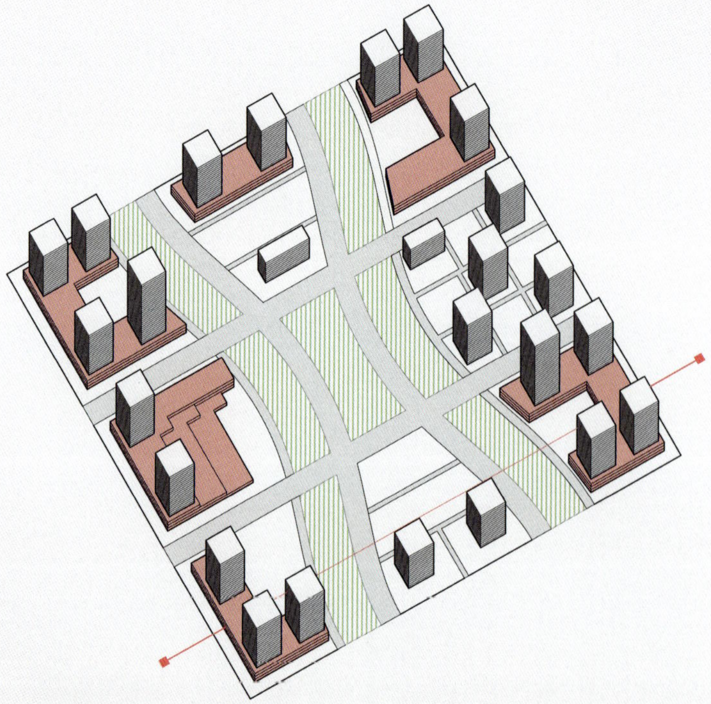

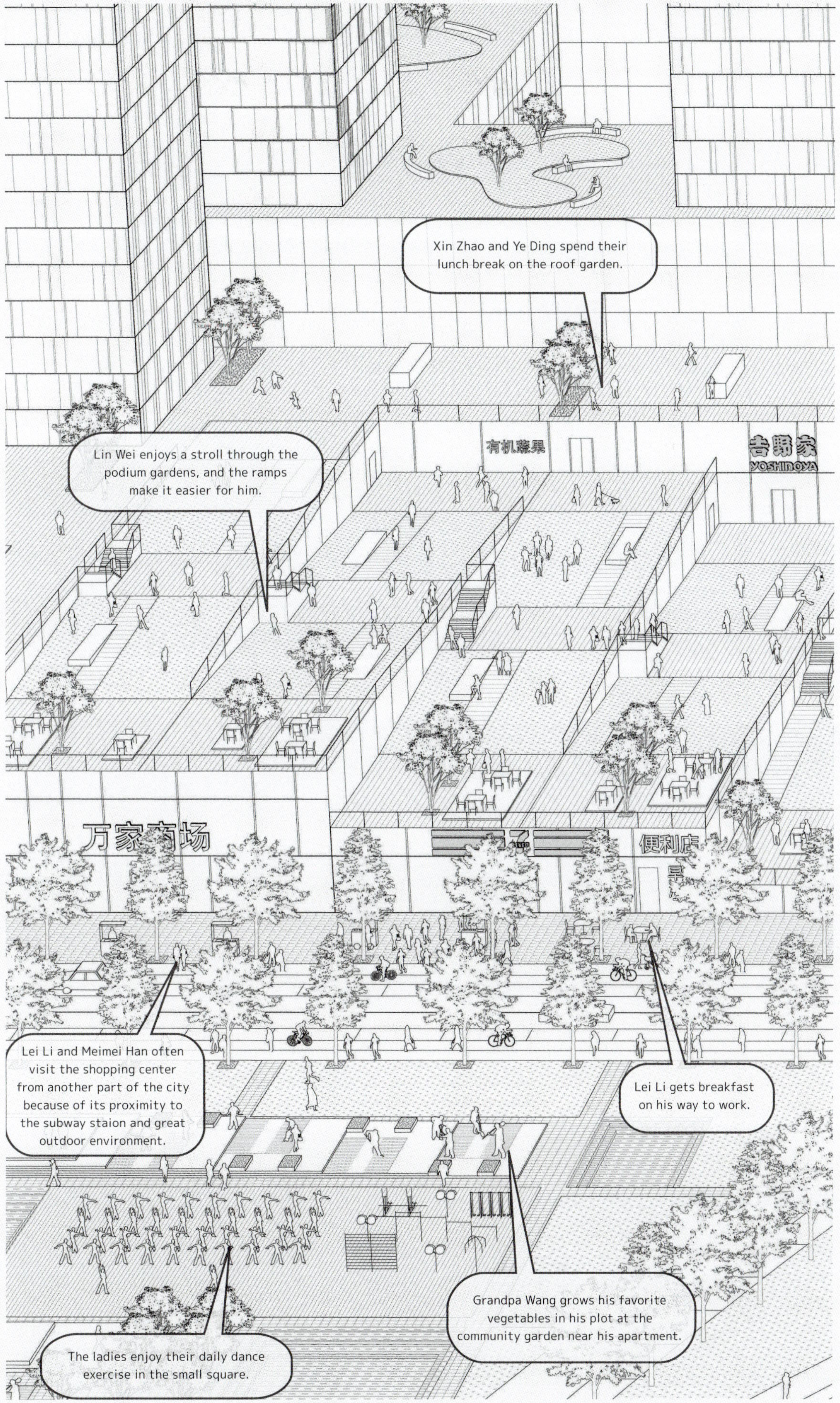

Block Comparisons

Scale comparisons between the typical Chinese (or more specifically, Songjiang) superblock show that it is equivalent to: 15 Midtown Manhattan blocks, 8 Boston Back Bay blocks, or 18 Hong Kong Central District blocks.

To offer a more permeable, walkable, and appropriately scaled urban grain, the team chose to propose subdividing the Chinese superblock.

15 NEW YORK MIDTOWN EAST BLOCKS

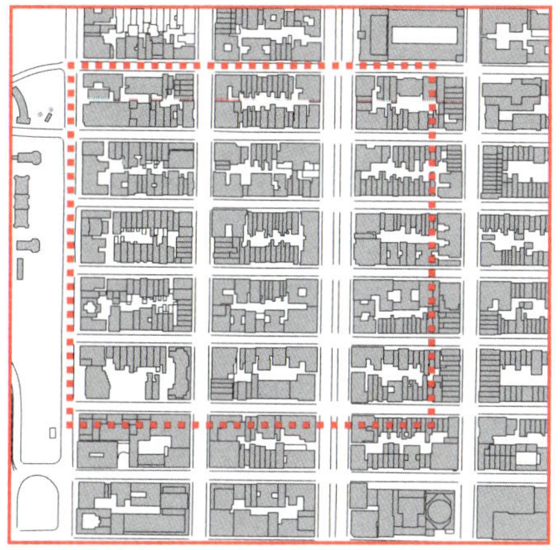

1 SONGJIANG BLOCK

8 BOSTON BACK BAY BLOCKS

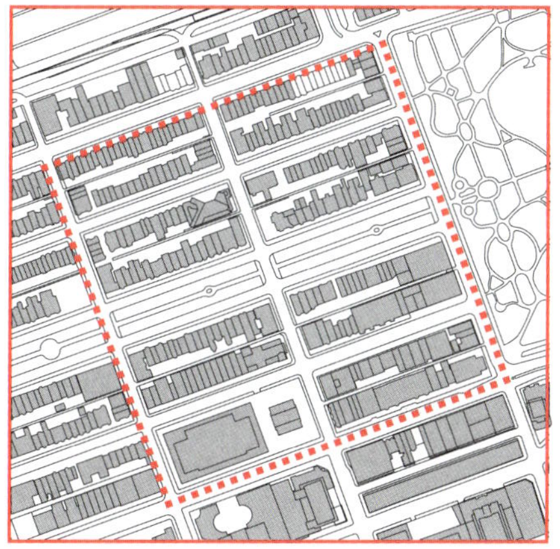

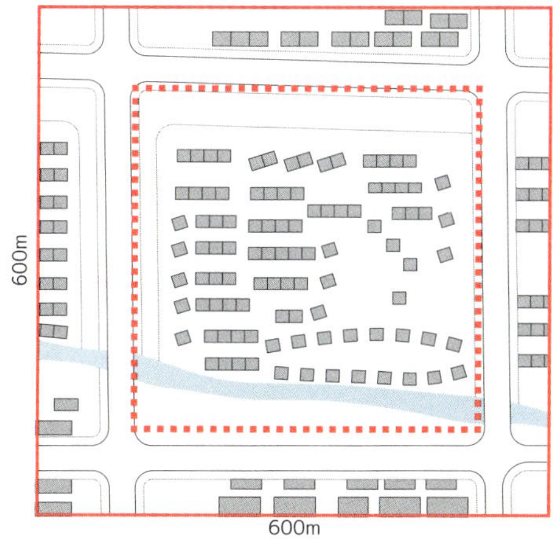

18 HONG KONG CENTRAL DISTRICT BLOCKS

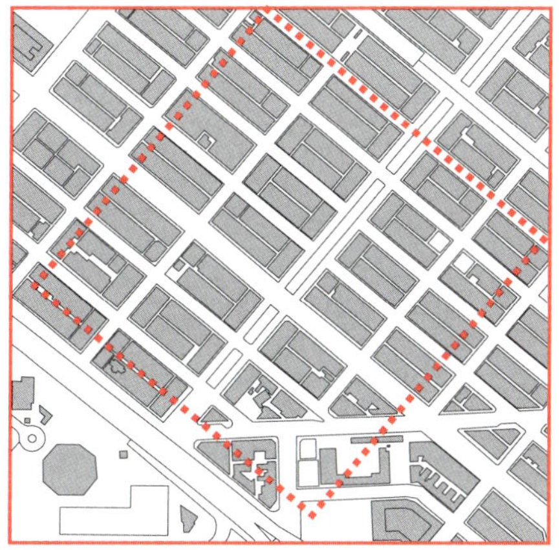

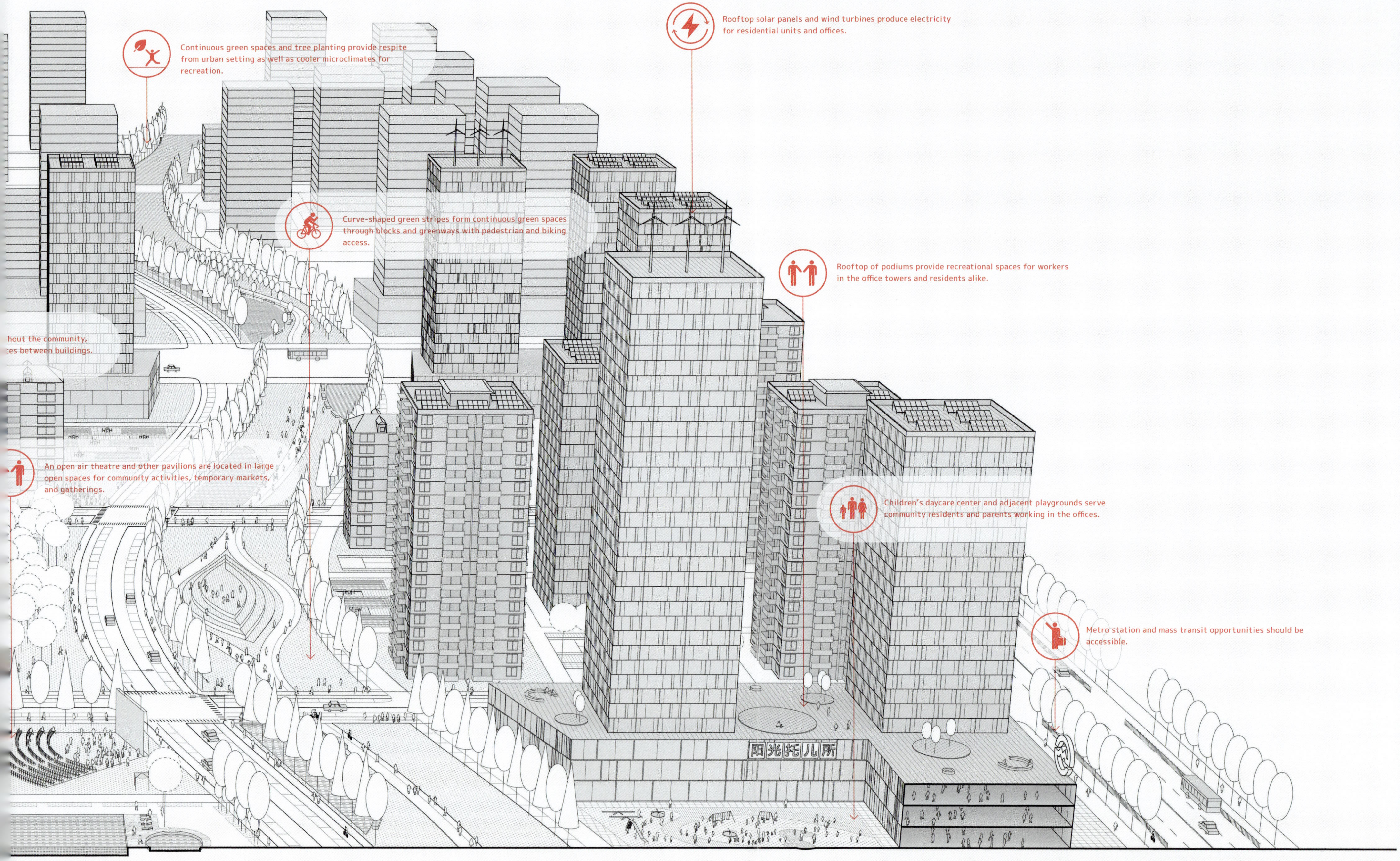
Continuous green spaces and tree planting provide respite from urban setting as well as cooler microclimates for recreation.
Rooftop solar panels and wind turbines produce electricity for residential units and offices.
Curve-shaped green stripes form continuous green spaces through blocks and greenways with pedestrian and biking access.
Rooftop of podiums provide recreational spaces for workers in the office towers and residents alike.
hout the community,
es between buildings.
An open air theatre and other pavilions are located in large open spaces for community activities, temporary markets, and gatherings.
Children's daycare center and adjacent playgrounds serve community residents and parents working in the offices.
Metro station and mass transit opportunities should be accessible.
阳光托儿所

Departing from the existing superblock with its low permeability, the design team chose to adopt an eight-entrance, nine-square grid subdivision as the basis for the next series of design analysis. This accounts for a number of walkability factors, such as walking distances and street connectivity. The next series of analysis and design iterations attempt to integrate an equivalent of nine square meters per person of open green space within the superblock, (as per World Health Organization recommendation), to ensure the provision of appropriate open green spaces for recreation and social activity.

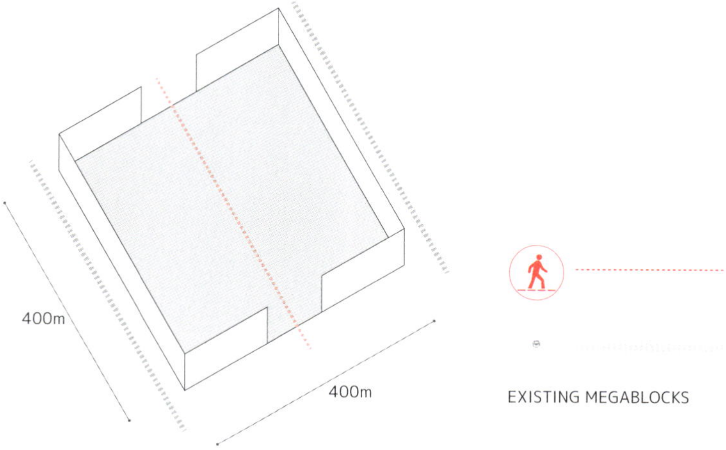

EXISTING MEGABLOCKS

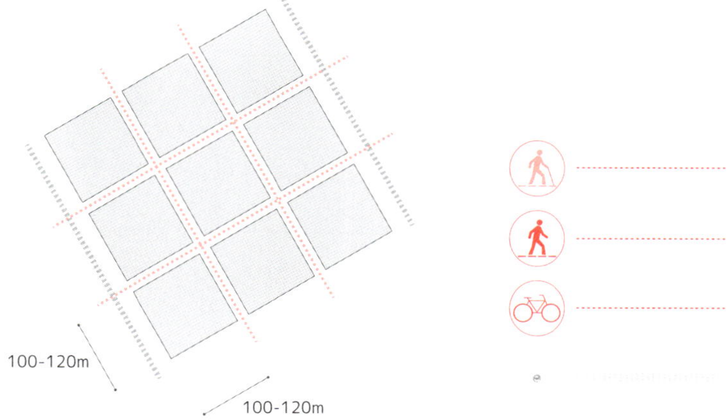

OPTIMUM BLOCK SIZE FOR WALKABILITY

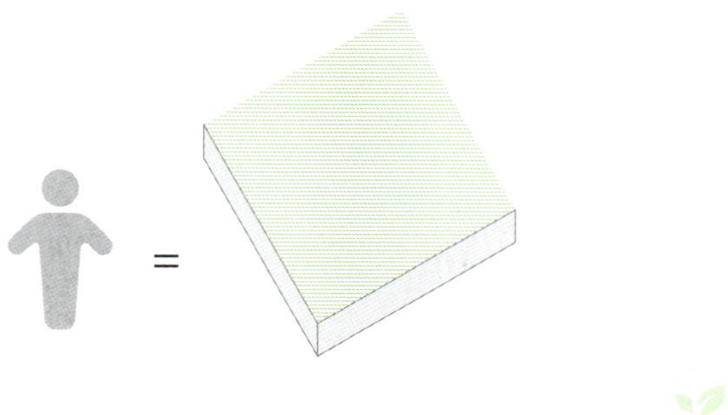

1 PERSON = 9 SQUARE METERS OF OPEN SPACE

Block Explorations
Generic Grids and Green Spaces

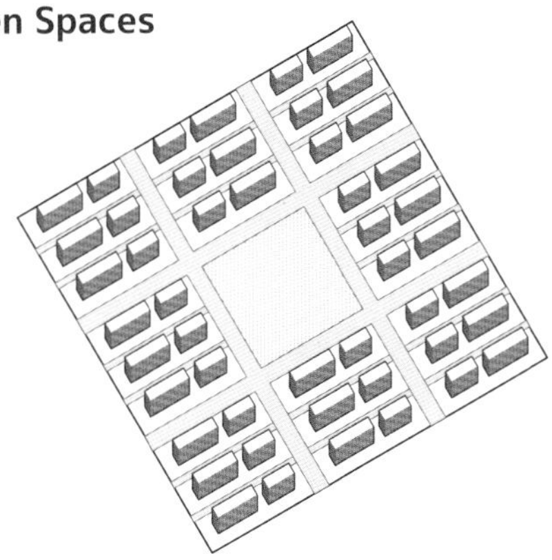

D13_Central Green Space

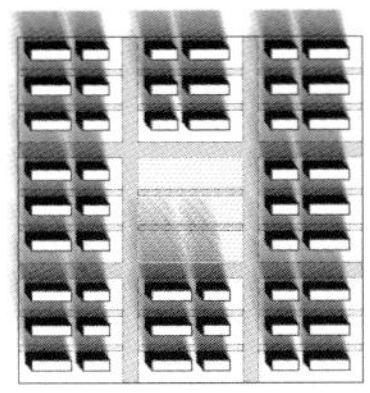

Annual Solar Study_11:00am

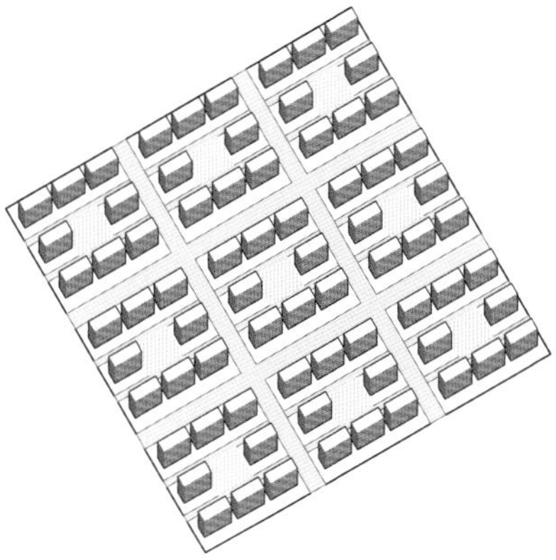

D10_Pocket Green Spaces

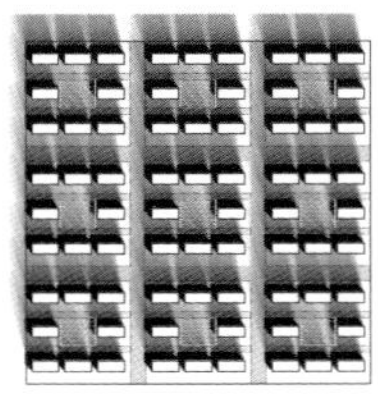

Annual Solar Study_11:00am

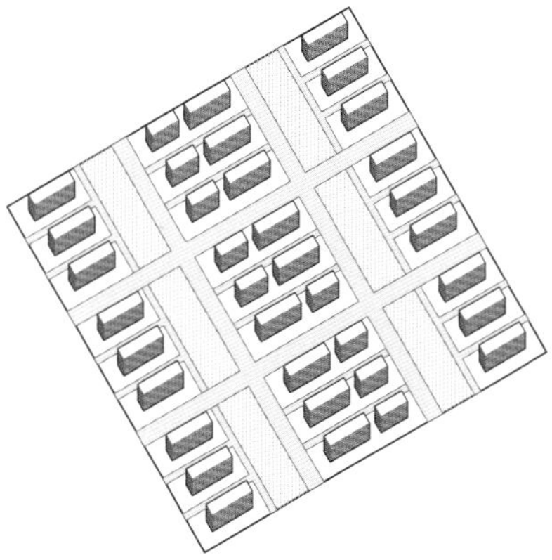

D16_Linear Strip Green Spaces

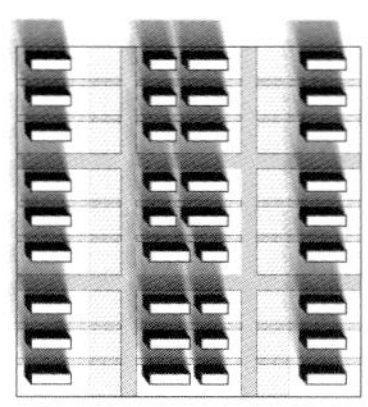

Annual Solar Study_11:00am

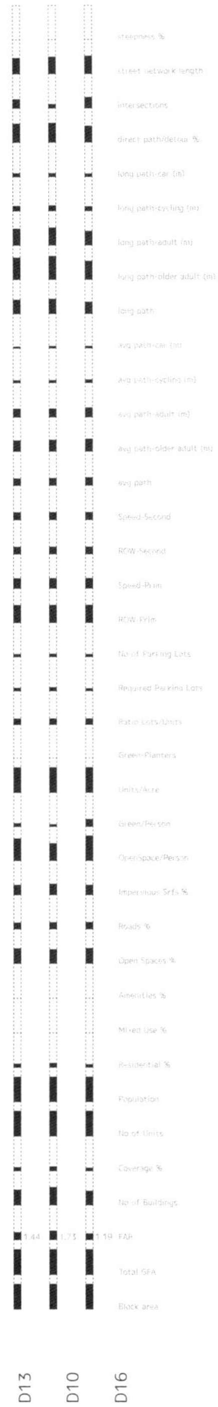

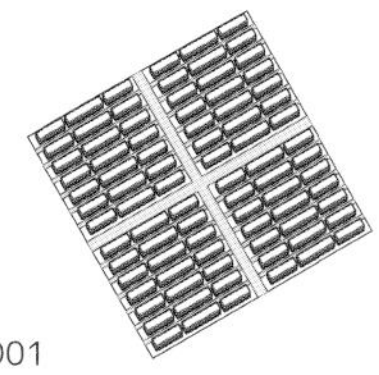
D01

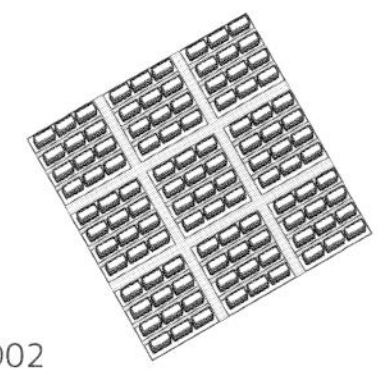
D02

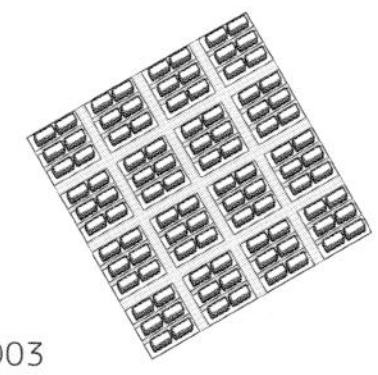
D03

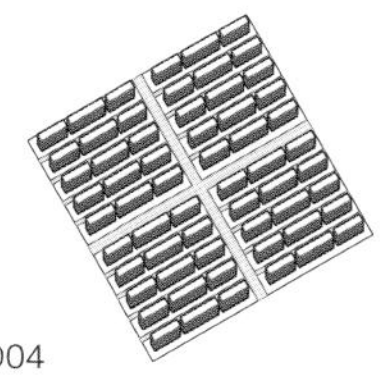
D04

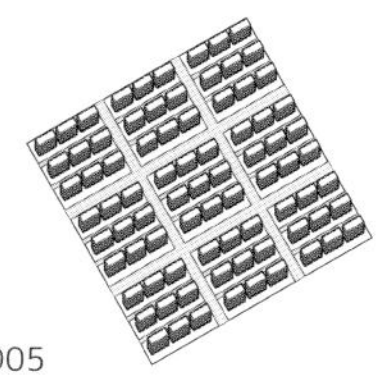
D05

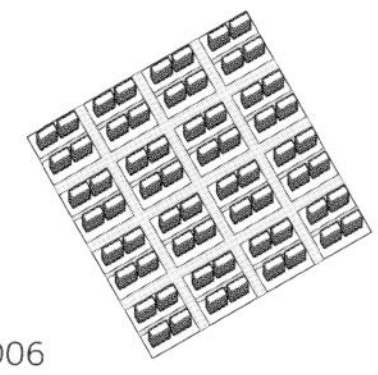
D06

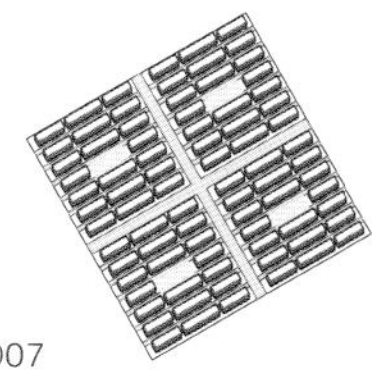
D07

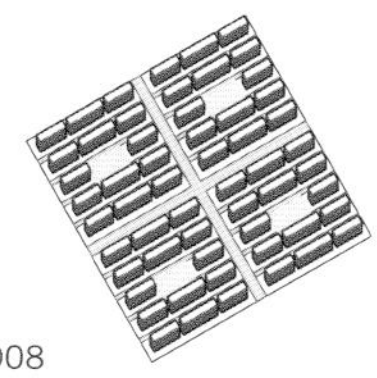
D08

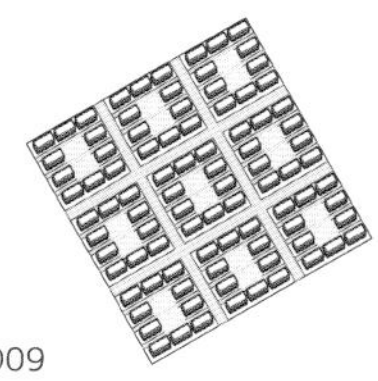
D09

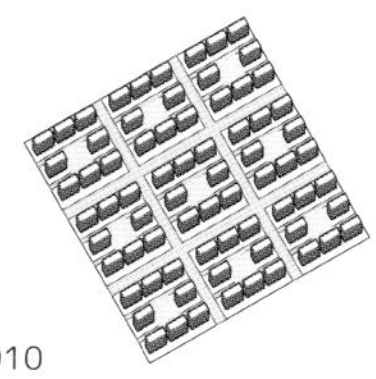
D10

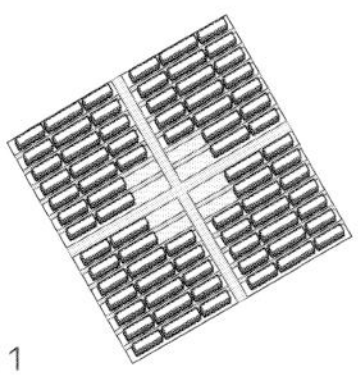
D11

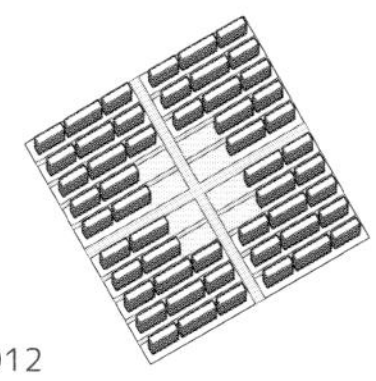
D12

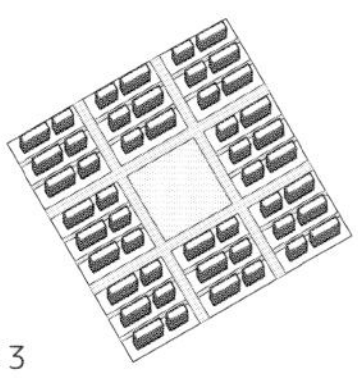
D13

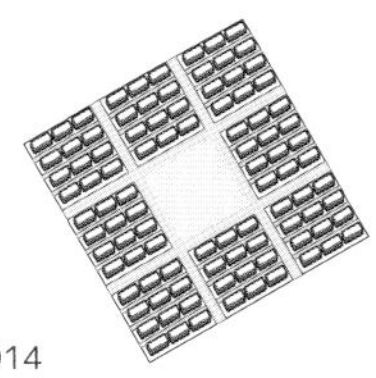
D14

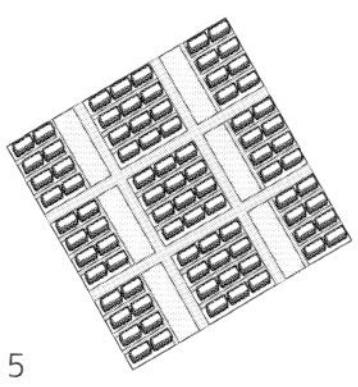
D15

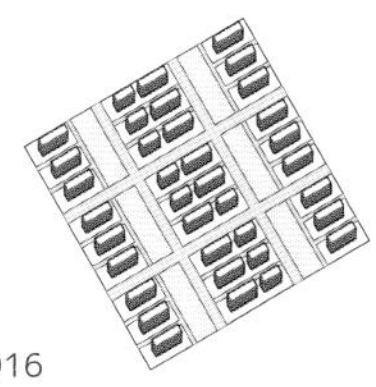
D16

A series of iterations of block types were generated to visualize and establish an appropriate sample of design options to analyze the open space patterns that may work well. A matrix of these iterations is represented here to offer an edited view of the range of variations that were studied.

Once the appropriate block-scale subdivision and permeability were determined, the generation of scenarios of the pattern of distribution of open spaces within the blocks were produced and subsequently evaluated according to a number of considerations.

The open space patterns were limited by the need to allocate nine square meters of open green space per person. This numbers were based on the projected residential population of the block. The generation of variations was pursued through the leveraging of associative modelling and design techniques. This permitted the rapid production of design iterations while keeping the green space to population ratio intact. The whole sample of studies was predicated on four simple schematic distribution schemes:

1. Open green space integrated only within the street grid pattern,
2. Smaller open green spaces distributed evenly throughout the block,
3. A large central open space, and
4. Greenways arranged in a north-south orientation.

While high ratios of open space per person may be seen to improve the health-related performance of these blocks, if not carefully balanced, a higher open space to population ratio may begin to produce some of the negative effects of low density on health including the absence of critical mass to sustain an active social community.

Shadow studies were conducted by the team to find the appropriate open space patterns in terms of access to sunlight. The distribution of open spaces within the street network alone was seen to underperform in relationship to the provisions of open spaces. The distribution of smaller designated open spaces also underperformed as large areas of these spaces would be overshadowed by adjacent buildings. Large central open spaces performed better in that respect. However, these would result in a section of buildings within the block with no immediate adjacency or frontage to open space.

The greenways were seen to provide more immediate adjacencies between nearly all the buildings and the main open spaces, while also ensuring that there would be minimal areas of its designated open spaces overshadowed by adjacent buildings. It was seen to perform the best in relation to a number of considerations, including the ease with which it may collect stormwater and runoff for treatment.

Block Explorations
Green Spaces and FAR

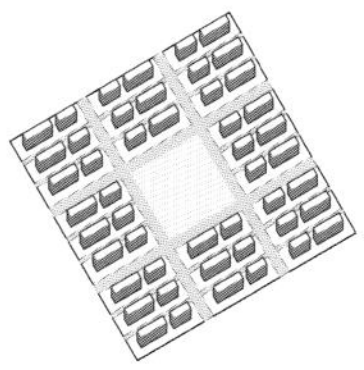

EC.01 13.31m^2 open space/person

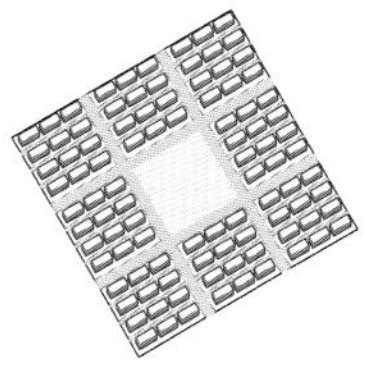

EC.02 13.00m^2 open space/person

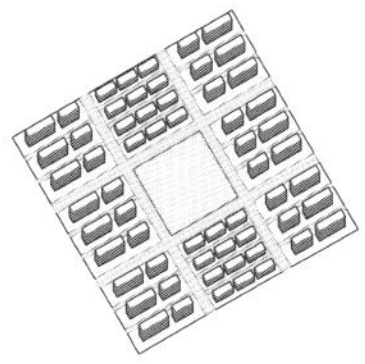

EC.03 13.24m^2 open space/person

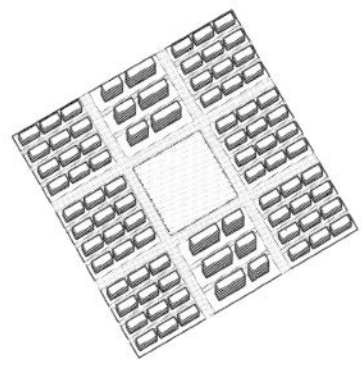

EC.04 13.09m^2 open space/person

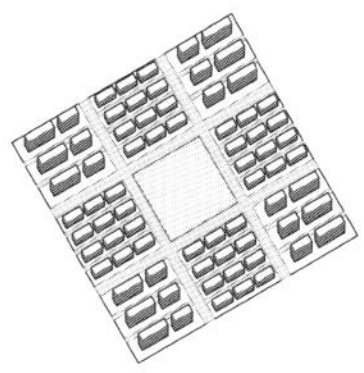

EC.05 13.17m^2 open space/person

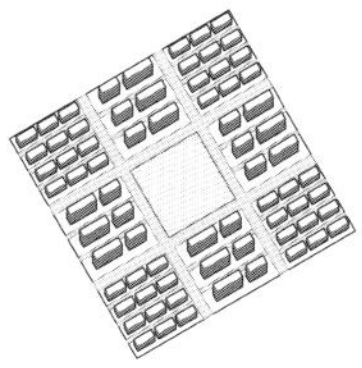

EC.06 13.17m^2 open space/person

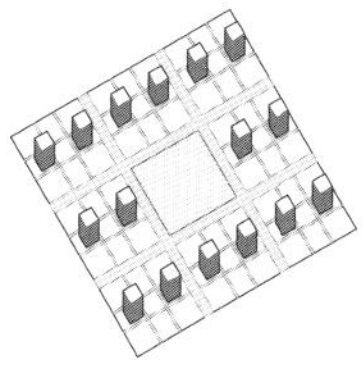

EC.07 24.27m^2 open space/person

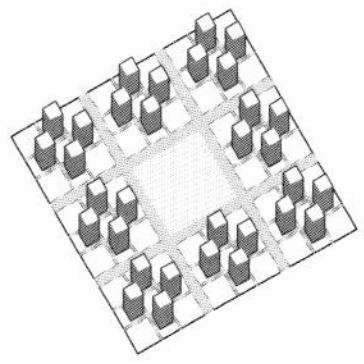

EC.08 11.31m^2 open space/person

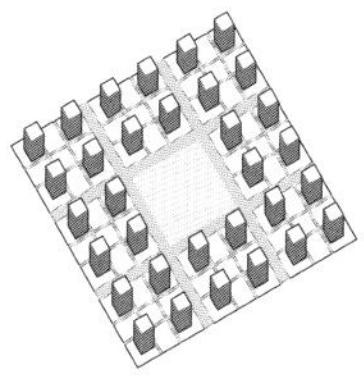

EC.09 11.31m^2 open space/person

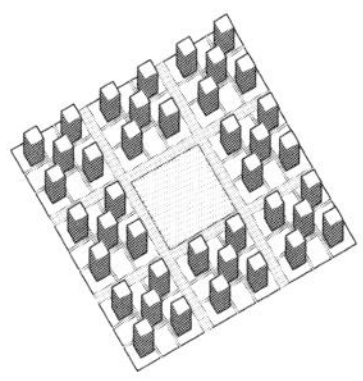

EC.10 8.72m^2 open space/person

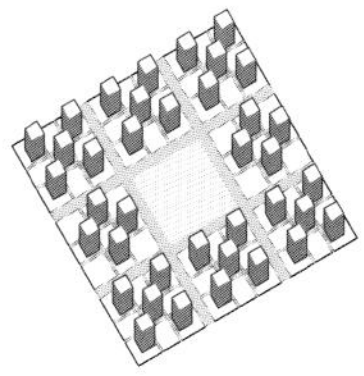

EC.11 9.27m^2 open space/person

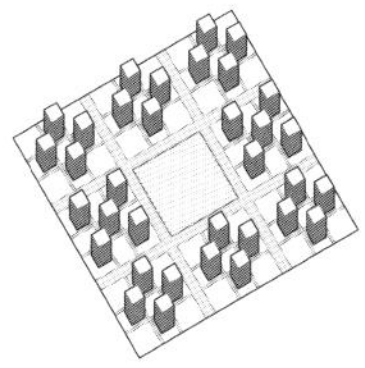

EC.12 10.55m^2 open space/person

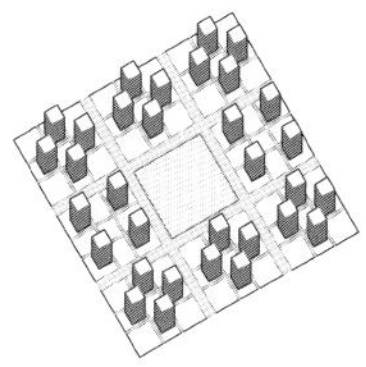

EC.13 11.31m^2 open space/person

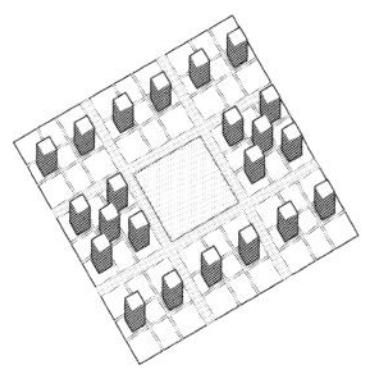

EC.14 17.21m^2 open space/person

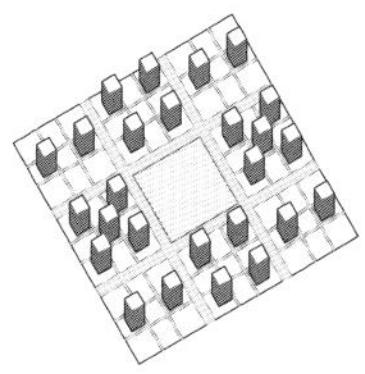

EC.15 14.30m^2 open space/person

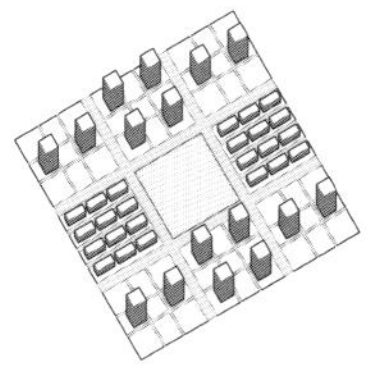

EC.16 16.74m^2 open space/person

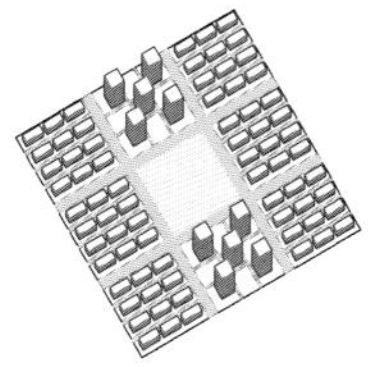

EC.17 11.17m^2 open space/person

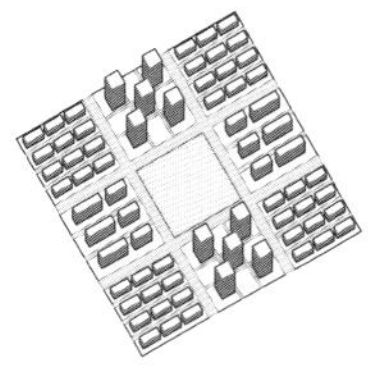

EC.18 11.33m^2 open space/person

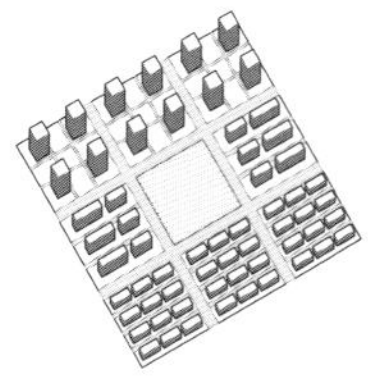

EC.19 12.24m^2 open space/person

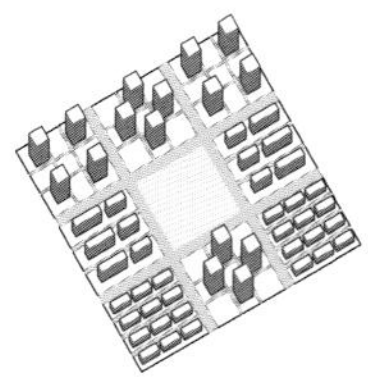

EC.20 12.03m^2 open space/person

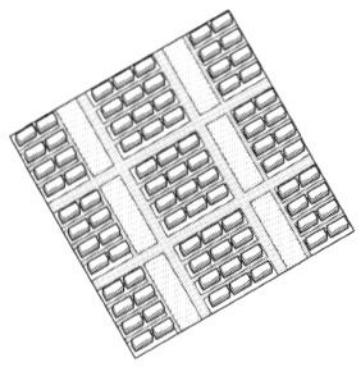

ES.01 15.33m² open space/person

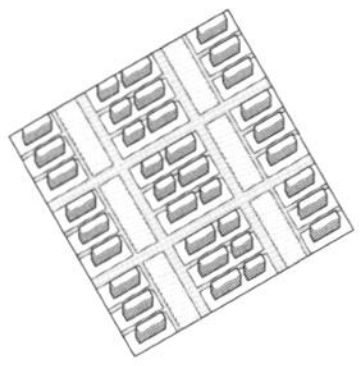

ES.02 16.26m² open space/person

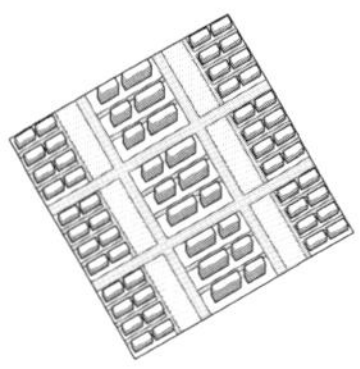

ES.03 15.26m² open space/person

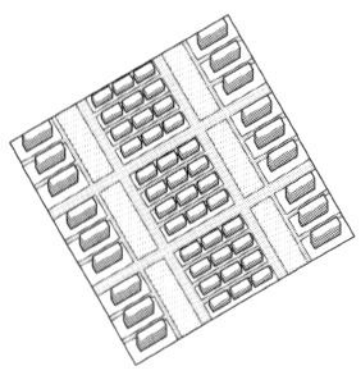

ES.04 16.43m² open space/person

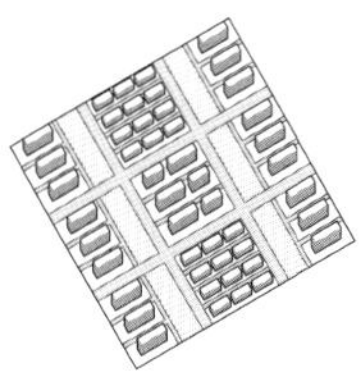

ES.05 16.37m² open space/person

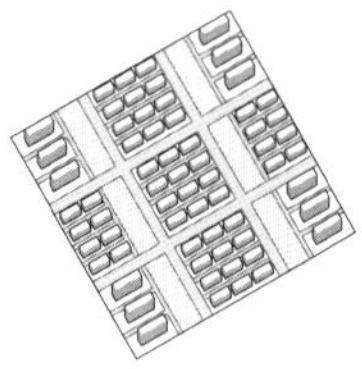

ES.06 16.08m² open space/person

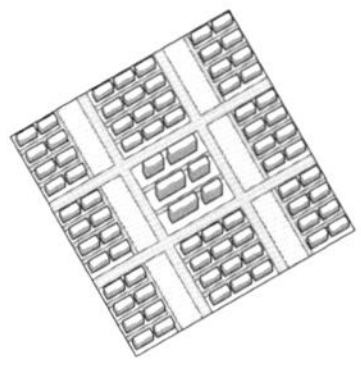

ES.07 15.31m² open space/person

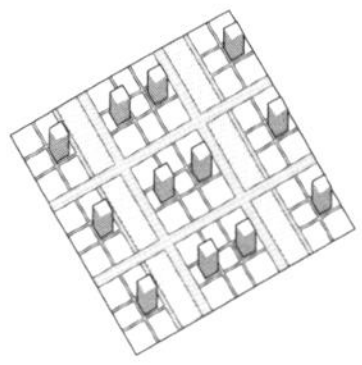

ES.08 29.86m² open space/person

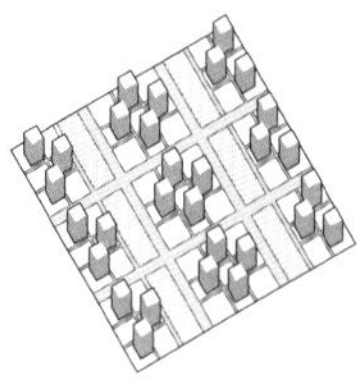

ES.09 10.95m² open space/person

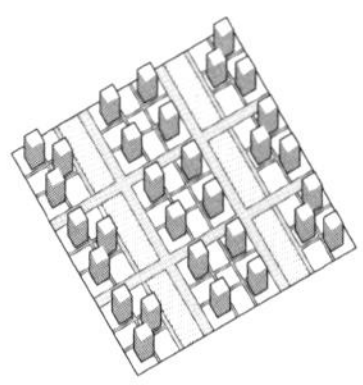

ES.10 10.95m² open space/person

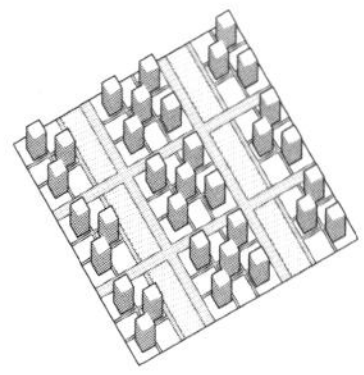

ES.11 9.81m² open space/person

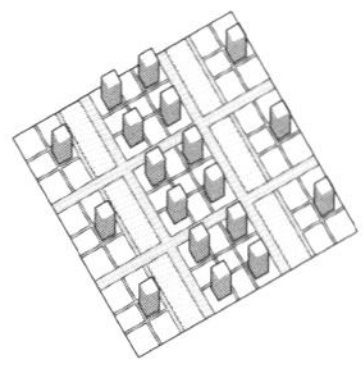

ES.12 19.35m² open space/person

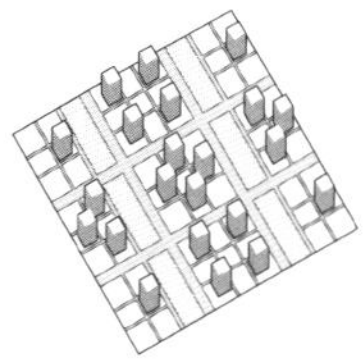

ES.13 15.54m² open space/person

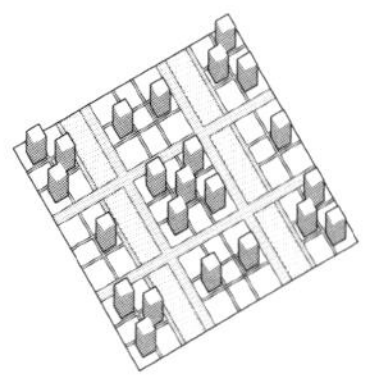

ES.14 14.79m² open space/person

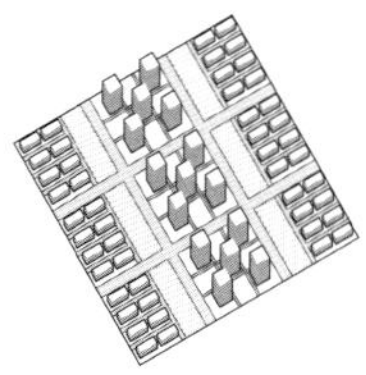

ES.15 11.85m² open space/person

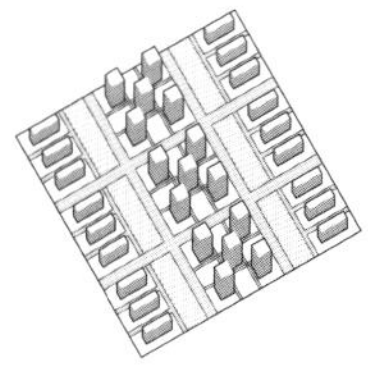

ES.16 12.75m² open space/person

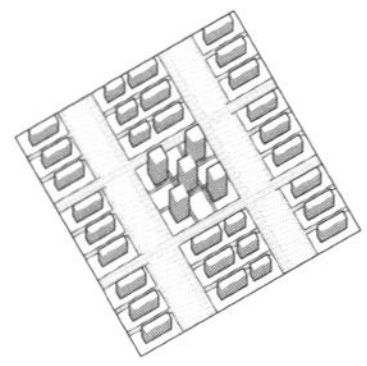

ES.17 14.84m² open space/person

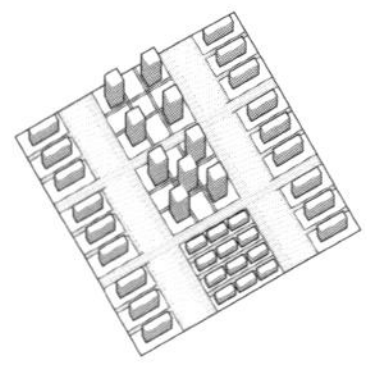

ES.18 14.39m² open space/person

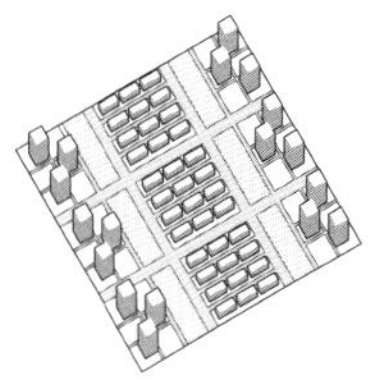

ES.19 11.33m² open space/person

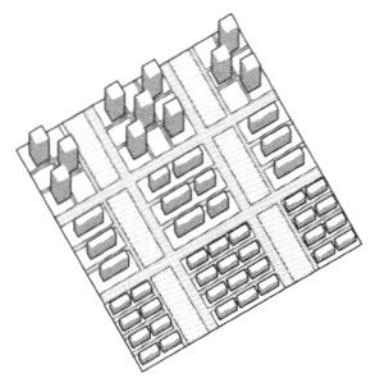

ES.20 12.88m² open space/person

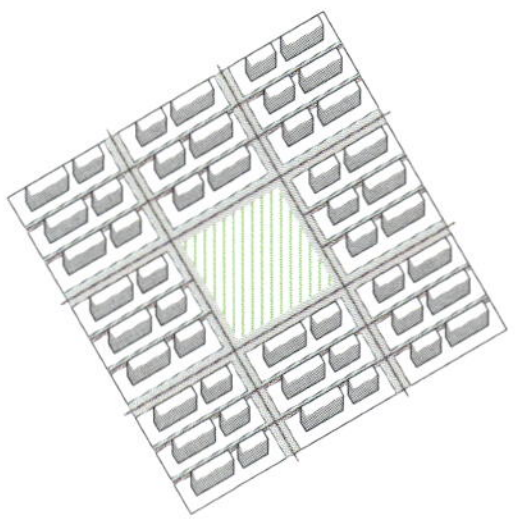
EC.01

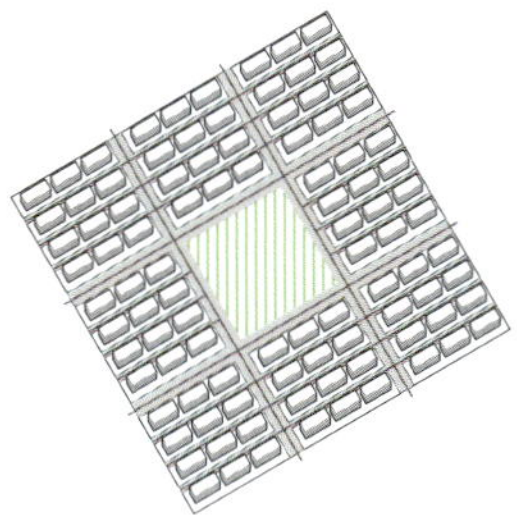
EC.02

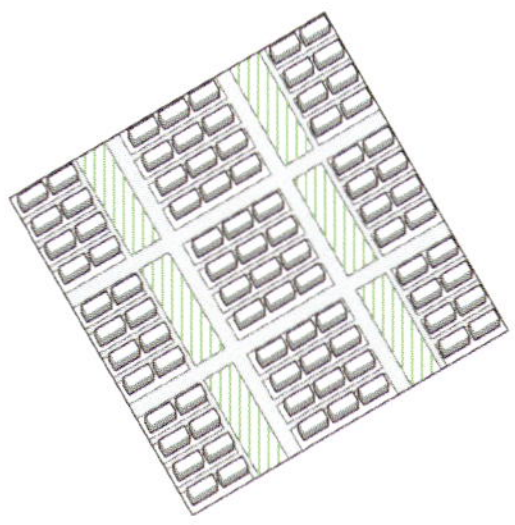
EC.01

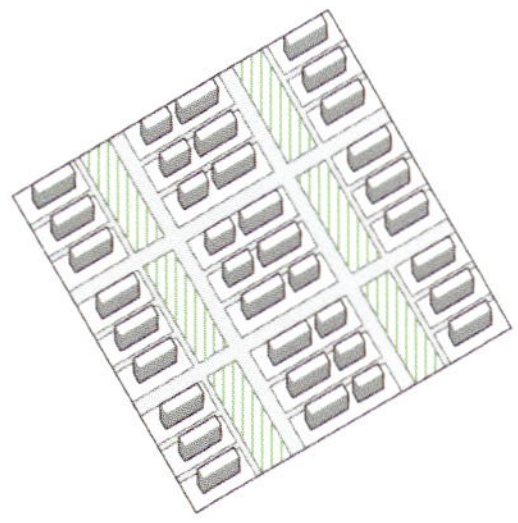
EC.01

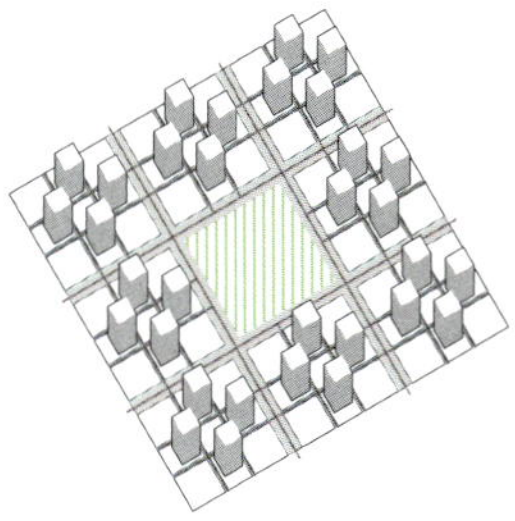
EC.08

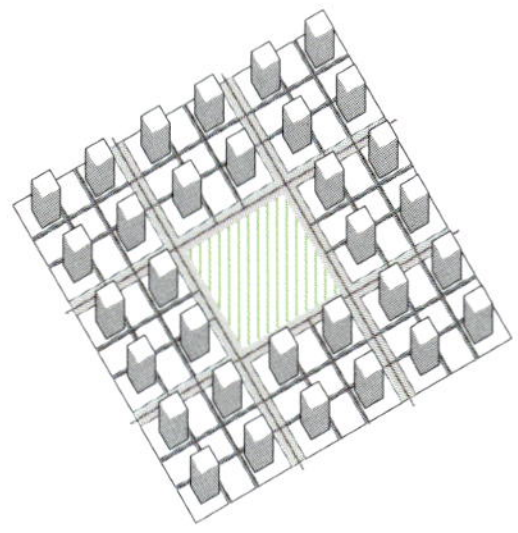
EC.09

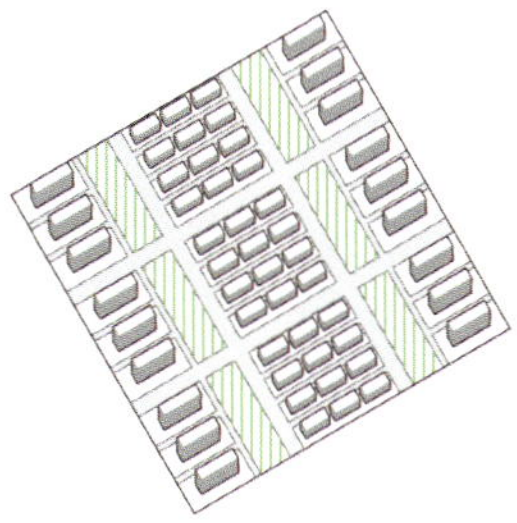
EC.01

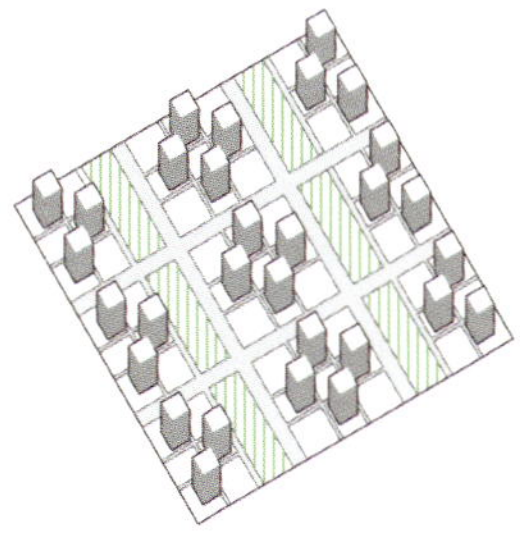
EC.01

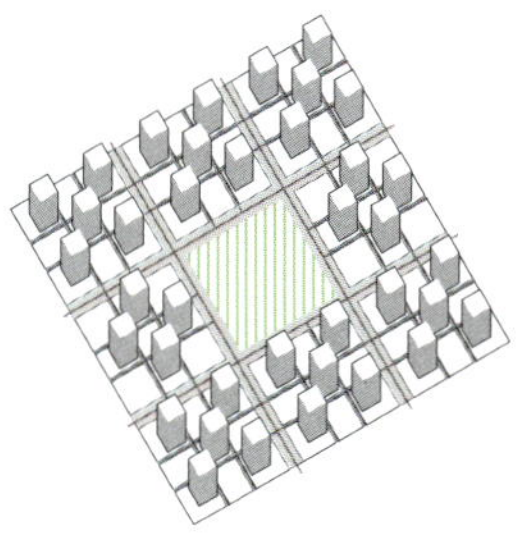
EC.11

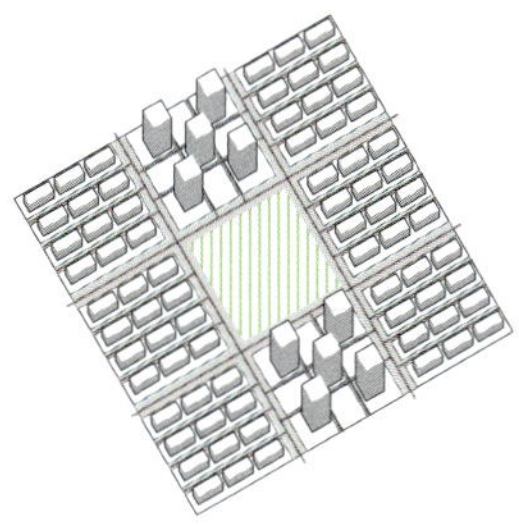
EC.17

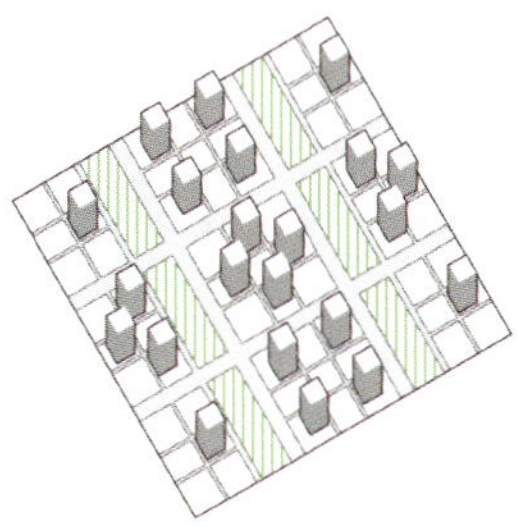
EC.01

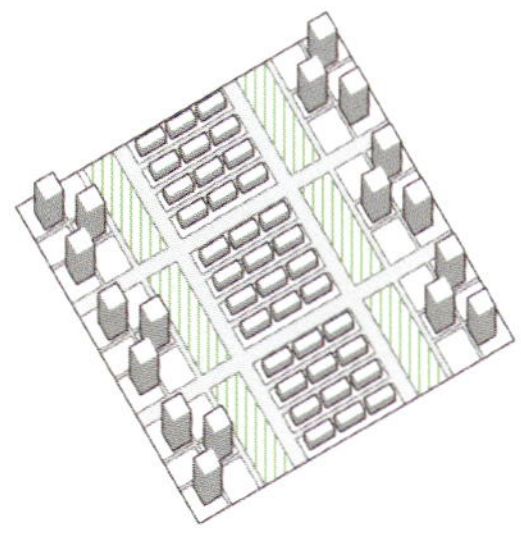
EC.01

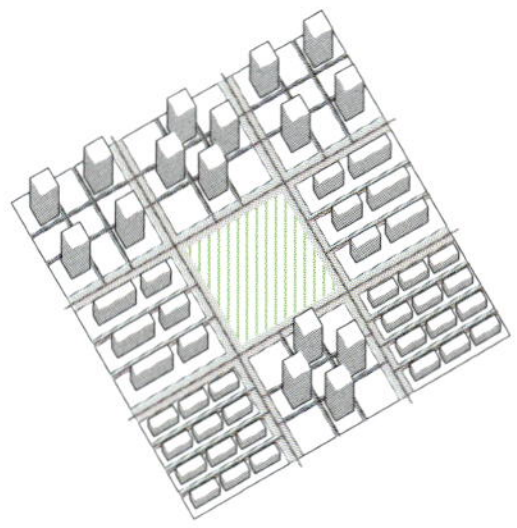
EC.20

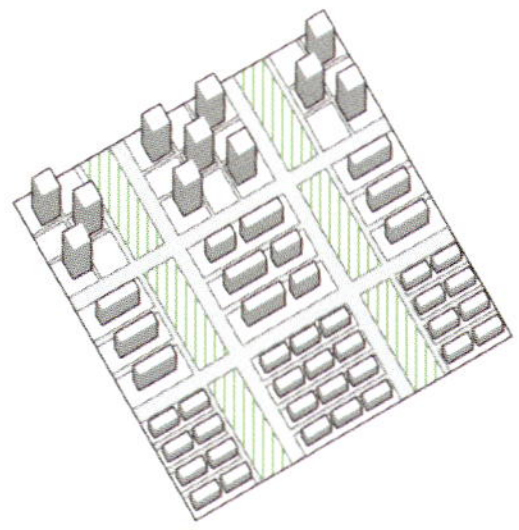
EC.01

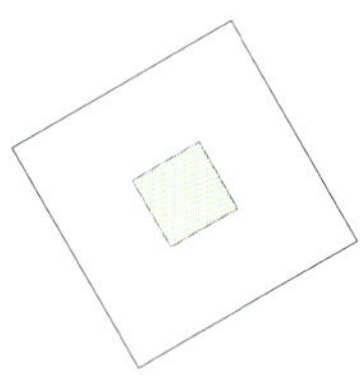

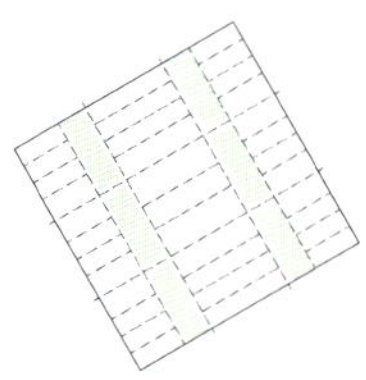

(Previous and Left) The preceding matrix of design iterations offer a wide range of schematic block organizations that satisfy the open space per person ratio. While some iterations satisfy a number of other constraints and parameters, none can be said to maximize all criteria. Other organizational factors could also be informed by considering additional conditions, such as accommodating a higher proportion of mixed uses, as well as diversity of building types.

The balance between open space provision and density was met in a wide range of iterations. According to these two criteria, a significant proportion of the sample set would "satisfice." A selection of design iterations were identified to perform well in specific circumstances. The collection was chosen for their maximization of density, based on constraints including the 'sunshine' laws, fire regulations, typical setbacks, as well as standard development and construction limits (such as construction systems and typical building floor plates, etc). These all satisfied or exceeded the open space per person ratio benchmark. The additional value of these iterations was in their role of visualizing hypothetical maximum densities of the block, based on the aforementioned constraints. These also provided a design process for identifying the basic open space and block pattern framework that would be needed to ensure a good open space provision even in the scenario of maximized building densities.

Other iterations included here were the variations with the highest open space ratios (those with the lowest densities). Finally, when planning for the design scenarios, blocks with mixed building types were also studied. A mix of building types was pursued as a strategy for providing a wider range of living arrangements and unit types. Additionally, it allowed for other programs to be integrated within the blocks, improving the amount of mixed use and potentially contributing to social diversity through the possibility of mixed tenure.

	EC.01	EC.02	EC.08	EC.09	EC.11	EC.17	EC.20
steepness %	0	0	0	0	0	0	0
street network length	3792	4853	5914	5914	5914	5096	5096
intersections	36	52	100	100	100	72	76
direct path/detour %	75	71	68	67	68	72	73
long path-car (m)	0.7	0.8	0.4	0.4	0.4	0.8	0.7
long path-cycling (m)	1.0	1.2	0.6	0.6	0.6	1.2	1.0
long path-adult (m)	3.3	3.8	1.9	1.9	1.9	3.8	3.3
long path-older adult (m)	4.4	5.0	2.5	2.5	2.5	5.0	4.4
long path	280.28	316.64	161.21	161.21	161.21	316.64	280.28
avg path-car (m)	0.3	0.4	0.3	0.3	0.3	0.4	0.3
avg path-cycling (m)	0.5	0.5	0.5	0.5	0.5	0.6	0.5
avg path-adult (m)	1.7	1.7	1.5	1.5	1.5	1.8	1.7
avg path-older adult (m)	2.2	2.3	1.9	1.9	2.0	2.4	2.2
avg path	139.69	145.78	123.03	121.96	124.02	151.49	140.43
Speed-Second	15.0	15.0	15.0	15.0	15.0	15.0	15.0
ROW-Second	7.3152	7.3152	7.3152	7.3152	7.3152	7.3152	7.3152
Speed-Prim	20.0	20.0	20.0	20.0	20.0	20.0	20.0
ROW-Prim	17.6636	17.6636	17.6636	17.6636	17.6636	17.6636	17.6636
No of Parking Lots	1084	1388	477	477	477	1160	856
Required Parking Lots	1200.0	960.0	1920.0	1920.0	2280.0	1320.0	1500.0
Ratio Lots/Units	0.5	0.5	0.5	0.5	0.5	0.5	0.5
[illegible]	0.0	0.0	0.0	0.0	0.0	0.0	0.0
[illegible]	60.70	48.56	97.12	97.12	115.34	66.77	75.88
Green/Person	2.05	2.57	1.44	1.44	1.21	1.96	1.77
[illegible]	13.31	13.00	11.31	11.31	9.27	11.17	12.03
[illegible]	40.17	53.25	27.46	27.46	29.45	47.46	37.09
Roads %	22.45	23.55	15.21	15.21	15.21	22.39	19.58
Open Spaces %	56.50	40.08	70.87	70.87	68.88	48.04	60.05
Amenities %	5.00	10.00	2.50	2.50	2.50	6.50	4.50
Mixed Use %	5.00	10.00	2.50	2.50	2.50	6.50	4.50
Residential %	11.06	16.36	8.91	8.91	10.89	16.08	11.78
Population	7195	5756	10259	10259	12183	7523	8368
No of Units	2400	1920	3840	3840	4560	2640	3000
Coverage %	14.39	23.03	10.58	10.58	12.56	20.58	14.64
No of Buildings	62	110	42	43	45	93	59
FAR	1.44	1.15	2.12	2.12	2.51	1.52	1.71
Total GFA	230256	184205	338560	338560	402040	243954	272895
Block area	160000	160000	160000	160000	160000	160000	160000

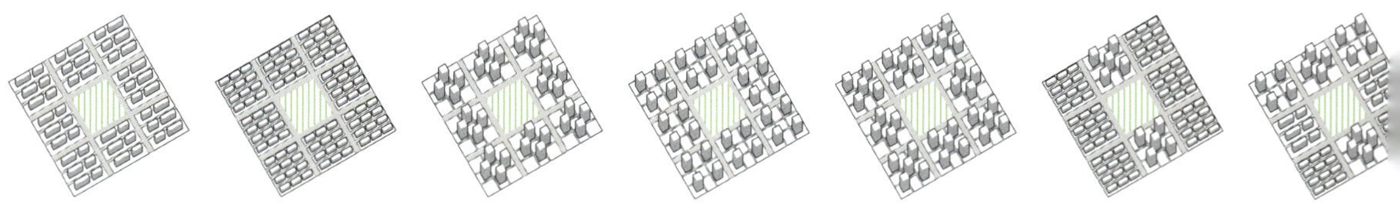

	ES.02	ES.04	ES.09	ES.13	ES.19	ES.20
steepness %	0	0	0	0	0	0
street network length	4277	4694	5877	5877	5494	5099
intersections	44	56	92	92	80	66
direct path/detour %	66	70	70	69	74	67
long path-car (m)	0.6	0.7	0.6	0.6	0.7	0.6
long path-cycling (m)	0.9	1.0	1.0	1.0	1.0	0.9
long path-adult (m)	2.8	3.3	3.1	3.1	3.3	3.0
long path-older adult (m)	3.7	4.4	4.1	4.1	4.4	3.9
long path	236.08	278.44	261.06	261.06	278.44	249.28
avg path-car (m)	0.4	0.4	0.3	0.4	0.4	0.4
avg path-cycling (m)	0.6	0.6	0.5	0.5	0.5	0.6
avg path-adult (m)	1.9	1.9	1.6	1.7	1.7	1.8
avg path-older adult (m)	2.5	2.5	2.2	2.2	2.2	2.4
avg path	158.48	156.41	137.10	140.73	142.24	152.10
Speed-Second	15.0	15.0	15.0	15.0	15.0	15.0
ROW-Second	7.3152	7.3152	7.3152	7.3152	7.3152	7.3152
Speed-Prim	20.0	20.0	20.0	20.0	20.0	20.0
ROW-Prim	17.6636	17.6636	17.6636	17.6636	17.6636	17.6636
No of Parking Lots	1008	1122	477	477	818	919
Required Parking Lots	990.0	900.0	1800.0	1320.0	1440.0	1270.0
Ratio Lots/Units	0.5	0.5	0.5	0.5	0.5	0.5
[illegible]	0.0	0.0	0.0	0.0	0.0	0.0
[illegible]	50.08	45.53	91.05	66.77	72.84	64.24
Green/Person	4.55	5.00	2.81	3.83	3.40	3.76
[illegible]	16.26	16.43	10.95	15.54	11.33	12.88
[illegible]	39.66	44.57	34.16	31.51	43.83	42.18
Roads %	24.46	24.79	22.57	22.57	26.24	24.60
Open Spaces %	57.01	50.76	64.17	66.82	53.17	54.55
Amenities %	5.00	7.00	2.50	2.50	4.50	5.00
Mixed Use %	5.00	7.00	2.50	2.50	4.50	5.00
Residential %	8.54	10.44	8.25	5.6	11.59	11.04
Population	5936	5397	9618	7053	7930	7184
No of Units	1980	1800	3600	2640	2880	2540
Coverage %	11.87	15.11	9.92	7.27	14.59	14.31
No of Buildings	57	75	41	29	69	63
FAR	1.19	1.08	1.98	1.45	1.62	1.46
Total GFA	189961	172692	317400	232760	259517	233427
Block area	160000	160000	160000	160000	160000	160000

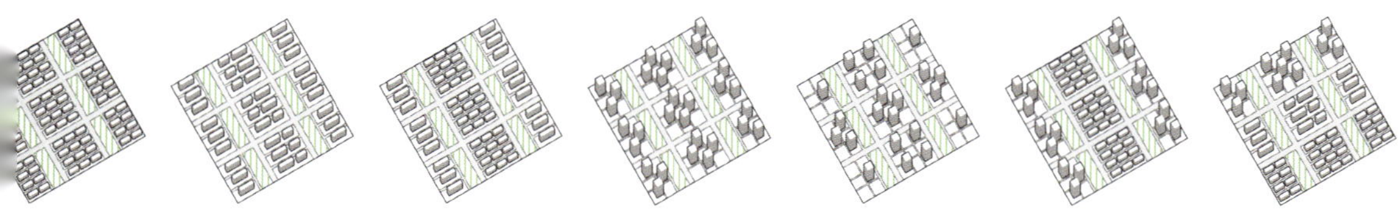

Block Explorations Variability

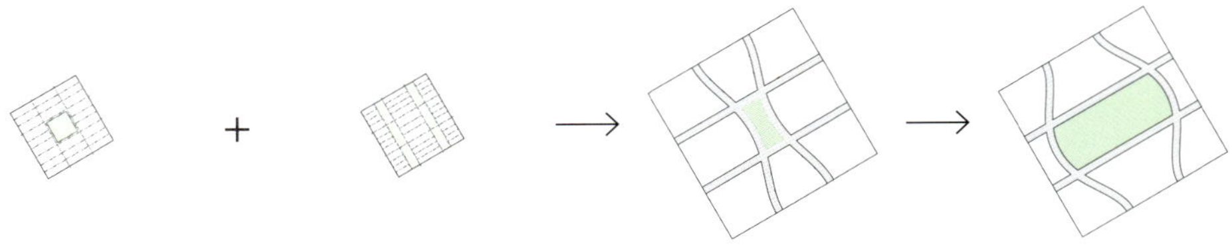

The schematic design iterations already offer a large selection of possible block organizations that work well or satisfactorily in relation to a number of health issues. The basic open space and grid patterns operate as frameworks, within which, a larger number of possible configurations of building densities may be composed. However, the initial normalized models can be further altered in order to expand the range of possible iterations, and more importantly, to achieve other benefits that may be integrated within the blocks.

01 Parcel Variability
While the schematic blocks already allow for a large number of variations, the blocks are standardized. In order to introduce block variation and to allow for the possibility of introducing programs and uses that benefit from smaller or larger blocks, such as schools, the greenway and grid framework can be modified.

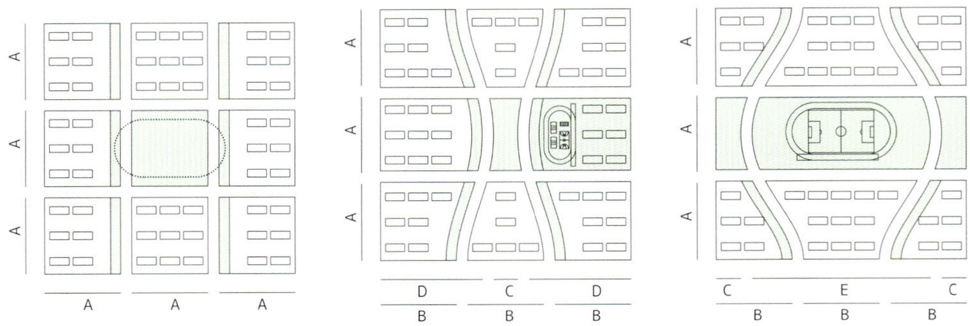

02 Greenway Interface
Additional benefits include the increase in linear meters of the greenways, adding a longer interface between urban block and green recreational spaces. It also provided a longer trajectory for the water treatment process.

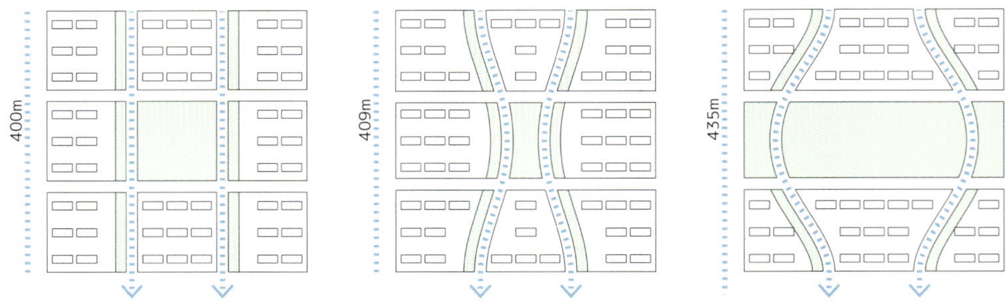

03 Vehicular Management
The differentiated block lengths that result also contributes to the management of vehicular traffic speed through the neighborhood by decreasing distances between intersections at key points in the block.

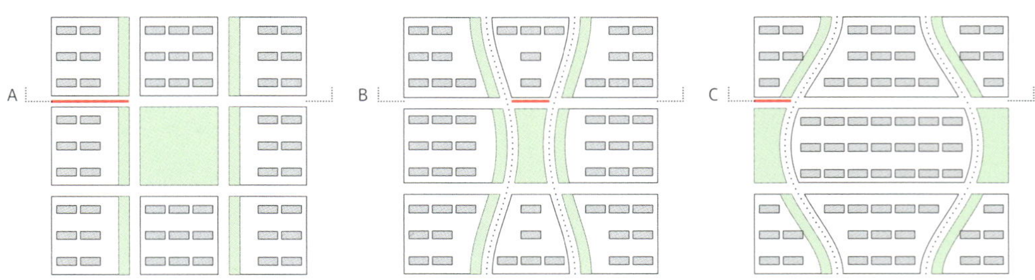

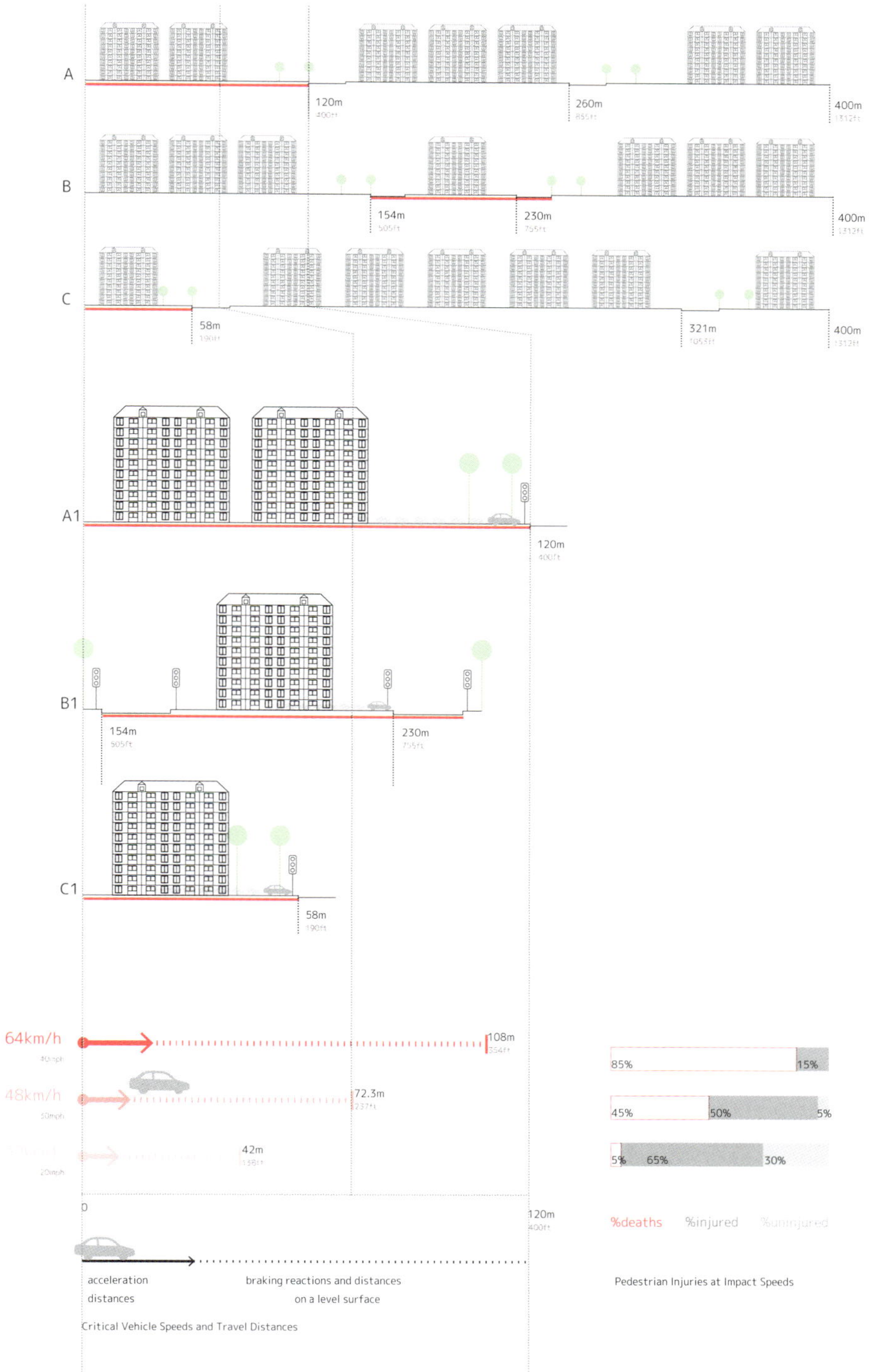

Road Safety

By pairing block length with acceleration and deceleration rates for vehicles, the team was able to identify the manner in which block sizes could operate as mechanisms to manage vehicular speeds. This identified areas that operated well by virtue of distances between intersections alone and areas where additional interventions could be deployed. Road safety, brought about by a management of traffic speed through block configurations was seen to coincide with a range of other health-related factors (street connectivity, open space provisions, etc.) and was influenced by lessons learned from other city grid precedents (such as downtown Portland, Oregon).

Block Explorations Connectivity

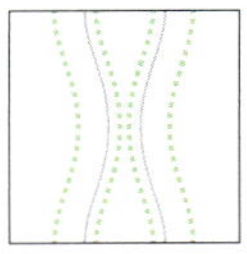

01: GREEN STRIPES CENTERED ON BLOCK
BOTH SIDES OF PRIMARY ROAD

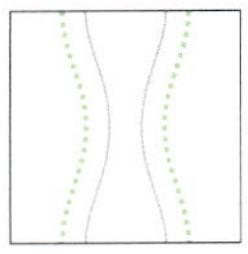

02: GREEN STRIPES CENTERED ON BLOCK
OUTSIDE OF PRIMARY ROAD

SLAB

S-01
FAR: 1.32
COVERAGE: 13.19%

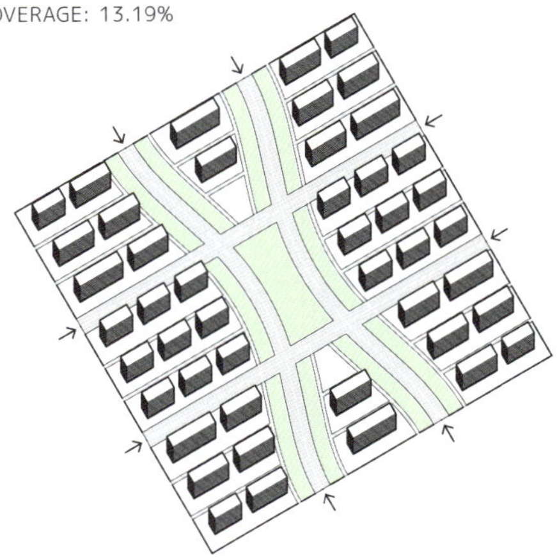

S-02
FAR: 1.27
COVERAGE: 12.74%

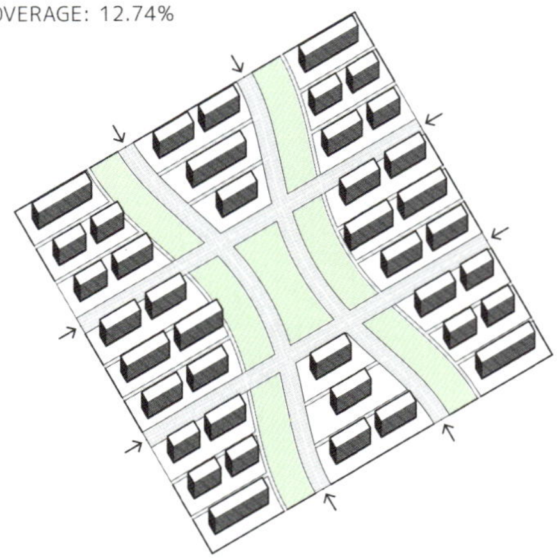

TOWER

T-01
FAR: 2.12
COVERAGE: 10.58%

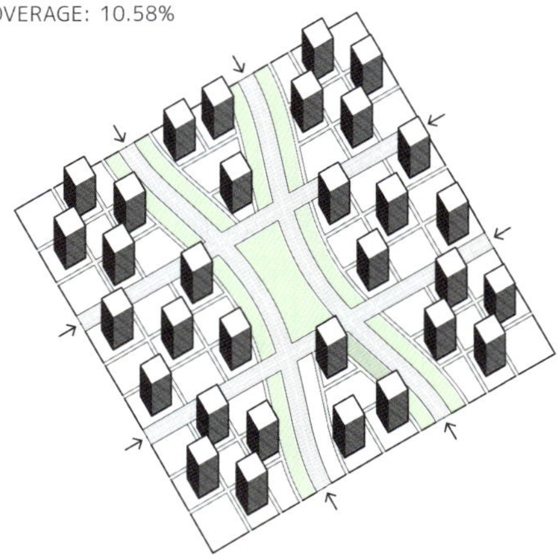

T-02
FAR: 1.85
COVERAGE: 9.26%

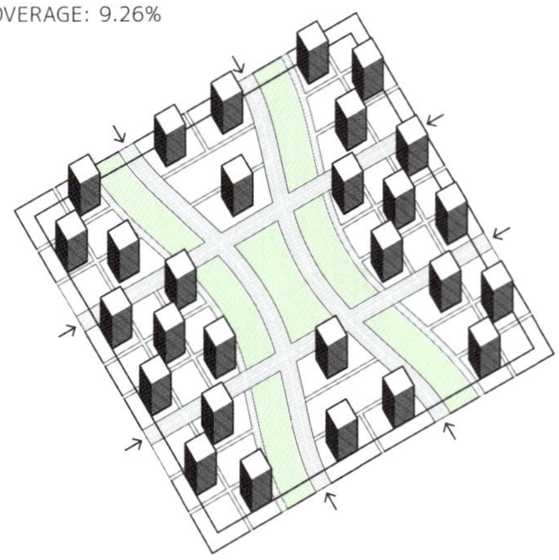

HYBRID

H-01
FAR: 1.6
COVERAGE: 9.08%

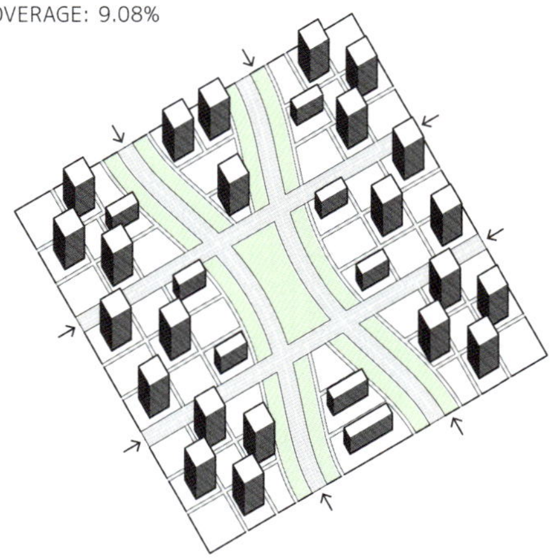

H-02
FAR: 1.65
COVERAGE: 9.12%

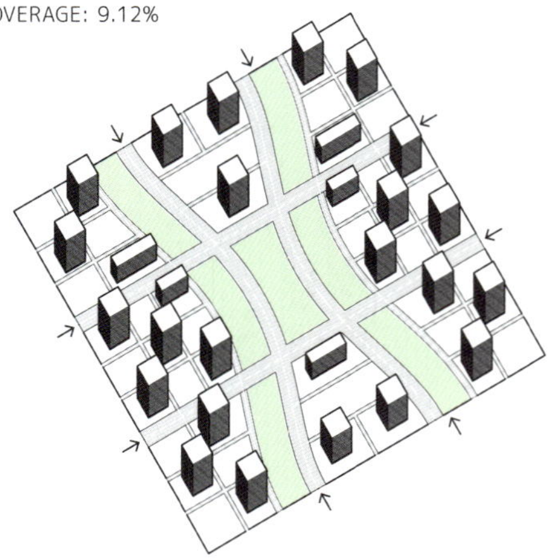

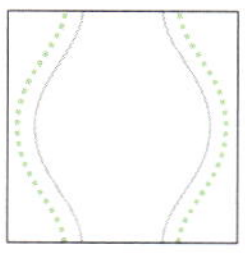

03: GREEN STRIPES PERIMETER OF BLOCK
OUTSIDE OF PRIMARY ROAD

S-03

FAR: 1.20
COVERAGE: 11.99%

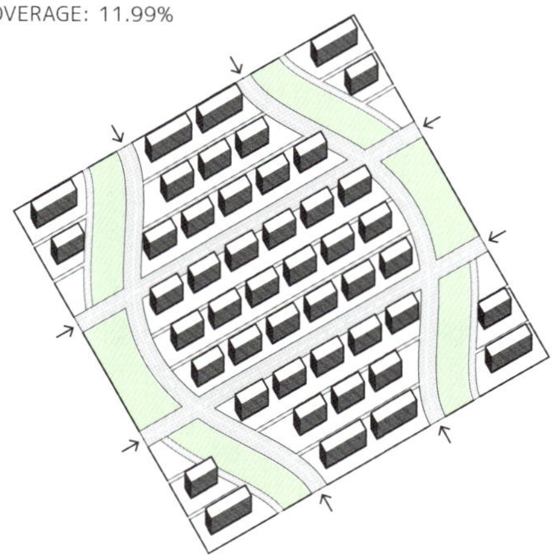

T-03

FAR: 1.79
COVERAGE: 8.93%

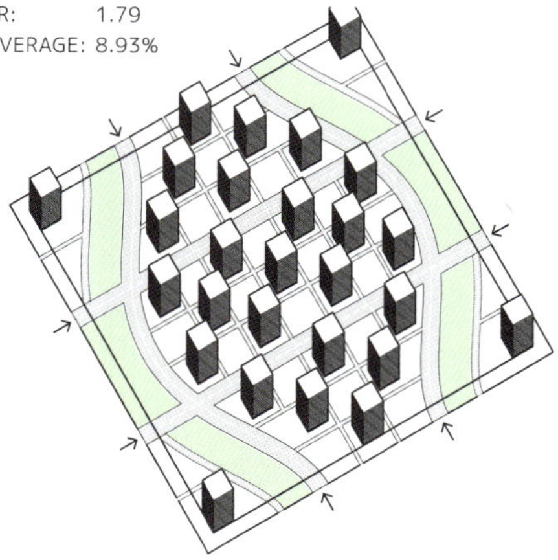

H-03

FAR: 1.58
COVERAGE: 9.10%

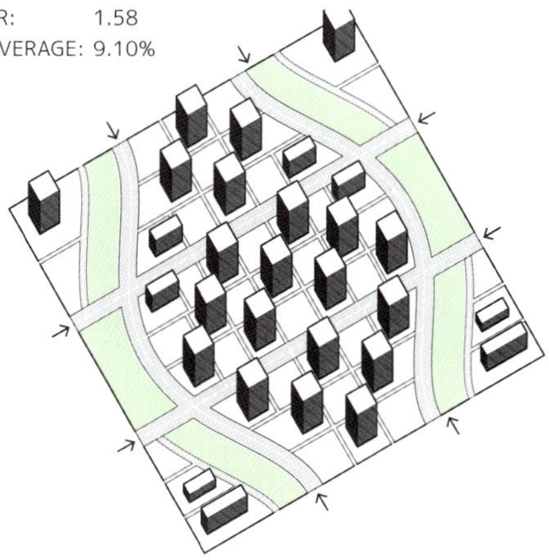

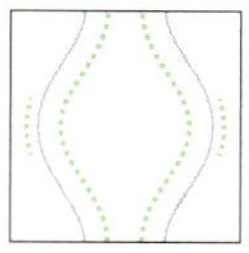

04: GREEN STRIPES PERIMETER OF BLOCK
BOTH SIDES OF PRIMARY ROAD

S-04

FAR: 1.18
COVERAGE: 11.80%

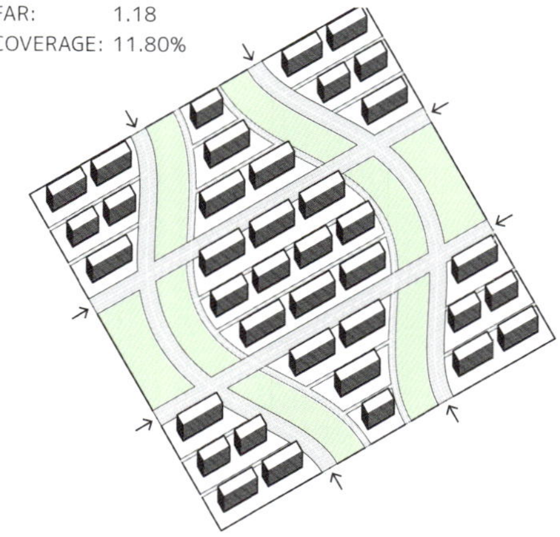

T-04

FAR: 1.98
COVERAGE: 9.92%

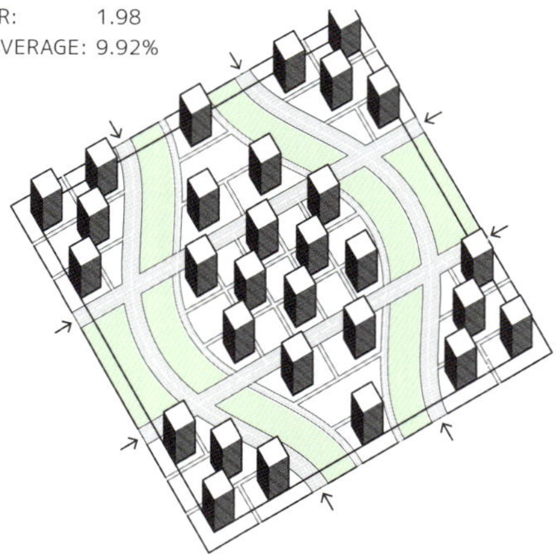

H-04

FAR: 1.68
COVERAGE: 9.88%

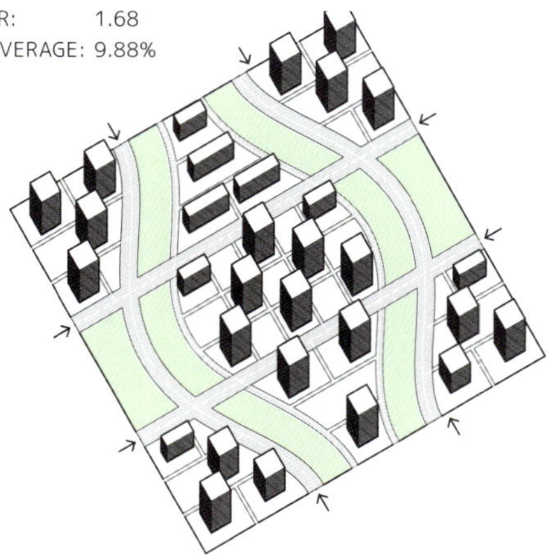

Solar Analysis

The existing blocks were studied for shadow and solar patterns in order to guide the organization of buildings. These also helped to inform us on the quality of the open spaces in between buildings. The subsequent analyses of the design iterations allowed us to strategically define the configuration and density of building types in the blocks. From this, we identified the different microclimate qualities of the open spaces. Predictably, the greenways and most north-south oriented spaces had better consistent exposure, while most east-west oriented spaces were often shaded by adjacent buildings. These helped to guide decisions at the scale of smaller neighbood landscapes and street level treatments as well as programming.

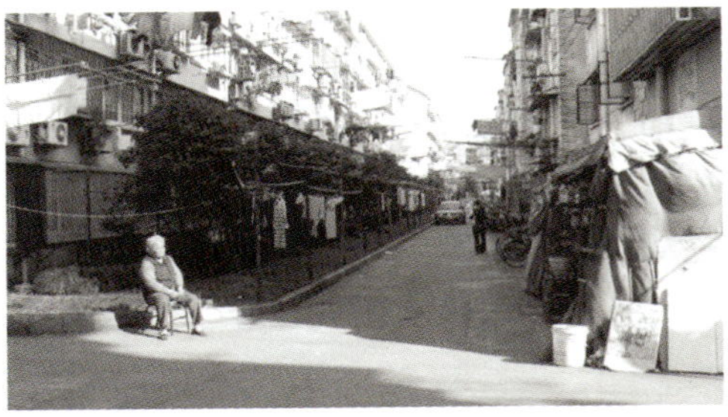

Figure 1 (Above) An elderly man in Shanghai "chases" the sun throughout a winter day. (Image courtesy Yu Yifan)

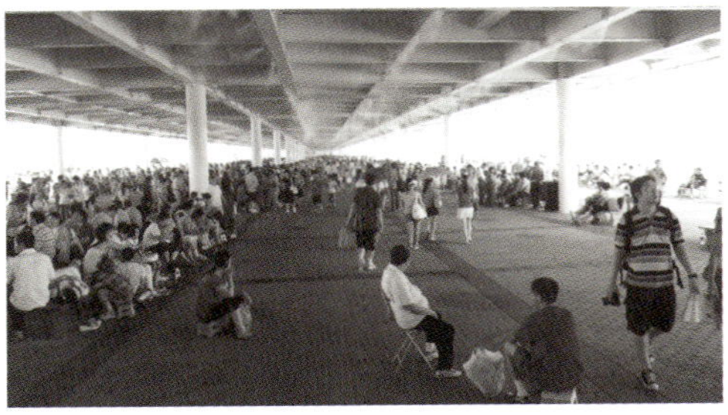

Figure 2 (Above) Shanghai experiences heat waves from time to time. Providing some shaded and cooler outdoor spaces offer citizens respite. (Image courtesy Reuters/WSJ.com)

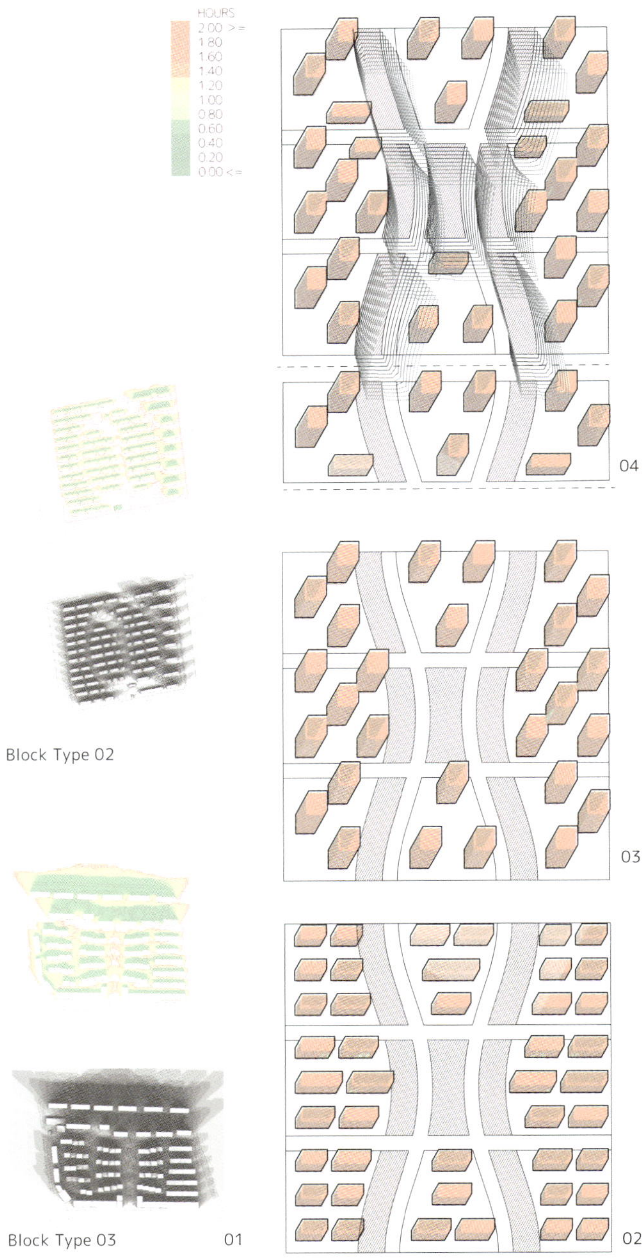

Solar Design Evaluation Process
[01] Solar and Shade Analysis of Existing Block Typology.

[02] Solar Analysis of Slab options
Verify that buildings receive minimum of 2 hours of sunlight a day.

[03] Solar Analysis of Tower options
Verify that buildings receive minimum of 2 hours of sunlight a day.

[04] Solar Analysis of Hybrid options
Certain areas adjacent to towers did not receive minimum hours of sunlight. Surrounding buildings are re-evaluated and replaced with slab typology.

Strategic Location of Amenities

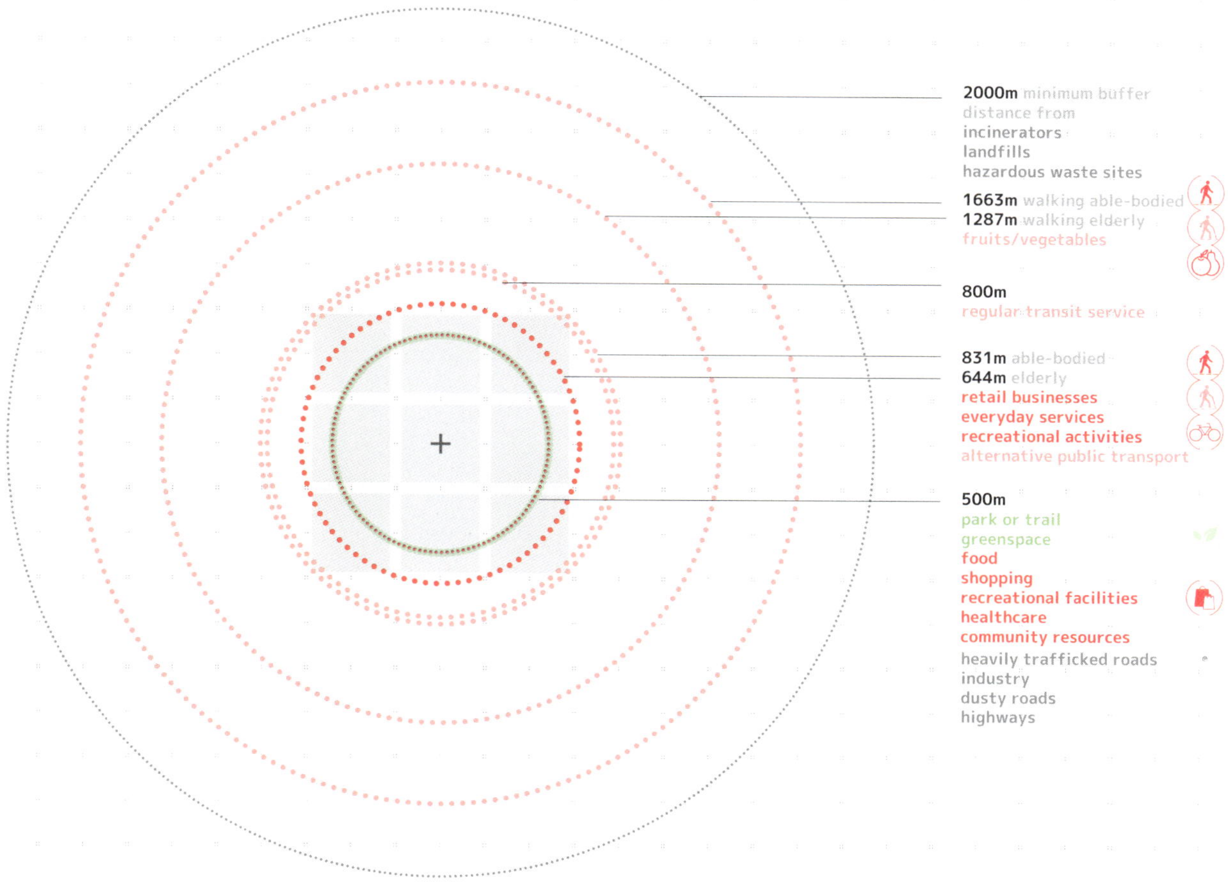

Walkability based on location of Amentities and Entrances

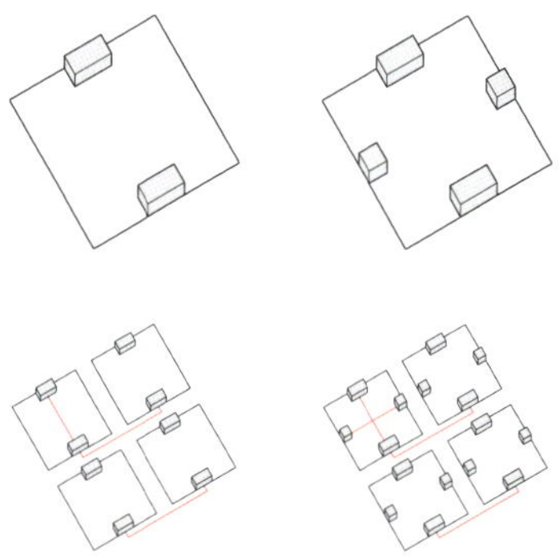

Testing Variations in Number of Block Entrances

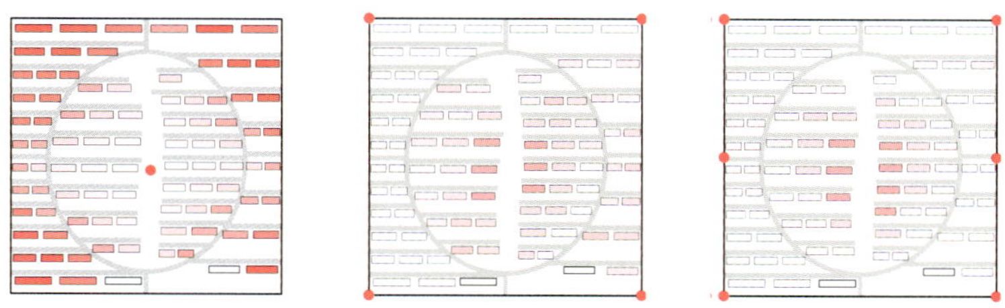

The location of amenities was informed by recommendations from the Health Impact Assessments. Many of the catchment zones for locating specific services and amenities were identified based on walking times or on assumed population densities. In parallel to these recommendations, a series of design evaluations, studying the relationship between walking times from all buildings within the blocks to different distribution patterns of amenities and services, were carried out. This was examined for one-block and multi-block configurations.

Together, these would inform the location of amenities at the larger scale of a nine-block aggregation. The nine-block arrangement was determined by the catchment zones, where all the necessary services and amenities were encapsulated within this larger area.

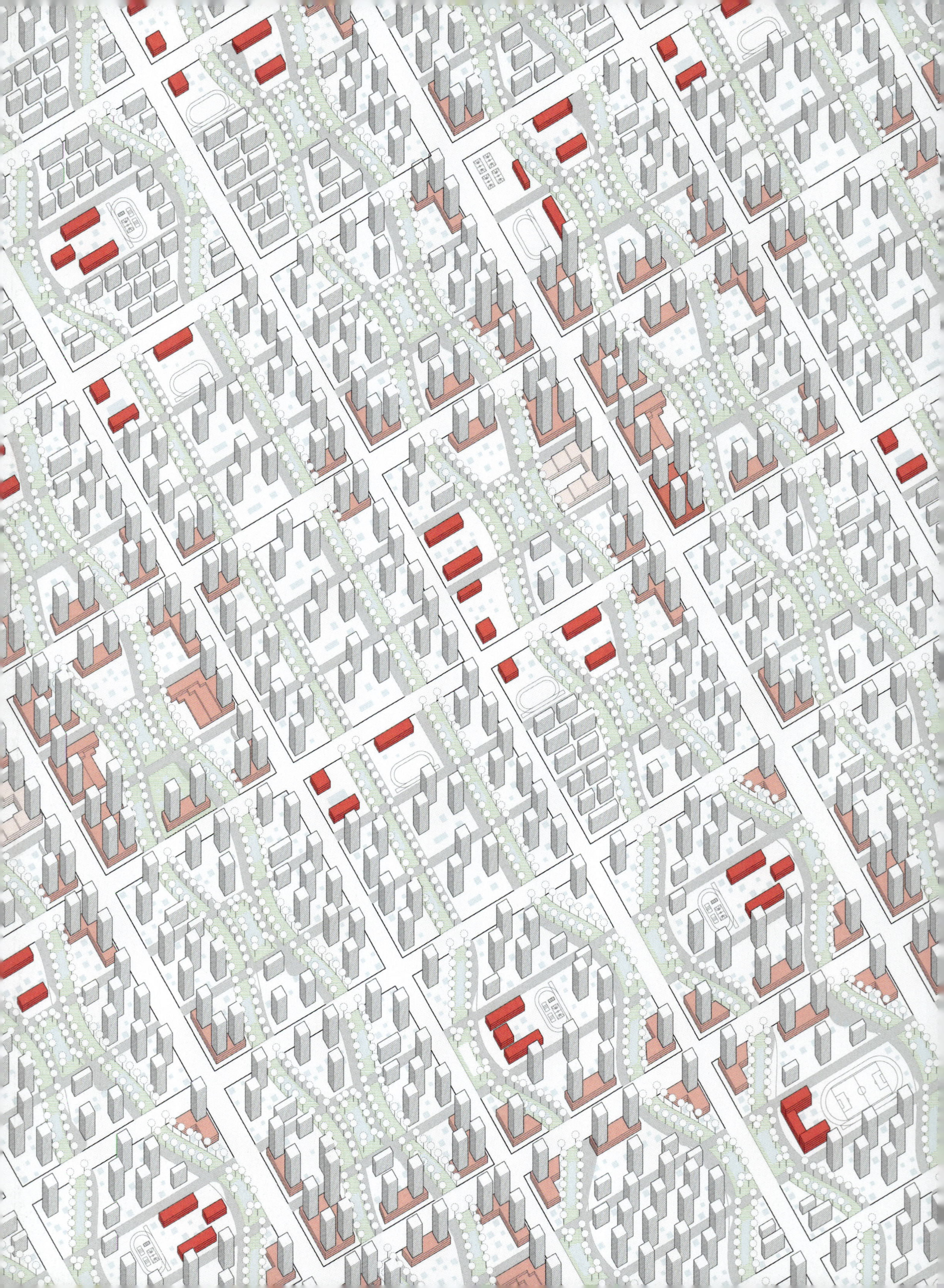

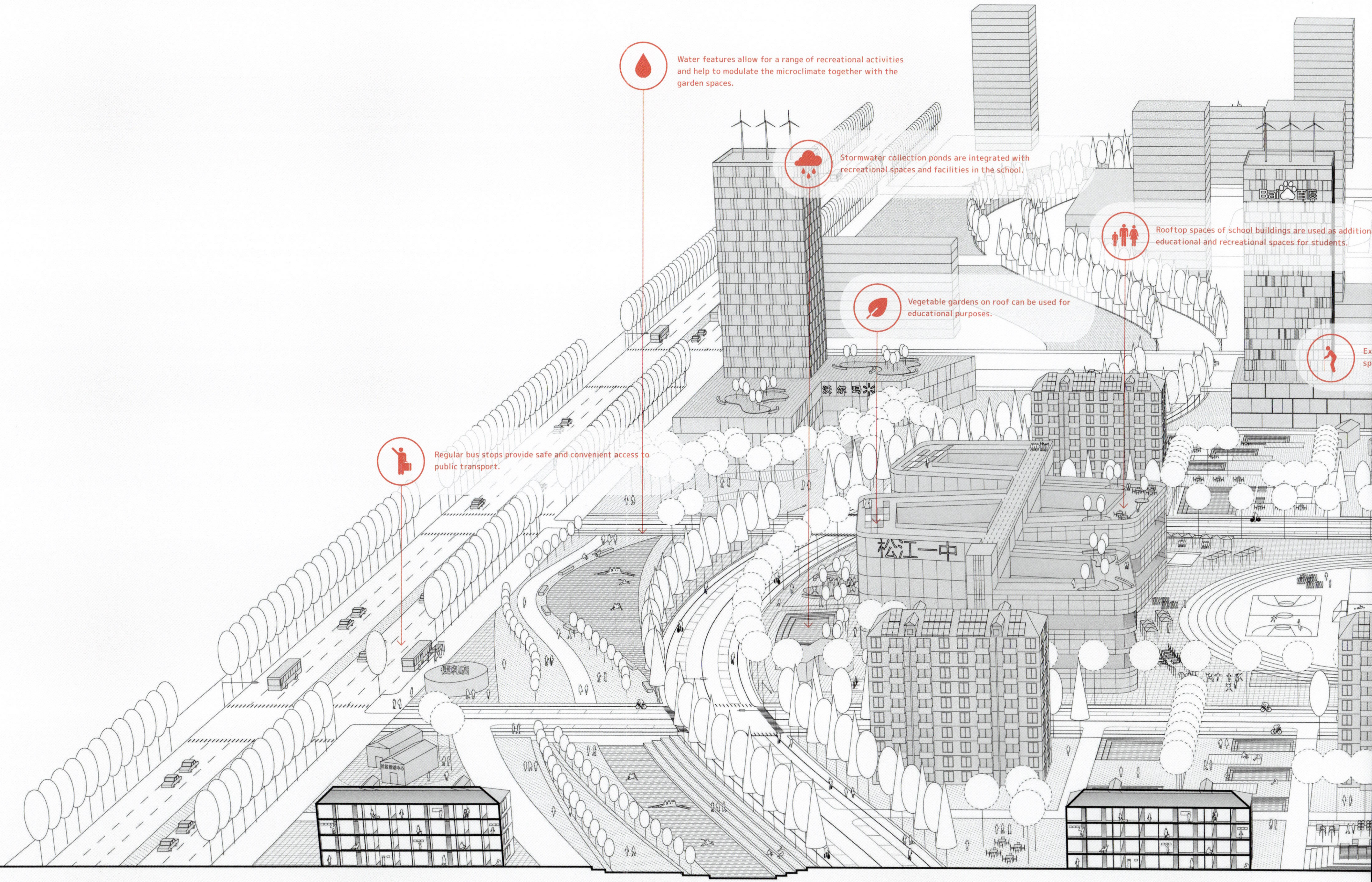

Water features allow for a range of recreational activities and help to modulate the microclimate together with the garden spaces.
Stormwater collection ponds are integrated with recreational spaces and facilities in the school.
Rooftop spaces of school buildings are used as additional educational and recreational spaces for students.
Vegetable gardens on roof can be used for educational purposes.
Regular bus stops provide safe and convenient access to public transport.
松江一中

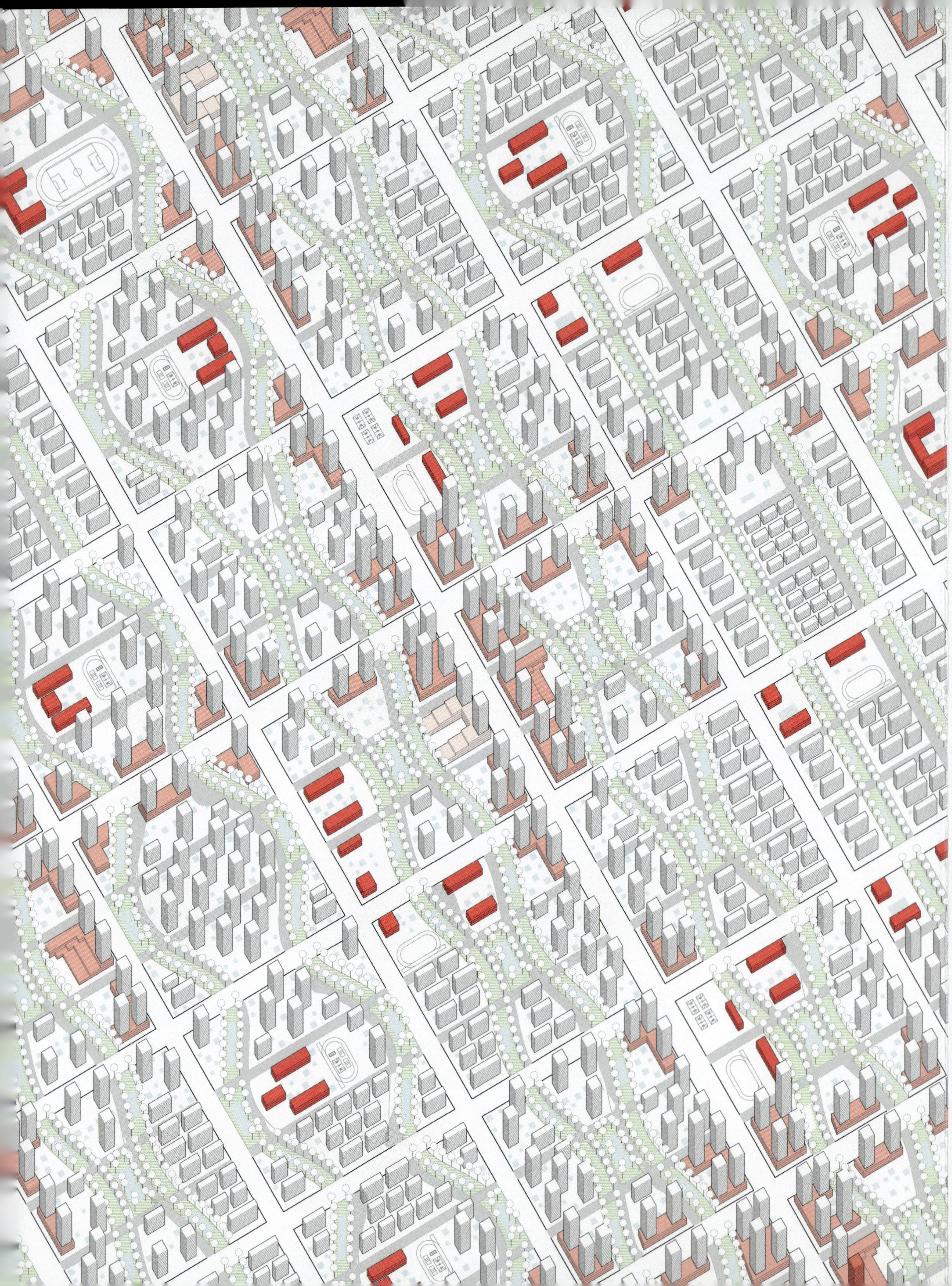

Scenario 2

Mixed Building Types and Large Institutional Building Scenario

This scenario represents the integration of important amenities within the neighborhood block. In this particular case, a school and sports field take the central location, providing social and recreational opportunities for the block as a whole. The greenway configurations are adjusted to accommodate the school grounds, while together with the rain gardens and small squares they offer opportunities for a range of different social spaces. Other programs, such as smaller retail or recreational pavilions may be scattered throughout this landscape framework.

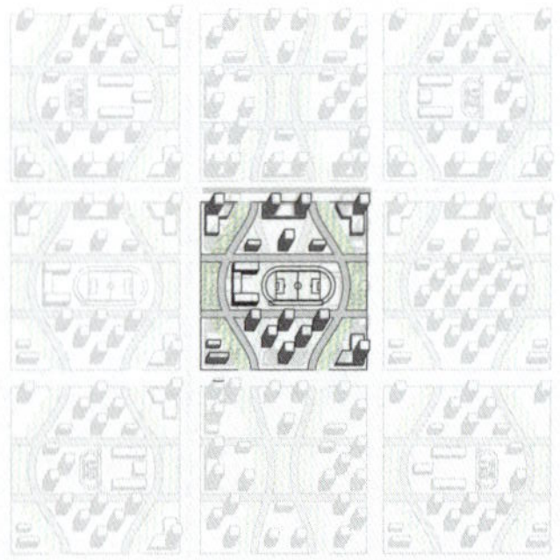

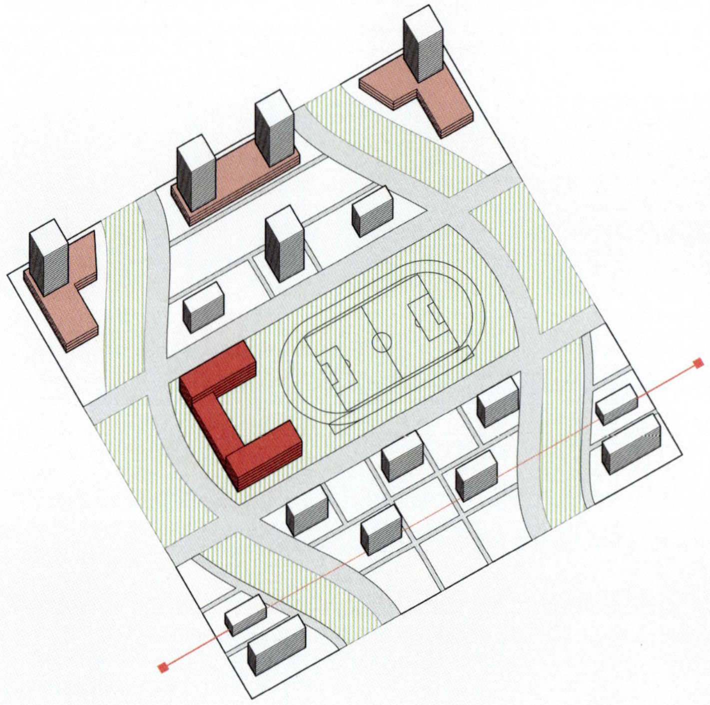

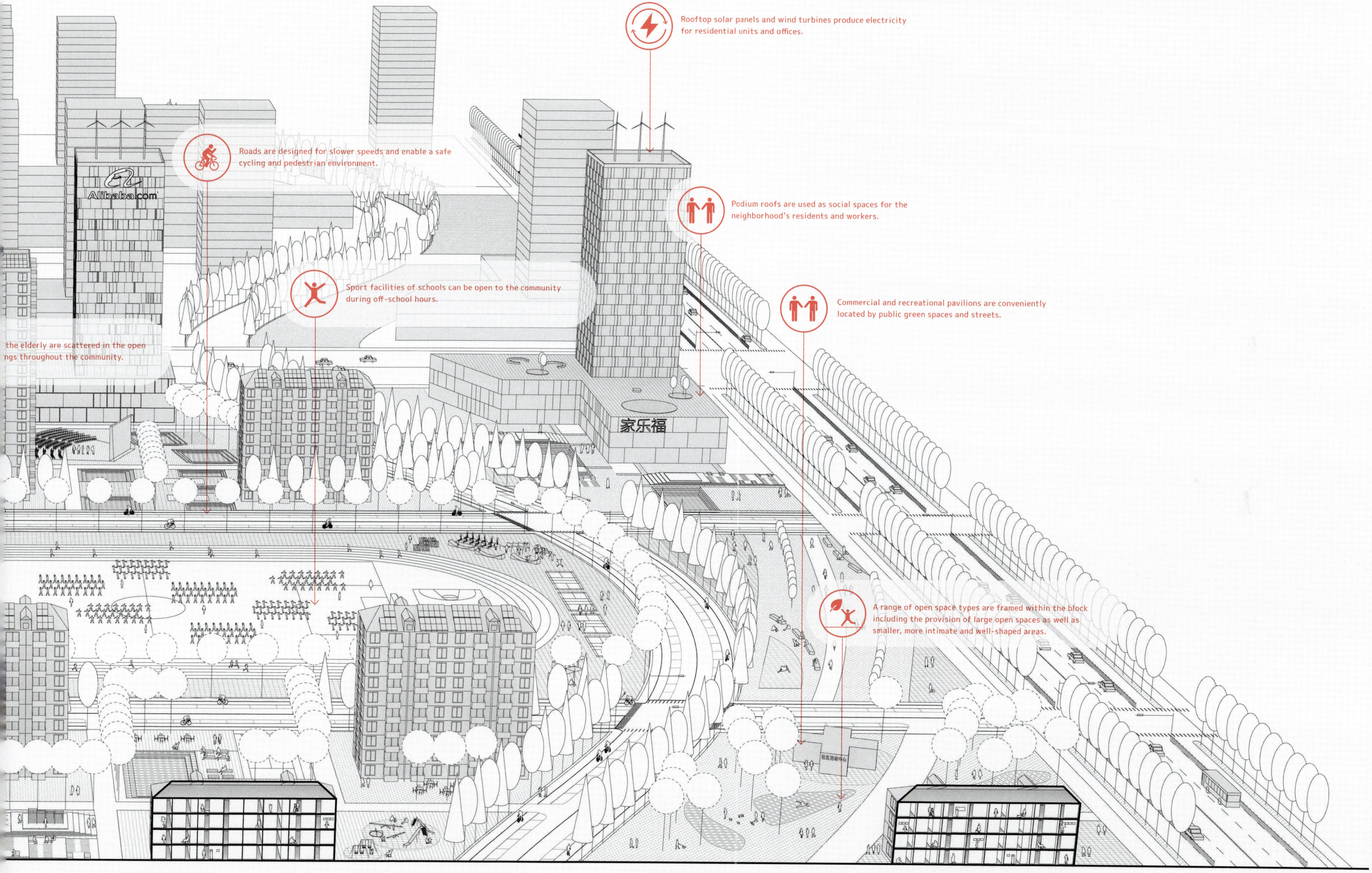

Alibaba.com
家乐福
Rooftop solar panels and wind turbines produce electricity for residential units and offices.
Roads are designed for slower speeds and enable a safe cycling and pedestrian environment.
Podium roofs are used as social spaces for the neighborhood's residents and workers.
Sport facilities of schools can be open to the community during off-school hours.
Commercial and recreational pavilions are conveniently located by public green spaces and streets.
the elderly are scattered in the open
ngs throughout the community.
A range of open space types are framed within the block including the provision of large open spaces as well as smaller, more intimate and well-shaped areas.

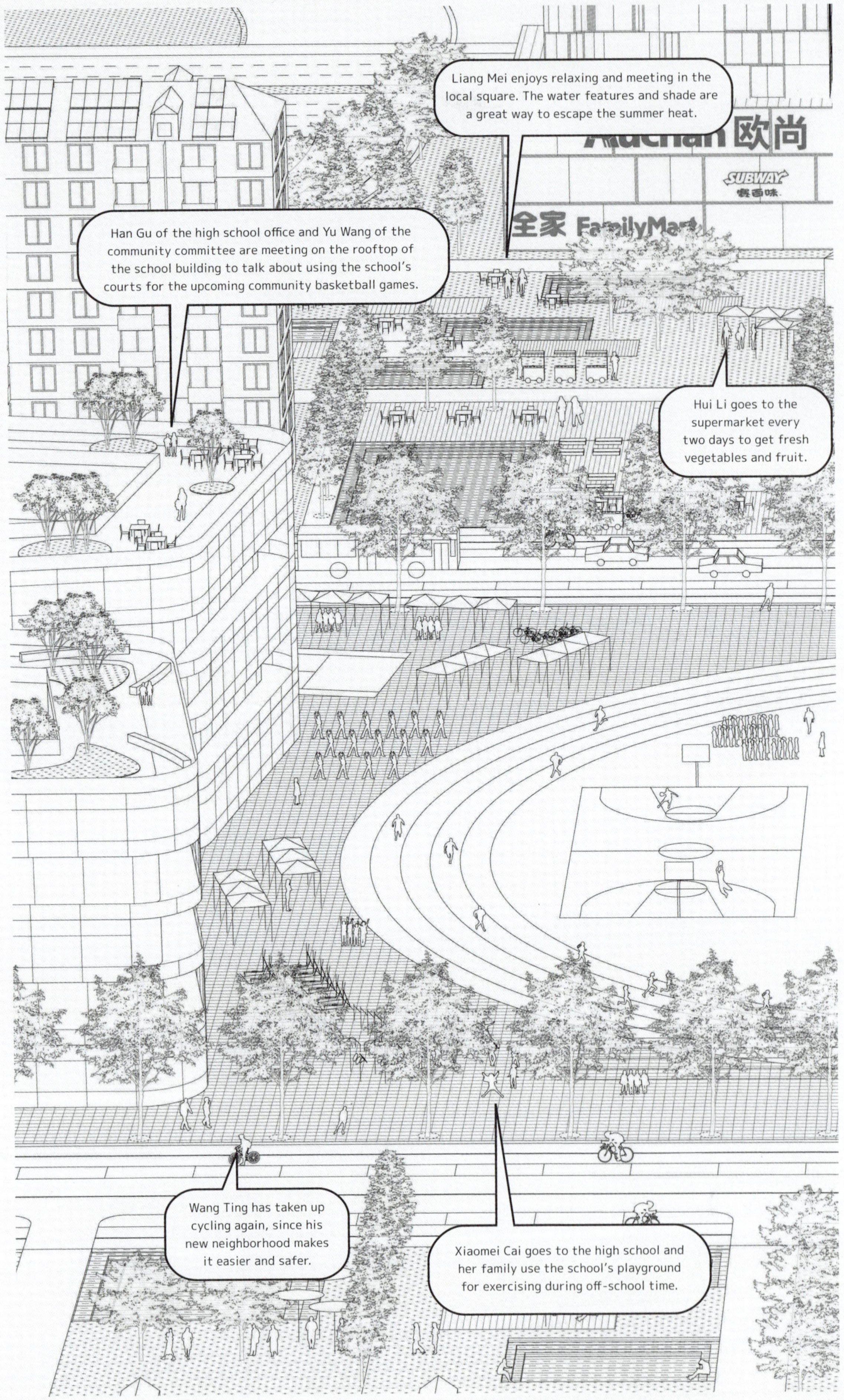

Liang Mei enjoys relaxing and meeting in the local square. The water features and shade are a great way to escape the summer heat.
Auchan 欧尚
SUBWAY
全家 FamilyMart
Han Gu of the high school office and Yu Wang of the community committee are meeting on the rooftop of the school building to talk about using the school's courts for the upcoming community basketball games.
Hui Li goes to the supermarket every two days to get fresh vegetables and fruit.
Wang Ting has taken up cycling again, since his new neighborhood makes it easier and safer.
Xiaomei Cai goes to the high school and her family use the school's playground for exercising during off-school time.

Greenway Systems

The nine-block arrangement allows for a number of combinations of greenway configurations, allowing for a differentiated open space pattern. This enables the definition of different organizations as well as characters for blocks within the nine block arrangement. The resulting framework allows for a variegated pattern for distributing functions and uses. At a smaller scale, the greenway section was also investigated to embed multiple functions and character within the open spaces.

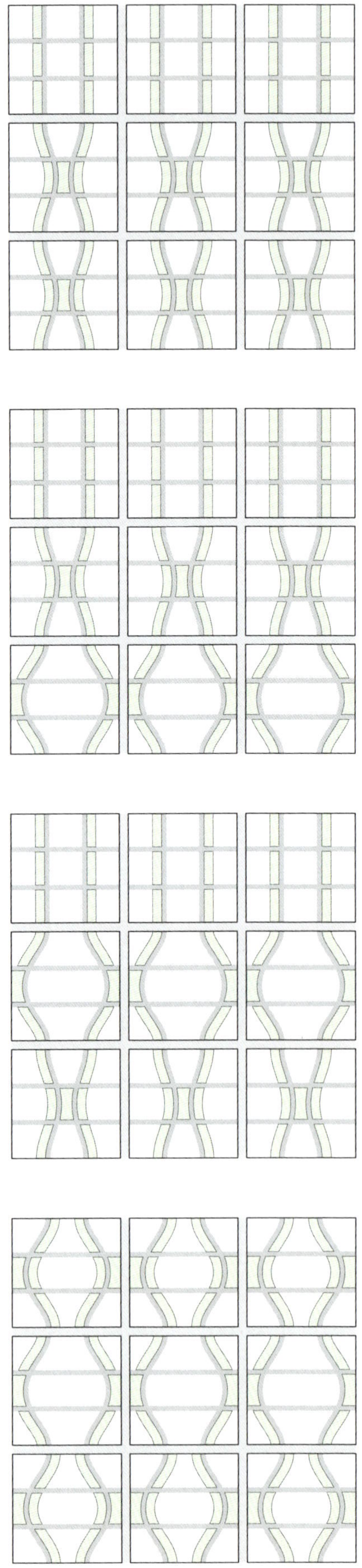

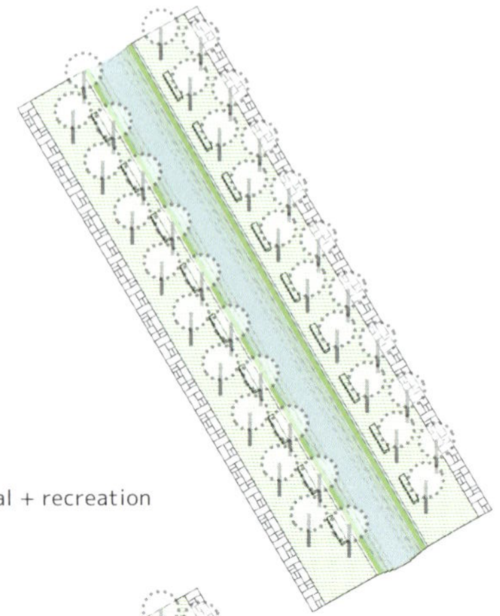

A. canal + recreation

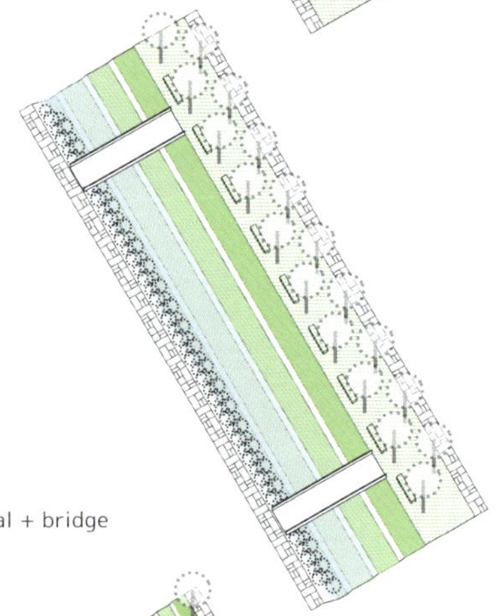

B. canal + bridge

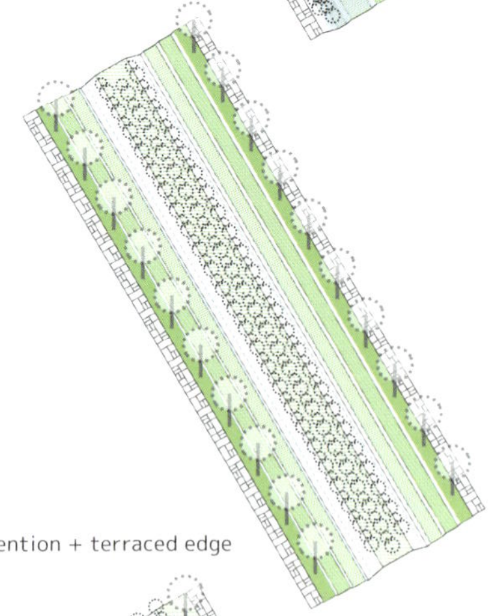

C. retention + terraced edge

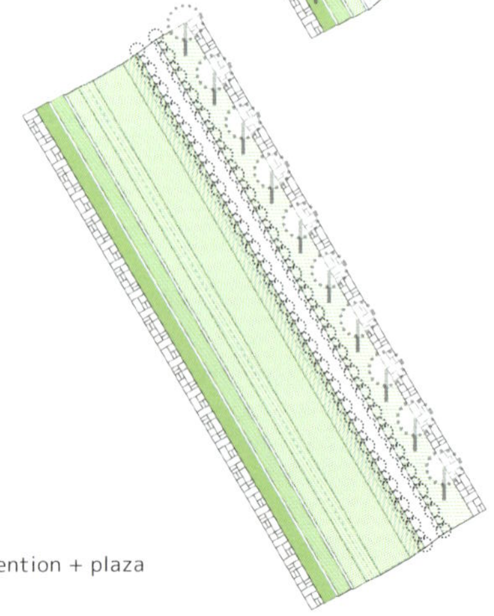

D. retention + plaza

Open Space Systems

Treatment of storm and rain water was integrated into the greenway as well as the open spaces in between buildings. This addressed the safeguarding of environmental health by proposing to utilize the block's landscape systems as a form of hydrological infrastructure for the neighborhood. Rain water is proposed to be collected and treated on site rather than being released to the general water network without treatment, limiting the local-scale pollution of the water system.

The multiple functions associated with these open spaces emphasize the importance of these framework elements, while ensuring the provisions of social spaces, green infrastructure, and biotic infrastructure for water treatment and management, making them an integral aspect of the blocks.

Stormwater Treatment Process

WET MEADOW **Swale** ⟶ OPEN DEEP WATER **Storm Water Sediment** ⟶ OPEN WATER **Containment Removal** ⟶ SHALLOW MARSH **Treatment Wetland** ⟶ SHALLOW MARSH **Treatment Wetland** ⟶ MUD FLAT **Enhancement Marsh**

Containment Removal:
Wetlands as chemical traps
Loading rate of chemicals (BOD, phosphorus, nitrogen)
Long detention times

Treatment Wetland:
Natural process
Wetland Plants Treatment

Treatment Wetland:
Natural process
Wetland Plants Treatment

Enhancement Marsh:
Natural process
Wetland Plants Treatment

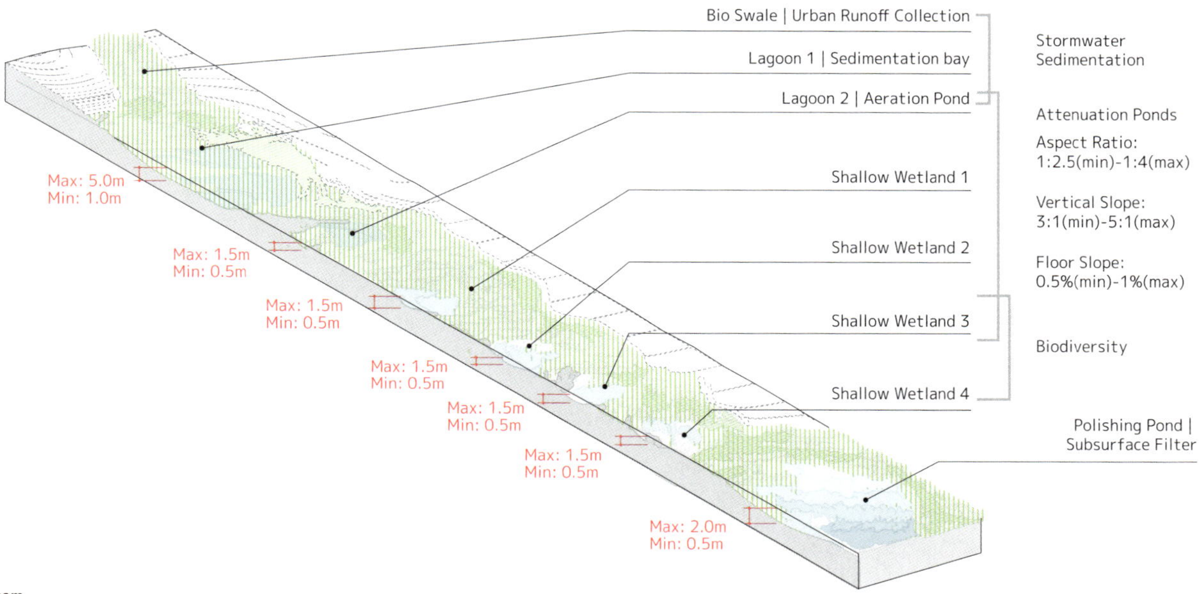

System

"Tanks in series" is proved to provide higher quality effluent.

FWS Ponds Shapes

Rectangle, polygon, oval, kidney shapes, and crescent shapes.

Size

Factors: Surface (permeable, non-permeable), local precipitation, runoff coefficient
Design: 20 -year rainfall intensity in 2h duration of storm rainfall
General: 2%-4% of contributing watershed area
The efficacy of created wetlands generally increases with size.
Most treatment wetlands that have been constructed range in size from 2.5-25 acres

Source: Wetland Design: Principles and Practices for Landscape Architects and Land-us Planners. Robert L. France.

Hydrology Systems

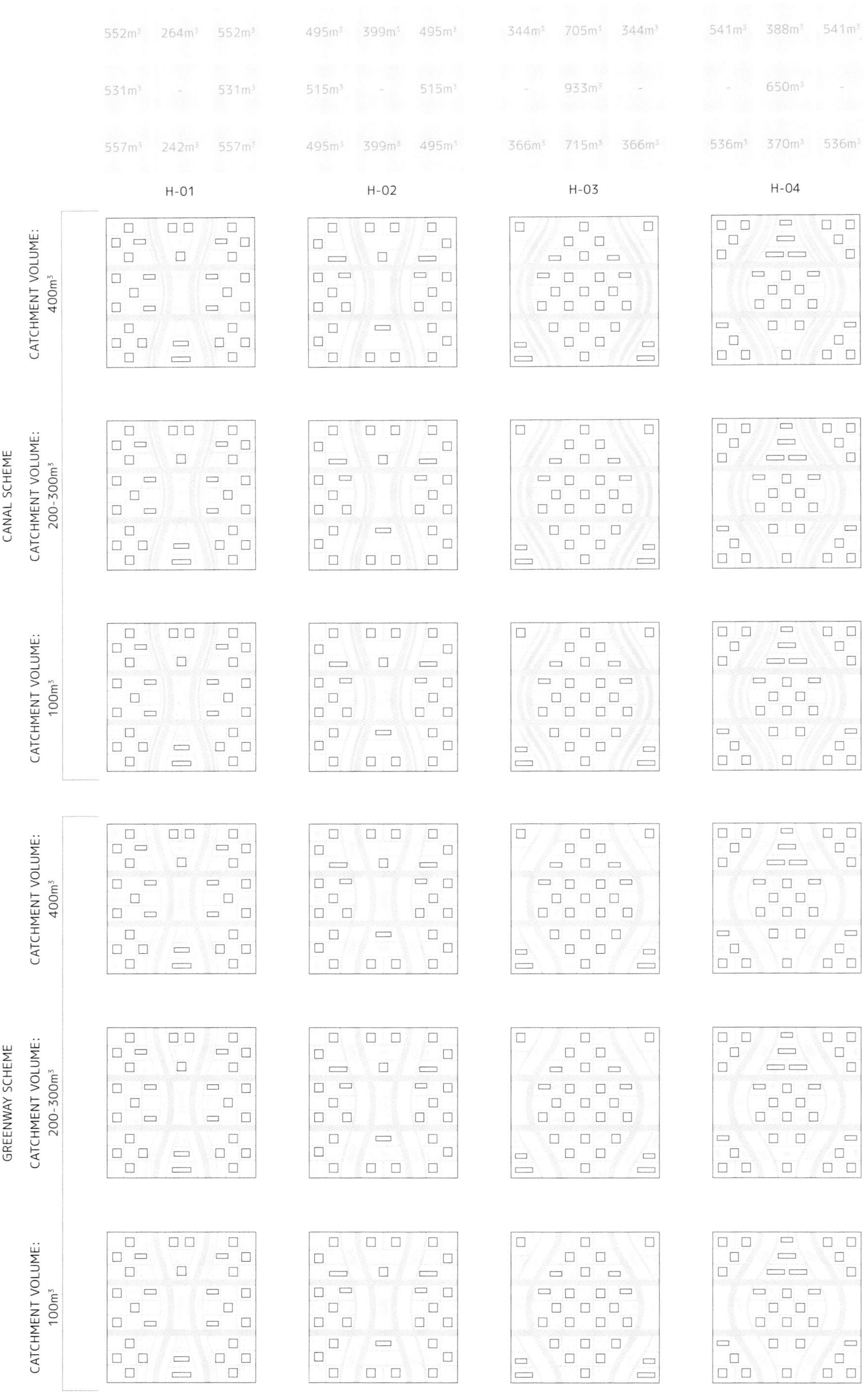

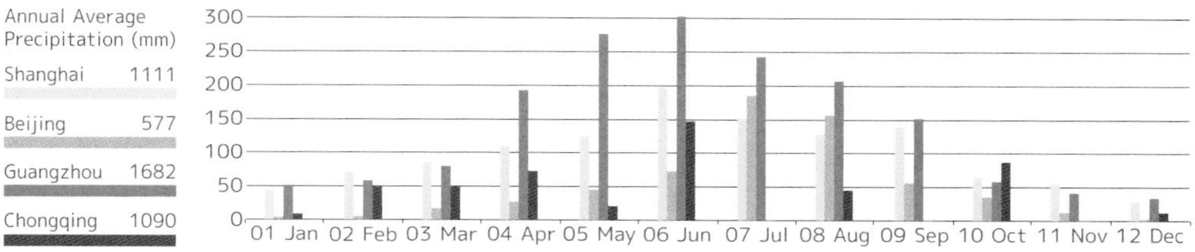

REGIONAL PRECIPITATION

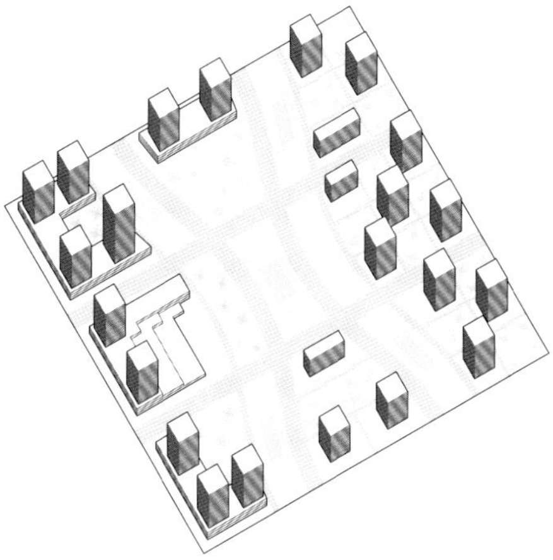

H-02 WITH PODIUM BUILDINGS

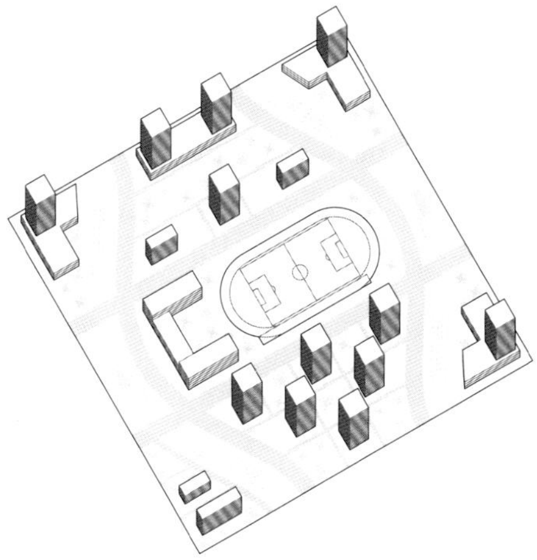

H-04 WITH PODIUM BUILDINGS

CATCHMENT VOLUME

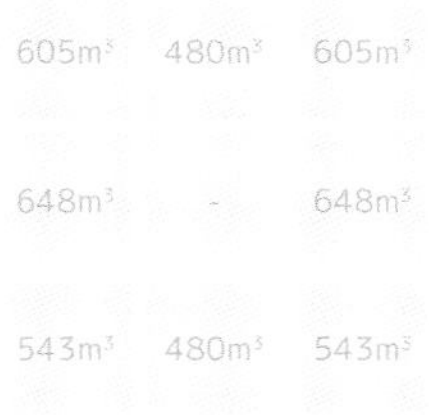

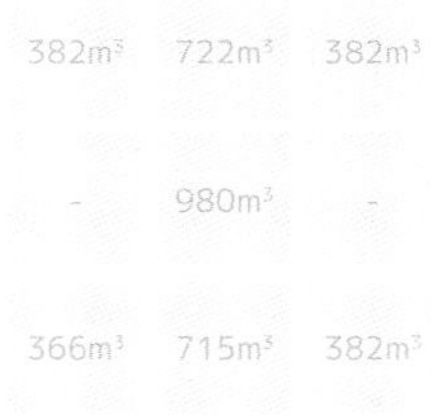

Each sub-plot material areas were calculated to determine total stormwater run-off volume.

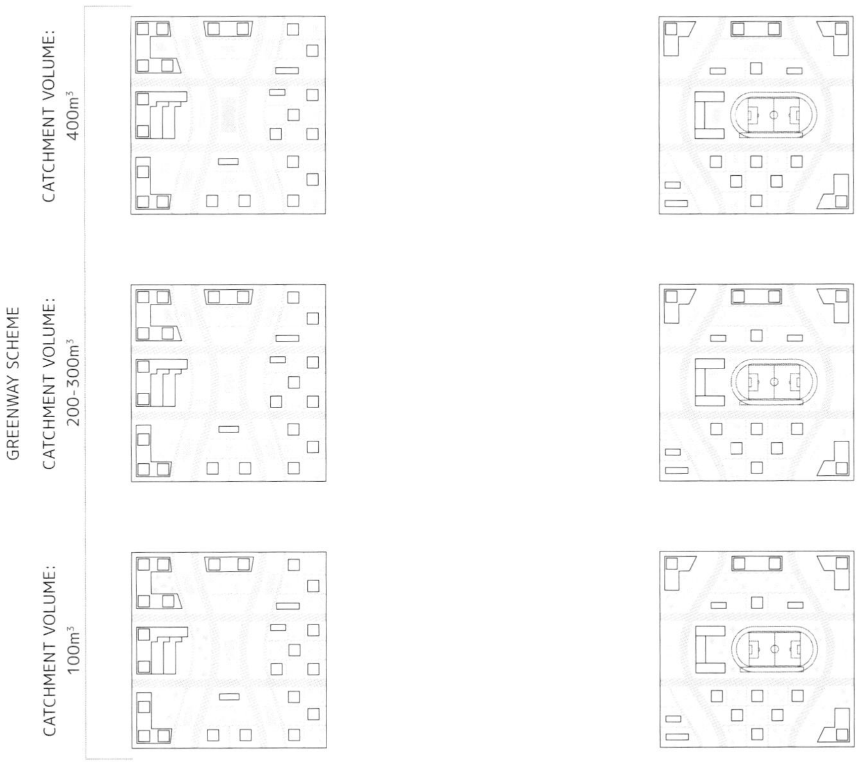

Utilizing the greenways as canals and larger swales and the interstitial spaces between buildings as sites for rain gardens and attenuation ponds, volumes of each hydrological feature were calculated to accommodate average to peak volumes, offering a systematic method for arranging "blue spaces" within the neighborhood block.

Greenway Types

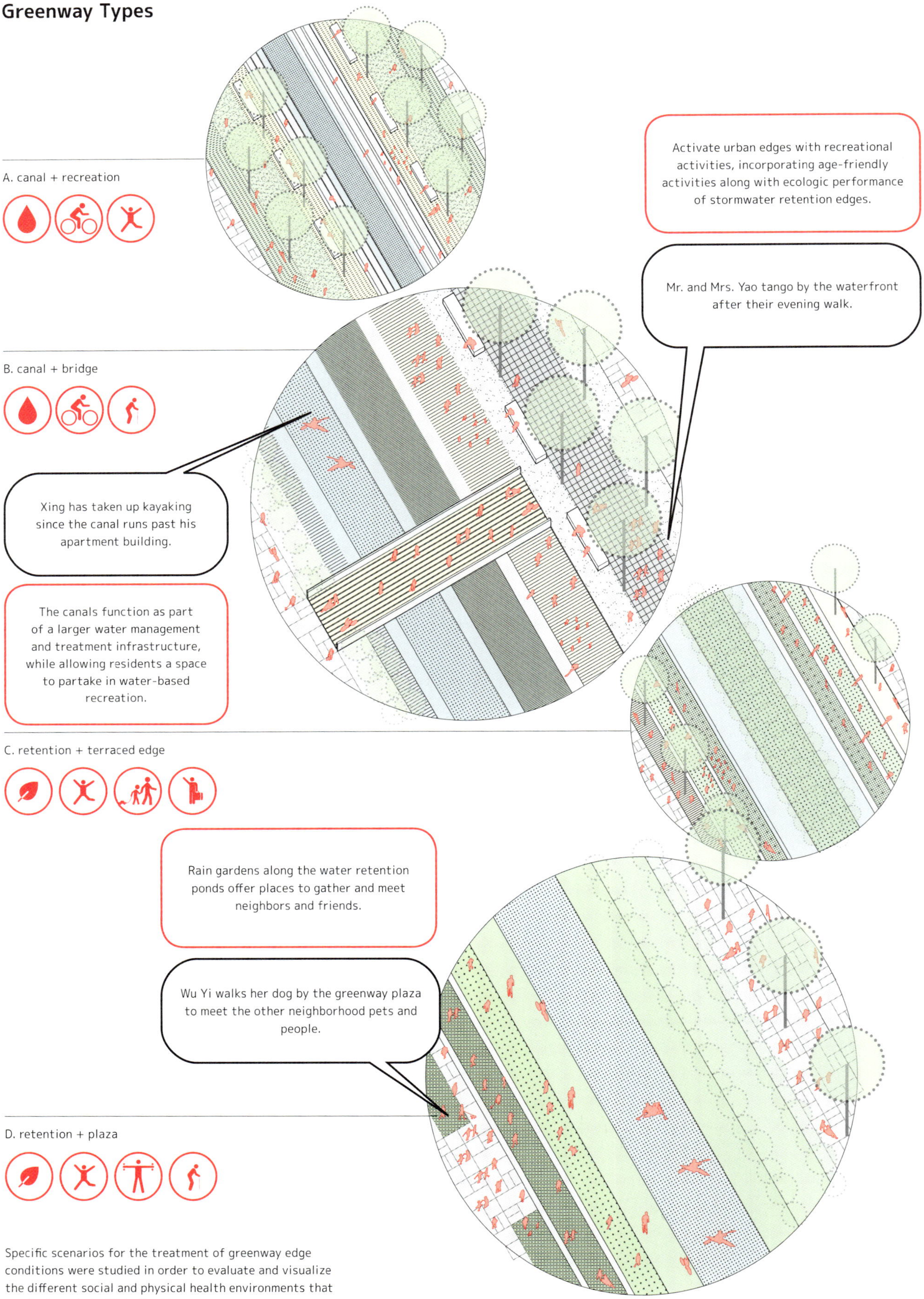

Specific scenarios for the treatment of greenway edge conditions were studied in order to evaluate and visualize the different social and physical health environments that may be inserted within the blocks.

Rain Garden Types

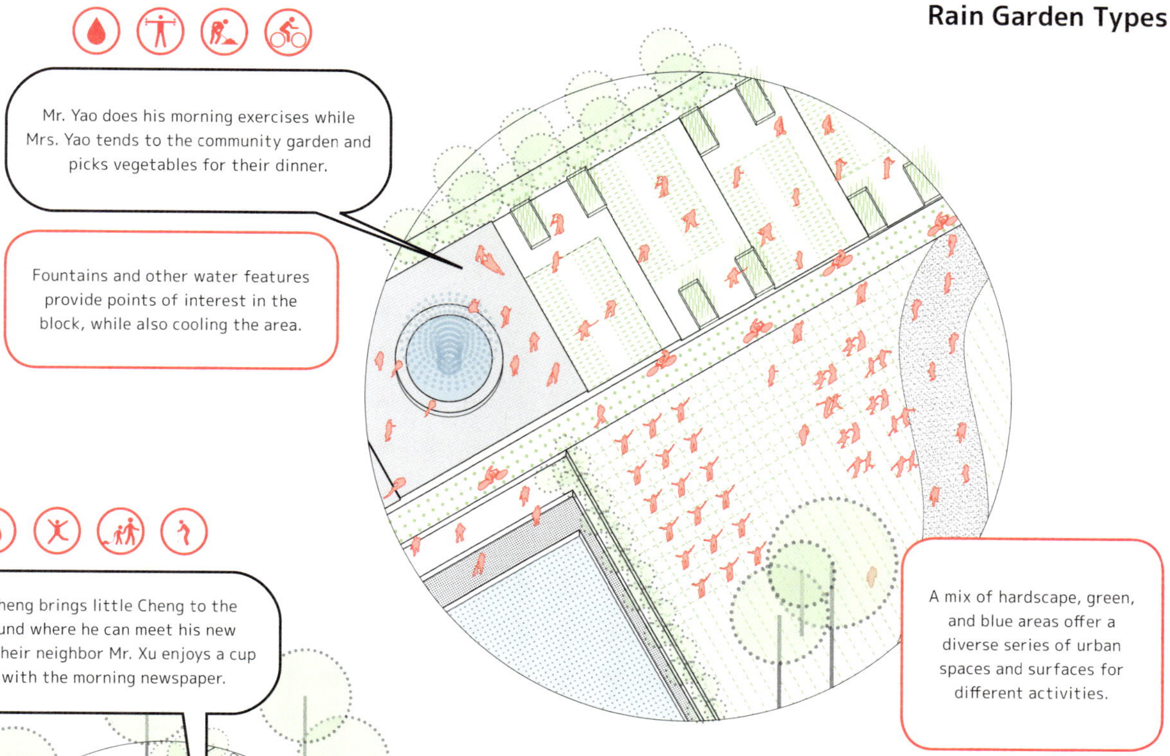

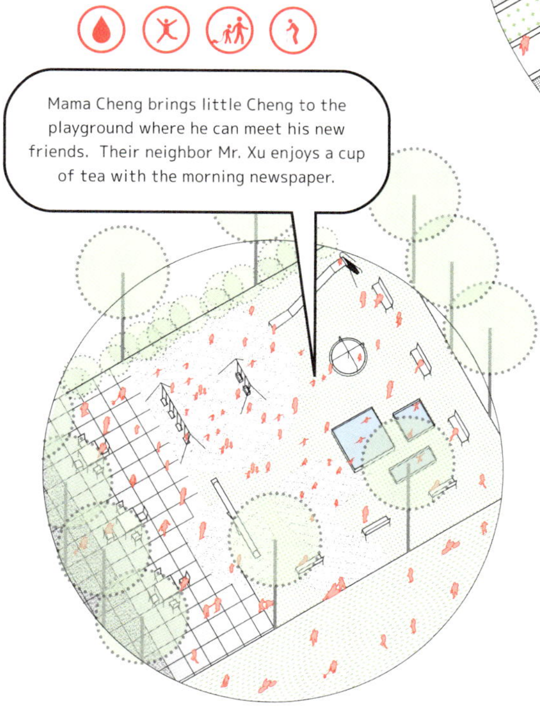

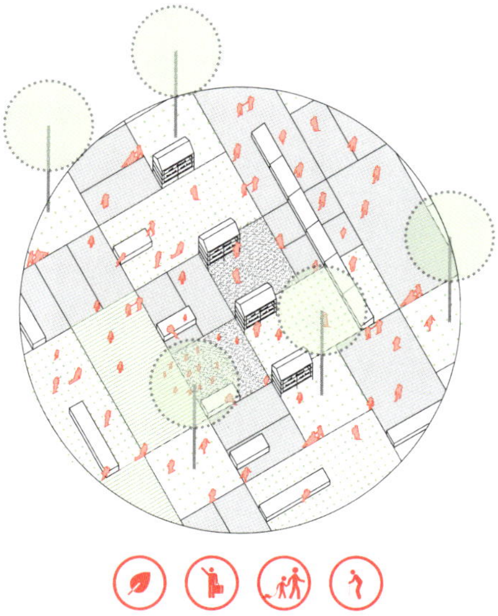

RAIN GARDEN TREATMENT SCENARIOS

[1] $400m^3$ catchment volume	[1] $200m^3$ catchment volume	[multiple] $100m^3$ catchment volume

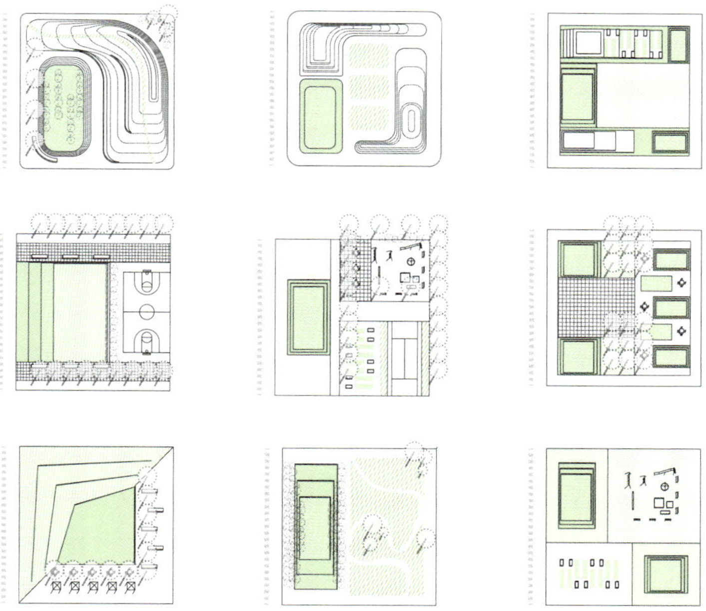

FLEXIBLE PROGRAMMING SCENARIOS

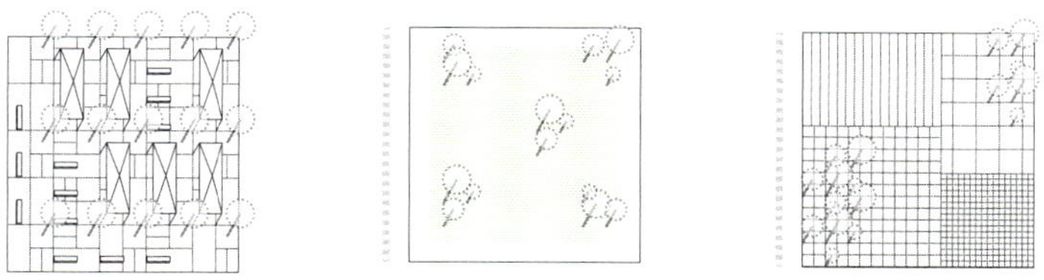

Block Aggregation

DISTRIBUTION OF AMENITIES ON A 9-BLOCK SAMPLE SITE
01: CENTRAL CORE

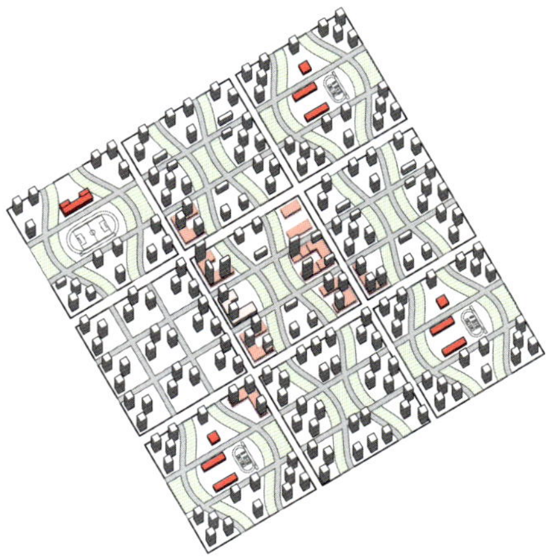

FAR: 1.585

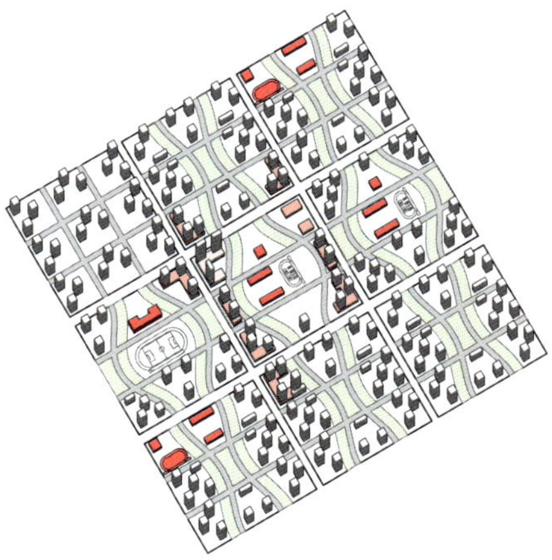

FAR: 1.633

02: CORRIDOR

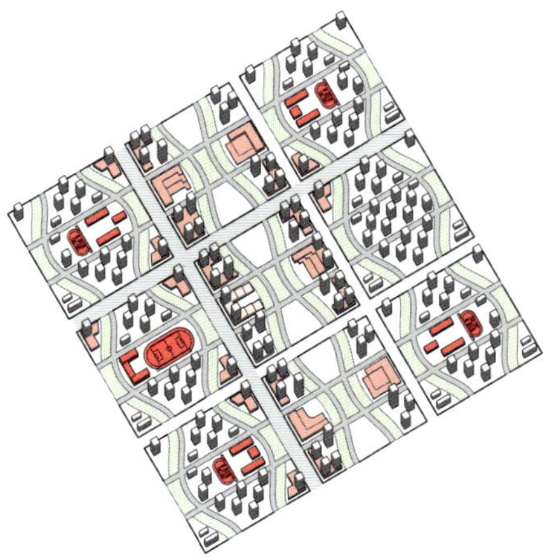

FAR: 1.438

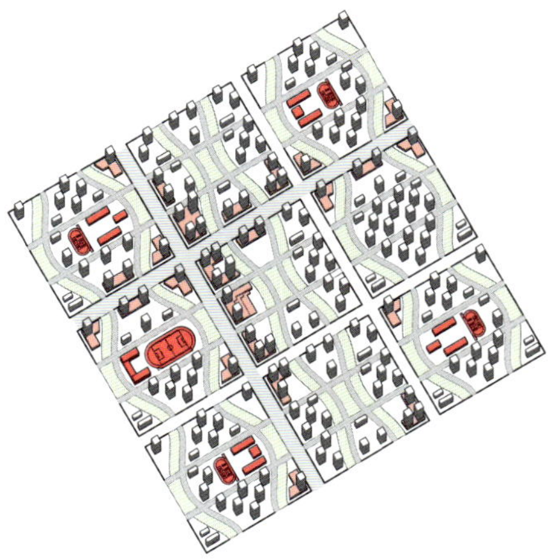

FAR: 1.506

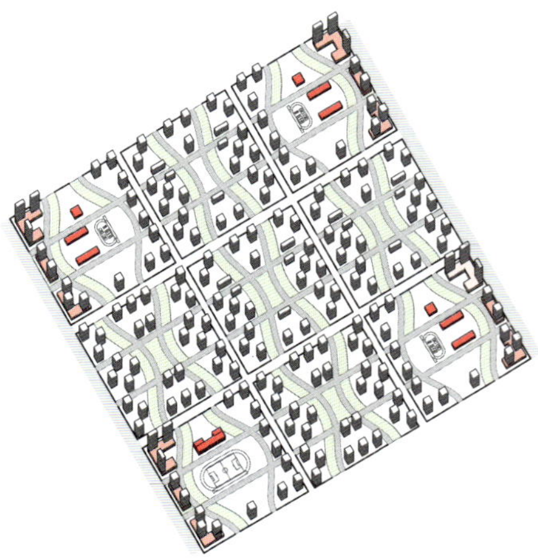

FAR: 1.580

OPEN SPACE
BLOCK STREETS
SUPERMARKETS
RETAIL/RECREATION/HEALTH CARE
SCHOOLS

03: CORRIDOR + CENTRAL

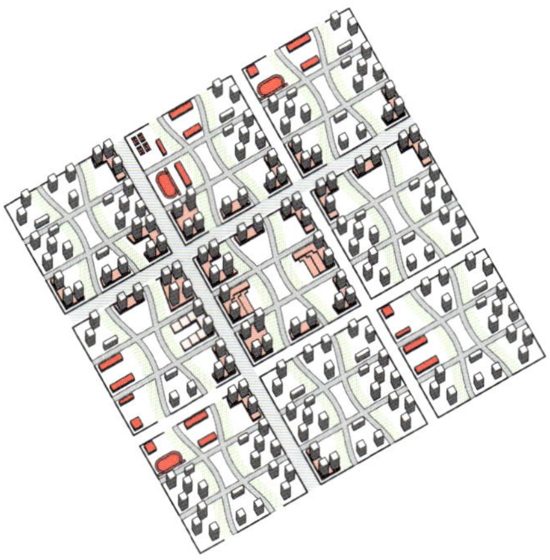

FAR: 1.840

04: EVENLY DISTRIBUTED

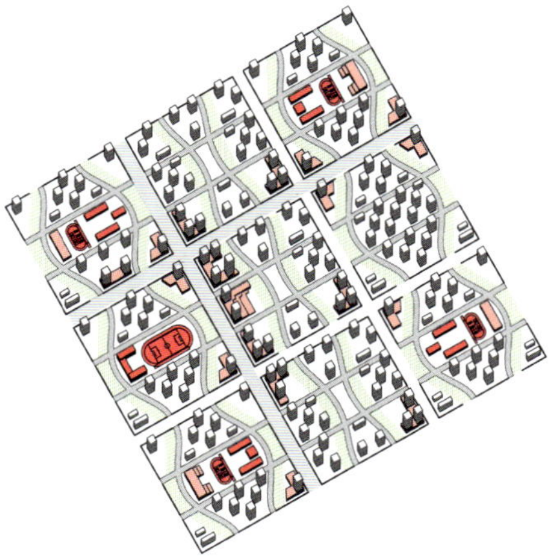

FAR: 1.461

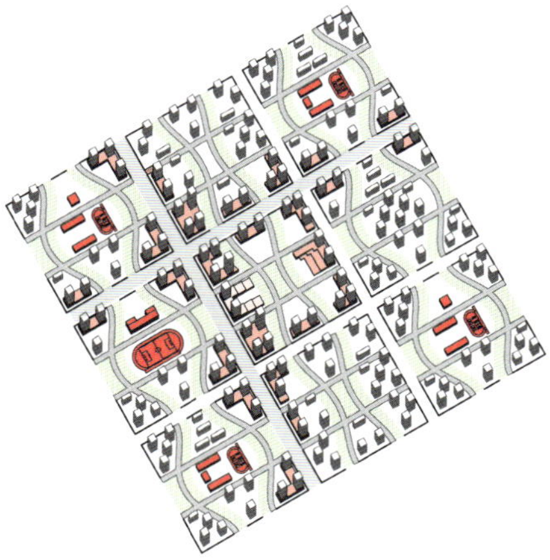

FAR: 1.598

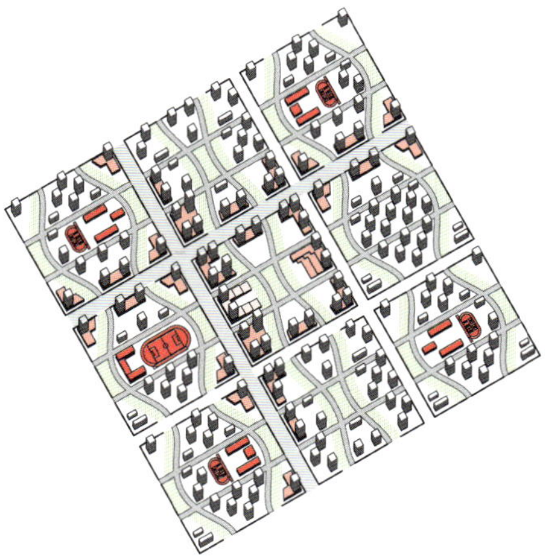

FAR: 1.559

Based on the catchment zones for amenities and services, the nine-square-block aggregation was found to be the appropriate scale to accommodate most of the identified facilities that are necessary for healthier living.

This aggregation can operate as the appropriate scale for the implementation of *shequ* (社区, community) organizations. The *shequ* is a community institution, intended to replace the *danwei* (單位, work unit) model that existed as the basic social institution in China prior to the housing reform of the 1990s. It is a local social institution of residents and citizens that oversee the management of the necessary neighborhood facilities and amenities, relieving the central state government of these particular responsibilities.

A series of possible configurations are depicted here that run through the gradient between concentrated to dispersed models of programmatic distribution. Based on the distribution configurations, the block framework could be guided by the specific location of key facilities and institutions. The location of building density and other programs is more flexible as these may be located and subsequently relocated in any number of blocks. The distribution patterns have a bearing on the emergence of different scales of street elevations, while also determining the infrastructure hierarchy as density is often used as a measure for the allocation of public transportation and services.

Building Types

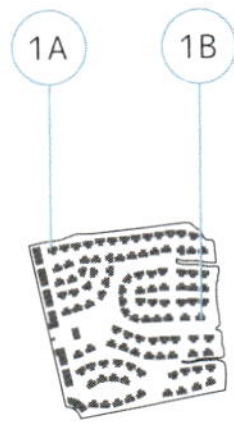

Block Type 1

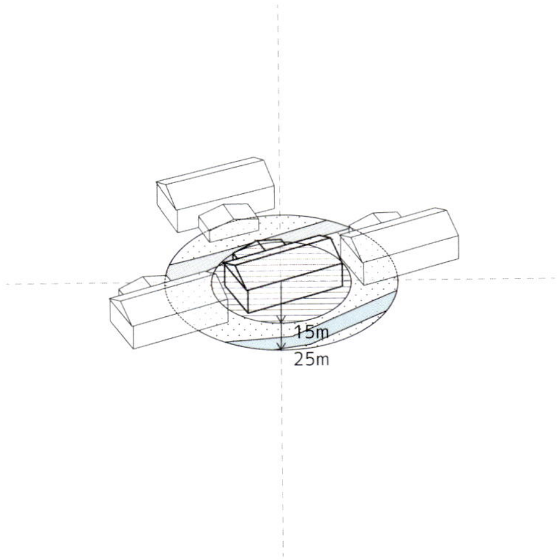

Building Type A

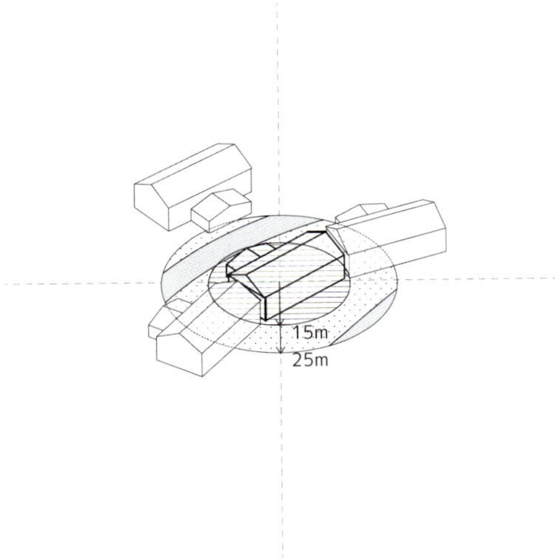

Building Type B

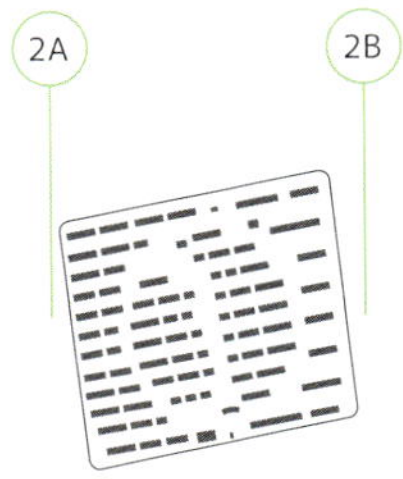

Block Type 2

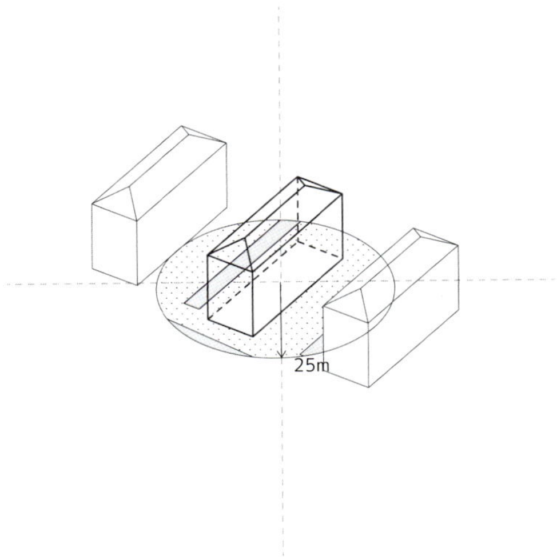

Building Type A

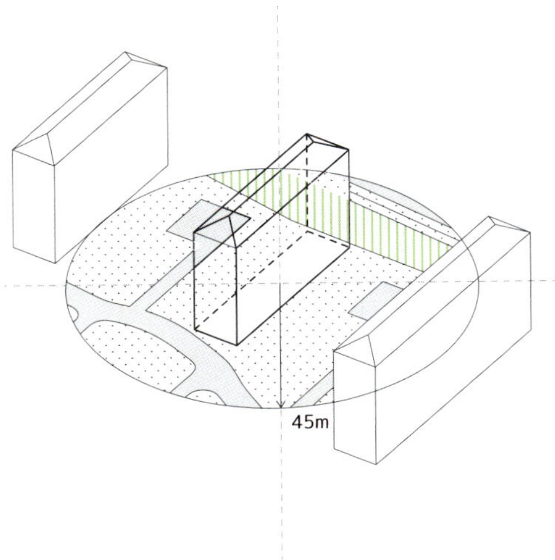

Building Type B

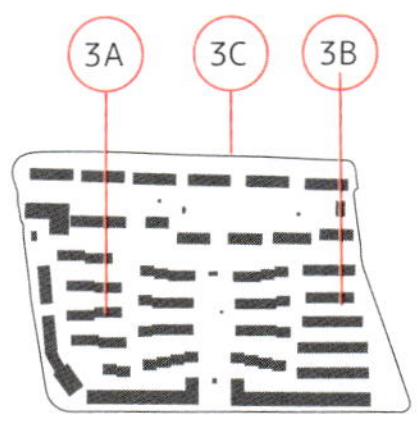

Block Type 3

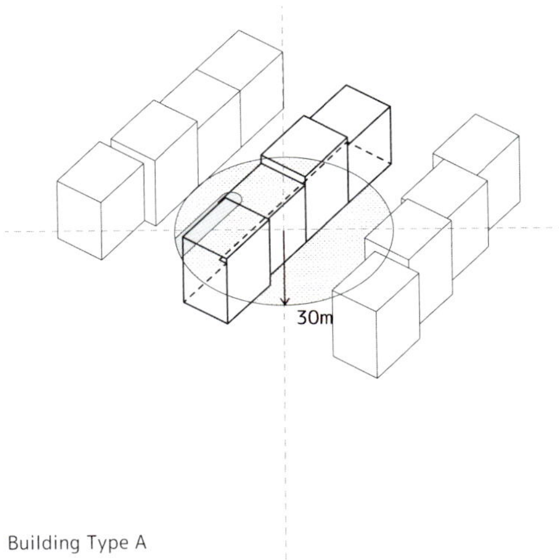

Building Type A

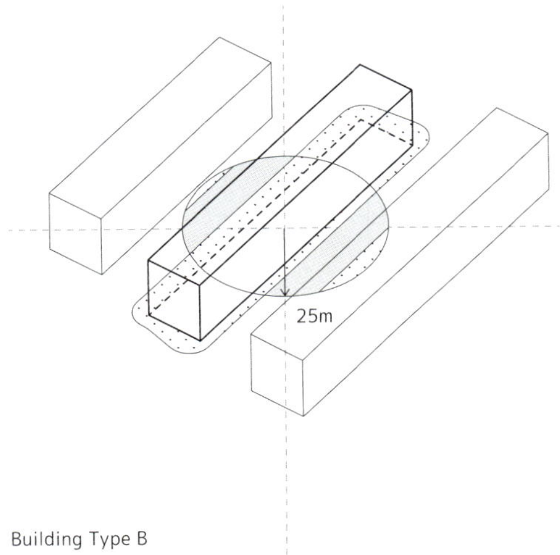

Building Type B

The existing buildings in the typical development blocks tend to be discrete, pavilion structures. These adhere to the "sunshine" law but result in a sharp differentiation between building figure and the leftover ground. There is a noticeable distinction between the buildings' and landscapes' as leftover spaces.

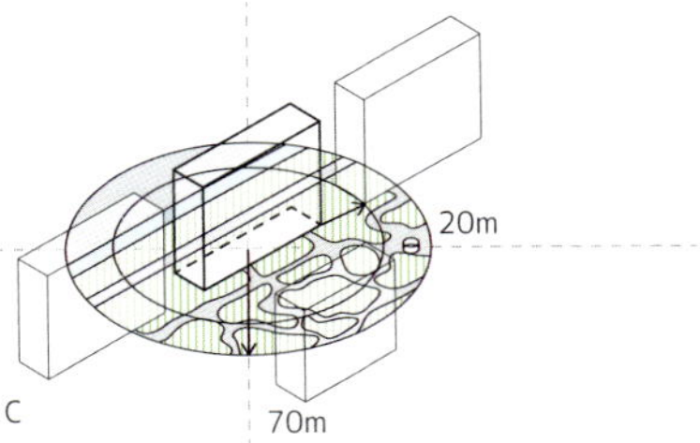

Building Type C

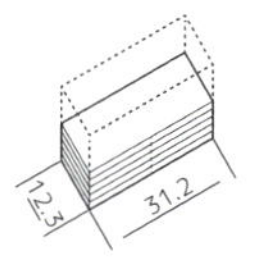

Slab Type 1
5 / 8/ 10 floors

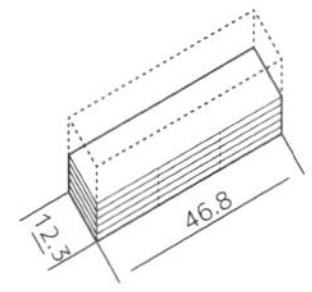

Slab Type 2
5 / 8/ 10 floors

Slab Buildings
Residential GFA per Person: 32m²/person
Residential GFA per Unit: 192m²/unit
Ratio of Parking Lots to Residential Units: 0.5
Parking: 75% of gross available area

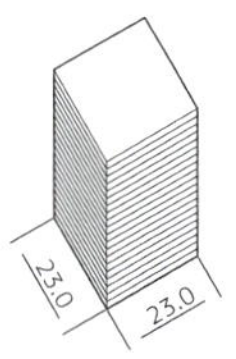

Tower Type 1
20 floors

Tower Buildings
Residential GFA per Person: 33m²/person
Residential GFA per Unit: 88.15m²/unit
Ratio of Parking Lots to Residential Units: 0.5
Parking: 75% of gross available area

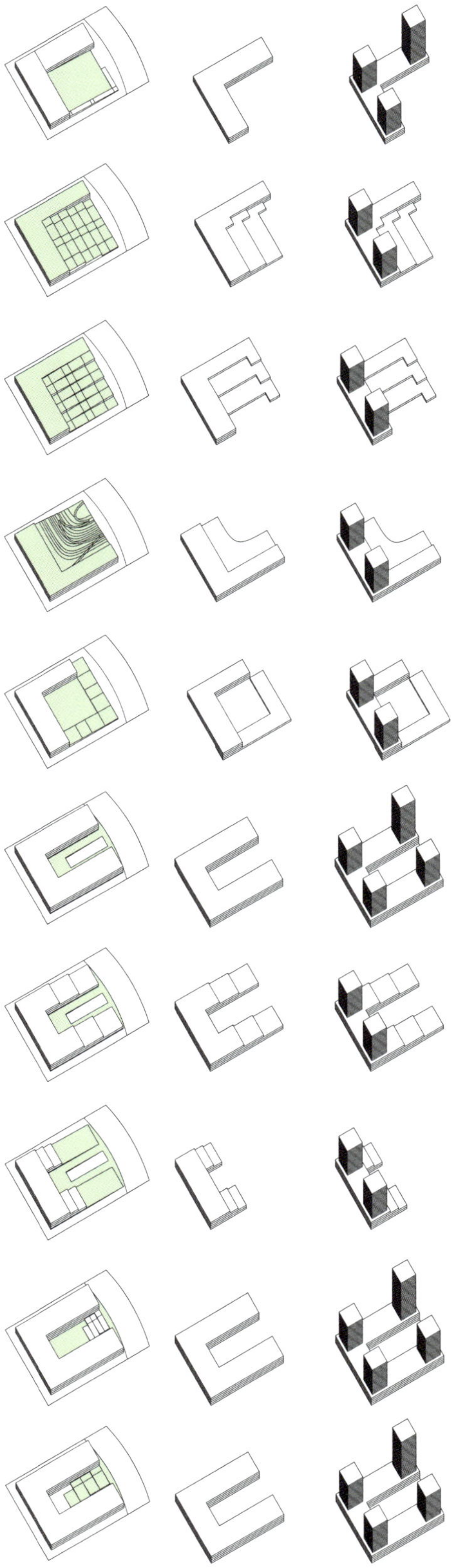

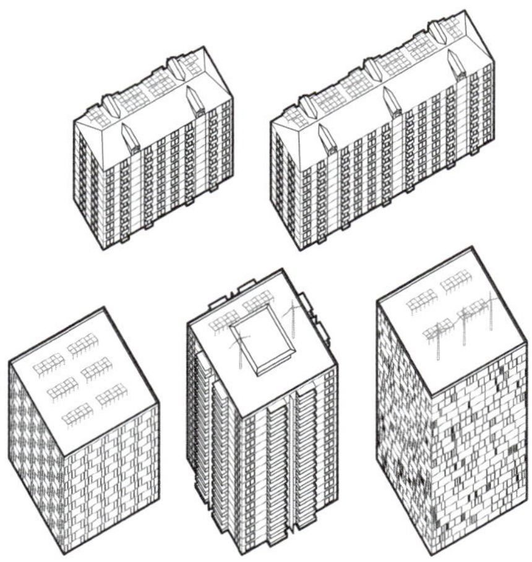

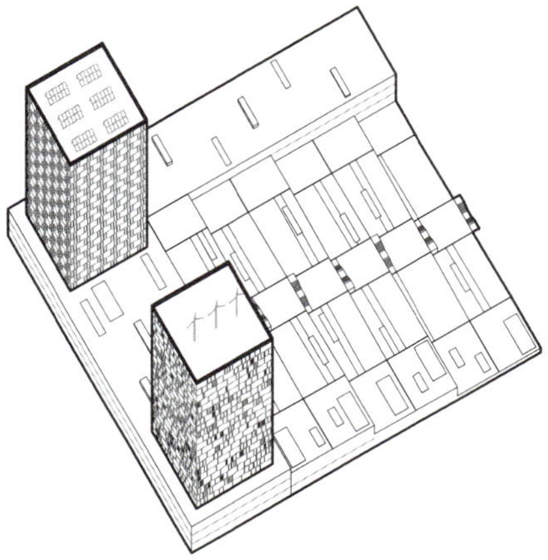

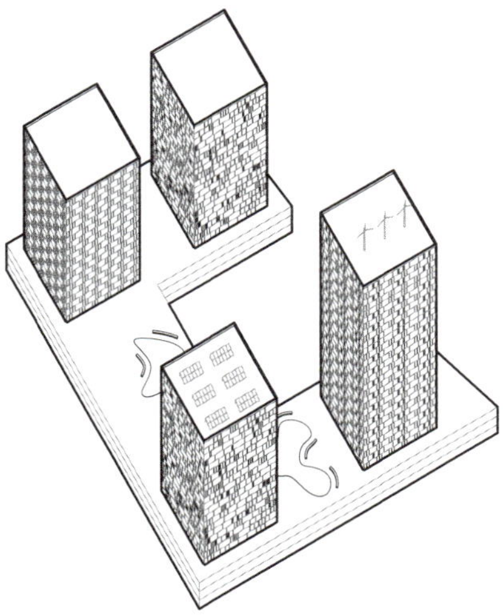

To account for the large areas of open and green spaces allocated for each block, many of the buildings utilized for the study were higher density models. This was done to ensure meeting existing block density, and in some cases, to offer higher densities. Podium bases were utilized to allow for different treatments of the relationship between the building and the ground. Multiplying the ground in order to accommodate more public spaces and programs (including community facilities, parking, retail, etc.), the podium and base building arrangements were defined to offer a variety of open spaces within the building parcel itself, from podium roof terraces to sheltered courtyards.

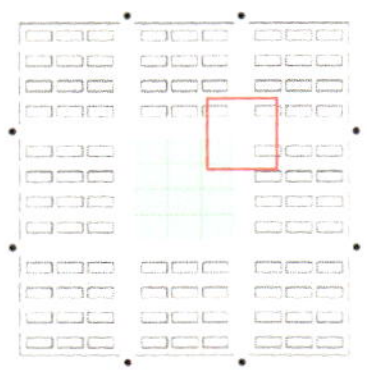

5-FLOOR BUILDINGS	Dimensions
A: ROADWAY	3.1m
B: PLANTER	1.8m
C: SIDEWALK	2.1m
D: BIKEWAY	1.8m
E: PARKING	2.4m / 2.1m
F: SHARED LANE	5.2m

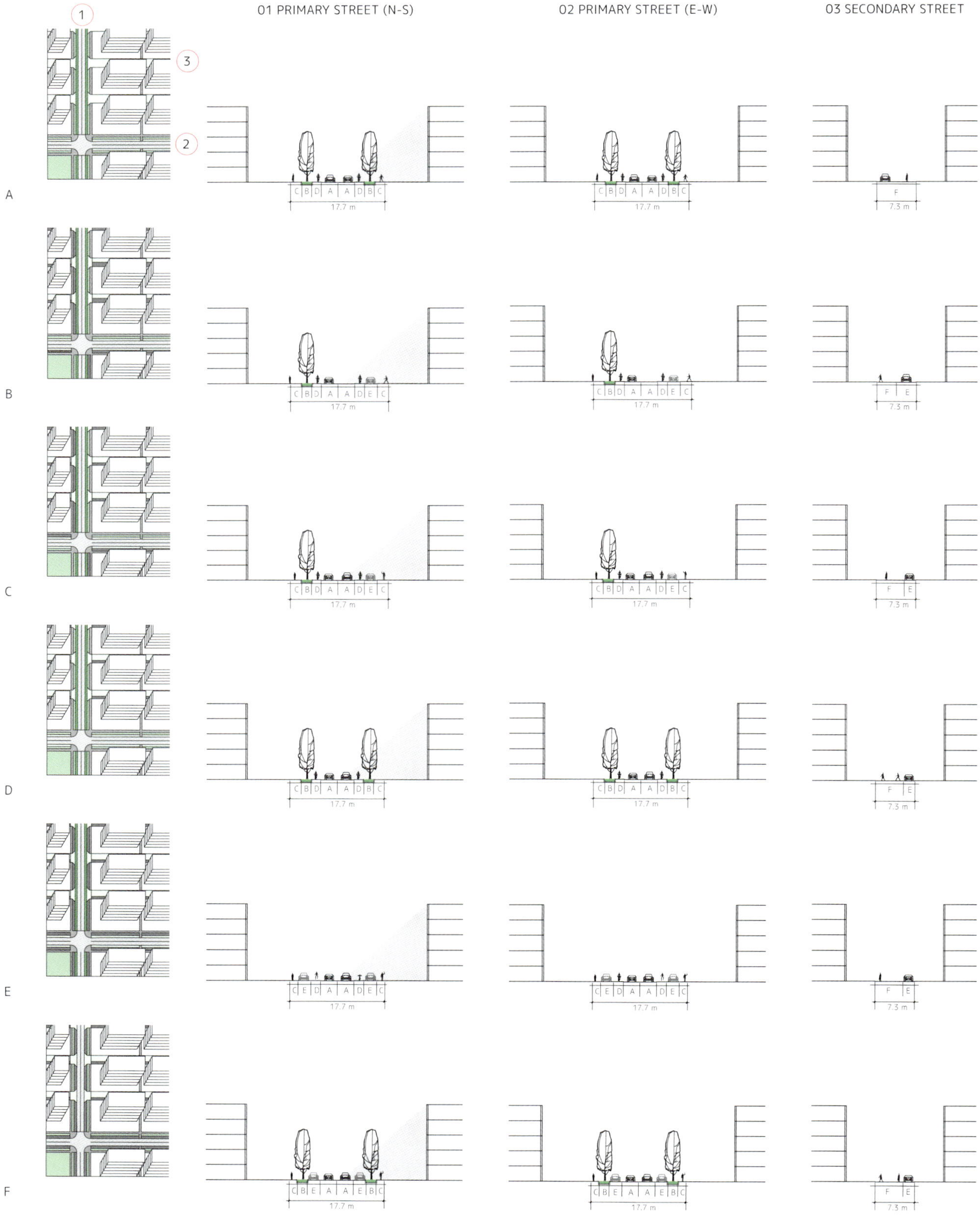

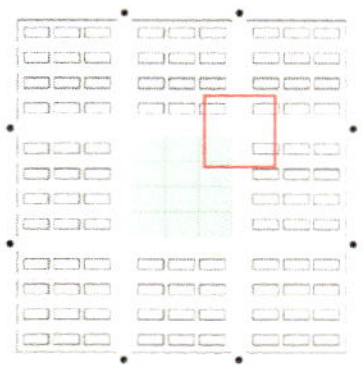

10-FLOOR BUILDINGS	Dimensions
A: ROADWAY	3.1m
B: PLANTER	1.8m
C: SIDEWALK	2.1m
D: BIKEWAY	1.8m
E: PARKING	2.4m / 2.1m
F: SHARED LANE	5.2m

Street Types

At the smaller scale, street arrangements were studied to achieve varying balances between allocation for parking, street planting, and providing ample spaces for pedestrian and bicycle activity. The shading of the street section and managing safety and traffic speeds were considerations.

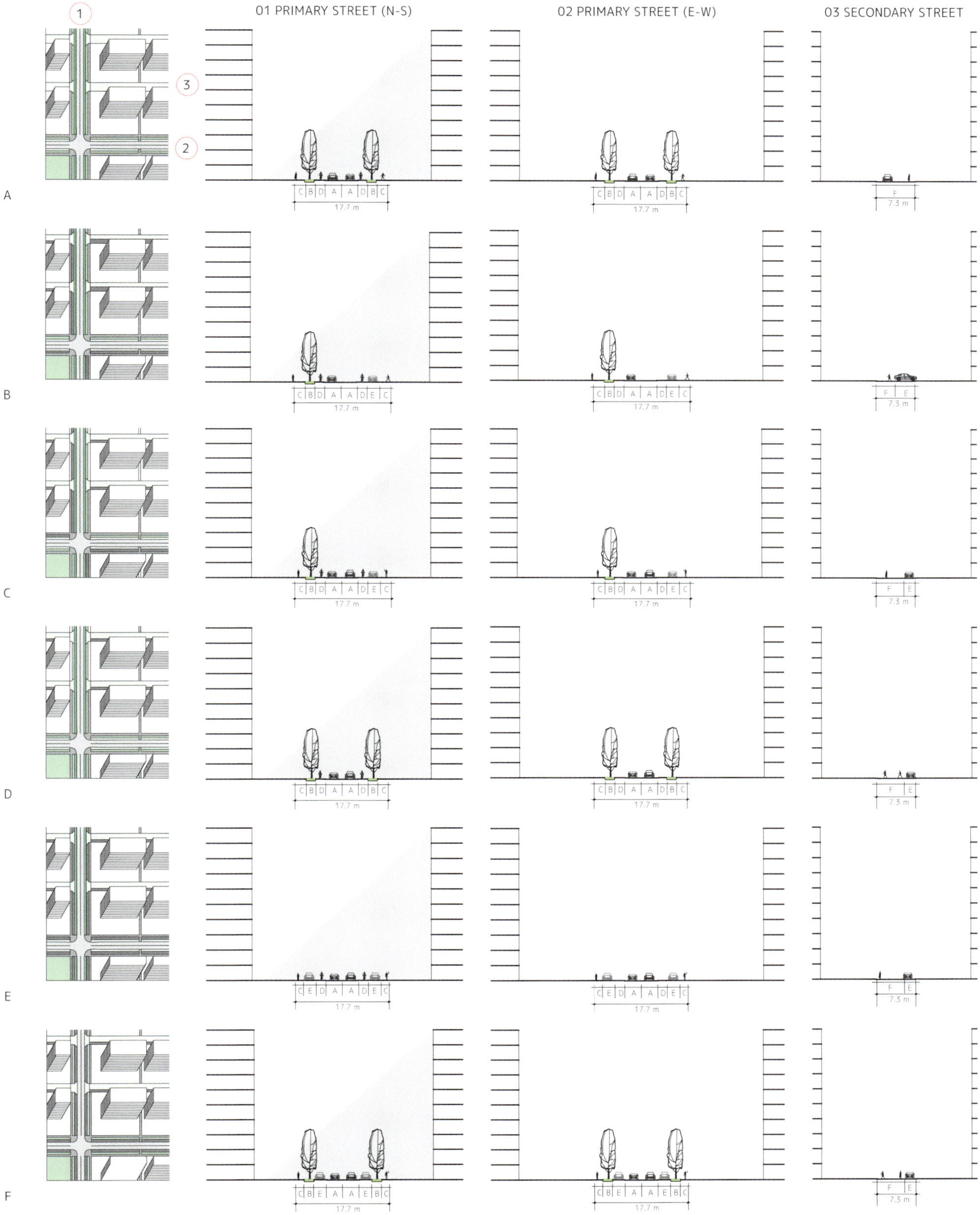

Street Trees
Regional

A range of tree and vegetation species were identified based on their regional suitability within China as well as for their capacity to achieve a range of ecological functions. These were utilized as a catalogue of landscape treatments for different aspects of the blocks.

North China_Wetland
Residential Green Space
01 Prunus
02 Photinia serrulata
03 Jasminum nudiflorum
04 Salix babylonica
05 Antirrhinum majus
06 Typha orientalis Presl
07 Lythrum salicaria
08 Phragmites

Road Buffer
09 Zoysia sinica Hance
10 Buxus megistophylla
11 Kerria japonica
12 Albizia julibrissin
13 Syringa
14 Cedrus
15 Ginkgo biloba
16 Euonymus fortunei

Residential Green Space

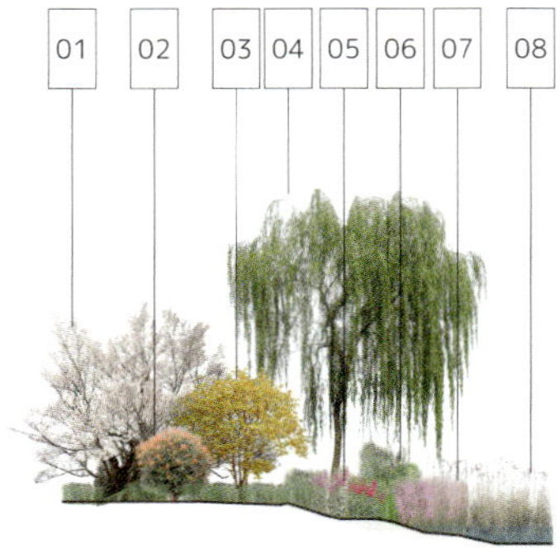

Road Buffer

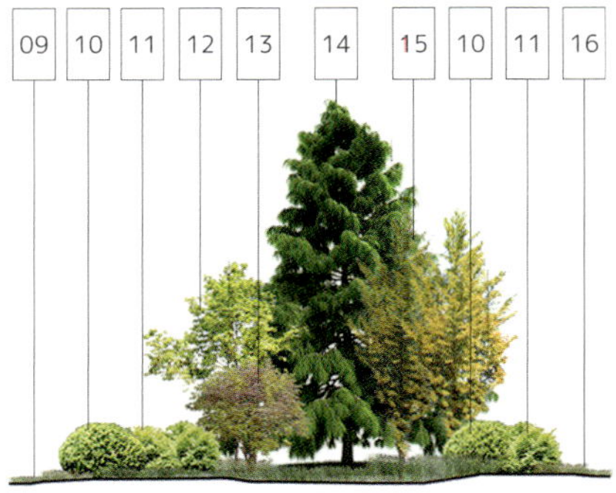

South China_Wetland
Residential Green Space
01 Taxodium distichum
02 Metasequoia
glyptostroboides
03 Hibiscus mutabilis Linn
04 Bauhinia blakeeana
05 Lythrum salicaria
06 Typha orientalis Presl
07 Acorusgramineus
08 Phragmites

Road Buffer
09 Buxus megistophylla
10 Kerria japonica
11 Livistona chinensis
12 Cinnamomum camphora
13 Camellia japonica L.
14 Podocarpus
macrophyllus
15 Ginkgo biloba
16 Euonymus fortunei

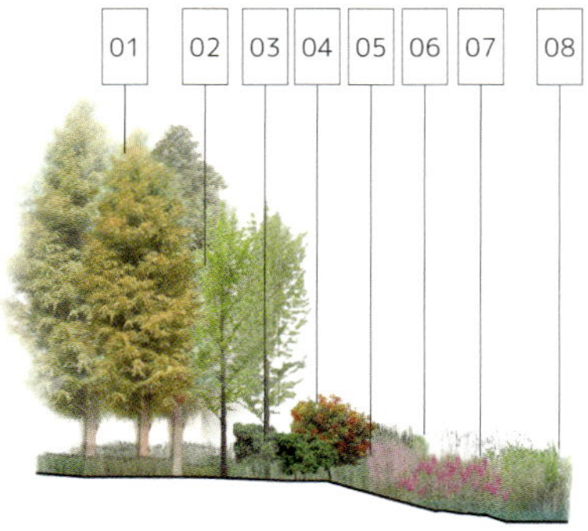

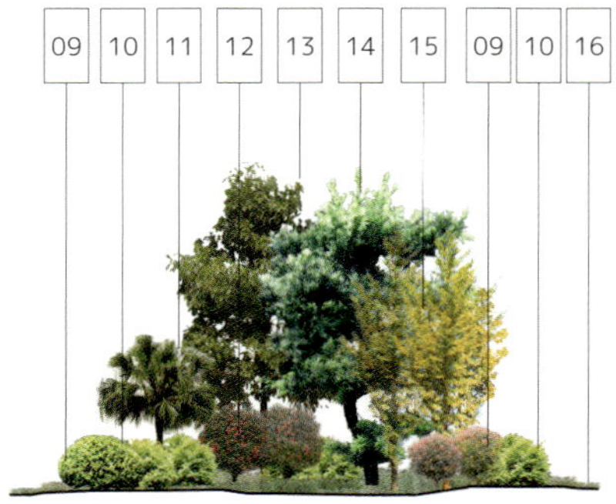

Common Plant List
01 Taxodium distichum
02 Metasequoia
glyptostroboides
03 Podocarpus
macrophyllus
04 Ficus microcarpal
05 Michelia alba DC
06 Camellia japonica L.
07 Livistona chinensis
08 Buxus megistophylla
09 Kerria japonica
10 Euonymus fortunei

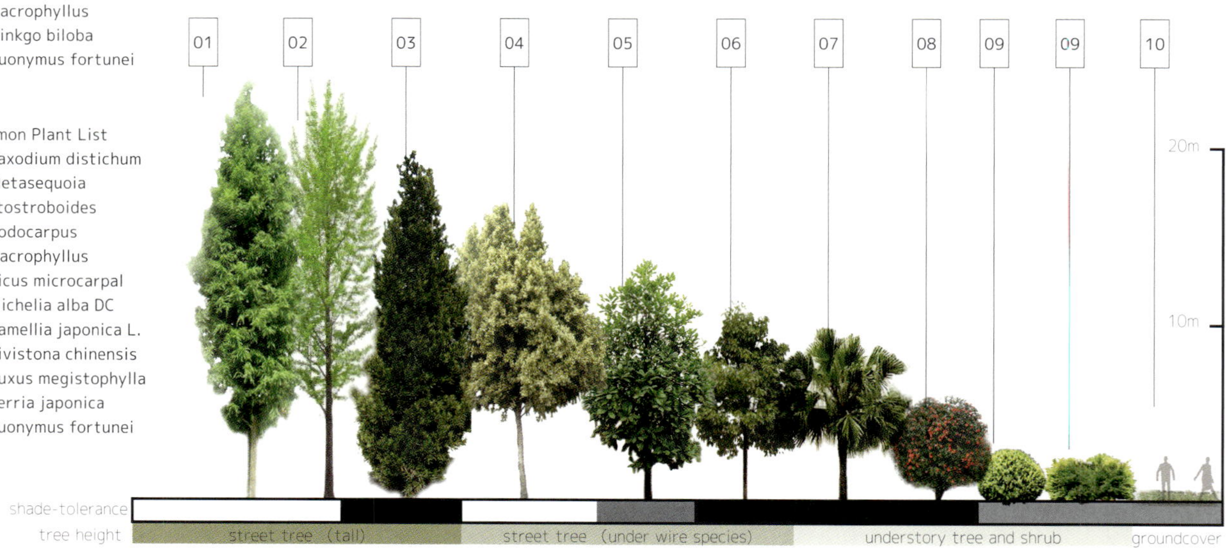

Street Trees Ecology

Street Plants Ecological Function

01 Wind Canyon: create good ventilation near building facades

02 Energy Saving: provide summer shading and winter windblock

03 Improve Air Quality: provide natural filtration of air pollutants

04 Shading: cool streets, sidewalk, and building envelope with tree corridor

05 Stormwater Control: increase permeable surface area and vegetal roots to receive runoff

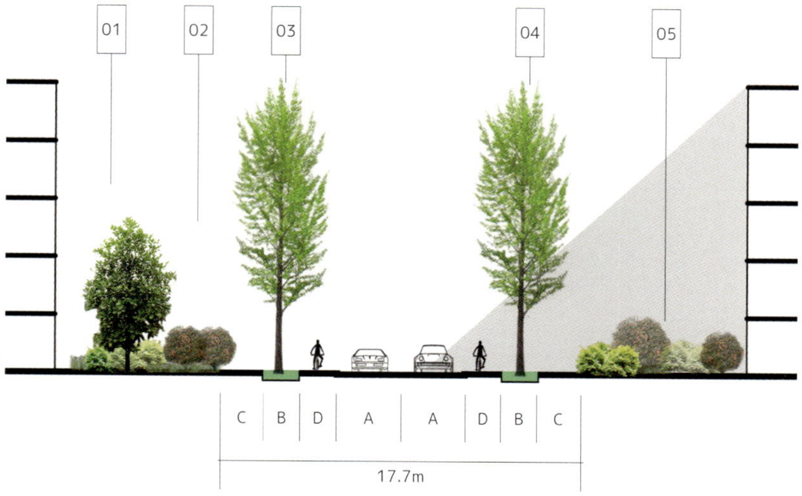

Primary Street (N-S) 5-floor Buildings

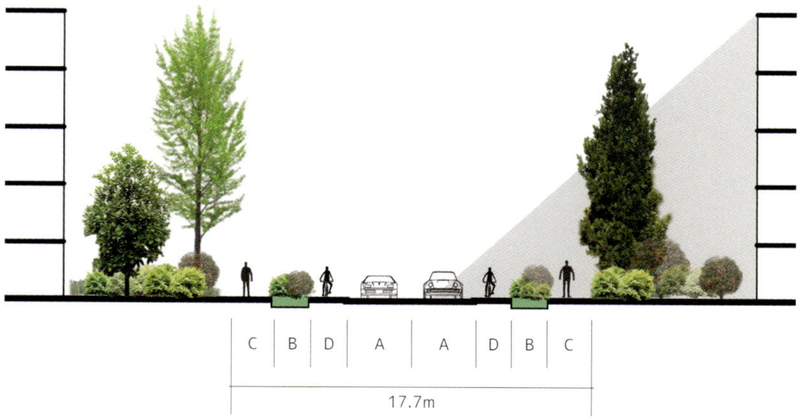

Primary Street (N-S) 10-floor Buildings

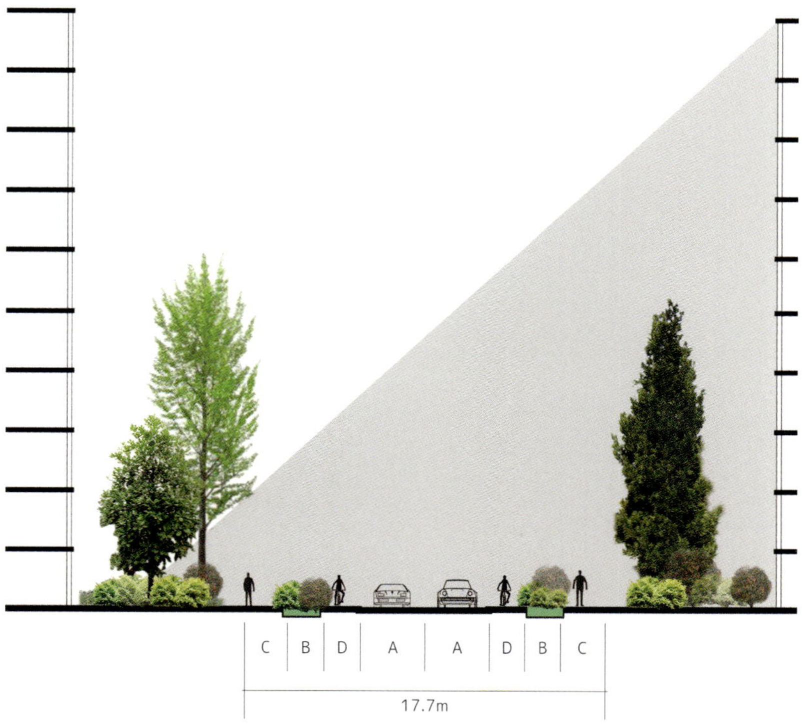

Phasing

The block configurations developed by the research project may be implemented either as newly built blocks or through the renovation of existing neighborhoods. A series of scenarios for how some of Songjiang's existing blocks may be gradually transformed and enhanced in phases are described here.

The phasing analysis represents the flexibility of the proposed open space framework and the possibilities of applying different spatial configurations through a phased process.

Based on the building compositions of the existing block types, different open space frameworks may be applied to different blocks. Both **Block Type 2 Transformation A** and **Block Type 3 Transformation A** are tested with open space frameworks that coincide with their original urban fabrics, while **Block Type 3 Transformation B** offers a large centralized open space in the first phase. The results normally consist of two types of community organizations with the same level of population density: one with more dense but lower buildings and the other one with high-rises but more open spaces.

The phasing strategy emphasizes the possibility of applying the enhanced urban prototypes in a gradual, incremental way. This was a deliberate strategy to address the potential of economic constraints and the large number of resident relocations that may be involved.

Block Type 2 Transformation A

Convex Open Space Framework

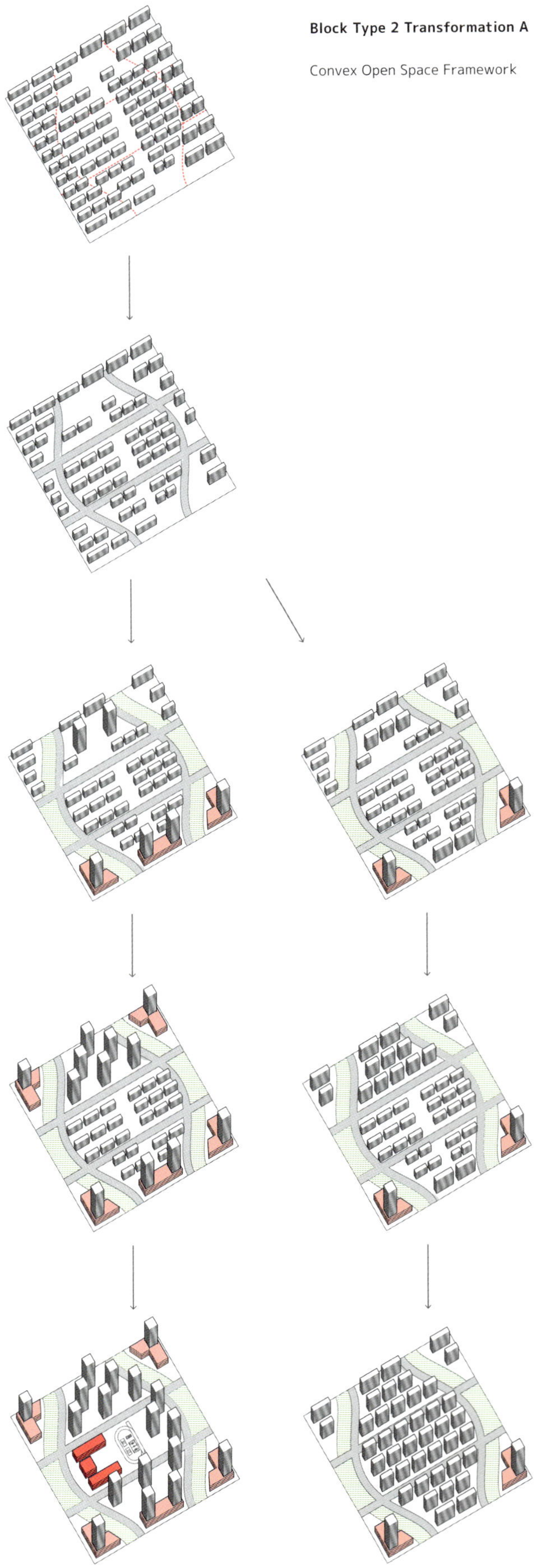

Block Type 3 Transformation A

Straight-lined Open Space Framework

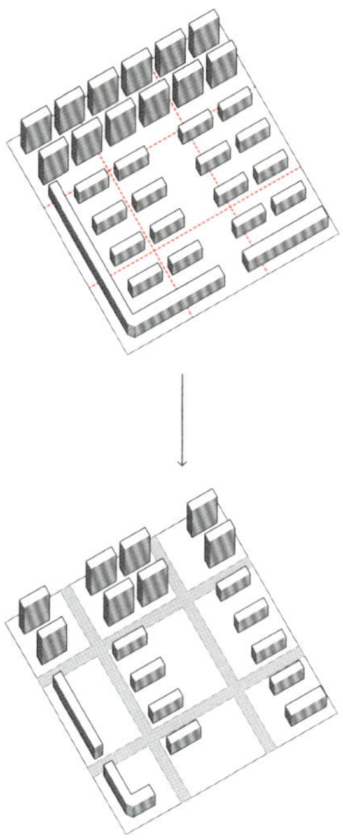

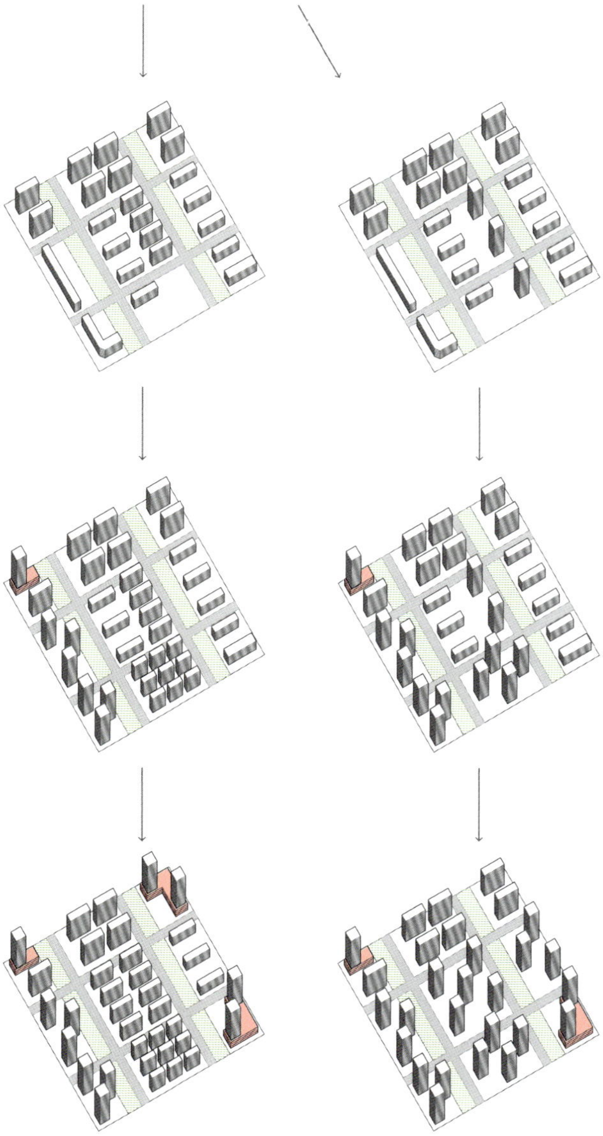

Block Type 3 Transformation B

Concave Open Space Framework

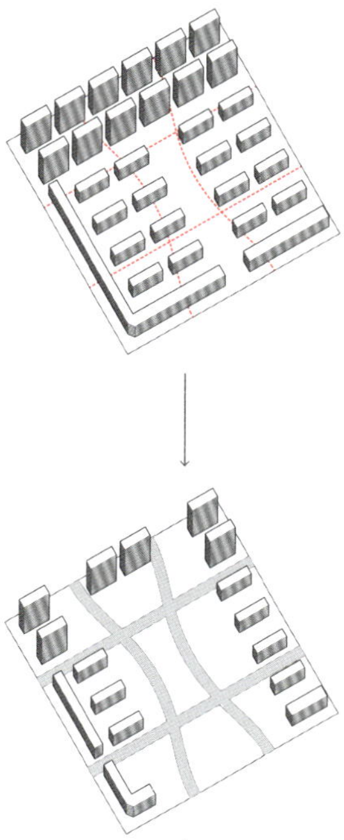

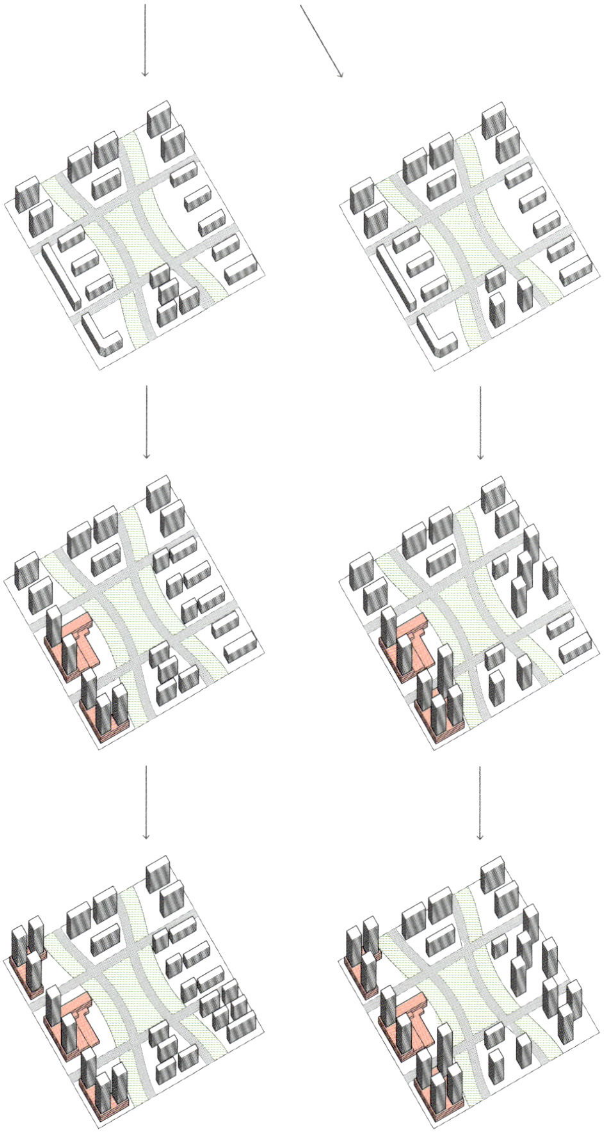

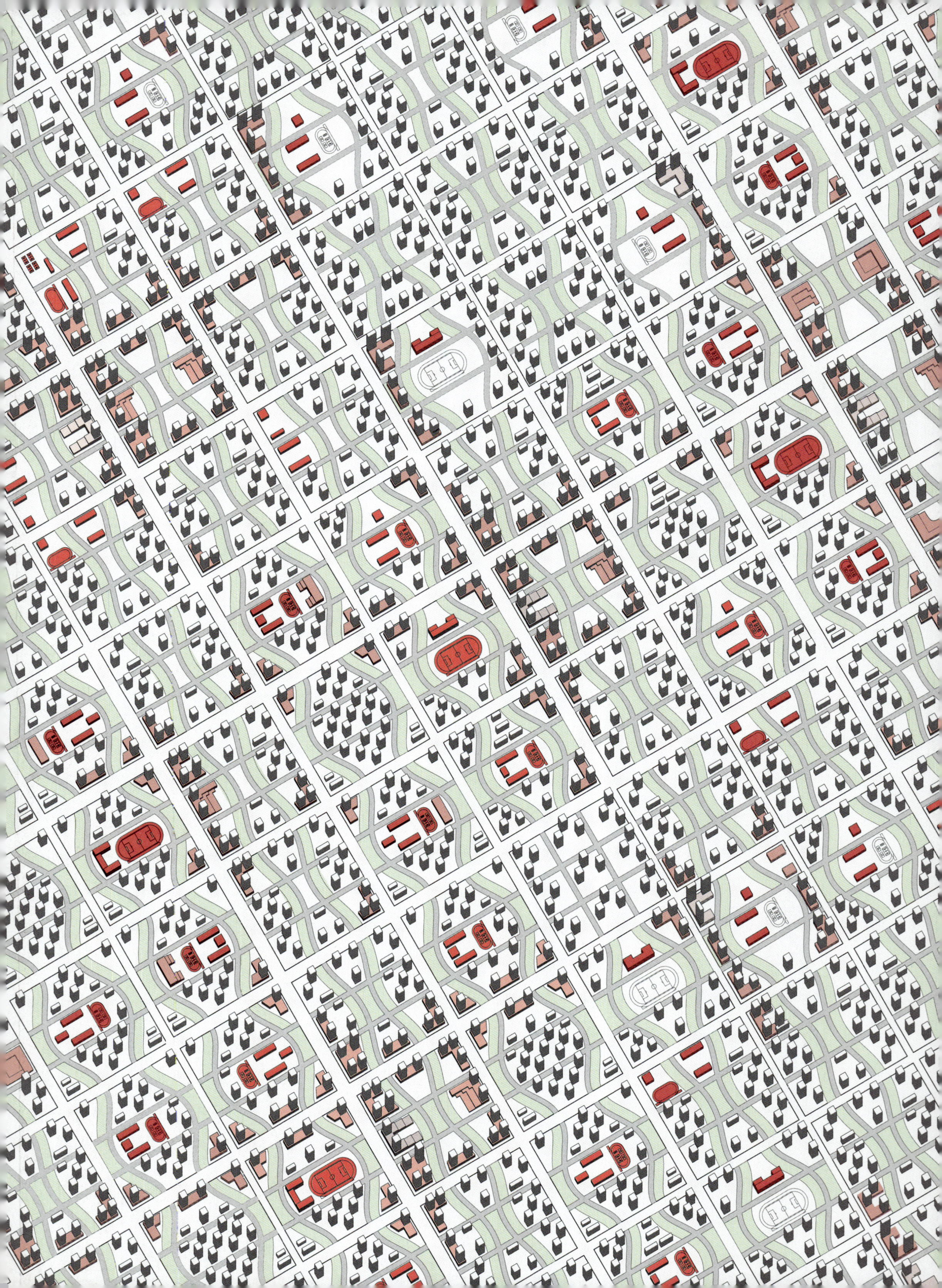

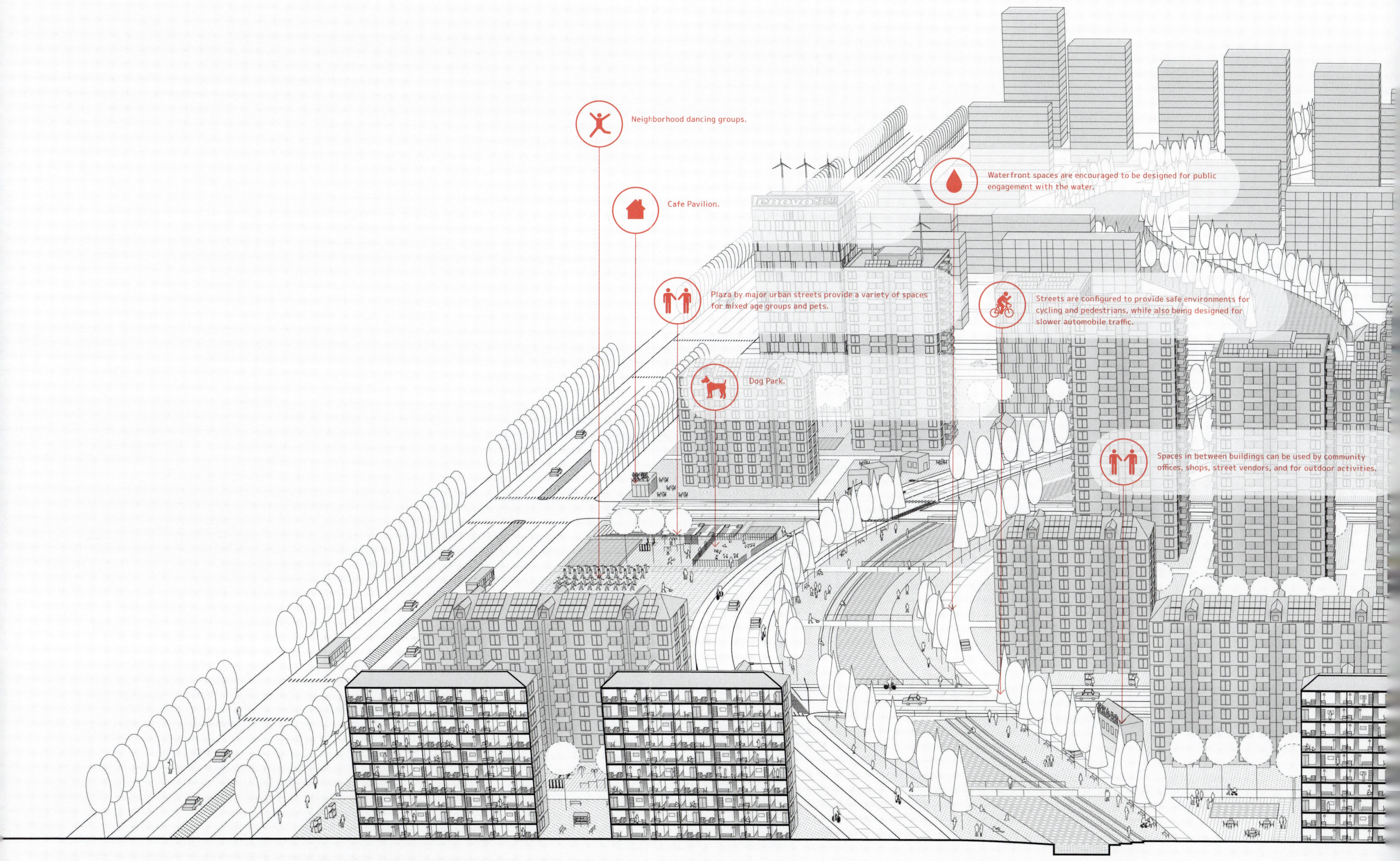
Neighborhood dancing groups.
Cafe Pavilion.
Plaza by major urban streets provide a variety of spaces for mixed age groups and pets.
Dog Park.
Waterfront spaces are encouraged to be designed for public engagement with the water.
Streets are configured to provide safe environments for cycling and pedestrians, while also being designed for slower automobile traffic.
Spaces in between buildings can be used by community offices, shops, street vendors, and for outdoor activities.
lenovo

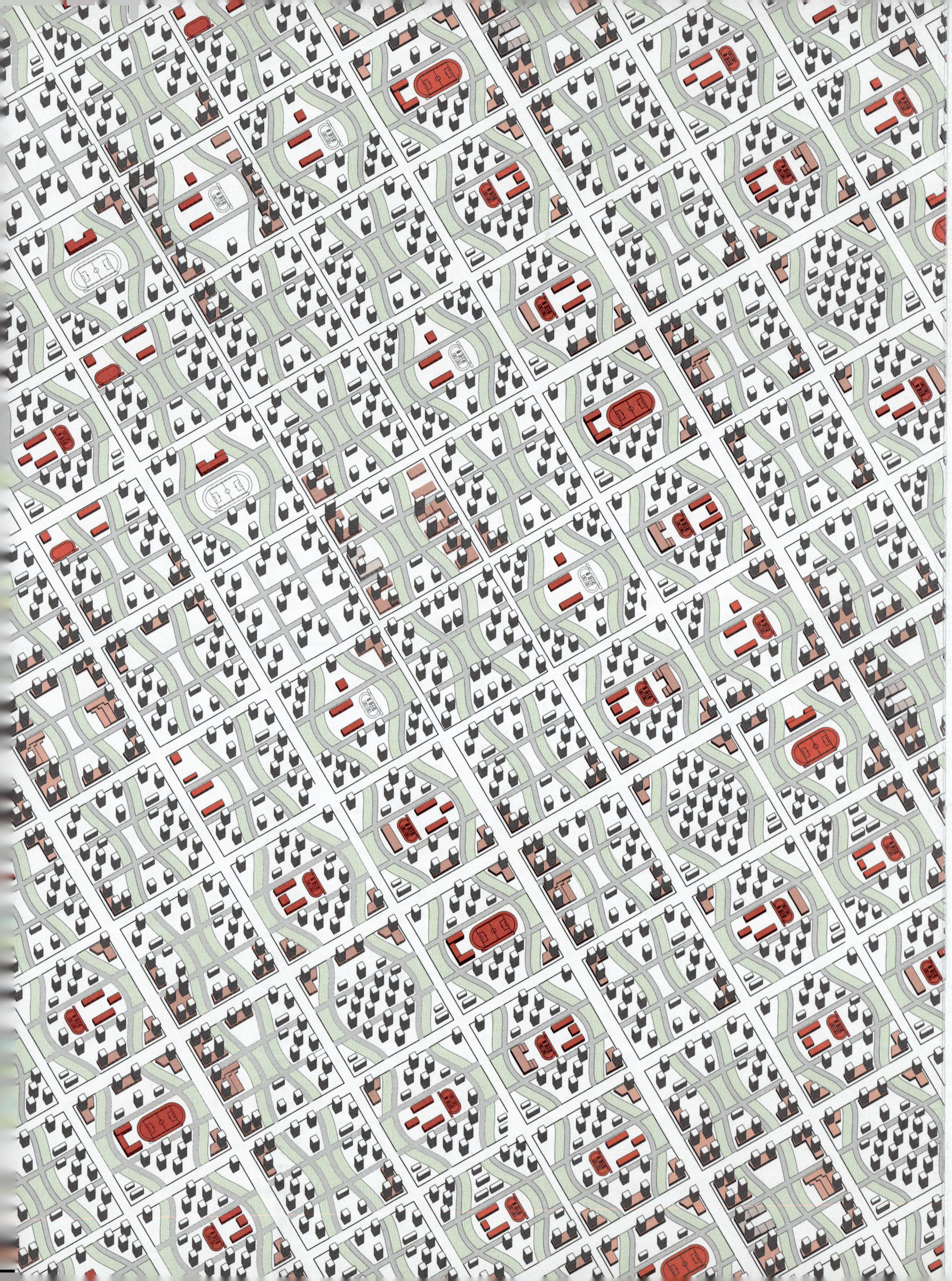

Scenario 3

Mixed Building Types and Canal / Greenway Scenario

This scenario depicts a different iteration of the block that utilizes the greenways as water canals which offer its residents and workers an enjoyable recreational and social space. It introduces a consistent element that spans through the block, treating stormwater and cooling the urban environment in addition to its role as an amenity for the neighborhood. The mix of building types also allows for the possibility of a mix of units and tenures, that may accommodate a cross-section of residents, from single, elderly, retirees to large extended families, promoting a diverse neighborhood.

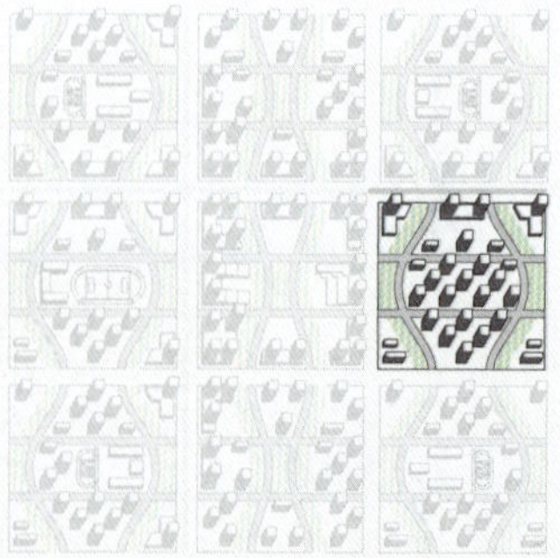

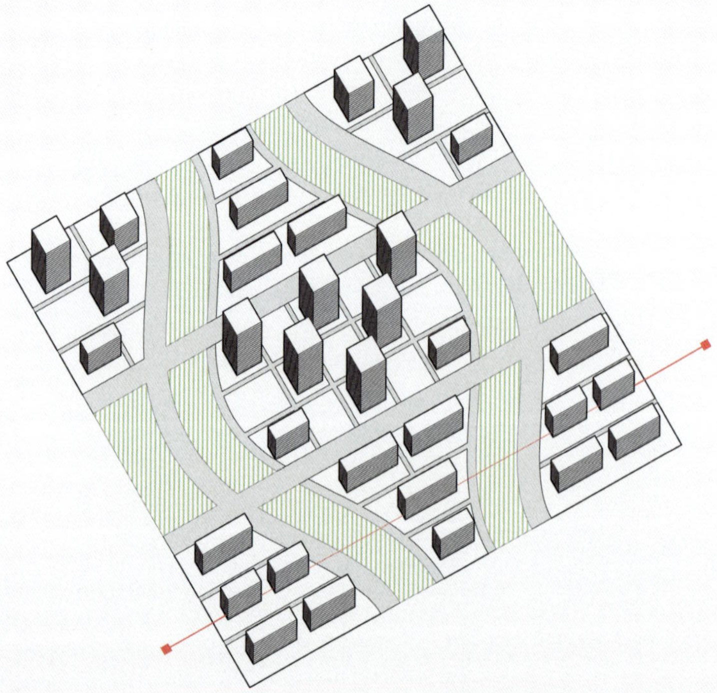

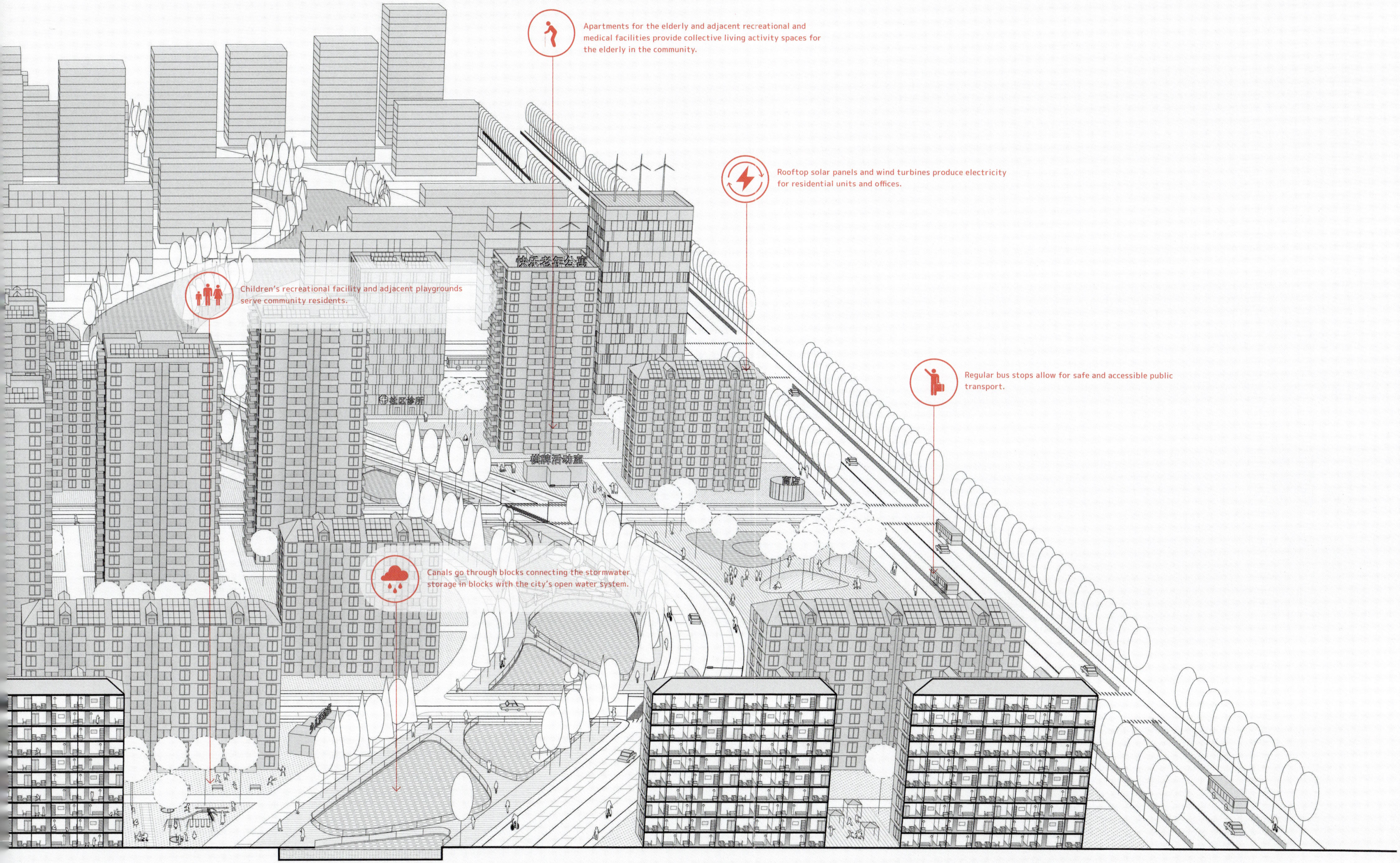

Apartments for the elderly and adjacent recreational and medical facilities provide collective living activity spaces for the elderly in the community.
Rooftop solar panels and wind turbines produce electricity for residential units and offices.
Children's recreational facility and adjacent playgrounds serve community residents.
Regular bus stops allow for safe and accessible public transport.
Canals go through blocks connecting the stormwater storage in blocks with the city's open water system.
快乐老年公寓
社区诊所
商店

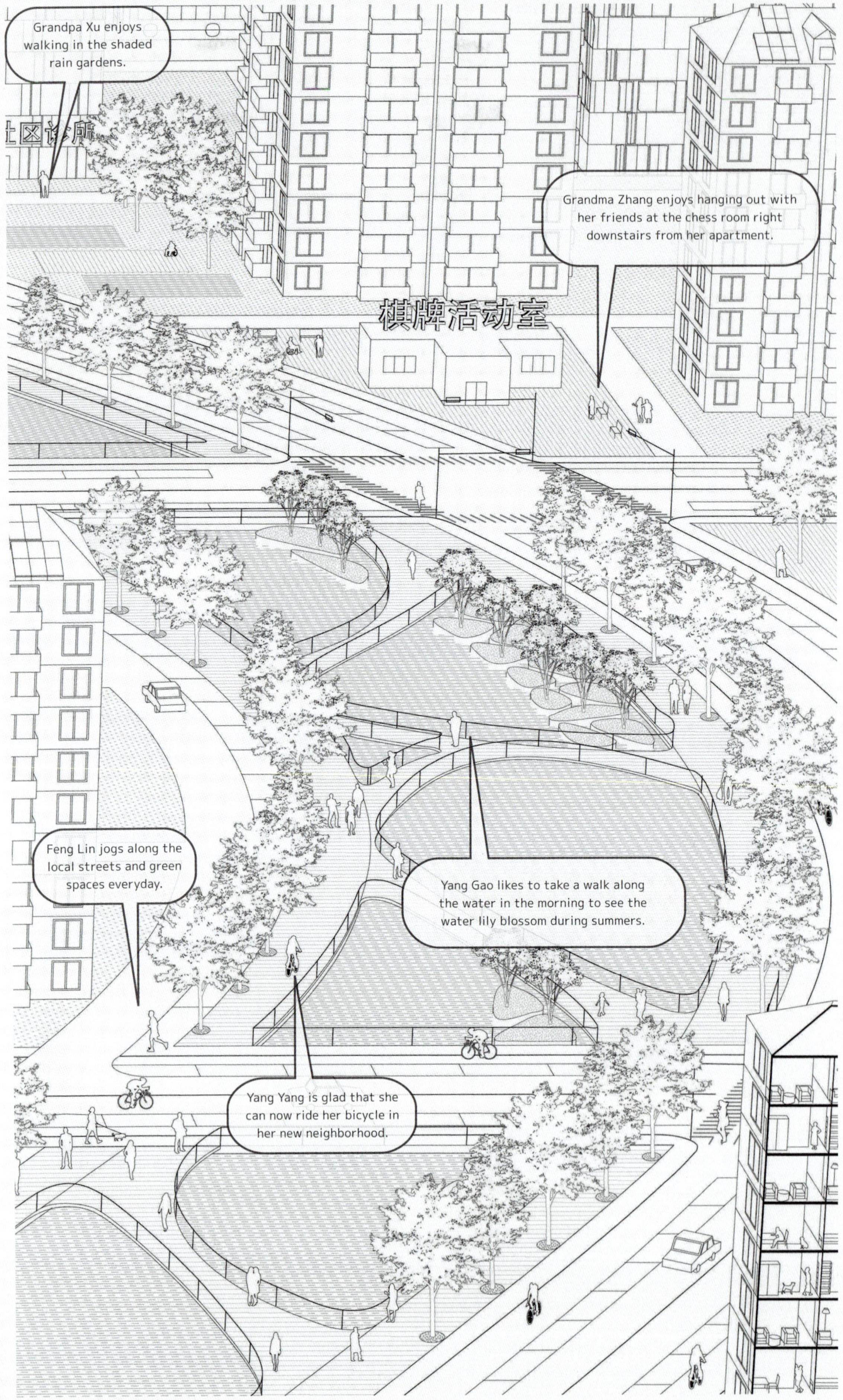

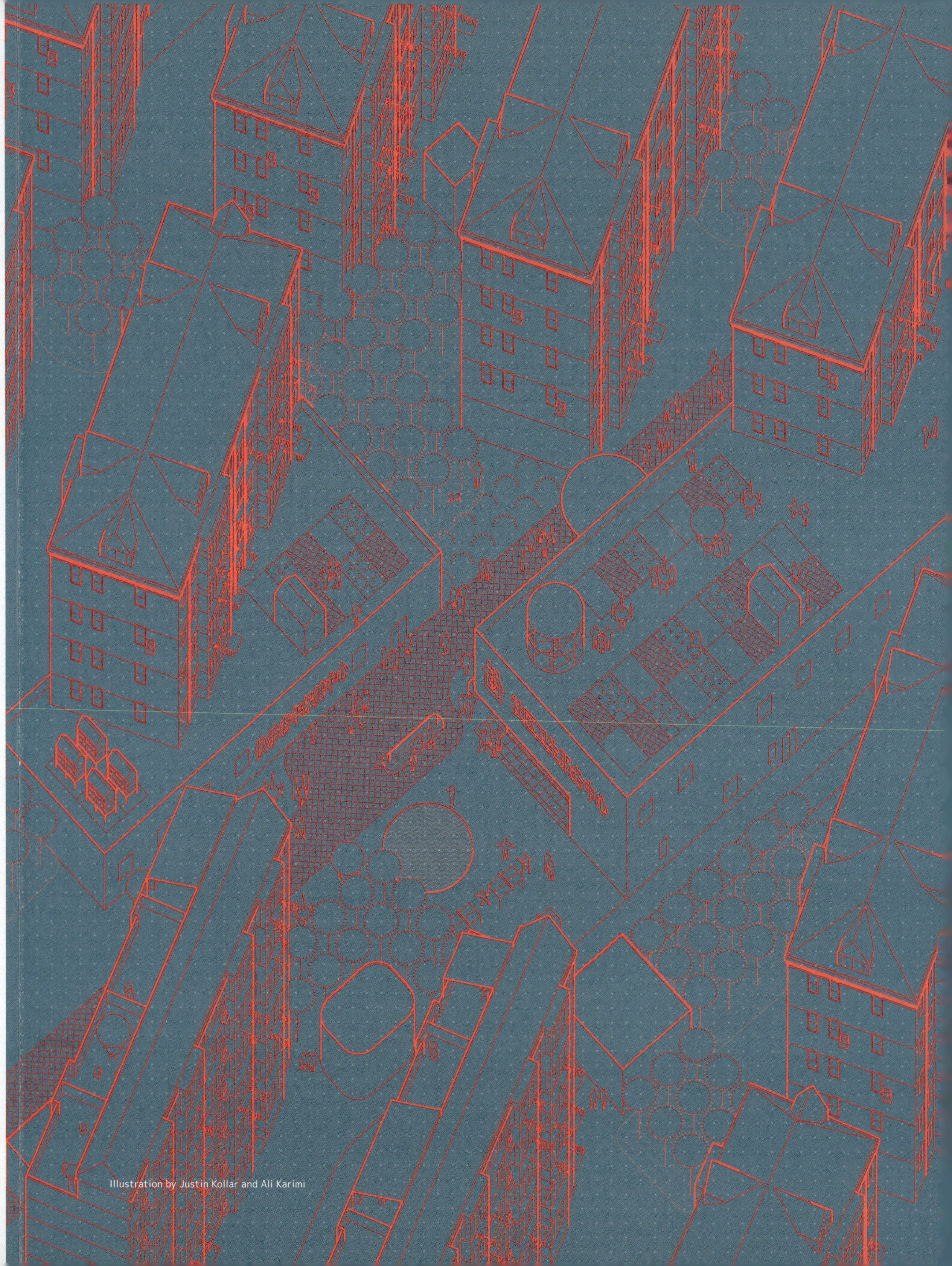

Illustration by Justin Kollar and Ali Karimi

Lifestyled – China-Town

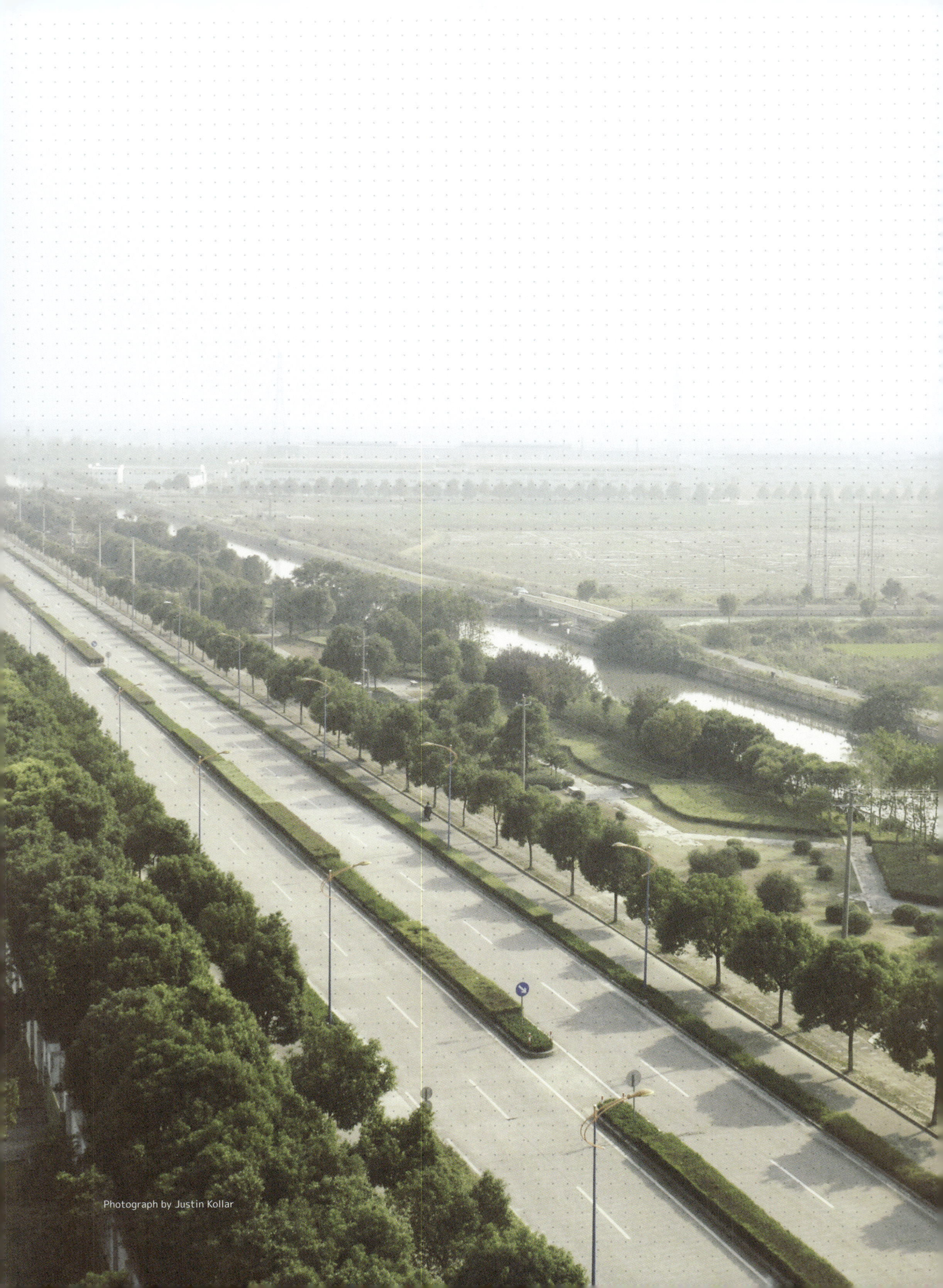

Photograph by Justin Kollar

Chapter 5

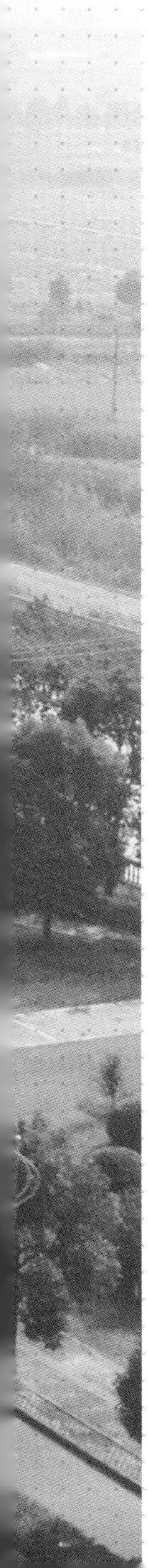

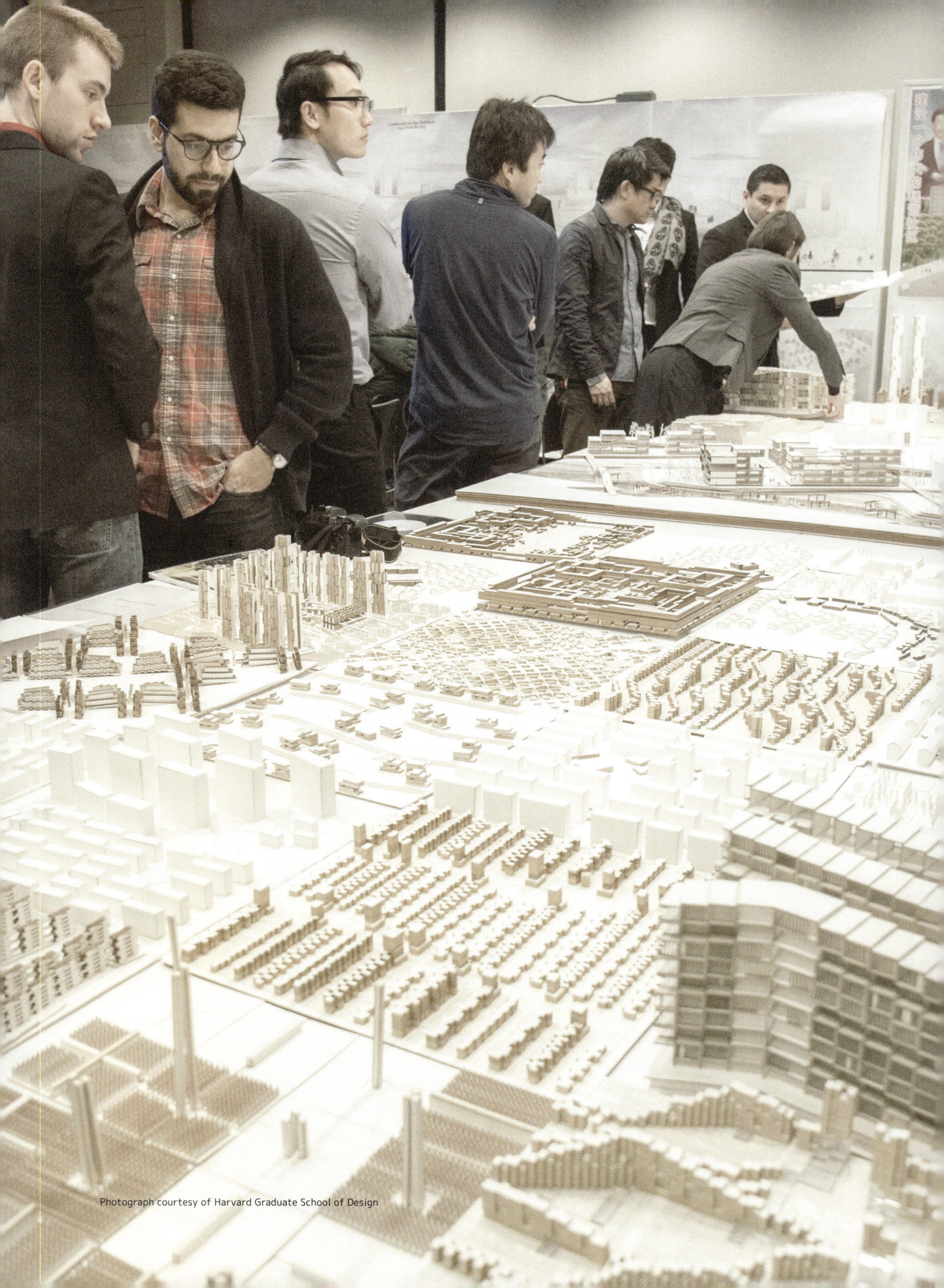

Photograph courtesy of Harvard Graduate School of Design

Lifestyled – China-Town Studio Themes

Leire Asensio Villoria, David Mah, Justin Kollar, Elizabeth Wu, Xinhui Li, Han Yang

The Lifestyled – China-Town advanced option studio was conducted at the Harvard Graduate School of Design in the Fall of 2014. The studio was led by Leire Asensio Villoria and David Mah, with participating students coming from the Harvard Graduate School of Design's three different departments (architecture, landscape architecture, and urban design). Similar to the research project conducted by the HAPI core design team, it was structured as a multidisciplinary studio with a focus on the development of propositions for Chinese superblock neighborhoods that account for health-related issues as the main design consideration.

The studio was framed to allow students to situate their projects within a very specific context; that of Songjiang New Town, a city (originally designated as a town) located on the outskirts of Shanghai. While this offered students, the capacity to situate their projects within a very particular site, it also allowed them to address more general issues concerning a particular development type, the superblock as models for new neighborhoods. Their proposals offer projections for how particular sites in Songjiang may be configured to accommodate a new healthy neighborhood, while also being models for how the normative approaches towards superblock developments in general may be reconsidered.

Their projects were, to differing degrees, situated within the social, economic, cultural, political as well as environmental context of China. While measures and recommendations from health impact assessments and guidelines developed by the HAPI research group were consulted during the studio, many of the students also chose to learn from and immerse their projects within the Chinese milieu. A series of important themes and considerations specific to China's situation emerged within the studio. These can be broadly grouped into

1) notions of the collective or different models of "family,"
2) governance and policy,
3) and environmental concerns.

While each project engaged with these issues in differing ways, the mandate of the studio was to return to the task of designing or developing projections for how the relationship between these themes and health concerns may be addressed through the organization of the physical environment of the Chinese superblock. The studio was underpinned by the ambition to offer design proposals, that leverage the diverse disciplinary knowledge and skills of the students. While they were encouraged to address the wider concerns of health and place by learning from the public health field, the students also applied their own disciplinary specific knowledge in architecture, landscape as well as urban design. As a result, the association or connection between ideas of the collective, governance, the environment and public health with particular block types from Chinese history were also studied as a means to offer some background knowledge for the studio. The block/building types, the *siheyuan* courtyard, the *Lilong*, the *danwei* complex and the contemporary *xiaoqu* were chosen primarily for their status as having been the building block or basic unit of urbanization in China during different periods in its history.

Figure 1 (Opposite page) Photograph of studio models at final review.

家 The Collective – The Family

The social organization of China's people has undergone significant transformations over time and none more so than in recent history which has seen a shift from a largely feudal structure through a Communist society to its current status brought about by its shift towards a market economy. We can see a population that has undergone consistent change over a relatively short period in history, prompting adjustments to the notions of collective life.

Throughout Chinese history, we have seen the evolution and adaptation of the organization of the population into simple units of collective living. These have ranged from traditional family households (*jiating* 家庭) to family clans (*jiazu* 家族),[1] work units (*danwei* 单位), and more recently, towards nuclear family models. Many factors have exerted influence over the formation of these social organizations, from traditional bloodline bonds to administrative systems and prevailing philosophies or ethics (such as Confucianism). In turn, these social organizations have been a large part of the foundation from which reform, and even revolution, has taken place.

1 **Family Clan (*jiazu* 家族):** The family system provided a strong and rigid foundation for much of pre-industrial Chinese society. Family networks formed through conjugal and blood relations could become particularly strong and far-reaching—even challenging state administrative powers.

The Traditional Family

In pre-republican times the traditional family was a self-enclosed economic unit. It was hierarchical, with a strong patriarch and subsequent levels of productive members divided along gendered lines. Members of the family unit would usually pool their incomes which would be redistributed by the head of the family, usually the most senior male. Within this common economic distribution, the interests of the individual were subordinate to that of the family as a collective. Under the Confucian tradition, the longevity of the family unit was given primary value and as such, strict patriarchal authority and filial piety were the cornerstones of productive life.

Throughout pre-republican history, this form of the family unit was very much the foundation of

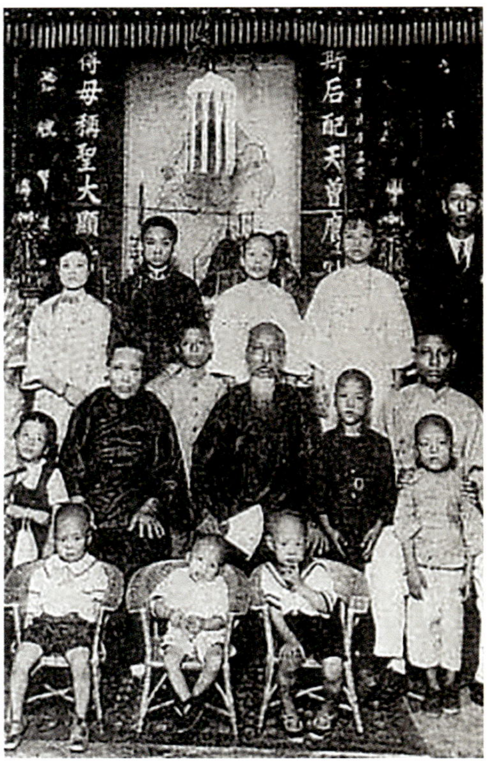

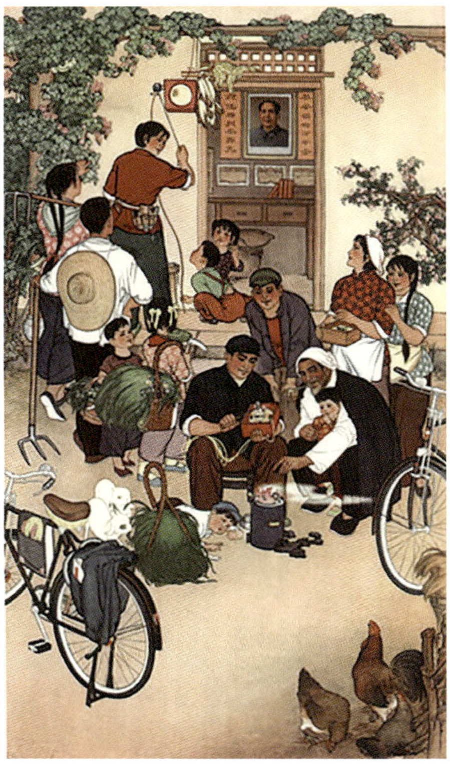

Figure 2 (Left) A photograph of a traditional family.

修身，齐家，治国，平天下
"Self, Family, Nation, World"

In traditional Confucian philosophy, this was the cosmic order whereby there was a direct link from the family to the nation and the world. To achieve peace and harmony in the nation, one had to find order in the family.

Figure 3 (Right) People celebrate the People's Commune—where the collective becomes a new foundation for productive life as opposed to the traditional family.

state organization and local administration. It has been the subject of much thought, contemplation, and administrative reordering. As the primary unit of wealth accumulation, the large joint-family unit operated through a system of blood relations. Ties between members of the same bloodline and through conjugal relationships stretched a tight network of families into a rigidly hierarchical community with shared benefits. These clans (*jiazu* 家族) had the potential of expanding into larger networks of relationships at the township level, or even to a racial or ethnic identification. This form of organization places a heavy burden on the state, as the strength of family-clans could rival and even challenge state control and administration. Nepotism was commonplace and stretched into crucial positions within society and administration. To combat this, the government would frequently assign officials to positions far away from their family networks.

While there were many different formations of local networks, each with their own administrative system, a common theme in the attempt for increased centralized control was the implementation of the *baojia* system (保甲制度).[2] Within this system, each household would typically be responsible for overseeing the manner and actions of the other households, keeping social conduct in check with collectively held ideals.[3] The *baojia* system also allowed for efficient galvanization of the population in the needs of defense, and likewise, also offered a strong administrative base for localized clans that could also rival the power of the state; a problem that would be felt strongly during the early republican era.

In the republican era, the rising Nationalist government also attempted to extend and consolidate their power throughout the countryside,[4] a form of the *baojia* system was adopted in the County Organization Law of 1929. It attempted to galvanize existing clans, and family networks into a more-coherent, top-down administrative system. Under the counties (*xian* 县) there were several layers similar to the *baojia* system: 5 households (*hu* 户) would be incorporated into a *lin* (邻), five *lin* would make up one *lu* (闾), at least 100 households or four *lu* would comprise a rural or urban township (*xiang* 乡, *zhen* 镇), and twenty to fifty townships made up a district (*qu* 区) which were organized under the county. This organizational restructuring had a minor effect in expanding reform into the countryside despite the factional tendencies, ethnic conflicts, warlordism, and the turmoil of the late 1930s, resulting in several wars up until the exile of the Nationalist Party and the founding of the People's Republic in 1949.

2 ***Baojia* System (*baojia zhidu* 保甲制度):** Originally formulated during the Song dynasty, the *baojia* system organized families into family groups of around 10 households called a *pai* (排) where a leader was designated as a representative that would carry out state or larger administrative decrees within the community. Every 10 *pai* constituted a *jia* (甲), and every 10 *jia* made up a *bao* (保).

3 Wang 2006.

4 Harris 2013, Bedeski 1981.

The Nuclear Family

In the early years of the new republic, under the influence of foreign and local cosmopolitanism, the Nationalist government sought to reconstruct the traditional family unit (household), reducing its size in an attempt to realign people's interests toward the state. Through the mandate of the economic goals of modernization, and a new entrepreneurial spirit under Chinese Nationalism, the traditional family would be stripped down to a newly introduced concept of the family. The nuclear family (or small household: *xiao jiating* 小家庭)[5] was promoted as being integral to building a modernized society. The nuclear family was considered more economically adept in an industrializing society allowing for a smaller, tighter concentration of wealth instead of its distribution amongst unproductive members of a family. The 'New Culture Movement' of the mid 1910s and 1920s under the Nationalist government advocated for smaller families, free marriage, individual independence, and above all, the individual devotion to the party and state to the exclusion of local affiliations.

> "The old form of repressing individuality, for the sake of the well-being of the whole, is swept aside. The individual is released from the collective responsibility of the whole family, and assumes his rights and duties as an independent member of a larger society-the nation."[6]

However, even as this idealism remains even today, the fight against patriarchalism would be put off and subordinated to the attempts of the state to reorganize and formulate its power in local administration.[7] The Nationalists failed to attain sufficient influence over the countryside, given the turmoil of the 1930s which continued up to their expulsion. Because of this, much of the countryside remained un-enamored by

5 **Nuclear Family/Small Household (*xiojiating* 小家庭):** In Nationalist propaganda, the small family was more economically viable, and better suited to industrial and consumer society. In Communist propaganda, the small family helped to place focus on a stronger collective base that was not predicated strictly on blood-relations in order to promote stronger allegiance to the party-state.

6 Chen 2007.

7 Johnson 1983.

家 *The Collective – The Family*

房 政
天 家

1845 British Concession in Shanghai
Based on Shanghai Land Regulation (上海土地章程), about 830 acres of land in the north of Shanghai was designated to the British as the British residence. For the following century, Shanghai International Settlement developed into the largest in China and had a great influence on local history.

1910s New Culture Movement
The 'New Culture Movement' of the mid 1910s and 1920s under the Nationalist government advocated for smaller families, free marriage, individual independence, and above all, the individual devotion to the party and state to the exclusion of local affiliations.

1929 Lǘlin System
During the republican era, as the Nationalists attempted to extend and consolidate their power through the countryside, a form of the *baojia* system was adopted in the County Organization Law of 1929.

1929 Clements Apartments
This Adam-style *Lilong* Housing was built by French businessman Clements to provide apartments for rent to foreigners.

1949 Marriage Registration
The state itself required registration of all marriages after 1949. Even the arrangement of marriages was to be carried out by local party-state administration.

1950s Administrative Villages
Under Mao in the early 1950s, administrative villages (xinzhengcun 新政村) were set up in a similar manner as the Nationalist's *lǘlin* system, however, family ties and village relationships were largely ignored.

1910 1920 1930 1940 1950

1845 - 1910 Late Qing + Treaty of Nanjing
Internationalism + Cosmopolitanism

1911 - 1936 Early Republican Era
New Individualism

1937 - 1948 Late Republican Era
Wartime Depression

progressive policies and ideological propaganda. Even during the early Communist era, it was difficult to instill new conceptions of family in the countryside.[8] It wouldn't be until collectivization, that family life and the culture as a whole would experience profound and real 'revolutionary' change.

8 Glosser 2003.

The Socialist Family

With the founding of the People's Republic, the administrative systems were adjusted once again to refocus people's interests and production in line with the goals of the newly established party-state. Under Mao in the early 1950s, the first wave of collectivization was initiated with the establishment of administrative villages (*xinzheng cun* 新政村). These collectivized units were built on much of the same existing social organizations—overlaying the historical foundations of the *baojia* and the Nationalist's *lulin* system. However, in this executive reordering of the population, many family ties and village relationships were largely ignored. Because of this, many officials were in charge of a collection of villages which they had no incentive to prioritize over their own. During this time, the Communist Party organization was also integrated into the administration. Party secretaries oversaw village branches, and once again, local interests were subverted as party secretaries' and officials' interests were aligned with the party-state rather than the village. This organization allowed for the penetration of mass line ideology into all corners of society enacting a more efficient attempt at refocusing energies and sentiments toward the nation as a whole. Building up an efficient socialist organization was the top priority, as it was to be the foundation of further progress.

Many of the reforms brought about by collectivization sought to level out society into one harmonious proletarian class. However, while change was brought about by the People's Commune Movement, existing social ills were replaced by other problems. Under the auspices of land reform and redistribution, the 'previous' classes of landowners and rich peasants were pitted against the poor. The former group was often stigmatized under the new regime, their property redistributed or seized.

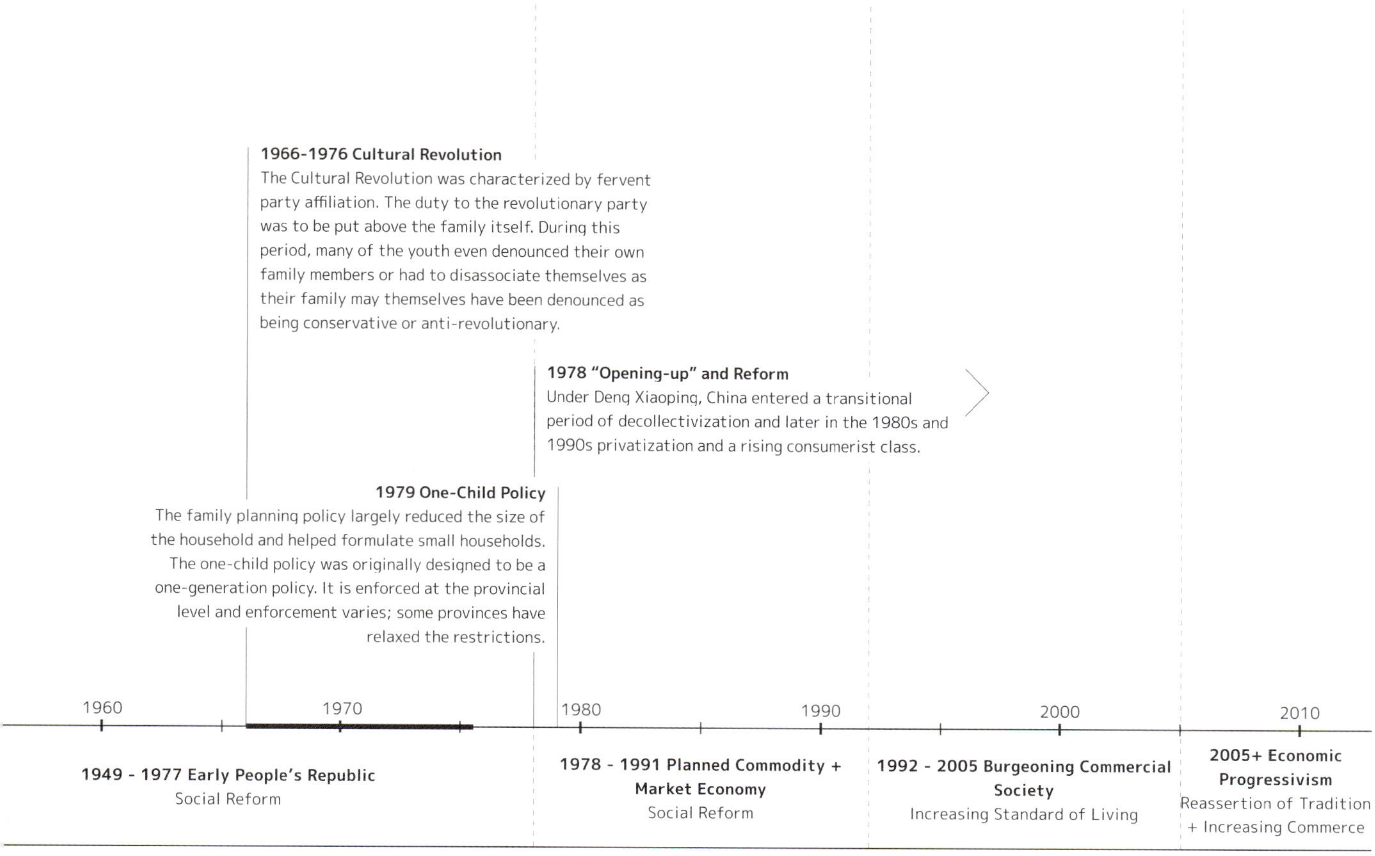

As the People's Commune Movement moved into the cities, effectively transplanting different segments of society (workers and peasants) and combining the cities with the countryside, many of the communes were established on the foundations of existing social organizations, enterprises, factories, schools, and neighborhoods, etc. With increased collectivization formalized through the establishment of work units (*danwei* 单位)[9], citizens were assigned a role within the new society under the *hukou* registration system. Farm groups, factories, armies, and governmental offices made up the landscape of work-unit organization. The *hukou* system established a firm divide between urban and rural populations and was introduced to control migration. A citizen is born to a specific locale and can only receive educational and healthcare benefits from their registered location. Even though families may have been broken up, there were still many rural work units comprised of large family units. The age-old issues of nepotism and concentrations of localized power would continue to persist even through revolutionary reform. Many customs and rituals were prohibited, and property was transferred to the control of the party branches—effectively disassembling much of the cultural activities revolving around the traditional family.[10]

9 **Work Unit (*danwei* 单位):** The work unit is a hybrid of Soviet-style central administration and the existing (or somewhat-existing) systems that evolved from the *baojia* or *lǚlin* systems. Work units were formed during the People's Commune Movement which established self-sufficient, isolated production units, and in many cases off of the foundations of existing social organizations.

10 Zhang 2009, 94-95

The most basic of the party branches and the lowest level of administration were Resident Committees (*jumin weiyuanhui* 居民委员会). These were a direct extension of the Central Party Committee as policies and agendas were transferred down to the members of these committees. This administrative arm oversaw all local issues, carried out internal reform, and oversaw the implementation of the marriage laws and family planning. During this period, committees ran much of social life, and parents were no longer the matchmakers. In the early years of reform, even the marriage system saw the arranged marriage of individuals from different classes with the aim of "diluting all 'inherited' class origins."[11] Members from the landlord, rich, and right-wing classes were to be wed with members of the revolutionary classes.

11 See "Big Family of Socialism" Urban China: Work in Progress 2009, 77.

Following the massive social upheavals of land reform and collectivization into work units, much of the revolutionary zeal from the Great Leap Forward fell into despair as one-size-fits-all policies led to famine and depression. In the subsequent years of the Cultural Revolution, family ties were put to the test. The Cultural Revolution was characterized by fervent party affiliation. In the late 60s and early 70s, many factions claiming to represent the ideals of the revolutionary vanguard, as set forth in the ideas of the late-Mao Zedong, ravaged social life, upending families and dissolving links. Once again, the link and affiliation with the revolutionary party was to be put above the family itself. During this period, many of the youth even denounced their own family members or had to disassociate themselves as their family may have been castigated as being conservative or anti-revolutionary.[12] Though the main deleterious effects were felt within the cities, even to this day many elderly have lost links with their children, or even suffer from complete estrangement.[13]

12 Glosser 2003, 167-195.

13 Ibid.

Contemporary Family Relationships

With the "opening up" of China and its economic restructuring, the remnants of the *danwei* were reorganized into various kinds of enterprises. Many were even made up of and controlled by large families—especially in the countryside and in remote areas. Many of these enterprises still retain much of the large-family network organization. The work unit system played a large role in social segregation and maintaining a certain degree of isolation during the formation of these enclaves of family-controlled enterprises. After the implementation of the *danwei*, many communities became even more isolated, ensuring the continual repositioning of families within the bureaucratic structure.[14] After economic reform, as many migrated away from their principle residence for work in the 80s and again in the 90s, the *hukou* system also played a large role in attempting to restrict worker circulation. A result of this mass urban migration and the *hukou* system is that many parents chose to leave their children back in their hometown with their grandparents so that they could retain access to healthcare and schooling. Many migrants from the countryside are not granted an urban *hukou* and lack the rights afforded to those with urban residency. On the flipside, if these migrants forgo their existing rural *hukou*, they also lose access to these rights and services in their hometowns. Other issues arise when parents migrate with their children to regions outside of their official residence. Many of these children are denied (to a certain degree of effectiveness) healthcare and schooling. As a result of these trends, many types of family compositions, such as families of children without parents, the fracturing of families from their local communities, or other complicated family relationship forms have emerged.

14 Zhang 2009, 96.

Now family networks can be said to take on a variety of 'types' of family compositions, from those of a single-person household, empty nests, multiple children, isolated grandparents, etc. On the other hand, today, two different ideals of family life are on the 'rise': Confucian 'traditions' and family attachments, as well as increased individualism and small households proliferate. There are contradictory tendencies in the rise and fall of extended families[15]. The differences are typically seen along the urban/rural divide. There is a family culture that emphasizes independence between family members in the urban communities, whereas extended families tend to be popular in rural communities. With the development of social services, the rise of the two-person family and the single-person household are also becoming more prevalent in the city[16].

15 Chesnes 2008, 222-233.

16 Ibid.

While the state-centric society attempted to harness, or even dominate the familial relationships with collectivized/socialist organizations, clans and blood relationships still played essential roles in the organization and administration of communities to different degrees all along the spectrum. The processes of organizational reform and administrative patterns across China were far from homogeneous and the uniform compliance to mass line ideologies far from complete. The use of socialist organizational policies and ideological propaganda was often a front for the underlying blood-related, familial networks as much as it was a complex re-organization of social life for others. But the organizational systems are far-reaching and continue to play an important role in the formation and continuing reproduction of family life. Policy and built form still influence family relationships, while, at the same time, both new and traditional conceptions of the family influence the nature of the built environment and policy.

政 Governance

Historically, China's governing power over its citizens has had extensive reach and repercussions across the country's social and cultural landscape. In this section, the governance enacted from the Mao period to the present will be broadly outlined to describe how different policies have influenced the current trends of urbanization (including its current tendency towards sprawl) as well as neighborhood structures, urban migration, and health policies (in particular the ways in which health care is delivered and embedded within different scales of the city).

Sprawl

With the implementation of the *danwei* in 1958, the workplace became the administrative unit for domestic and social activities. The close association between place of work and place of residency had a self-regulating effect on the inhabitants, reinforcing a sense of belonging to a productive community.[17] Using the traditional Chinese spatial language of enclosures to demarcate living areas, the *danwei* took the form of a walled unit with secure entry gates. The wall suggested a sense of security, a protected area where the interactions and activities within were safe and exclusive to its members. The sense of enclosure reinforced the goal of place-identity[18]—entry in to the *danwei* was regulated, and there was little need to venture out when major social and domestic activity all unfolded within the community bounds. On the other hand, with six-day work weeks, so much time spent within the *danwei* also drove members, particularly the younger workers, to seek entertainment outside. Access to regional shopping and entertainment centers were equally important in sustaining the lifestyle of the *danwei*.[19]

Initially the proliferation of the *danwei* model had little impact on city transportation infrastructure. Preferring to develop on readily available land, *danwei* were typically constructed on the city periphery.[20] Along with a history of large urban complexes (probably most emblematically exemplified by the Forbidden City in Beijing and the *Siheyuan* courtyard typologies), subsequent rapid urbanization led to their prevalent replication.[21]

In the 1990s, employees were no longer assigned free housing; instead they could choose to buy or rent state-owned housing, although they were still limited in their rights to sell their property. Further evidence of the waning power of the *danwei* came in the early 2000s, when citizens were no longer required to obtain permission from employers to sell their property.[22] However, the legacy of the *danwei* exists as a neighborhood infrastructure, where low-density superblocks provide a basis for housing developments.

17 Bjorklund 1986, 21.

18 Ibid, 21.

19 Ibid, 28.

20 Chang 2008.

21 See also Chapter 3 of this book, Peter Rowe and Har Ye Kan's essay on "China's Modernist Superblocks."

22 2003 'Danwei people become citizens,' *Economist* 4 September 2003. Accessed August 18, 2015, http://www.economist.com/node/2043197.

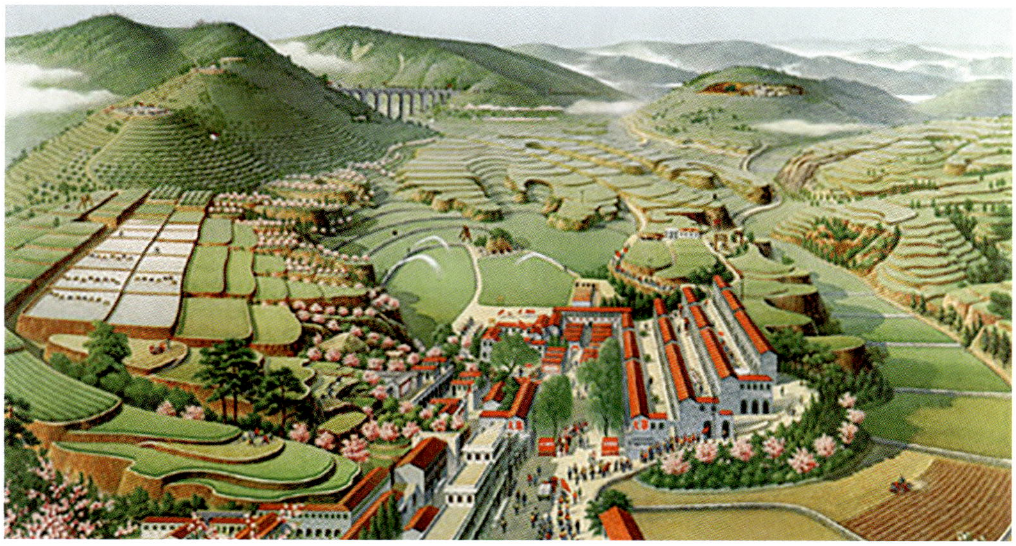

Figure 4 (Left) A Dazhai poster from the 1970s. Mao Zedong advocated for the emulation of this model of self-reliance which turned out to have disastrous consequences for other communes. The model was officially discredited by the 1980s.

Figure 5 Diagram of Administration: Hierarchies + Healthcare

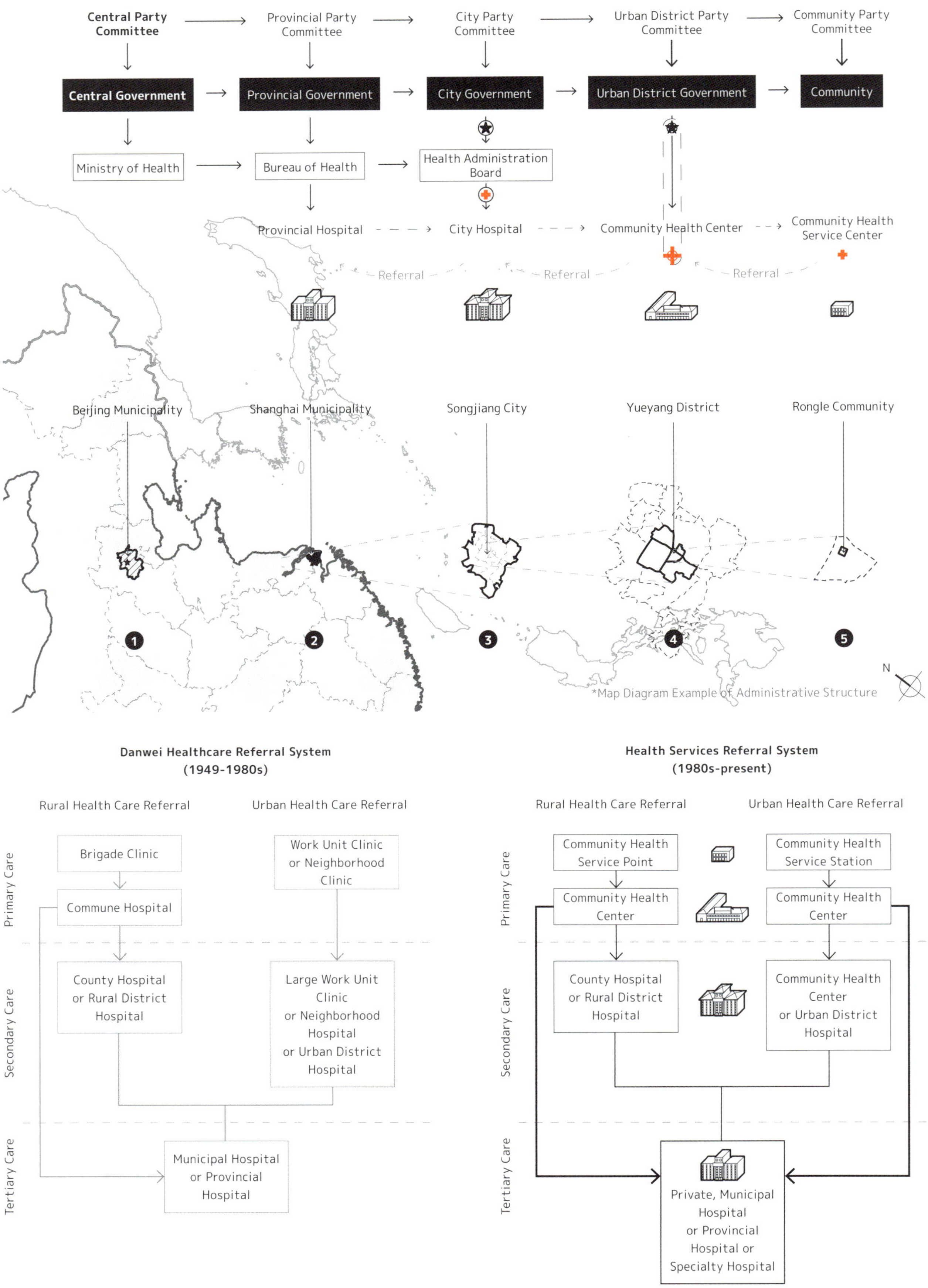

This structure had put in place the tendency towards sprawling urbanization through the replication and adoption a Soviet model of wide roads circumscribing an urban mesh composed of large, bounded superblocks. Today, many of contemporary urbanization practices still persist with this basic organization, conflating it with other models from Garden City planning and adaptations of North American suburban models.

Social Administration

The *danwei* was comprised of administrative offices, to which resident's belonged and from which social services were supplied and regulated. The local residents' committees within this administration system had very little power, and were governed by district government outposts known as subdistrict offices (*jiedao* 街道).[23] Under this system, urban residents remained static, though, each was provided residential space and social services. With the dissolution of the *danwei* model, residents were free to move around—and as social life away moved away from the *danwei*, the administrative model has had to undergo change as well.

In the late 1980s and early 1990s, the experimental development model of the "microdistrict" or "block" (*xiaoqu* 小区) was made an official model of private residential development across the nation. Given the necessary structural shifts to accommodate this, the work unit administrative structure under the residents' committees was reconfigured into a more open administrative entity encompassing mostly community services, while lower level ('grassroots-level') administrative functions, such as disseminating party propaganda, lost their effectiveness. In the early 1990s, as the market expanded and models of neighborhoods grew in size and density, a new form of administration was proposed. Resident's Committees were to be combined into a larger administrative entity simply called a "community" (*shequ* 社区).[24]

The *shequ* is supposed to inherit all of the infrastructure and equipment of the residents' committees, but improving the scope of social services is the primary focus of what is called "community building" (*shequ jianshe* 社区建设): the program is expanded to include other administrative aspects such as health, environment, public security, cultural development, and party-building. This new organization may be seen to be a counterweight to the political, social, and cultural fragmentation brought on by increasing globalization.[25] The Ministry of Civil Affairs (MoCA) promotes it as being able to "expand grassroots democracy while improving/maintaining close ties with the party, to uphold social and political stability, and to promote coordinated urban economic and social development."[26] The program promotes social development and the maintaining of stability while giving the citizens a sense of self-government. The MoCA promoted the community concept to encourage the move from "*danwei ren*" (people of work unit) to "*shehui ren*" (people of society).[27] The service functions were still determined by the government, but the *shequ* was by definition a territorial zone. Residents of *shequ* were encouraged to sign a "resident's pacts" (*jumin gongyue* 居民公约) as a social contract to uphold their role in the *shequ*.[28] The *shequ* resident's committee was to act as a self-governing entity, while the city government maintained jurisdiction over the subdistrict offices.[29]

Though development models emerged as early as the 1980s, the MoCA did not release its "Ministry of Civil Affairs' Opinions on Advancing Urban Community Construction" until 2000. In it, the MoCA outlines how the *shequ* would fulfill five main goals:[30]

1 provide social welfare services to the elderly, disabled, unemployed, and families in need of assistance,
2 manage and maintain the urban sanitation and healthcare services,
3 organize and improve educational and cultural programs,
4 strengthen and uphold local security and public order,
5 and maintain beautification of *shequ* environment and community.

23 **Subdistrict Office (*jiedao banshichu* 街道办事处):** Usually translated as just "Street," the Street office is the highest administrative body within a district. The Street Office handles the governance of Communities (shequ) and other district-level civic

24 **Community (*shequ* 社区):** Covering 1,000-3,000 family units. The name can refer to "community" in general, but in official policy it has a more specific designation and definition.

25 David Bray, 2006.

26 Ministry of Civil Affairs, 2000.

27 Bray 2005, 182.

28 Ibid., 186.

29 Kojima and Kokubun 2002, 86.

30 Ministry of Civil Affairs, 2000.

政 *Governance*

1949 Industrialization in Cities
In the immediate post-1949 period, industrialization in cities was prioritized by Mao to the detriment of other sectors such as agriculture and the urban living.

1952 Patriotic Health Campaign
A widespread campaign to promote hygeine, and combat diseases through improving literacy in aspects of health.

1958 Land Reform and Land Tenure System
All land was confiscated and became either state or collectively owned.

1958 Hukou System Established
A system that segregated the rural and urban populations classifying a person's residence.

1980 "Regulation on Norm and Quota in Urban Planning" Implemented
First defined the urban land use amount, road categories and widths. It also set the norm that residential buildings should mostly be five- to six-storeys.

Early 1980s Land Leasing System Introduced
It allows companies to lease government owned land for fixed periods of time.

1985 Temporary Registration
The stringent restrictions around working in the city was relaxed by the newly introduced temporary registration.

1986 Land Administration Law Passed
Legalizes the private use of state-owned land by private companies and individuals. The Bureau of Land Administration was established to oversee plans and implementation of land-use laws.

1986 Promotion of Shequ Services
The first proposal for the expansion of the residents' committees and responsibilities of the street offices is promoted by the Ministry of Civil Affairs.

1950 1960 1970 1980

1949 - 1977 Early People's Republic
Social Reform

1978 - 1983 Early Reform
The Planned Commodity Economy

1984 - 1991 Economic Reform
Market Economy

Urban Migration

Registered Residence (*hukou* 户口): It is a residential license, or permit, to ensure that people only lived and worked in places designated by the state.

The CCP used the *hukou*[31] system to limit the growth of urban centers, and to allow the government to keep track of its citizens. While the system worked in limiting urban slums,[32] the social implications of the *hukou* system are far reaching. The *hukou* essentially created a separation between urban and rural communities, or what critics have called a caste system. "Urban" citizens were given preferential treatment, receiving more government funding and benefits as a measure to limit dissent.[33]

Following the reform-era policies, in 1985 a temporary registration was introduced, relaxing the stringent work restrictions set by the *hukou*. This created a "rollover migration" effect, where many urban dwellers who were not permanent residents did not feel financially compelled to manage or contribute to maintenance of the urban infrastructure.[34]

In 2000, China had 121 million migrants, including 70 million citizens moving from rural to urban settings; in 2003, that figure jumped to 140 million migrants from rural to urban.[35] As urban migration continues to expand and contribute to the economic growth of the country, social reform measures will need to address migrant workers' rights and their access to housing, healthcare, and education.

32 Wang 2010, 335-364.

33 Chan and Buckingham 2008.

34 Chang 2008.

35 Wang et al. 2001, also cited in China Report, 7.

Health Policies

In the 1950s, Mao promoted a systematized form of traditional Chinese medicine (TCM), enshrouding a healthcare policy with national ideology. Following an ancient Chinese philosophy that the best doctors care for people without sickness, TCM encouraged a strategy of prevention, promoting healthy diet and exercise. Through propaganda and often sensational proclamations, the government promoted the efficacy of Chinese medicine.[36] Other public healthcare policies of the Maoist era adopted much of the Soviet Union model.

36 Levinovitz 2013.

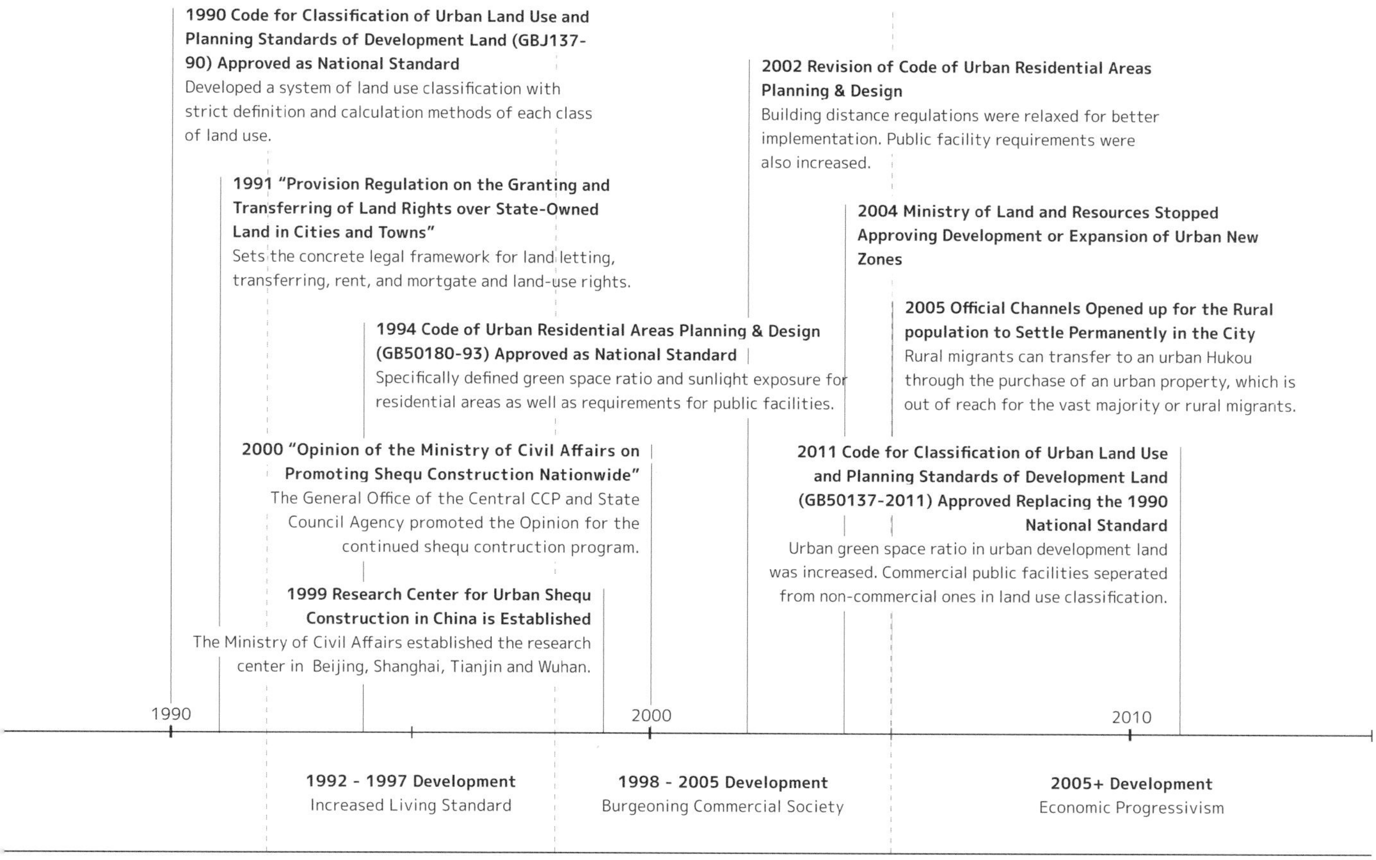

37 Lee and Lv 2009, 3.

In June 26, 1965, Mao famously suggested changing the name of the Ministry of Health to the Ministry of Health for Pampered Urbanites.[37] There was a subsequent shift in focus towards addressing the imbalance in health care provision between urban and rural communities. A three-tier system was implemented under the Rural Cooperative Medical System (RCMS) to provide rural healthcare access. At the rural tier, 'barefoot doctors' administered basic hygiene and TCM practices. Along with the Patriotic Health Campaign (PHC), which identified "four pests" to eradicate (flies, mosquitoes, mice, and sparrows), while proclaiming the value of preventative care associated with TCM, much of the actual public health campaigns of the Maoist era targeted the elimination of epidemics of communicable diseases.

38 Ibid, 2.

39 Kahler 2015.

More recently however, with agricultural reform and policy decentralization, rural healthcare services have received even less government funding during the shift towards a market economy. In 1993, government funding accounted for 34.9% in rural areas; in 1998 this percentage decreased to only 24.9%.[38] The growing disparity between rural and urban health care services prompted the formation of the 2003 New Rural Cooperative Medical Care System, the major difference being a voluntary plan which was extended nationally. To meet the growing need, the State Council's 2010 plan calls for establishing more hospitals, community health service centers, and healthcare clinics on all tiers.[39]

40 Xinhua 2015.

41 Lee and Lv 2009, 8.

42 Ibid, 9.

Current health care reform focuses on addressing the disparity of accessibility, with an effort to return to traditional Chinese medicine philosophy.[40] Changes in diet and nutrition, and lack of physical activity are major contributors to the increase of non-communicable diseases (NCDs). China faces a burden of 'double malnutrition.'[41] Together with cases of under-nutrition, the country is faced with growing over-nutrition. Along with long work hours and increased urbanization, commuting patterns have seen a shift from active commuting to motorized transport.[42] With public health trends showing an increase of non-communicable diseases (NCDs), Health China 2020 aims to provide universal healthcare access and treatment for all, by focusing on nutrition, agriculture, food, and social marketing policies. Chronic disease prevention is targeted by promoting better lifestyle choices, and eating habits.

天 The Environment

In the immediate post 1949 period, industrialization in cities was prioritized by Mao to the detriment of other sectors such as agriculture and urban living.[43] Learning from the Soviet Union, the Communist Party followed the principle of "transformation of cities of consumption to cities of production,"[44] which resulted in the formation of a larger population of an urban working class and the deployment of a socialist model of collective living. Even though many heavy industries had been placed inside or very close to citiy centers through this process, the environmental impacts of this spatial organization did not capture the public's attentions until China's recent economic boom.

43 Liu 2006.

44 Ibid.

Rapid industrialization took a significant toll on China's physical landscapes as well its cultural connection to nature. In earlier courtyard typologies, we see a close connection between places of inhabitation and places of natural scenery. The 'garden' is a space embedded within the private or semi-private domestic environment. From the classic examples of the Suzhou scholars' gardens to the widespread courtyard spaces that provided light and air, the notion of a balance between nature and the built environment persisted as a common cultural thread. As more and more urban centers expand across China, access to natural resources and public green spaces become more valuable and necessary. In order to address this, green open spaces are often being aggregated into larger entities, such as large, open, and undifferentiated green spaces located within new residential developments or the adoption of Garden City principles such as the zoning of green buffers or green belts.

China's government stated that environmental protection would become a state policy from as early as 1983, and the government repeatedly claimed that it should avoid the "pollute first, treat later" (*"xian wuran hou zhili"* 《先污染后治理》) path that many industrialized nations had taken[45]. However, the rapid pace of industrialization has inevitably caused widespread environmental and health concerns. Starting in the 1980s, China has followed necessary precautions for the protection of land and natural resources. However, like most protection policies, these are largely federally issued and rely on local governments to oversee their execution, with often mixed results as a consequence of this split. Many planning precautions such as Shanghai's greenbelt zones are now encroached upon by development, often as a result of lack of regulation or oversight at the local level, diminishing the initial safeguards for green space set up by the planning authorities.

45 Environmental Protection Leadership Group 1978

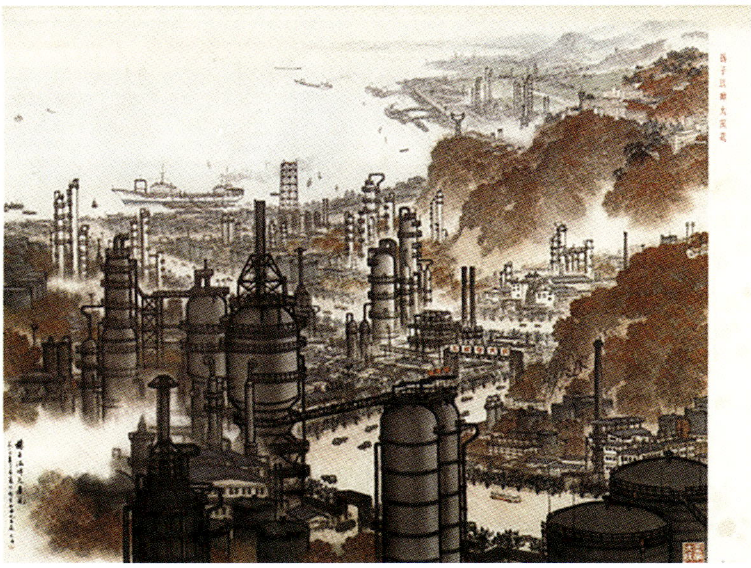

Figure 6 (Left) Poster of Daqing. While Dazhai was the model for agricultural collectivization, Daqing was the model for collectivized industrialization around the same period.

Pollution

According to the annual publication of the *Environmental Status of China* (*"zhongguo huanjing zhangkuang gongbao"*《中国环境状况公报》), the total emissions of sulfur dioxide grew more than 50% from 1991 to 2006.[46] Due to the recent occurrence of several severe smogs and the widespread dissemination of results from the US Embassy in Beijing's air quality index, the Ministry of Environmental Protection has started to publish hourly PM2.5 (particulate matter) concentrations in all major cities from 2012, along with establishing a major revision of the Ambient Air Quality Standards.

In Northern China, where the heavy industries are concentrated and coal is used for winter heating, the air pollution index frequently goes beyond the healthy limit. According to an article in the Economist published in August 2015, Berkeley Earth's scientific director Richard Muller, says, "breathing Beijing's air is the equivalent of smoking almost 40 cigarettes a day and calculates that air pollution causes 1.6 million deaths a year in China, or 17% of the total."[47]

Growing awareness of the potential health risk of exposure to polluted air has impacted the lifestyle of many people. Many changes in behavior have resulted including the adoption of private automobile transport over the previous widespread use of bicycles which can often be motivated by a desire to reduce exposure to the pollution. People have also started to prefer higher floors when purchasing apartments as a desperate measure to safeguard their personal health.

46 Ministry of Environmental Protection 2014.

47 "Mapping the Invisible Scourge" *Economist* 15 August 2015. http://www.economist.com/news/china/21661053-new-study-suggests-air-pollution-even-worse-thought-mapping-invisible-scourge.

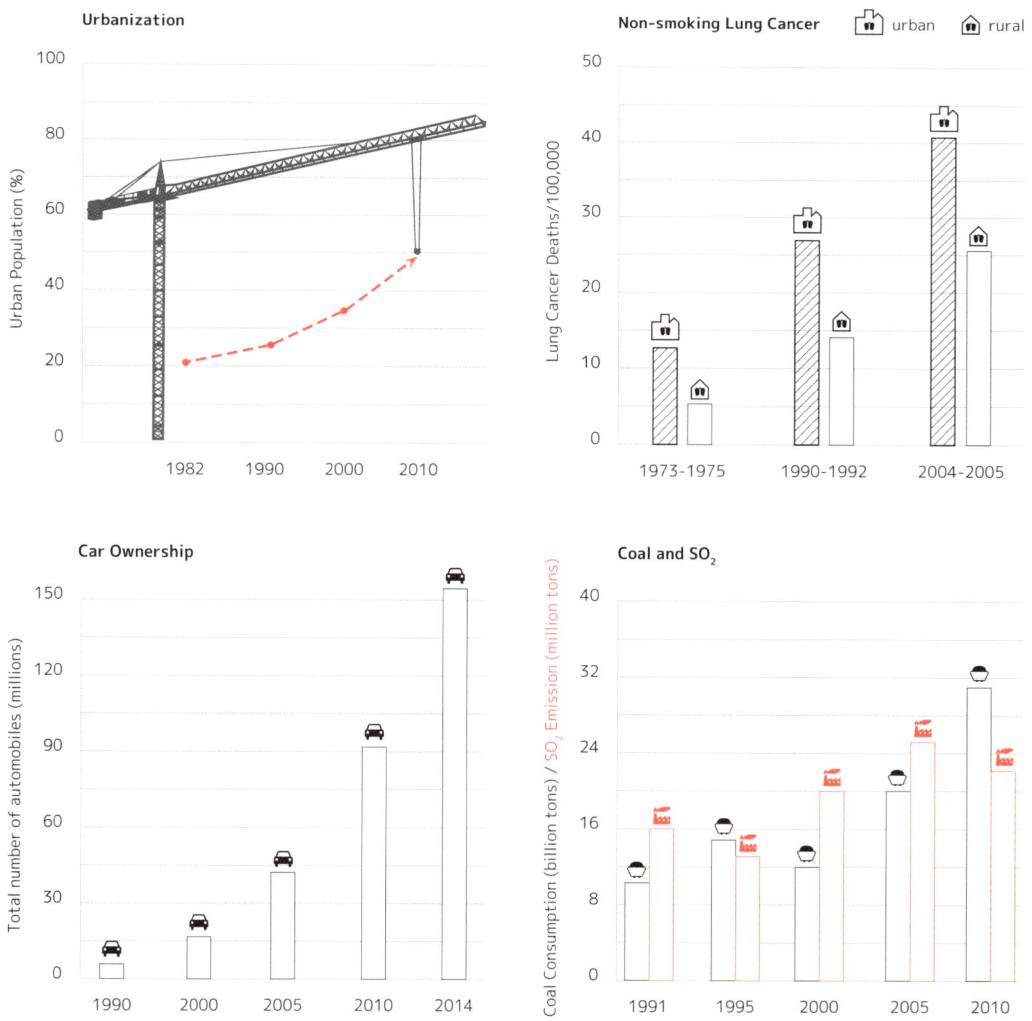

Figure 7 (Left) Sources: State Statistics Bureau, Ministry of Health (now National Health and Family Planning Commission), and Ministry of Environmental Protection.

天 *The Environment*

房 政
天 家

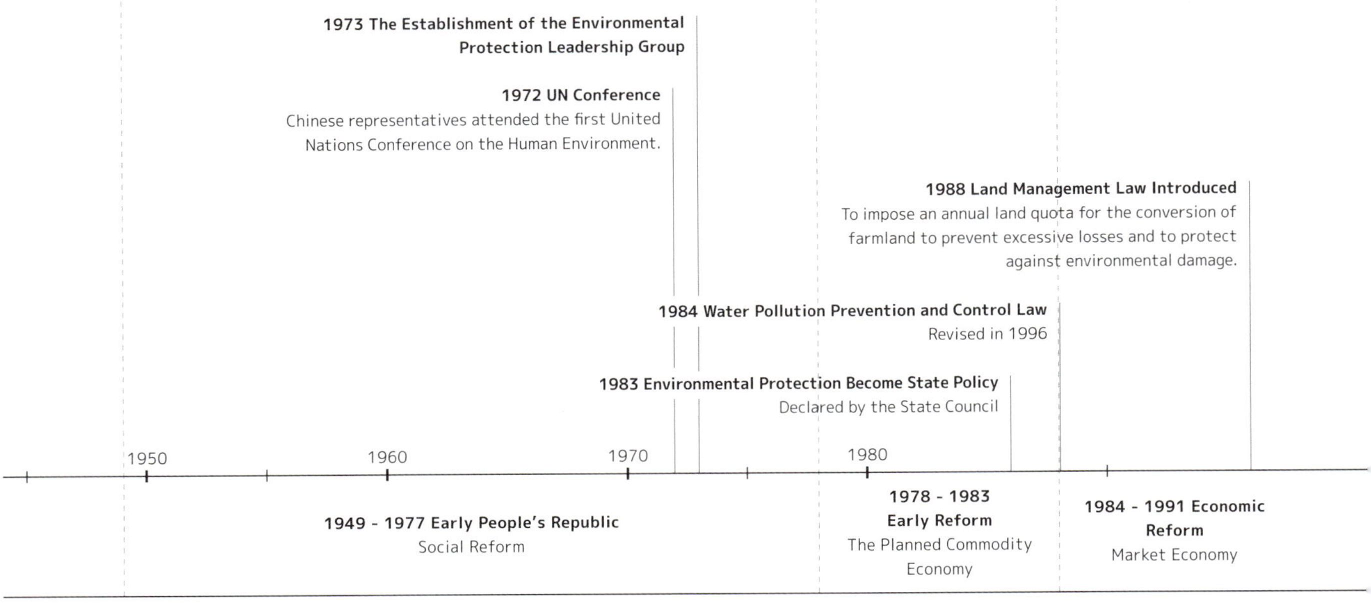

Figure 8 (Right) Source: Caixin.com

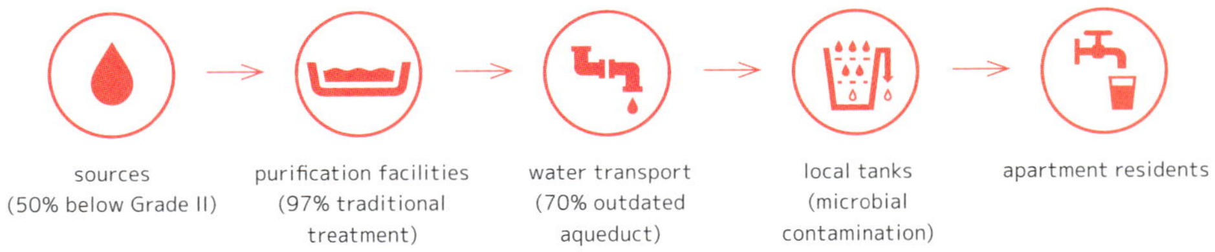

Water Systems

The annual China Environmental Status reports documented a four-fold increase of industrial solid waste output and a three-fold increase in water chemical oxygen demand from 1991 to 2014.[48] Even though relevant laws and regulations have existed since 1984, the untreated and badly managed discharge of waste has greatly affected the water quality of the groundwater as well as the major water bodies including reservoirs. The deteriorating quality of tap and drinking water is as harmful as air pollution for the health of the population but less visible, resulting in much less public debate. The freshwater quality varies significantly across the nation, and more than 50% of the drinking water sources are said to be polluted. Many densely populated urban areas are susceptible to drinking water pollution because of the presence of unregulated discharge from heavy industries. In developed cities, tap water is produced following high standards yet these can still be polluted by the outdated aqueducts and water tanks running between neighborhoods and water purification facilities.

Untreated urban runoff and stormwater compounds these problems with water quality. Many things can be done at the neighborhood level to address the issues related to urban runoff treatment and release. Despite not being able to address other sources of contamination such as industrial waste, the reconsideration of how stormwater is managed within our urban environment can contribute towards limiting the extent of water pollution.

48 Ministry of Environmental Protection, 2014.

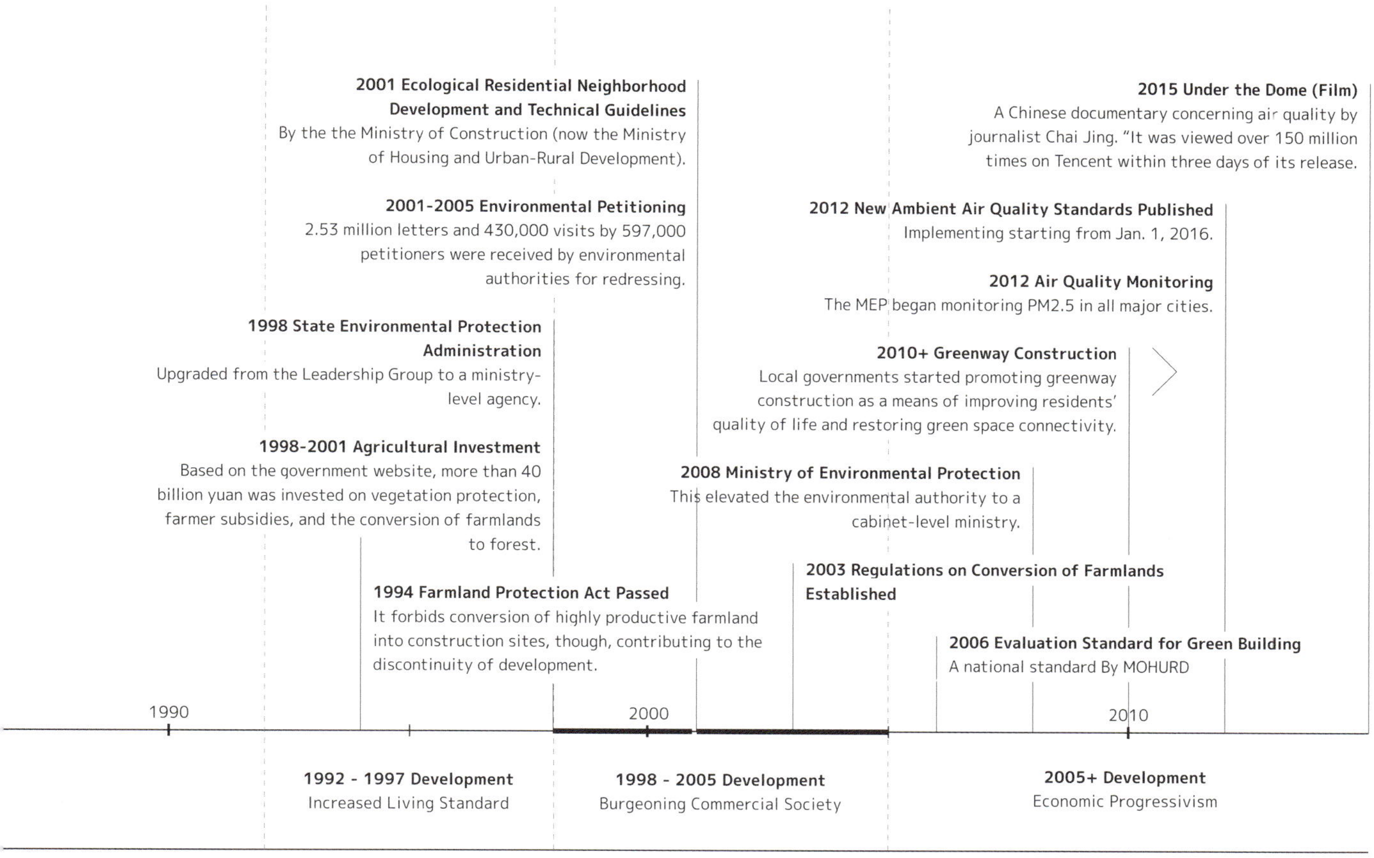

Figure 9 (Right) Source: State Statistics Bureau and China Customs

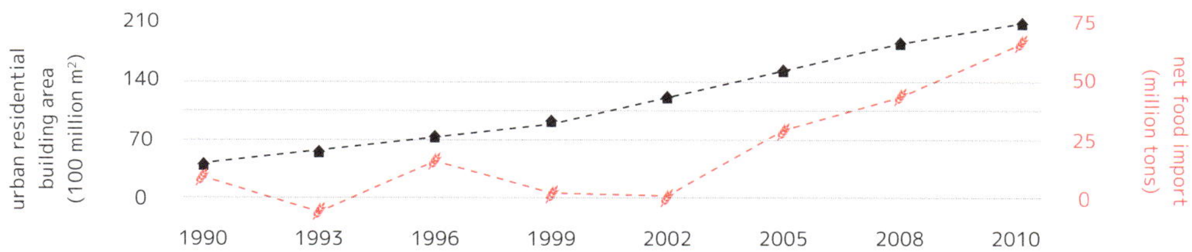

The Food Environment

After economic reform, the State Land Administration was established and integrated with other land authorities to form the Ministry of Land and Resources. This authority regulates all land-related activities including real estate development and farmland surveys. According to its second National Land Survey in 2009, the per capita arable land has dropped since 1996,[49] despite the rapidly growing appetite of the Chinese population. The changing dietary preference has resulted in the need for more food imports, which may lead to a greater influence on the global food market and more severe environmental impacts.

It is reasonable to expect that the conflation between even more demand for quality foods and a gradually diminishing amount of arable land due to future urban expansion is likely to produce a crisis. Urban agriculture and organic farming have been trending topics on social networks and online shopping platforms, but very little has been done at the administrative levels to address the problems associated with food security, including broken cold chains and inadequate access to nutritious food.

49 Ministry of Land and Resources, also see Xiao et al. 2015.

房 The Block

China's breadth of housing and living styles is vast and diverse. It would take much space to elucidate the particularities of the kinds of living environments that have existed in China throughout history. Because of the scale and pace at which China is urbanizing, it is relevant to look back at part of this legacy. As background information, we chose to focus on four emblematic models for collective living: (i) the *Siheyuan* courtyard house, (ii) the *Lilong*, (iii) the *dayuan* and (iv) the contemporary *xiaoqu* development. To get a glimpse of the changing lifestyles and its effect on housing conditions, a look back to the traditional courtyard style of house is warranted. Even as the traditional family has undergone many changes, its regular adaptation and retrofitting has produced new types of private urban spaces and a connection with the ground—a feature lost in today's high-rise development. The *Lilong* is also an important typological precedent as it was one of China's first mass produced housing styles for the market, but it also contained notable social characteristics afforded by the lane and alleys between the units where children would play, residents would cook, and neighbors would interact. These types were then abandoned as models for urbanization with the revolutionary rupture of 1949 and the founding of the People's Republic. As housing was considered a social necessity under the new government, the preoccupation with development and production led to a new wave of collectivized, mass-produced development types associated with the organization of work units. Later, as the socialist project accommodated an open market, much of the social and administrative machinery remained intact. A new development style tasked with creating an effective community in a superblock (referred to as *xiaoqu* 小区)[50] while operating under market conditions has characterized much of China's building boom. There are still many problems to tackle, and the large scale of residential building is an important aspect to be considered from social, political, and environmental perspectives.

50 **Microdistrict (xiaoqu 小区):** A typical large-scale plot of land development that involves a large community and the provision of services as a complete unit.

The development of the *xiaoqu* in China is usually done with a repetition of building units. Type is a useful concept to begin to structure a large array of residential units, equipped with services and amenities at the scale of a small town or very large neighborhood. Type allows for the categorization of elements and the ability to break apart and recombine them in the design process. By categorizing, we develop and assign a value system. It is here where values such as living styles, family life, and health come into play. Regulations, rules, and frameworks also structure living patterns and in turn inform the organization and form of a type.

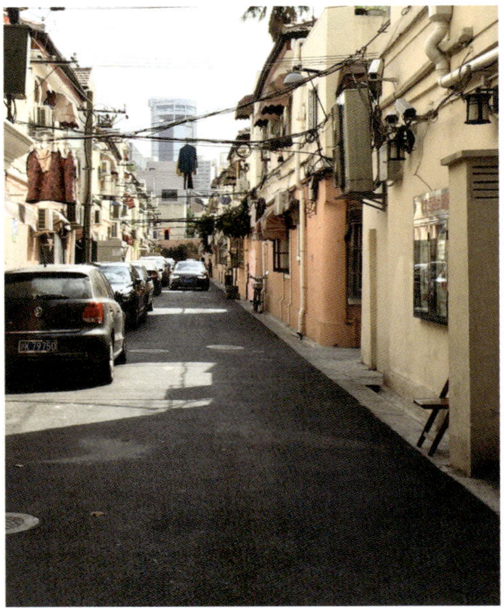

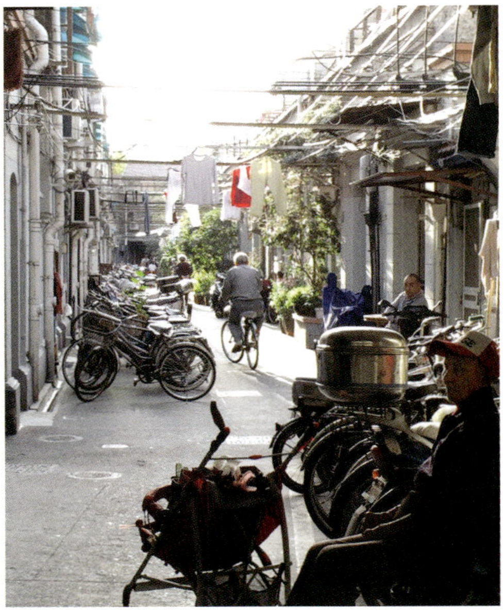

Figures 10, 11 (Left) Photographs of typical Shanghai *Lilong*.

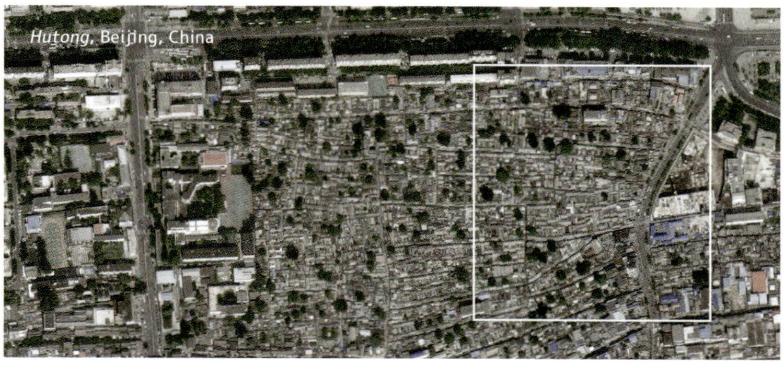

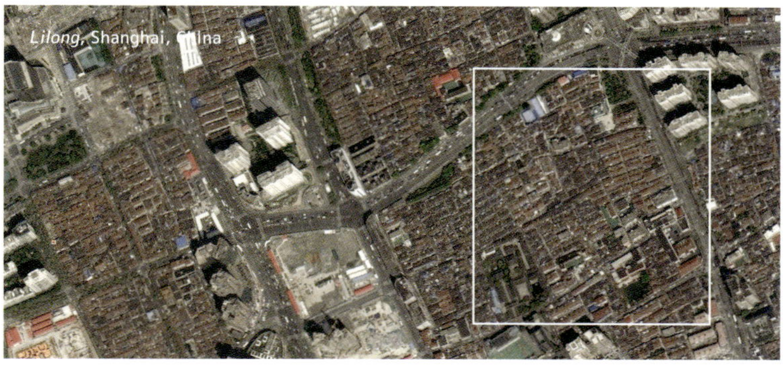

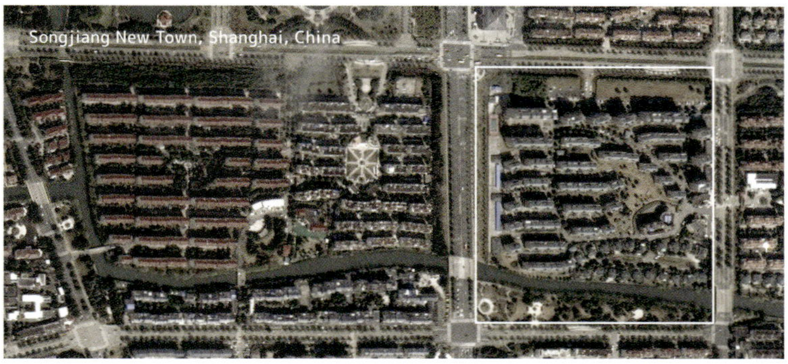

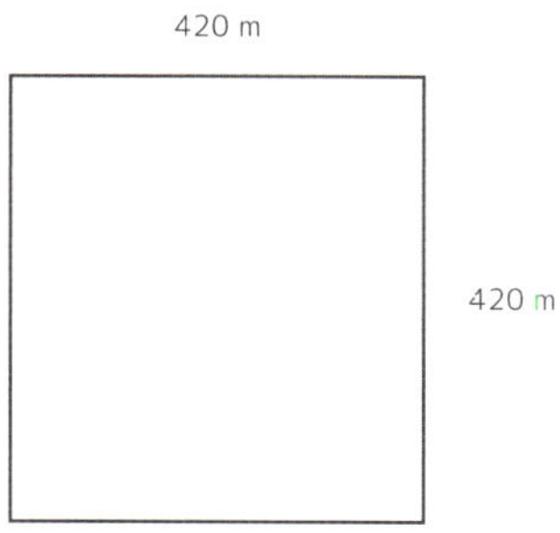

Figure 12 (Above, Left) A size comparison between the present development type of the xiaoqu (below) where the area of development reaches around 400 m by 400 m. The scale of land coverage is comparable, however, the population densities of the various types vary greatly.

Figure 13 (Below) Residential typologies

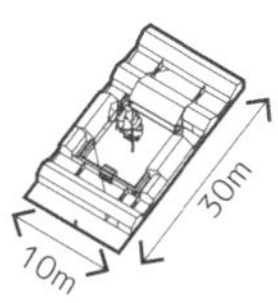

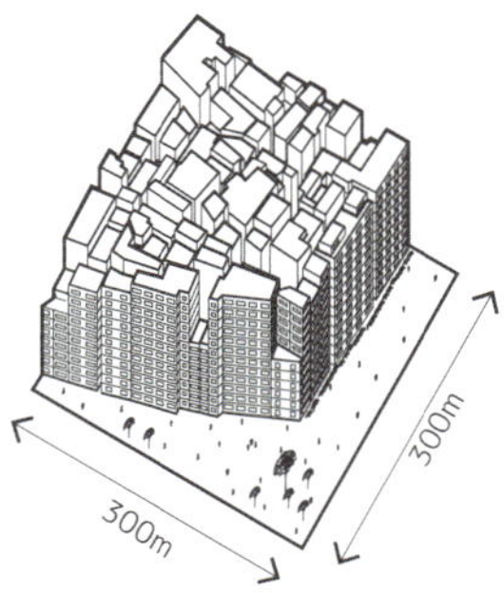

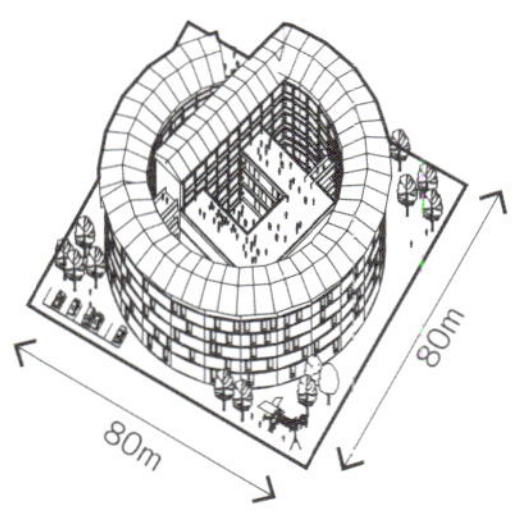

Courtyard House

Building Area: 250-300 sqm
Floors: 1
Public Space Area: <100 sqm
Units: 1
FAR: 0.5
Residents: 5-10
Average Area: 30-45 P/sqm

Kowloon Wall City

Building Area: 32,000 sqm
Floors: 10
Public Space Area: <500 sqm
Units: 400
FAR: 8-9
Residents: 1,000-1,200
Average Area: 10-15 P/sqm

Tulou

Building Area: 10,000 sqm
Floors: 6-7
Public Space Area: <3,000sqm
Units: 160
FAR: 6
Residents: 300
Average Area: 10-20 P/sqm

房 *The Block*

房 政
天 家

1854 "Rules on Land Leasing in the British, French and American Concessions of Shanghai"
It was said that combustible building materials should not be used in the building of houses.

1865 Gas Supply in Shanghai
The Great Britain Gas Company—the first of its kind in China—started to supply gas in Shanghai's concessions

1869 "Rules of the Pidgin Beishou Concession in Shanghai"
promoted massive development and an orderly array of residential buildings.

1881-1882 Water and Electricity Supply
In 1881, the Shanghai Tap Water Company was established with British investment and, in 1882, the British-backed Shanghai Electric Light Company was established to supply electric power.

Early 1900s Urban Public Facilities Established
1905 Inland Tap Water Company; 1904 Belgian Merchants Power Plant for Streetcar and Electric Light; 1908 Hazhen Jiji Water & Power Company

1920s Large tracts of urban housing development in major cities

1930s Slum Issue
More than 20,000 households lived in slums outside the concession in Shanghai.

1860 1870 1880 1890 1900 1910 1920 1930

1845 - 1910 Late Qing + Treaty of Nanjing
Internationalism + Cosmopolitanism

1911 - 1936 Early Republican Era
New Individualism

Figure 14 (Below, Continued) Residential Typologies.

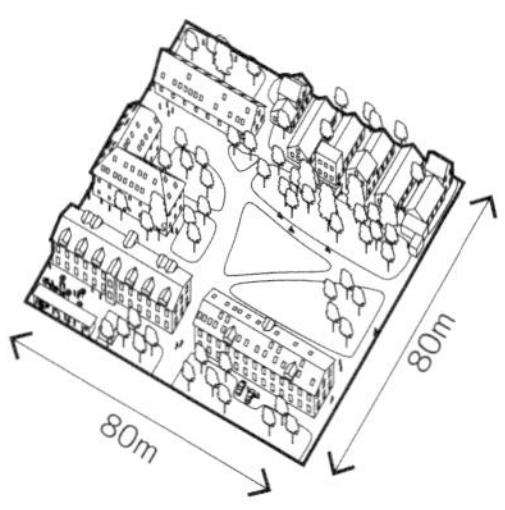

Xiaoqu Building

Building Area: 4,200 sqm
Floors: 5-7
Public Space Area: <5,000 sqm
Units: 30
FAR: 4
Residents: 120
Average Area: 35-40 P/sqm

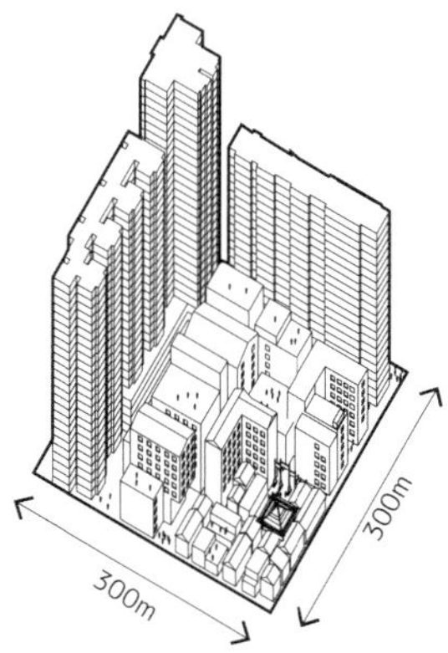

High-rise Residential

Building Area: 33,000 sqm
Floor: 30-33
Public Space Area: <2,000 sqm
Units: 240
FAR: 6-7
Residents: 700-850
Average Area: 25-30 P/sqm

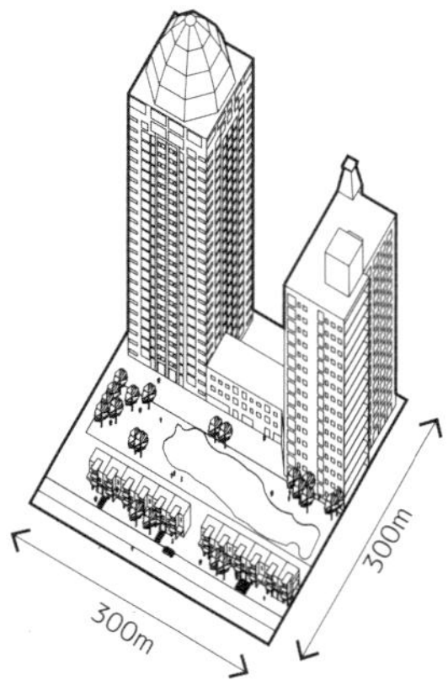

Mix-use Residential

Building Area: 37,000 sqm
Floors: 30-33
Public Space Area: <4,000 sqm
Units: 200
FAR: 8-9
Residents: 700-750
Average Area: 25-35 P/sqm

1950s Workers' Villages
Many semi-temporary, low-rise apartments and dormitory-like apartments were built as quickly as possible to accommodate large numbers of families. In Shanghai, the total floor space of housing was 4.8 million square meters more in 1957 than in 1950, and 57.7% of this was housing for workers.

1973 Standard Advanced
The State Construction Commission issued "Proposals for Revising the Building Standards of Apartments and Dormitories"

1977 Concrete Technology Development
A total of 1 million square meters of large concrete panel structures were constructed in Beijing, Nanjing, Kunming, Xi'an and Shenyang.

1978 Decline
A survey of 182 cities showed a decline of per-capita floor space from 1952 to 1978 and 6.89 million families almost didn't have a place to live.

1979 Prototype
The trial construction of a low-rise high-density integral living environment design by Tianjin University Department of Architecture was completed in Changjiang Street in the Nankai District of Tianjin.

1985 Blue Paper on Technological Policies of China
was concerned with large-scale residential construction standards and directions.

1987 Land Leasing
By taking advantage of its preferential treatment as a special economic zone, Shenzhen took the lead by leasing, for the first time, land under Chinese sovereignty, whereby a paid transfer of land-use rights was effected.

1991 "Opinions Concerning an All-Around Promotion of Housing Reforms in Cities and Towns"
was issued by the government.

2005 Urbanization
Official channels opened up for the rural population to settle permanently in the city.

1940 · 1950 · 1960 · 1970 · 1980 · 1990 · 2000 · 2010

1937 - 1948 Late Republican Era
Wartime Depression

1949 - 1977 Early People's Republic
Social Reform

1978 - 1991 Planned Commodity + Market Economy
Social Reform

1992 - 2005 Burgeoning Commercial Society
Increasing Standard of Living

2005+ Economic Progressivism

Courtyard House

The spatial configuration of the traditional Chinese courtyard housing reinforced the importance of a "harmonious hierarchy" of the family structure and filial piety in traditional society. The axial arrangement of halls surrounding an interior courtyard focused the family activities inward and allowed for multiple generations to live in close proximity. Southern facing halls on the central axis were dedicated to ancestral altars and the living spaces for the patriarch of the family. The eldest son and his family were privileged along the central axis, while younger sons and their families would live in outer courtyards. Separate guest halls served as intermediary spaces between the outside and internal family functions. As the family grew, additions grew from within the walls and even extending into courtyards.

The separation of domestic activities reinforced gender roles. Women had separate quarters to handle the care of the household and children. Men handled the financial and external relationships of the household from their own distinct quarters. As courtyard housing units expanded, interconnecting gardens and alleys provided additional spaces for women to socialize within their network as they often could not leave the compound unaccompanied by a male member of the family.

The courtyard allowed for more shared interactions between the domestic spheres. With multiple generations living together, the courtyard allowed for daily interaction. In warmer weather, cooking would occur here in order to reduce heat. Tables and chairs allowed for studying or games of chess. Children would play here under the watchful eyes of adults nearby. With typically single-story halls, the natural light and ventilation readily filtered in to the interior living spaces through the courtyard.

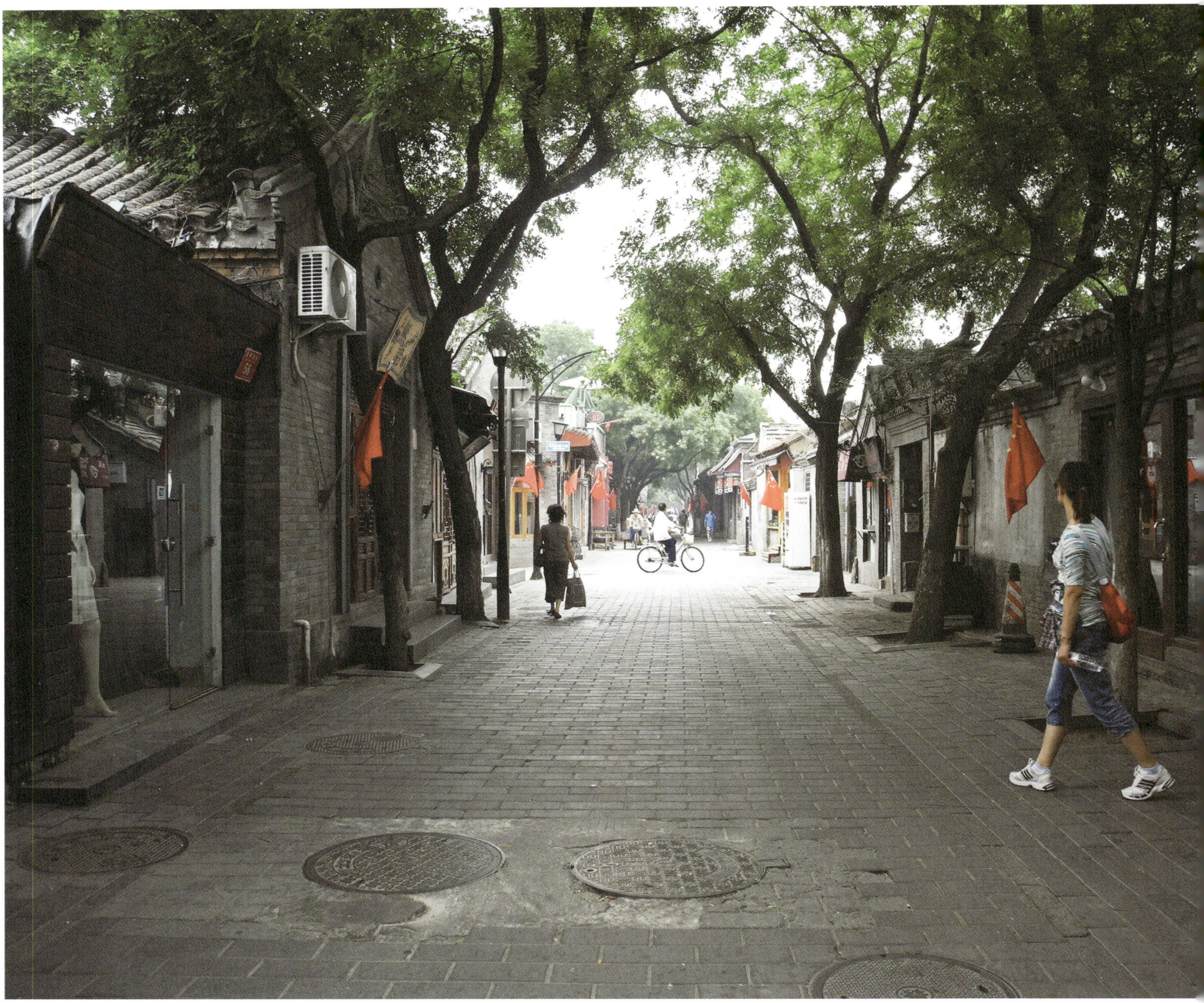

Figure 15 (Above) Recent photograph of a Beijing Hutong.

Figure 16 (Below) Primary elements of the courtyard house type.

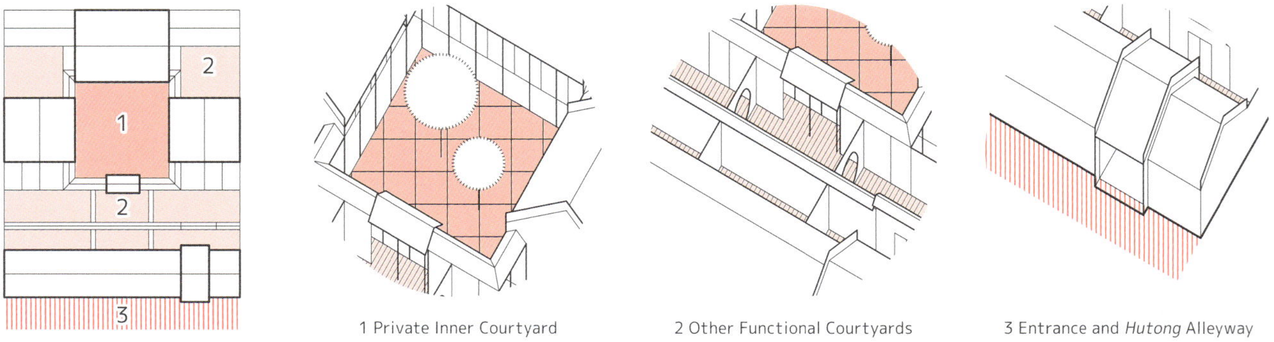

1 Private Inner Courtyard

2 Other Functional Courtyards

3 Entrance and *Hutong* Alleyway

Figure 1 (Below, Left) *Siheyuan* (四合院) Example courtyard house and Hutong aggregation pattern.

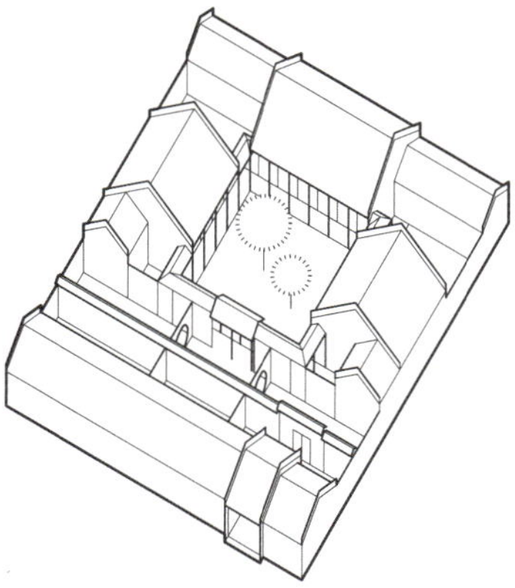

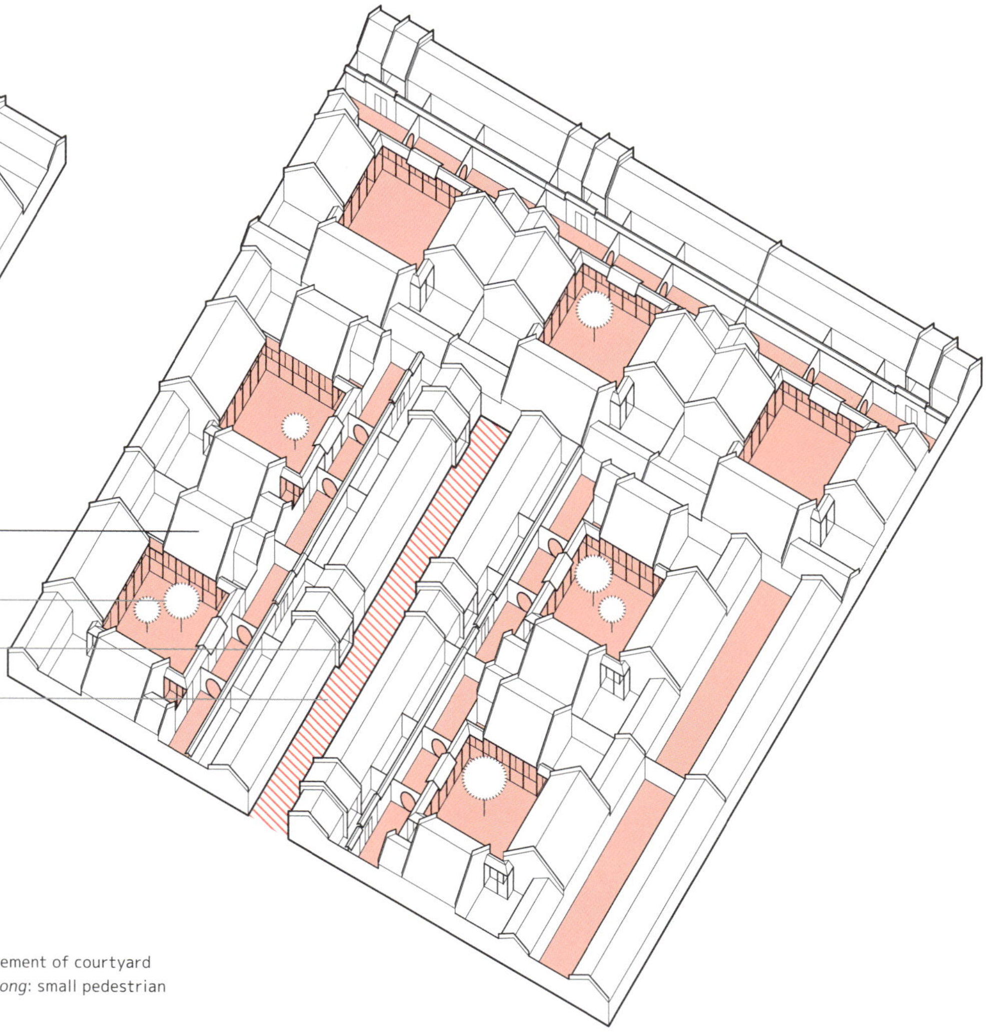

Figure 18 (Above, Right) The arrangement of courtyard houses fills in space to form the *hutong*: small pedestrian alleyways.

Changes in the family structure and property ownership demanded a re-thinking of the courtyard housing typology and its conservation. The shrinking of the family unit to nuclear family models has shifted emphasis away from preserving an extensive family structure. Private courtyard housing ownership was transferred to government ownership in the 1950s and 1960s. This changed the single-extended family function of the courtyard housing to multi-family compounds. Throughout the 1960s and through the 1980s, many courtyard houses were packed with a variety of migrant populations and partitions were put up that largely negated the older structure. Present day conservation and construction of new courtyard housing typologies address the preservation of the cultural heritage of the traditional courtyard house, even if traditional family functions have been lost.

Lilong Housing

With China's defeat in the Opium War of 1842, Shanghai was forced to open to European trade, and by the end of the 1840s, many foreign powers had already set up settlements in the city. According to the Land Regulation of 1845, these settlements were to be reserved for foreigners and their own housing. However, these regulations were far from effective as many migrants and refugees moved in to Shanghai's foreign settlements throughout the Taiping Rebellion, and by 1854, the segregationist policies were dropped. Under the new mixed-residence policy coupled with a surging population, property suddenly became one of the most valuable businesses.

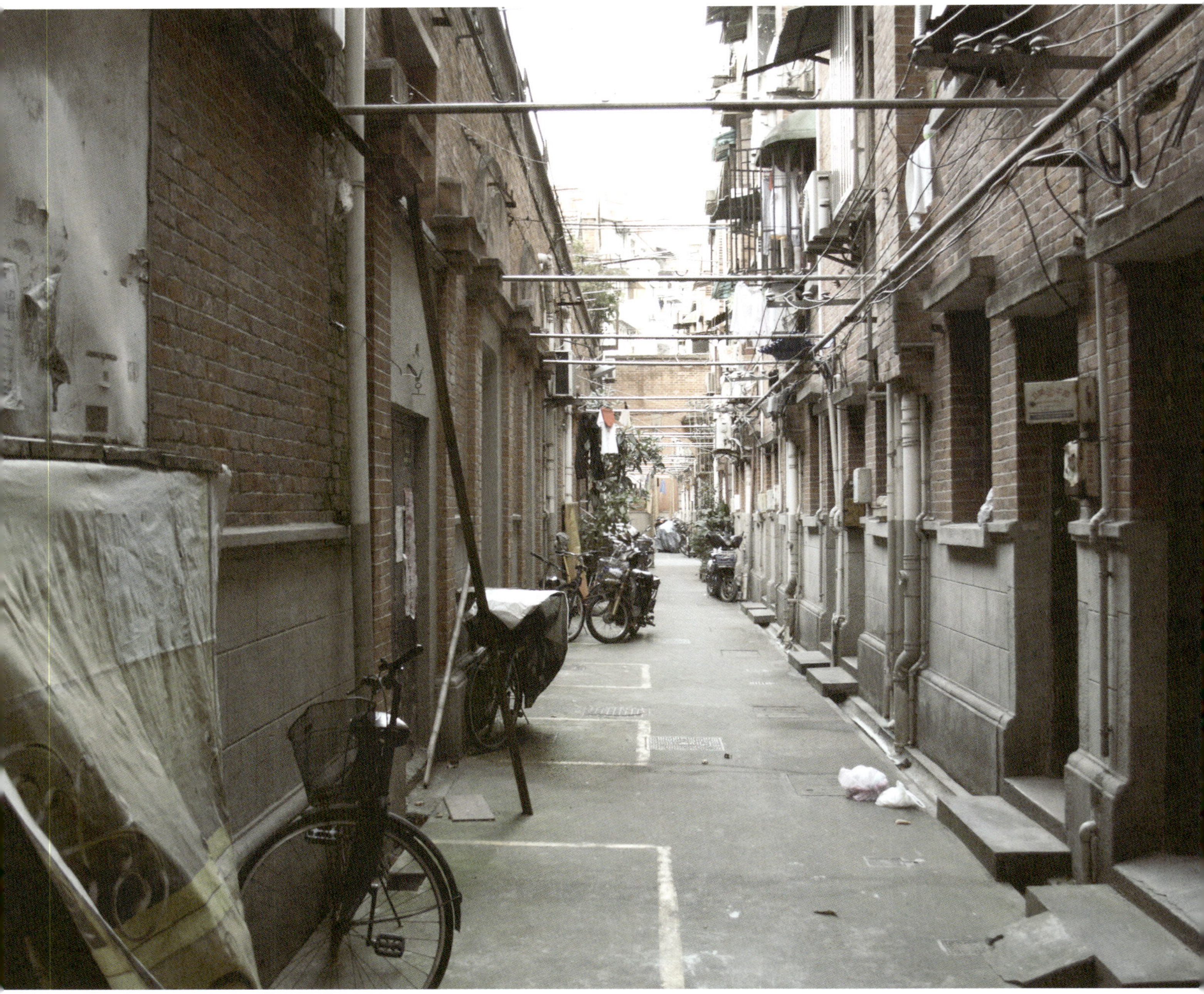

Figure 19 (Above) Contemporary photograph of a Shanghai *Lilong* alley.

Figure 20 (Below) Primary elements of the *Lilong* type.

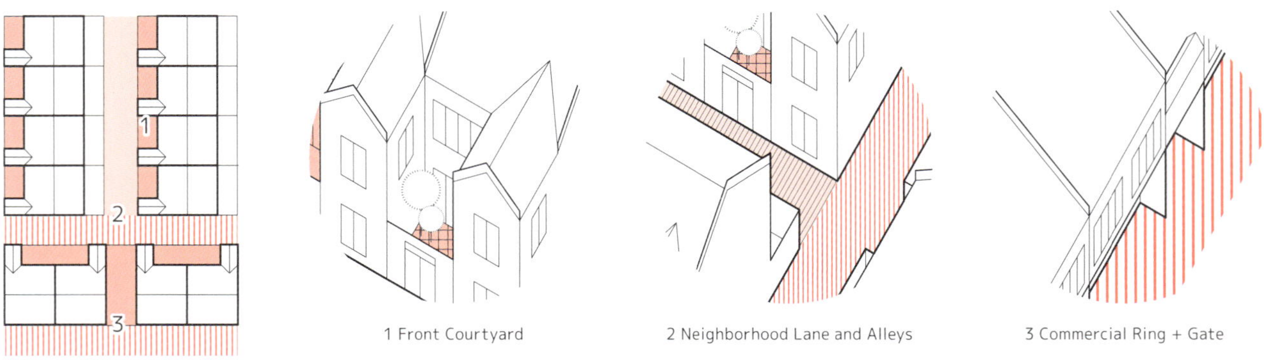

Figure 21 (Below, Left) Shanghai *Lilong* (里弄) example typologies and aggregation

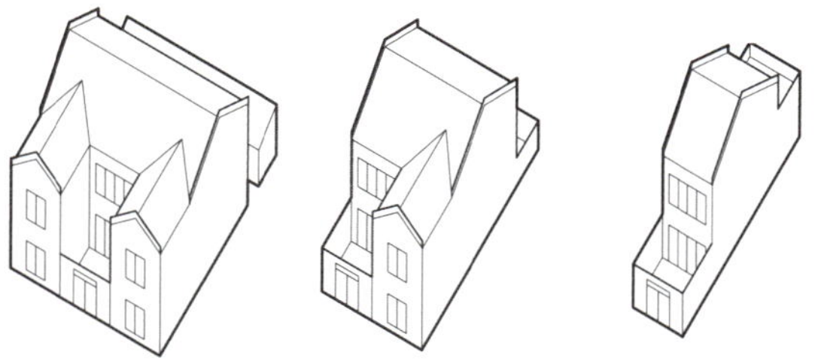

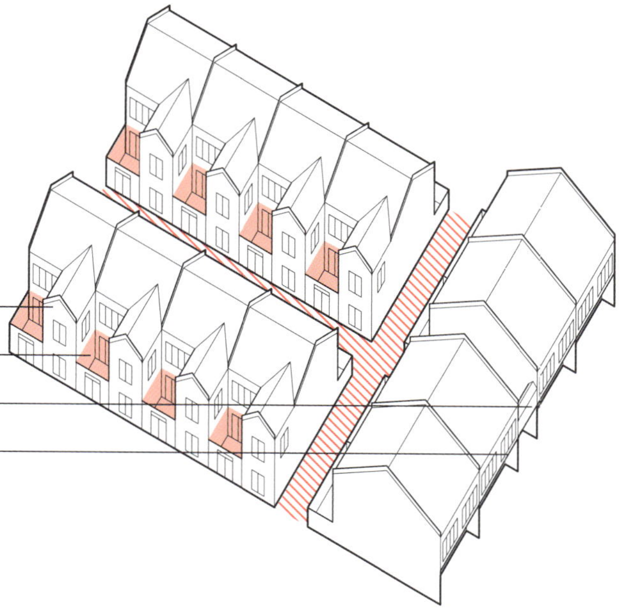

Figure 22 (Above, Right) The array of row-houses are oriented so that each entryway meets the alley at the rear of the house across from it. These alleys were much more intimate and the heirarchy of streets grew progressively wider away from the entryways.

The *Lilong* was first born as a series of wooden shacks aggregated in rows accessed by alleys and walled off with a gate for the control of entry and exit. It was simple and effective. *Li* (里) was the name given to these properties, simply meaning 'neighborhood.' By 1870, after more than 8,000[51] had already been built, the early wooden prototypes were banned due to their flammability. Nevertheless the type remained popular, and would proliferate in brick and concrete.

51 Wu Jiang 1997.

The early *Shikumen* (石窟們)[52] housing estates were rather small compared to later developments. These early neighborhoods included commercial and shop houses along the periphery of the streets while the units themselves could only be entered through internal alleys accessed by the gates. All of the houses within the neighborhood were replications—built of the same form and material. The layout had been inherited from the traditional three-sided courtyard house of the south (*sanheyuan* 三合院). It was typically a two-story building that enclosed a central courtyard near the front and adjacent to the alley. The early *Shikumen* house attempted to replicate what the courtyard house had: rooms that were laid out symmetrically with larger rooms and service spaces such as the kitchen at the ground level and bedrooms on the second. The rear lane became the service lane where the kitchen was located and used for cooking, or as an area for children to play.

52 **Stone Gate Housing (*shikumen* 石窟們):** A type of *Lilong* housing characterized by a prominent stone-gate entry into a small walled courtyard in front of each row-house.

While the early *Shikumen Lilong* could grow in size, accommodating many more rooms and larger families, many other factors also led to the evolution of smaller and more numerous units. With rising foreign influence, commerce, and a changing economic landscape, cosmopolitan life became a cornerstone and major attribute of a changing social and family structure. Larger families were difficult to manage, especially through difficult times such as war and migration. The cosmopolitan life of Shanghai offered a new model for the family that also adjusted well to the new dwelling style afforded by the *Lilong*. During the time that this style and neighborhood was built, family sizes began to reflect a changing lifestyle, moving away from the older feudal organizations and into the industrializing and entrepreneurial setting of the city.

The collapse of the Qing Dyansty in 1911 signaled the beginning of the end of traditional extended families. The new *Shikumen Lilong* was adapted to smaller and lower income families. The neighborhood developments grew larger and also allowed for more units to be subdivided within the existing building shell. There was little change to the overall aggregation of the units, although the rooms and sizes began to diminish, the courtyard remained a central feature, even as it began to occupy more space at the front of the building. While the courtyard brought the landscape into the life of the inhabitants of the courtyard house, the *Lilong* took it away. The courtyard's size was reduced only allowing for a few plantings or a paved private outdoor space and much of the active family life was forced into the lanes, shared with neighbors.

Newer types of *Lilong* housing began to alter their structure to allow for more variation than the earlier *Shikumen* styles. The peripheral shop houses and gated entries began to be relaxed where the periphery saw less commercial frontage and more porous entry. The new types were also produced to accommodate varying classes. The general form stayed the same while allowing for balconies, guest rooms, roof terraces and other amenities for wealthier residents. Many compact models grew to three stories and also lacked segregated circulation. The change in circulation access promoted the use of the alleys and service alleys near the kitchen allowing for more social contact. These lanes became the communal space for the residents, and arguably the most prominent social feature of life that characterized many of Shanghai's *Lilong*.

In recent years, private development has began to focus on the *Lilong* for its historical and cultural legacy. A recent redevelopment of the Jianyeli by Portman Holdings highlights the inherent qualities of interest with regard to the spatial type of the Shanghai *Lilong*. However, some of these developments replicate the forms of the *Lilong* but offer a very different internal organization scheme, whereas the Jianyeli development operates more as a series of exclusive and gated residences.

Dayuan: Spatial Manifestation of the Danwei

From 1949 to 1976, the socialist transformation of China was characterized by the nationalization of all urban institutions and enterprises. The *danwei* started to play an increasingly important role in urban areas as both the life and work of the urban population were planned based on it.

Translated as "work unit," a *danwei* not only offered stable jobs, but also provided dwellings and even other social services including hospitals and schools. After the land reforms of the 1950s, the State allocated large tracts of land with full land-use rights to the *danwei* at no cost, and the *danwei* began to construct offices, residential buildings, and service facilities based on their needs and their economic situations. Normally referred to as *dayuan* (大院, big yard), these enclosed communities became the spatial manifestations of the *danwei* systems and the main driving force of urban expansion at that time. Along with Mao's initiatives of transforming city consumerism into production, many industrial *danwei* emerged in cities to facilitate the land allocation processes.

Given the fact that the old city centers had already been filled up, the *danwei* tended to choose land that was deemed "remote" to avoid handling demolitions and relocations. Measuring up to eighty square kilometers, the *dayuan* were closed to outer traffic with sparsely distributed five- or six-storey buildings. Residents could find almost everything they needed (and even went to work) within their communities. However, such spatial organization increasingly became a problem as urban residents and traffic grew exponentially after the economic reform.

Under the *danwei* system, cities were efficiently subdivided into micro-administrative units and all the economic and social activities were tightly controlled. As urban dwellers normally developed lifelong relationship with their *danwei* and *dayuan*, the space of the *dayuan* became part of their social identity and class.

After the economic reform in the late 70s and 80s, the market economy housing development inherited many spatial characteristics of the *dayuan* and became a new generation of gated communities that steered the rapid expansion of cities. *Dayuan* today can be considered, and are commonly referred to, as *xiaoqu* (microdistricts). The linguistic interchangeability is an evidence of the similarities between the two. While the *xiaoqu* itself is commonly translated as a block or microdistrict, it will be referred to as a specific large-scale development type.

Figure 23 (Below, Right) *Dayuan* (大院) Example *Danwei* Typologies and Aggregation

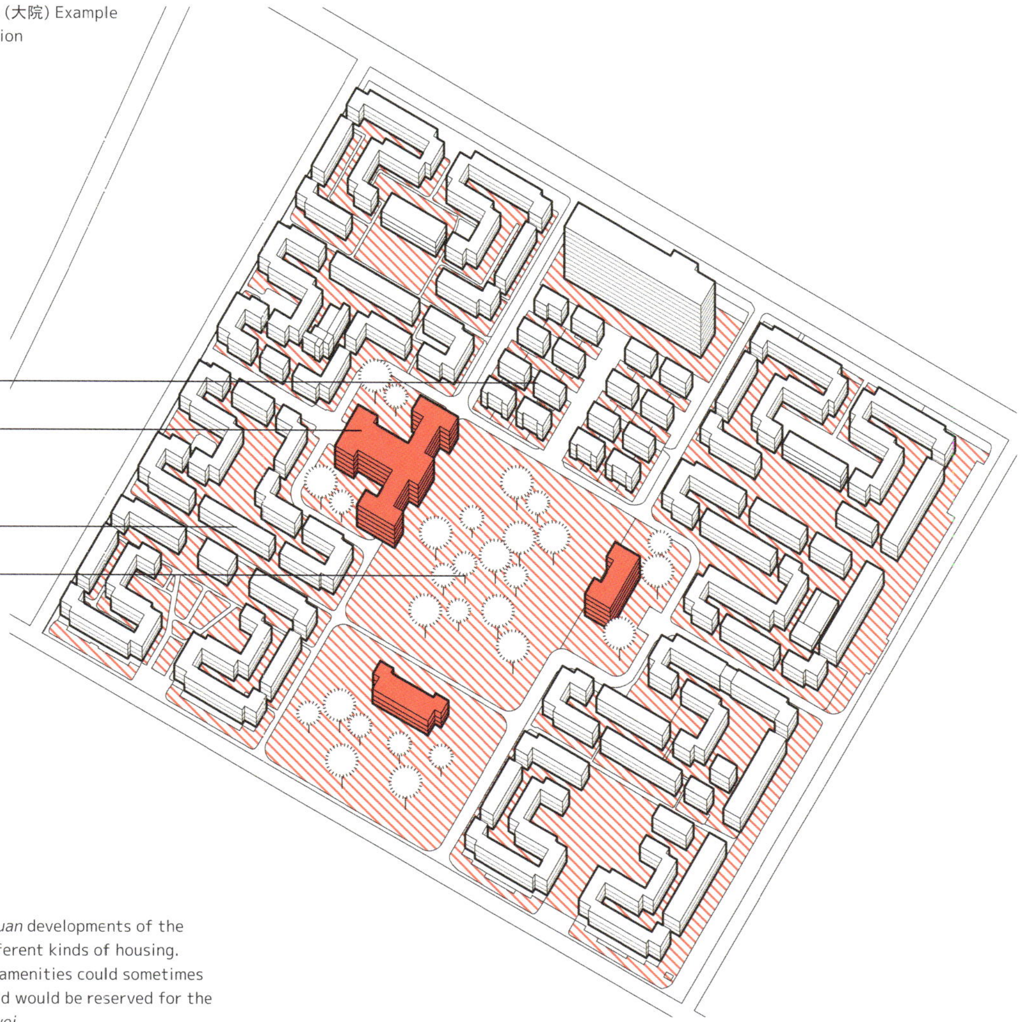

Figure 23 (above, right) The *dayuan* developments of the *danwei* system provided many different kinds of housing. Work spaces, services, and other amenities could sometimes be integrated within the block and would be reserved for the residents of that particular *danwei*.

Xiaoqu: New Market Development

With the reform era and the opening up of the economy, the *danwei* system that governed daily work and social life in Mao era no longer met the needs of a changing society. In the 1980s, the Central Party Committee began to shift focus from a socialist planned economy to a market-driven economy. Small-scale private businesses, *getihu,*[53] were allowed to set up based on 1981 guidelines for the expansion of small businesses. These *getihu* were often located along main commercial streets, or along back streets of residential blocks. With *getihu*, families could operate as "one family, two system" economic units. One partner could stay in the *danwei* system, ensuring provisions of social welfare services, while the other partner could focus on the financial gains of an entrepreneurial income. Additionally, the *getihu* allowed for a shift away from being tied to the bounded enclosures of the *danwei* to a focus on commerce on the exterior street.[54]

On the path to modernization, the Ministry of Civil Affairs (MCA) issued its "Decision on the Reform of the Economic Structure" in 1984, declaring one of its key objectives to relieve the *danwei* model of the welfare functions to allow them to pursue business functions.[55] The decision to join the international supply chain meant that many of the state-owned enterprises faced drastic operational overhauls.[56] By the 1990s, government policies encouraged employees to purchase housing from the *danwei* to ease their financial burden.

The open economy had two effects on housing development. With growing individual economic power and property rights, individuals were no longer tied to their place of work for their choice in residency. Secondly, the overhaul of *danwei* systems left many people unemployed and without a welfare

53 Individual Industrial and Commercial Households (*geti gongshanghu* 个体工商户): *Getihu* is short for many entities. It is officially defined as a small business as individual laborers are named *geti laodongzhe*.

54 Bray 2005, 167-169.

55 Chan 1993, 22.

56 Nguyen 2013, 215.

Figure 24 (Below, Left) *Xiaoqu* (小区) Development Example Typologies and Aggregation

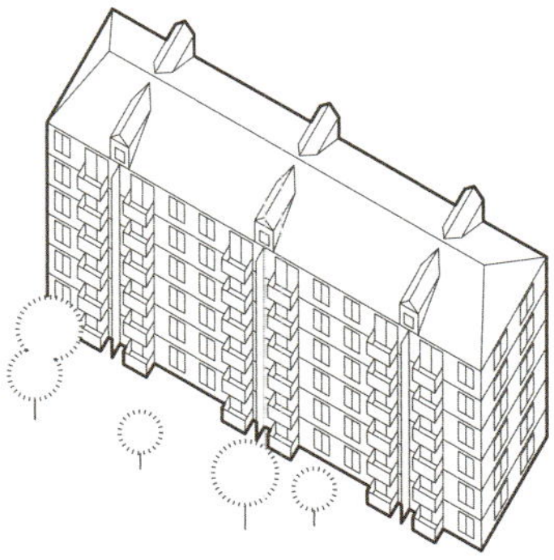

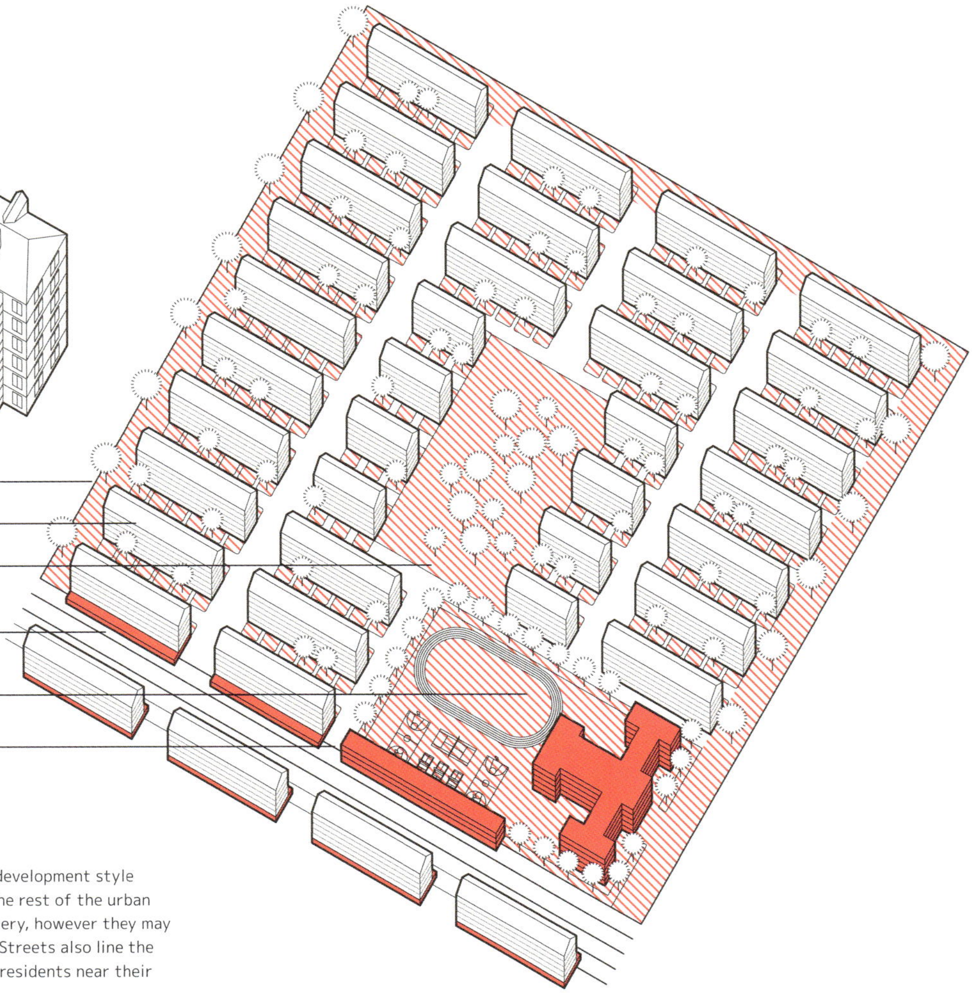

Figure 25 (Above, Right) The *xaioqu* development style typically segregates the block from the rest of the urban fabric. Services are kept in the periphery, however they may also be found within the block itself. Streets also line the *xiaoqu* and provide ample parking for residents near their unit.

support network.[57] As early as the 1980s, the MoCA began promoting the *shequ* model for development to fill the void of services created by the separation of work and living arrangements.

The size and designated territory of the *shequ* may vary . It can range from operating in a small compound, to encompassing multiple residential blocks demarcated by specific roads. The ideal model that is often referred to in MoCA's promotion of *shequ* building is Shenyang, Shanghai. The Organic Law of 1989 initially established Residential Committees to be 100-700 households. In Shenyang, the provision was increased to 1,000-1,500 households and renamed "*shequ* residents' committees." Activity centers were built close to the center of the *shequ* (as the old *danwei* was the focus of Maoist urban developments).

Since economic reform, the real estate market has gradually become one of the main contributors to economic growth and sources of local government revenue. Today, local governments hold auctions for land-use rights and developers buy the rights to use the land to develop the land into *xiaoqu*. Since the dissolution of the *danwei* system, the *xiaoqu* developments and subsequent "*shequ* construction program" have introduced a new social order to neighborhood planning. No longer tied to work, residences became a diverse collection of backgrounds. On the other hand, buying in to *xiaoqu* lifestyle required certain economic standing. Under the market-driven economy, the *xiaoqu* development has shown a great level of diversity in quality and amenities; rich urban dwellers can afford premium estates that offer world-class facilitties and management, but average *xiaoqu* may have shortsighted design and insufficient or poor services.

Even though the Ministry of Housing and Urban-Rural Development (MOHURD) and local authorities have detailed regulations and recommendations regarding residential development (Code

57 In the effort to reduce redundancy, many jobs were eliminated or consolidated. *Danwei* were supposed to provide service and support for up to three years. However, with fewer jobs and an influx of urban migration, *danwei* often could not meet the support demands. Bray 2005,178; Nguyen 2013, 216.

58 State Bureau of Technical Supervision and The Ministry of Housing Code of Urban Residential Areas Planning & Design Ver. 2002 (城市居住区规划设计规范, 2002年版)

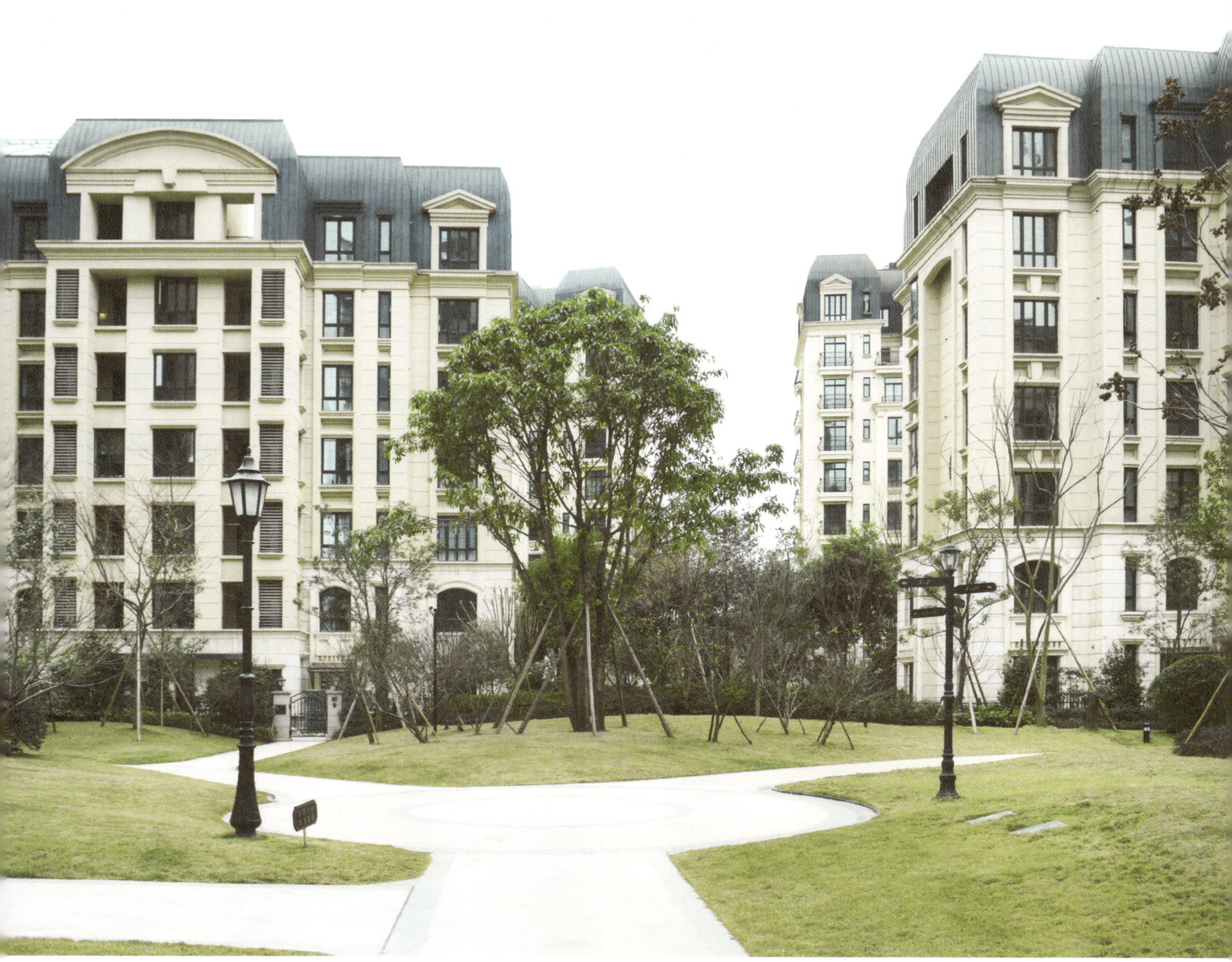

Figure 26 (Above) Interior of a *xiaoqu* development

of Urban Residential Areas Planning & Design),[58] many developers tend to fulfill the requirement quantitatively instead of qualitatively. The lack of consideration is especially evident in the design of open space and service arrangements within *xiaoqu* as most apartment buyers focus more on the unit quality, while services and amenities are not as profitable of an investment for developers. These auxiliary services are normally poorly managed after developers have sold all the units and employ cheap management teams. Minority residents such as the elderly, the disabled, and children normally suffer more in these processes as few design considerations highlight their extra needs.

In 2013, Beijing local authorities published the "Residential Exterior Design Guidelines,"[59] targeting building exteriors and the open spaces in residential neighborhoods. The MOHURD issued a special notice regarding accessibility improvements and elderly facilities in *xiaoqu* in 2014. Authorities have been targeting these issues from different levels and some reputable developers have accomplished quality neighborhoods that can be viewed as paradigms across the country.

There is, however, still a lag between the interests of developers under the market-driven economy and the necessary attributes in planning for healthy communities. What is needed most are ideas for the creation of spaces conducive to healthy lifestyles - whether it be the accommodation of diverse groups of people, the development of socially-connected communities, sufficient access to services and amenities, places for children to play, or families to interact. Designing for the qualitative aspects of life is a less specific process that may require a more nuanced approach than afforded by calculations of the return on investment, the percentage of open space, or the size of individual rooms. This is particularly pertinent in light of the consideration that social and individual well-being is likely to be effected by the design and quality of the city blocks in which one lives.

59 Beijing, Residential Exterior Design Guidelines, (http://www.mohurd.gov.cn/dfxx/201308/t20130823_214822.html).

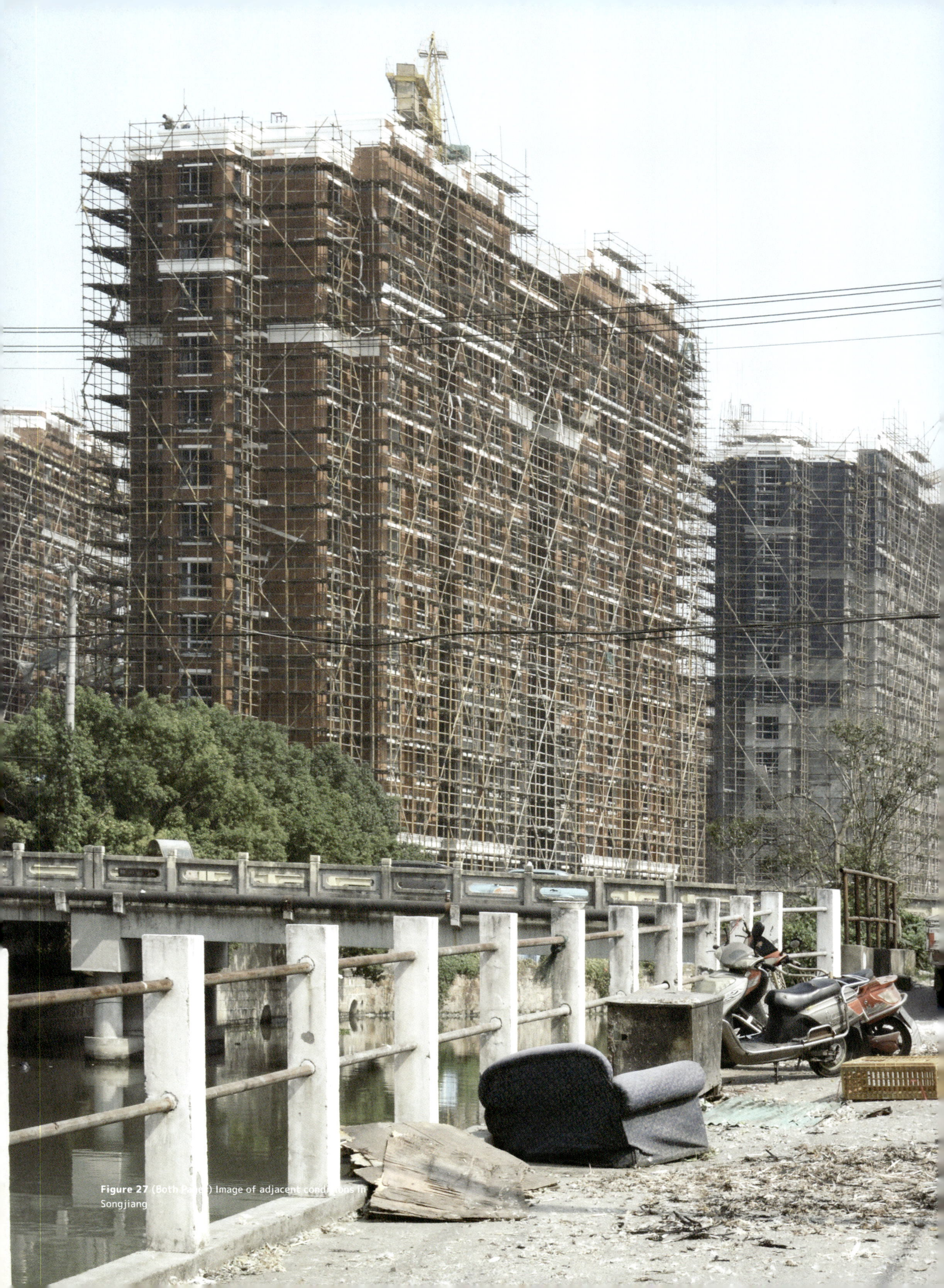

Figure 27 (Both Pages) Image of adjacent conditions in Songjiang

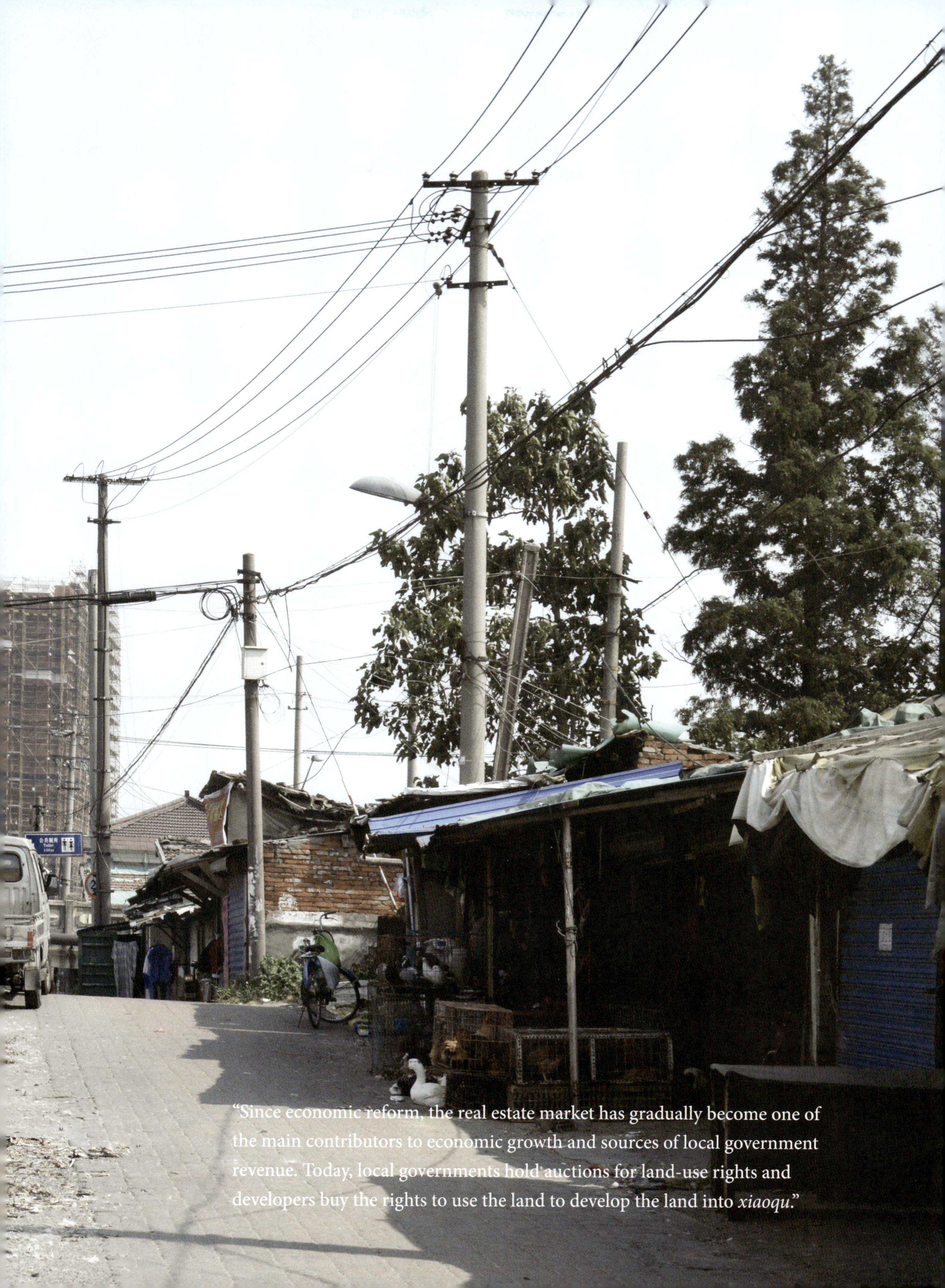

"Since economic reform, the real estate market has gradually become one of the main contributors to economic growth and sources of local government revenue. Today, local governments hold auctions for land-use rights and developers buy the rights to use the land to develop the land into *xiaoqu*."

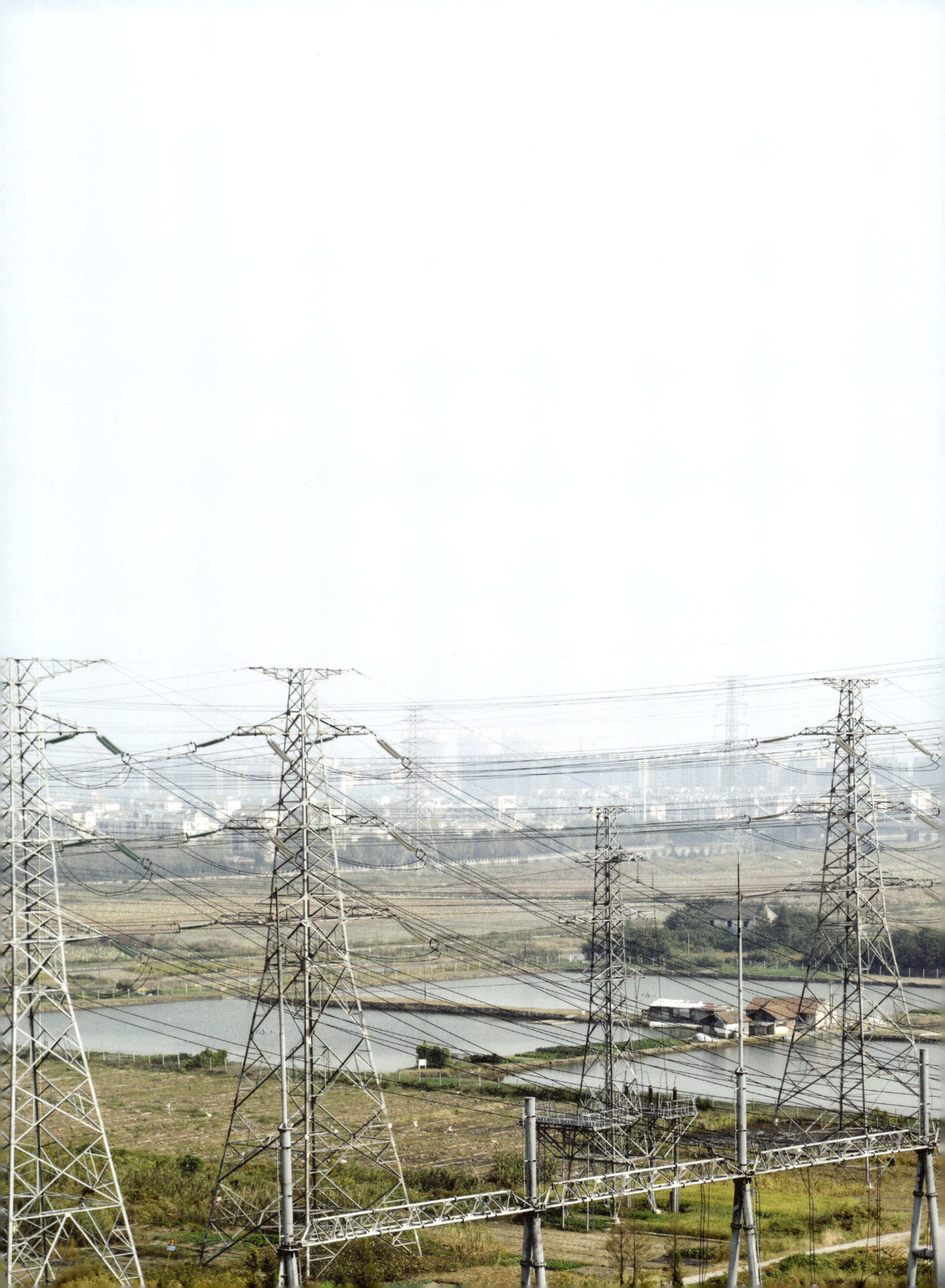

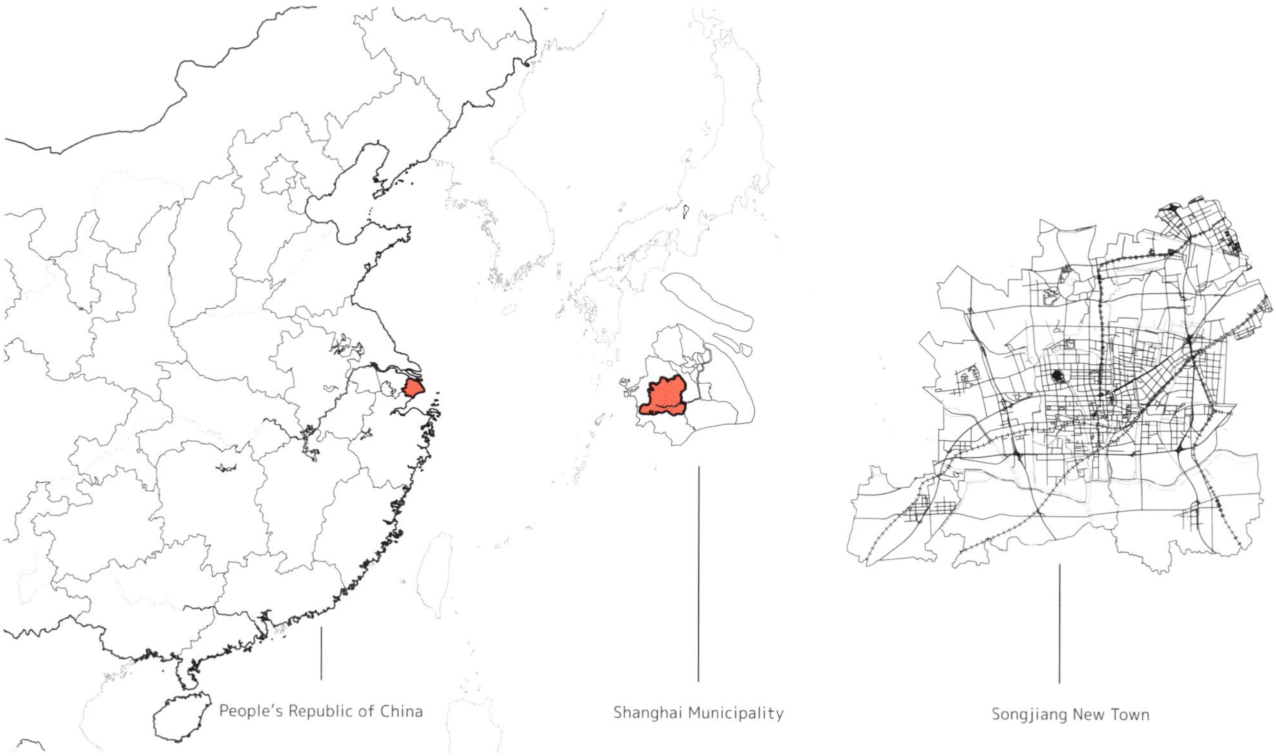

Figure 28 (Opposite Page) Patchwork of urban concitions in Songjiang.

Figure 29 (Above) Geographic diagram of Shanghai and Songjiang.

Songjiang New Town

Adopting the 1-9-6-6 model (one central city, nine new cities, 60 new towns and 600 central villages), Shanghai's 1999 "One City, Nine Towns Development Plan" and its tenth five year plan (2001-2005) contributed to the rapid development of a number of satellite locations in the city's rapidly urbanizing outskirts. Songjiang New City, one of nine towns pegged for conversion into a satellite city for Shanghai underwent a dramatic transformation in this period. Its role as a means to alleviate pressure on the main Shanghai city center was reflected in its conceptualization not as a dormitory town but as a city center able to sustain itself both socially and economically. It also reflected an ambition for projected lifestyles that manifested itself in the transplantation of various development and neighborhood types that would borrow and adapt from numerous global sources, with the sprawling Thames Town (a one-square-kilometer residential development replicating English towns) being among the most visible exemplars. Part of this wider ambition, Songjiang University Town was also initiated to operate as the largest tertiary education hub in the country, offering Songjiang a clear role within this constellation of new towns and cities.

As part of the Health and Places Initiative research group at the GSD, the studio engaged with Songjiang New City as a means to speculate on the construction of urban environments that respond to the projected and emerging lifestyles that are anticipated for Songjiang's citizens. While being informed by broader scales, the studio was invested in the systematic definition of urban environments at the smaller scale, focusing on the development of neighborhood models restrained to the scale of the typical Songjiang superblock. Through a focused study and investment at the neighborhood scale, the studio generated proposals that offer urban models and prototypes with the potential to operate as tools for restructuring the wider urban development patterns practiced within a number of Chinese contexts. Projects developed in the studio strategized the ways in which architecture, landscape, and urban design elements may be arranged to enable and express various projected and emerging lifestyle and health-related concerns, such as quality of life, the impact of chronic diseases, and the rapid "graying" of Shanghai's citizens.

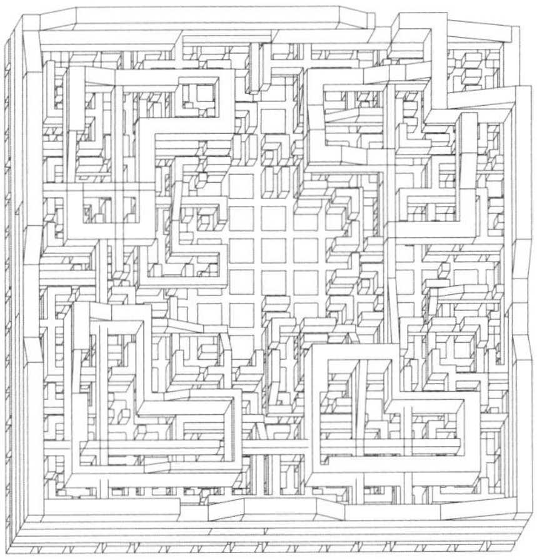
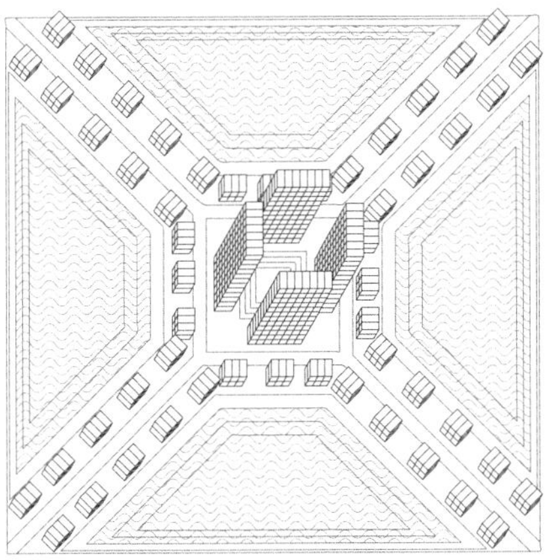
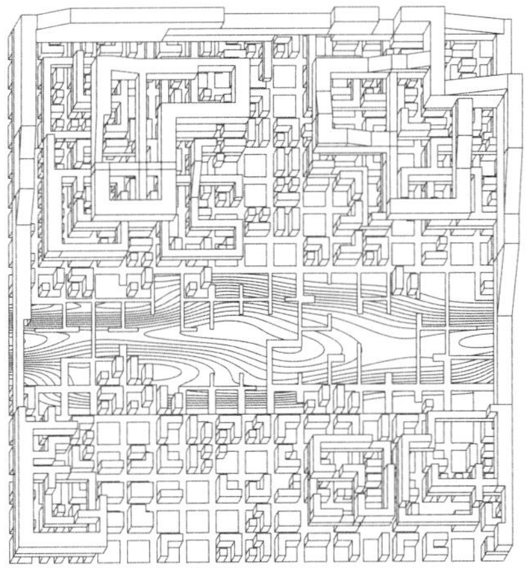
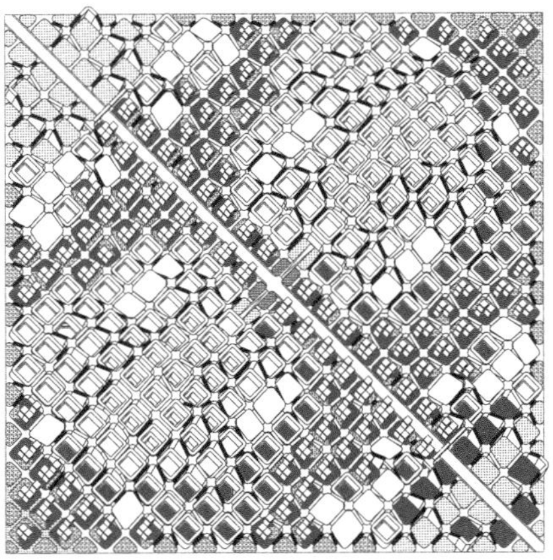
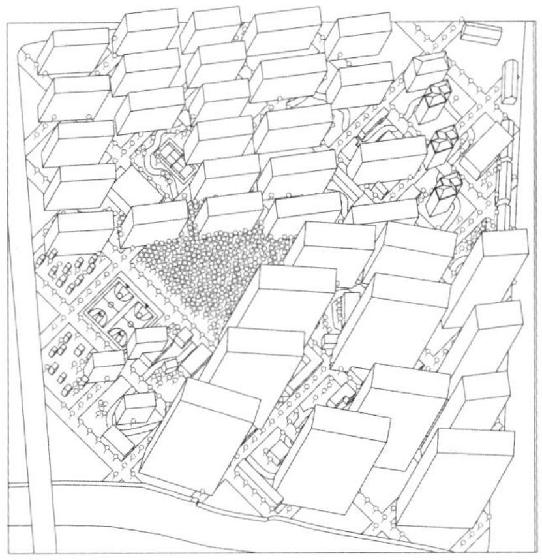
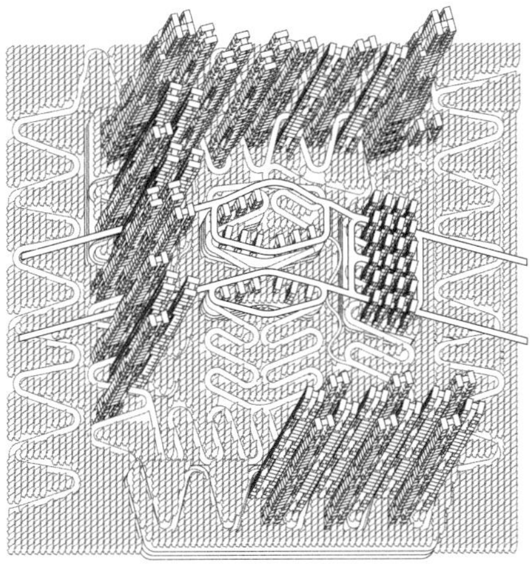
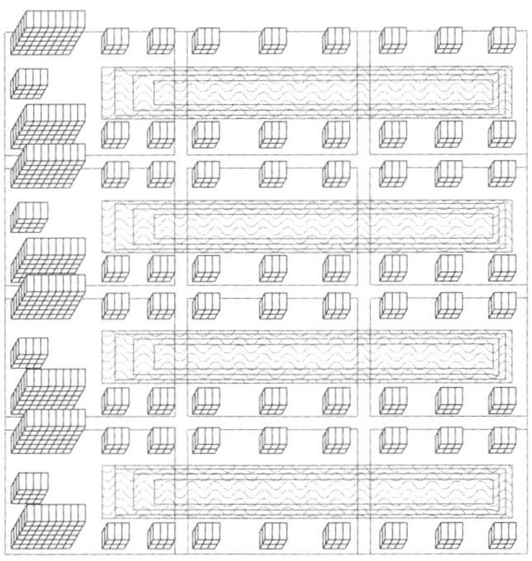
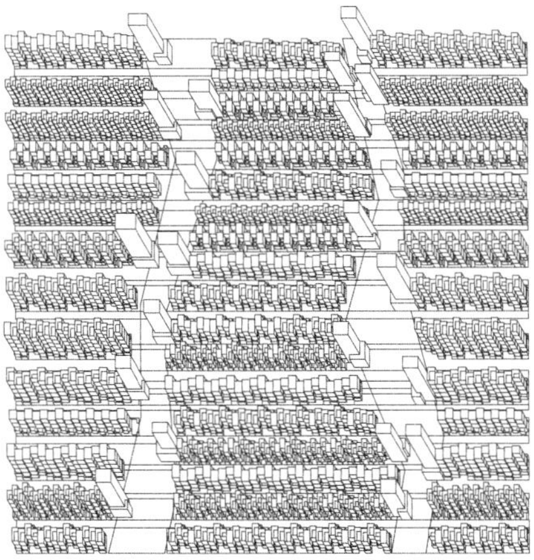
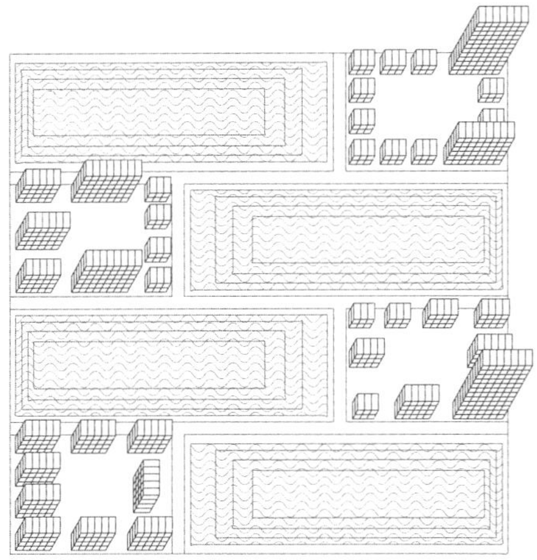
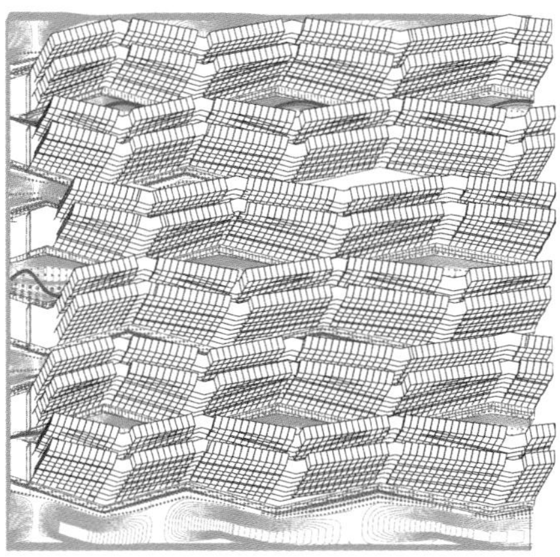
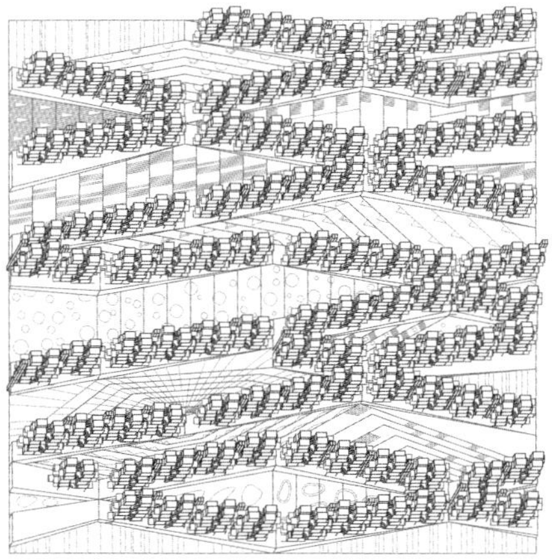
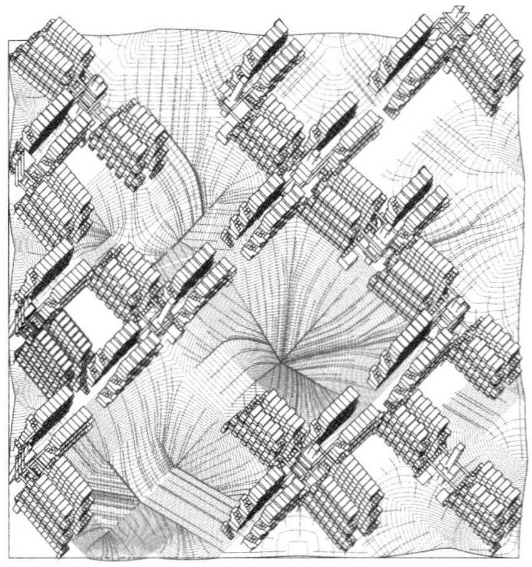

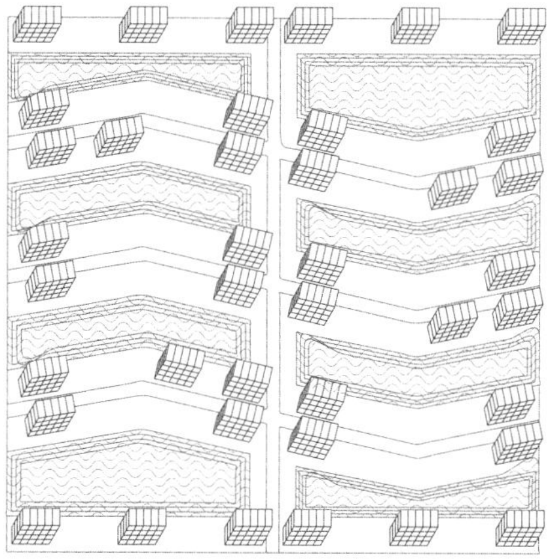
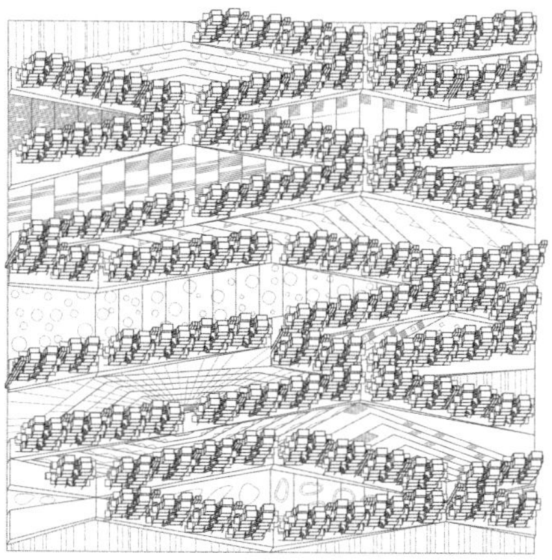
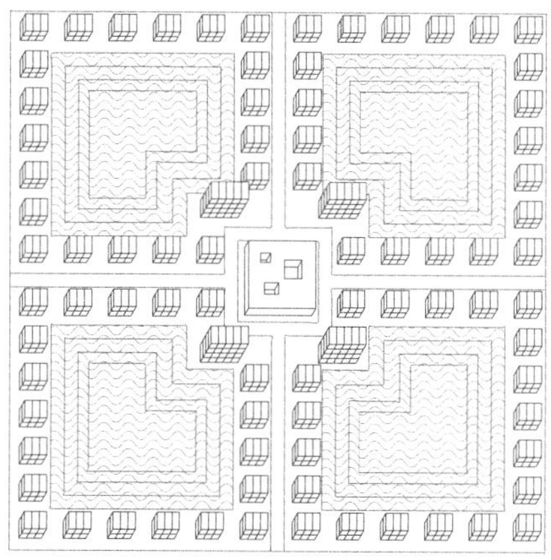
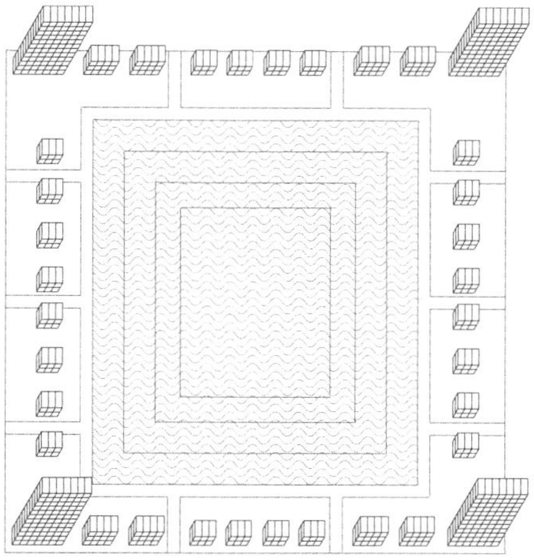
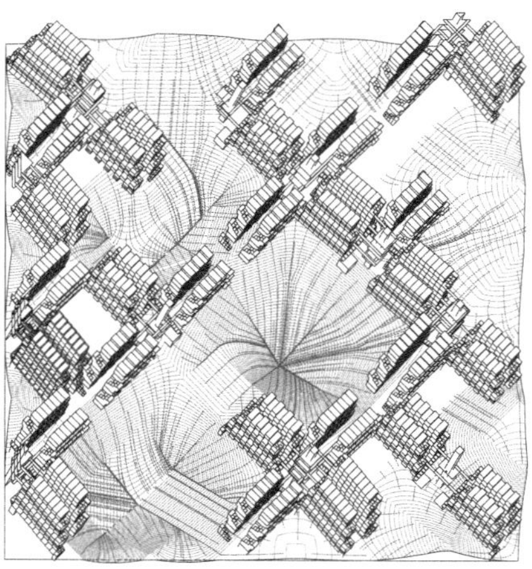
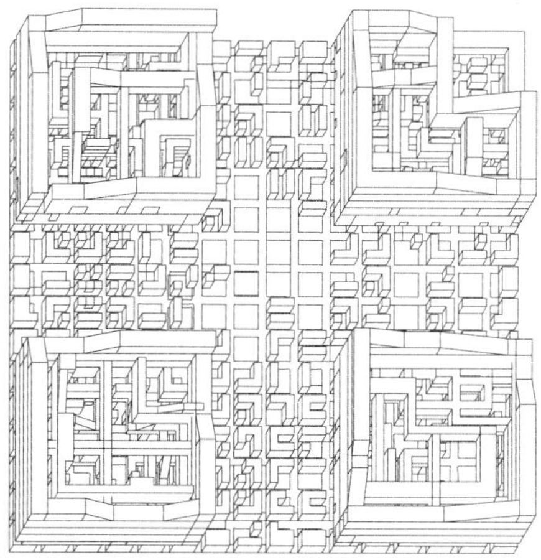
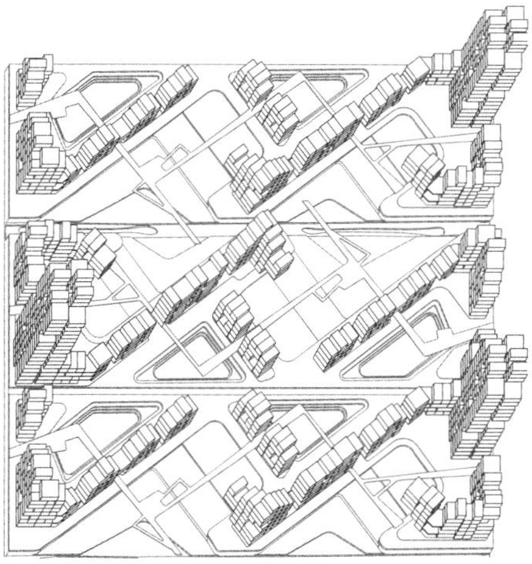
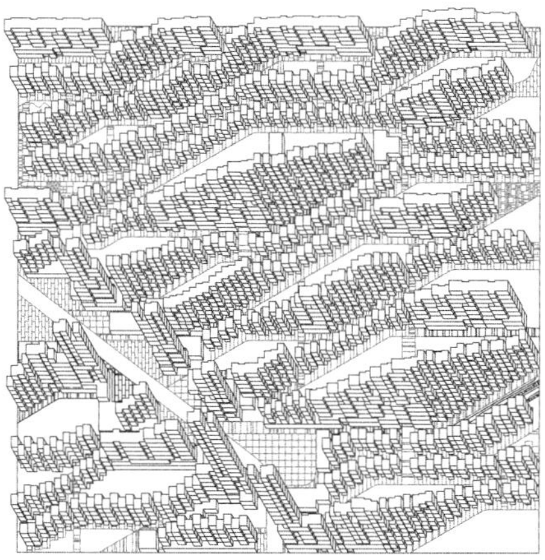
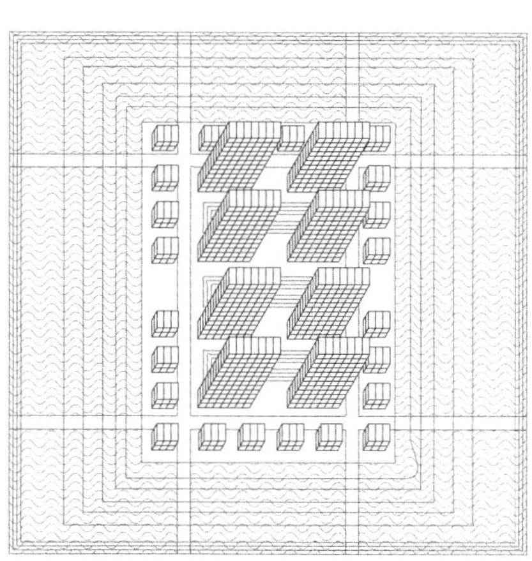
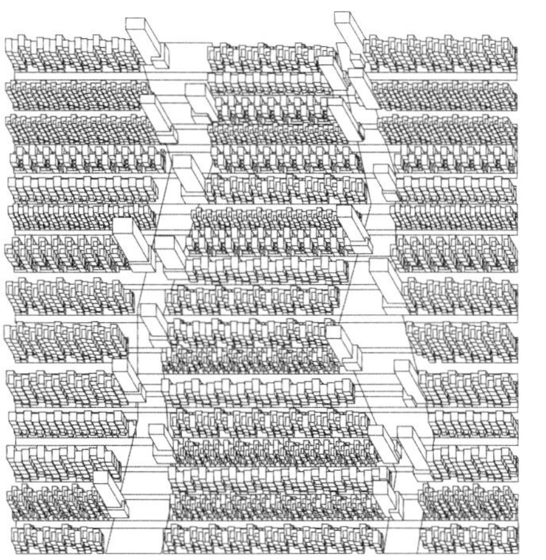
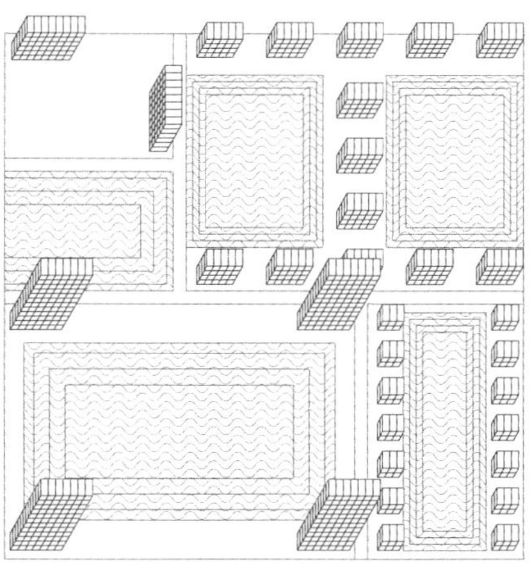
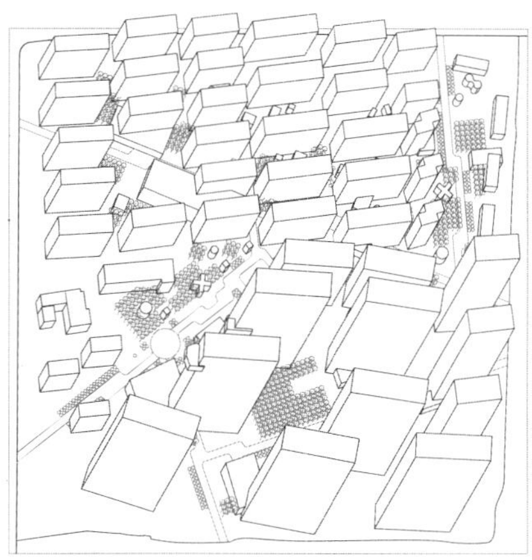

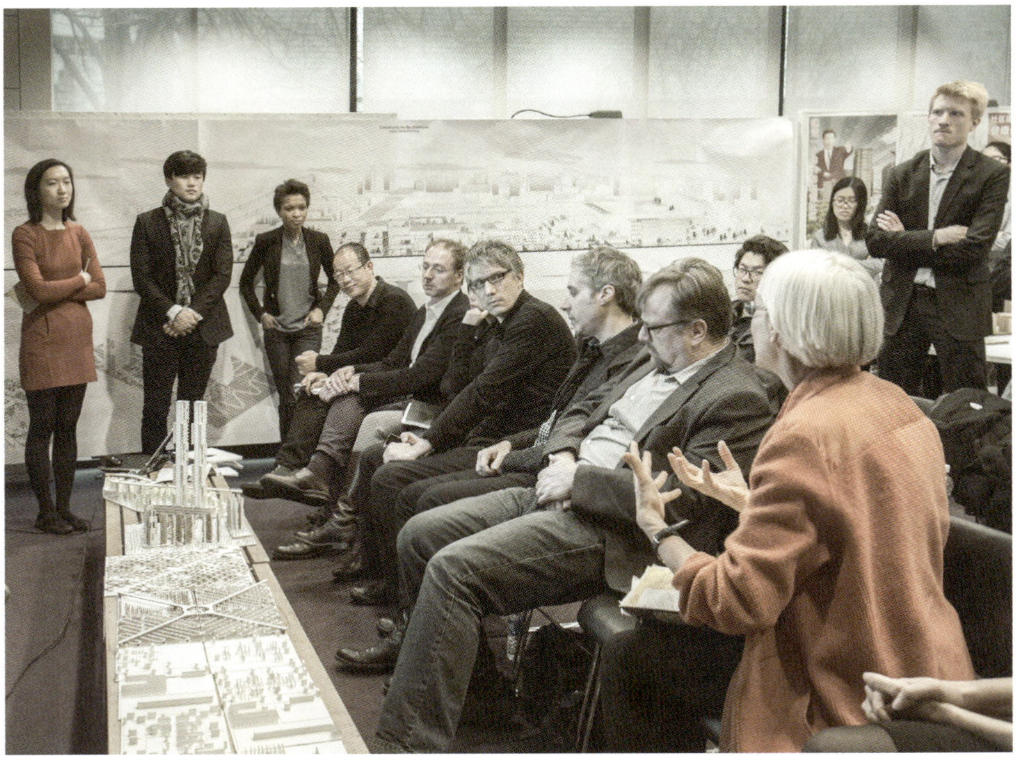

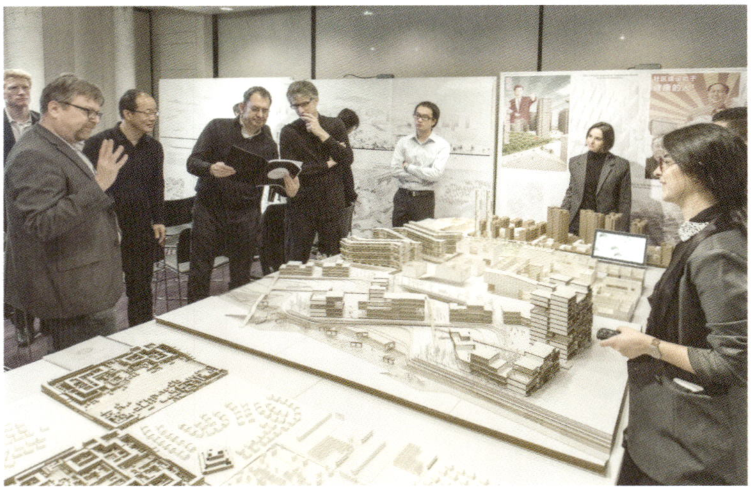

Figure 30 (Previous Page) Studio block prototypes

Figure 31, 32 (Left, Bottom) Photographs of studio final review

Figure Credits

All images are created by Life-Styled China Town Studio unless otherwise noted.

Figure 1, 31, 32, Harvard Graduate School of Design 2014, *Studio Review*, photographs. In possession of: Harvard Graduate School of Design.

Figure 2, *Honto-Jin Chen Family*, 1930, photograph. Public Domain. https://commons.wikimedia.org/wiki/File:Honto-Jin_Chen_Family_circa_1930.JPG.

Figure 3, Huang Entao, 1972, *Red loudspeakers are sounding through every home*, poster, Beijing renmin meishu chubanshe.

Figure 4, *Dazhai*, early 1970s, IISH Landsberger collection. Shanghai renmin chubanshe.

Figure 6, Song Wenzhi, 1975, *On the banks of the Yangzi river, Daqing blooms*, IISH Landsberger collection. Jiangsu renmin chubanshe.

Figure 10, 11, Mah, David, 2014, *Shanghai Lilong*, photographs. In possession of: Author, David Mah

Figure 12, Images from Google Map interface. Map data: Google, DigitalGlobe

Figure 15, Angelard, Caroline, 2011, *Hutong Beijing - Ruelle Pékin*, photograph. Accessed 11 January 2016, https://www.flickr.com/photos/caro_angelard/6059423022/. Creative Commons Attribution 2.0 Generic license; Desaturated.

Figure 19, Kollar, Justin, 2014, *Shanghai Lilong*, photograph. In possession of: Author, Justin Kollar.

Figure 26, Kollar, Justin, 2014, *Interior of Xiaoqu development*, photograph. In possession of: Author, Justin Kollar.

Figure 27, 28, Kollar, Justin, 2014, *Songjiang*, photographs. In possession of: Author, Justin Kollar.

References

Bedeski, Robert E 1981, 'State-Building in Modern China: The Kuomintang in the Prewar Period', *China Research Monograph*, no. 18, Center for Chinese Studies, Berkeley: University of California.

Bjorklund E. M. 1986 January, 'The Danwei: Socio-Spatial Characteristics of Work Units in China's Urban Society', *Economic Geography*, vol.62, no. 1, pp.19-29. Accessed 18 August 2015, http://www.jstor.org/stable/143493.

Branigan, Tania 2014, 'China reforms hukou system to improve migrant workers' rights,' *The Guardian* 31 July. Accessed 18 August 2015, http://www.theguardian.com/world/2014/jul/31/china-reform-hukou-migrant-workers.

Bray, David 2005, *Social Space and Governance in Urban China: The Danwei System from Origins to Urban Reform*, Stanford University Press, Stanford

———2006, 'Building "Community": New Strategies of Governance in Urban China' in *Economy and Society*, vol. 35, no. 4, pp. 530-549.

Chan, Cecilia L. W. 1993, *The Myth of Neighborhood Help: The Contemporary Chinese Community-Based Welfare System in Guangzhou*, Hong Kong University Press, Hong Kong.

Chan Kam Wing & Buckingham, Will 2008, 'Is China Abolishing the hukou System?' *The China Quarterly*, no. 195, pp. 582-606.

Chang Liu 2008, 'Policy sprawl: the internal logic of spatial production', *The Chinese Dream: a Society Under Construction*, eds Neville Mars and Adrian Hornsby, 010 Publishers, Amsterdam, pp. 286-327.

Chen, W. P. 2007, 'The New Culture Movement in China' in *East Asian History*, no. 34, December 2007, Institute of Advanced Studies Australian National University.

Chesnes, Dora 2008, 'Family Structure' in *In the Chinese City: Perspectives on the Transmutations of an Empire*, ed Edelmann, Frederic, pp. 222-233.

Glosser, Susan L. 2003, *Chinese Visions of Family and State, 1915-1953*, University of California Press.

Harris, Lane J. 2013, 'From Democracy to Bureaucracy: the Baojia in Nationalist Thought and Practice, 1927-1949' in *History China*, vol. 8 no. 4, pp. 517-557.

Johnson, Kay A. 1983, *Women, the Family, and Peasant Revolution in China*, University of Chicago Press, Chicago.

Kahler, Christine 2015 'China's Healthcare Reform: How Far Has it Come?', *China Business Review*. Accessed 18 August 2015, http://www.chinabusinessreview.com/chinas-healthcare-reform-how-far-has-it-come/.

Kojima, Kazuko & Kokubun, Ryosei 2002, 'The Shequ Construction Programme and the Chinese Communist Party', *Copenhagen Journal of Asian Studies*, vol. 16, pp. 86-105

Lee Liming & Lv Jun 2009, 'Public Health in China: History and Contemporary Challenges', *Global Public Health: A new Era*, eds Robert Beaglehole and Ruth Bonita, Oxford Scholarship Online. Accessed 18 August 2015, http://www.oxfordscholarship.com/view/10.1093/acprof:oso/9780199236626.001.0001/acprof-9780199236626-chapter-9.

Levinovitz, Alan 2013, *Chairman Mao Invented Traditional Chinese Medicine*. Accessed 18 August 2015, http://www.slate.com/articles/health_and_science/medical_examiner/2013/10/traditional_chinese_medicine_origins_mao_invented_it_but_didn_t_believe.2.html.

Meng Qingyue, Shi Guang, Yang Hongwei, Gonzalez-Block, Miguel & Blas, Erik 2004, Health Policy and Systems Research in China, Special for Research and Training in Tropical Diseases. Accessed 18 August 2015, http://www.who.int/tdr/publications/documents/health-research-china.pdf.

Ministry of Civil Affairs 2000, *Opinions on Advancing Urban Community Construction* [关于在全国推进城市社区建设的意见] People's Republic of China Ministry of Civil Affairs. http://www.reformdata.org/.

Ministry of Environmental Protection 2014, *Environmental Statistical Yearbook for 2013* [2013年环境统计年报] Accessed 11 November 2014, http://www.mep.gov.cn/zwgk/hjtj/.

Wang L, Meng Q & Bian Y 2001, 'Reform of taxation and fee system in rural areas', *Health Economics Research*, 3:3-5.

Wang, Fei-Ling 2010, 'Renovating the Great Floodgate: The Reform of China's Hukou System' in *One Country, Two Societies: Rural-Urban Inequality in Contemporary China*, ed Martin King Whyte, Harvard University Press, pp. 335-364.

Wang Jianxun 2006, 'Village Governance in Chinese History' in *Political Economy of Village Governance in Contemporary China*, Dissertation Indiana University.

Xiao Linlin, Yang Xiaohuan, Cai Hongyan & Zhang Dingxiang 2015, 'Cultivated Land Changes and Agricultural Potential Productivity in Mainland China', *Sustainability*, vol. 7. http://www.mdpi.com/2071-1050/7/9/11893/pdf.

Xinhua 2015, 'Plan to promote traditional Chinese medicine unveiled', *ChinaDaily* 7 May. Accessed 18 August 2015, http://www.chinadailyasia.com/nation/2015-05/07/content_15260970.html.

Zhang, Donia 2013, *Courtyard Housing and Cultural Sustainability: Theory, Practice, and Product*, MPG Books Group, London.

Zhang Yi 2009, 'The Systematization of Danwei and Family' in *Urban China: Work in Progress*, pp. 94-95.

Life-Styled: China-Town

Studio

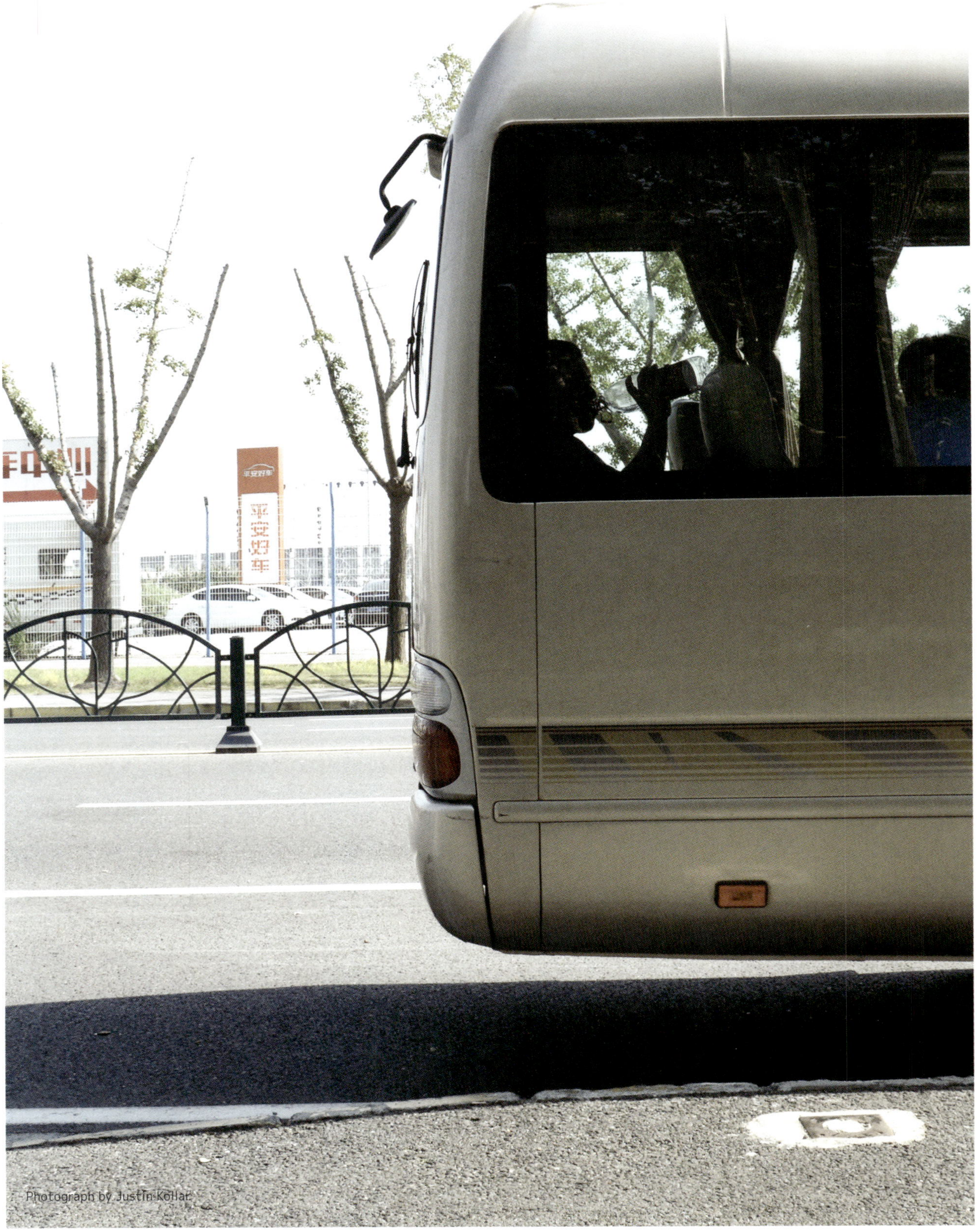

Photograph by Justin Kollar

The Glorious Manual for Community Health

Ali Karimi + Justin Kollar

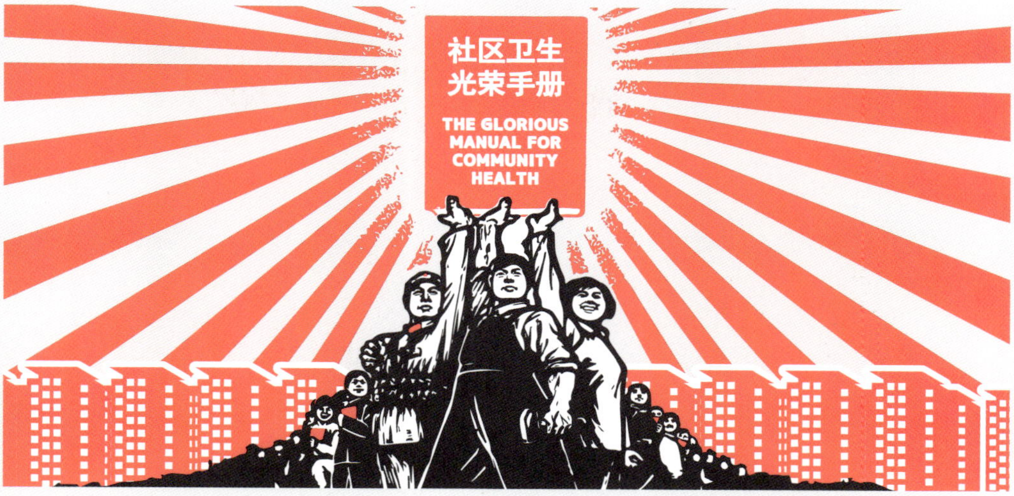

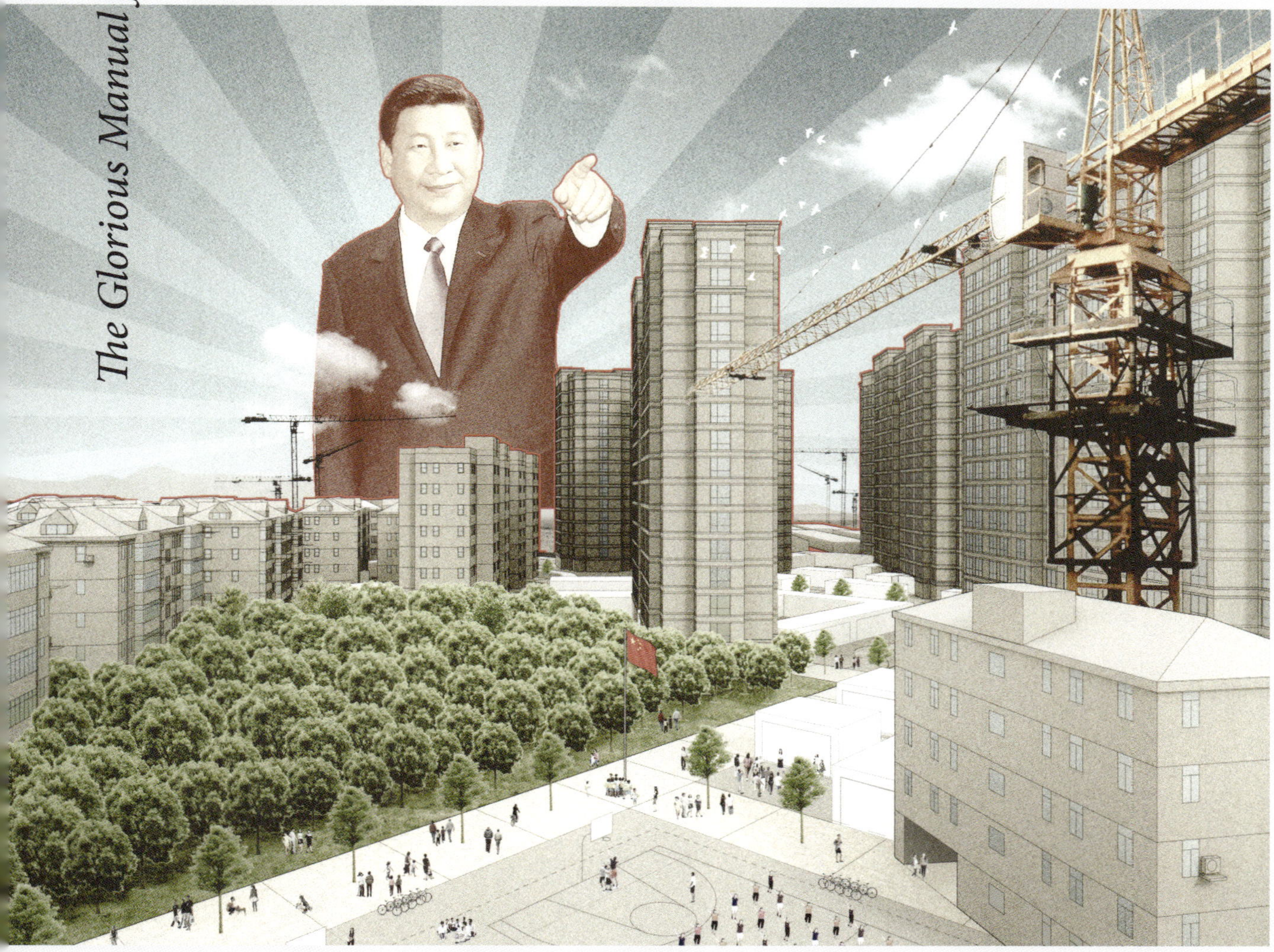

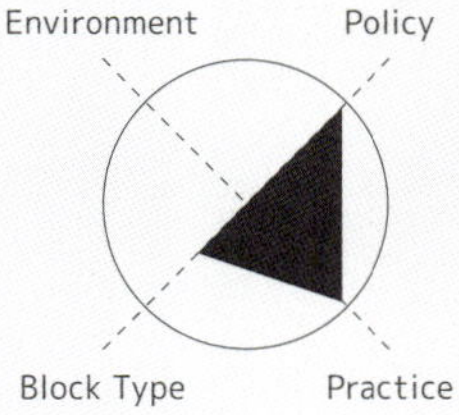

Looking through the lens of healthcare and health management, it is obvious that current urban conditions are unfit. This is due to the creation of an administration system designed to address a different order of life (*danwei* + residents' committees). The provision of services is typically an afterthought since the proliferation of the market-driven superblock development.

Using the community health center together with its associated programs and administrative functions as a vehicle for reviving the *xiaoqu*, we can also address the larger urban and lifestyle problems of Songjiang. By blending civic services into the fabric of the block, and providing support for its position, we can find an intermediate scale of urban life situated between the superblock and neighborhood, and provide a framework for a new administrative system (*shequ*/community) and for property negotiations.

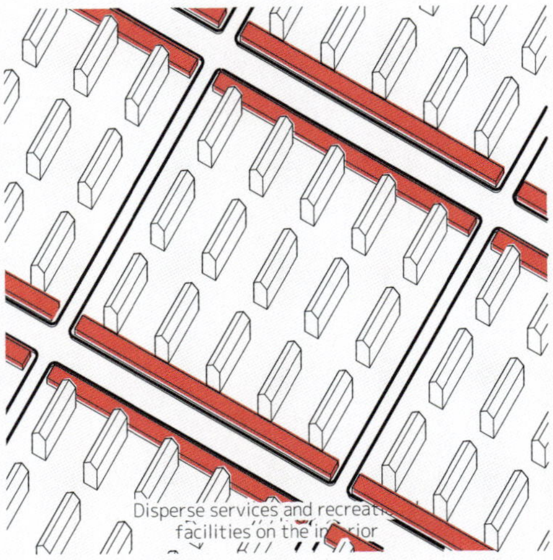

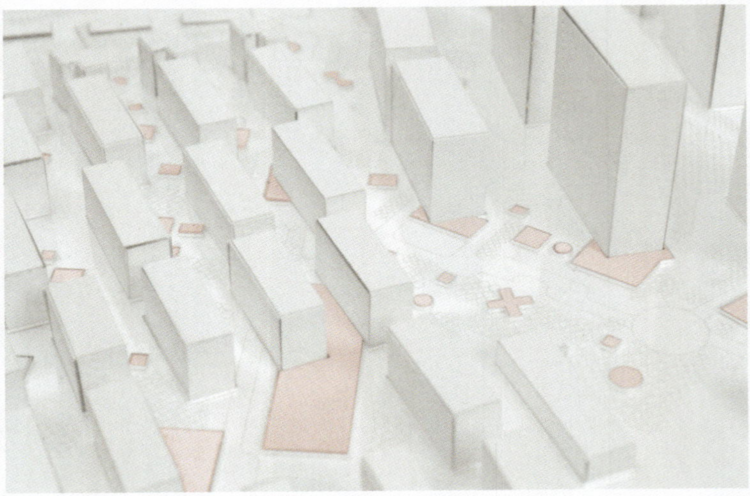

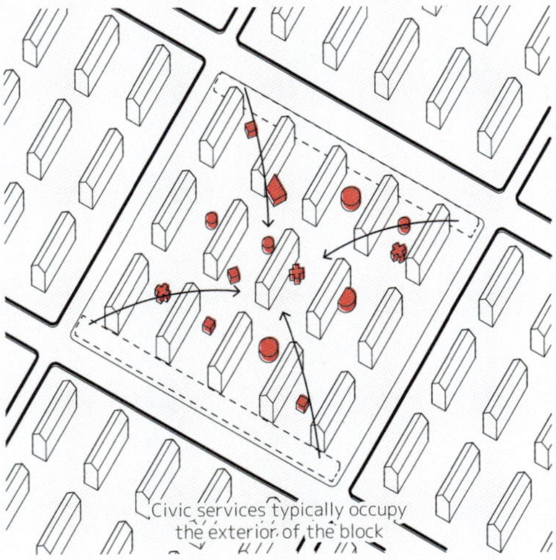

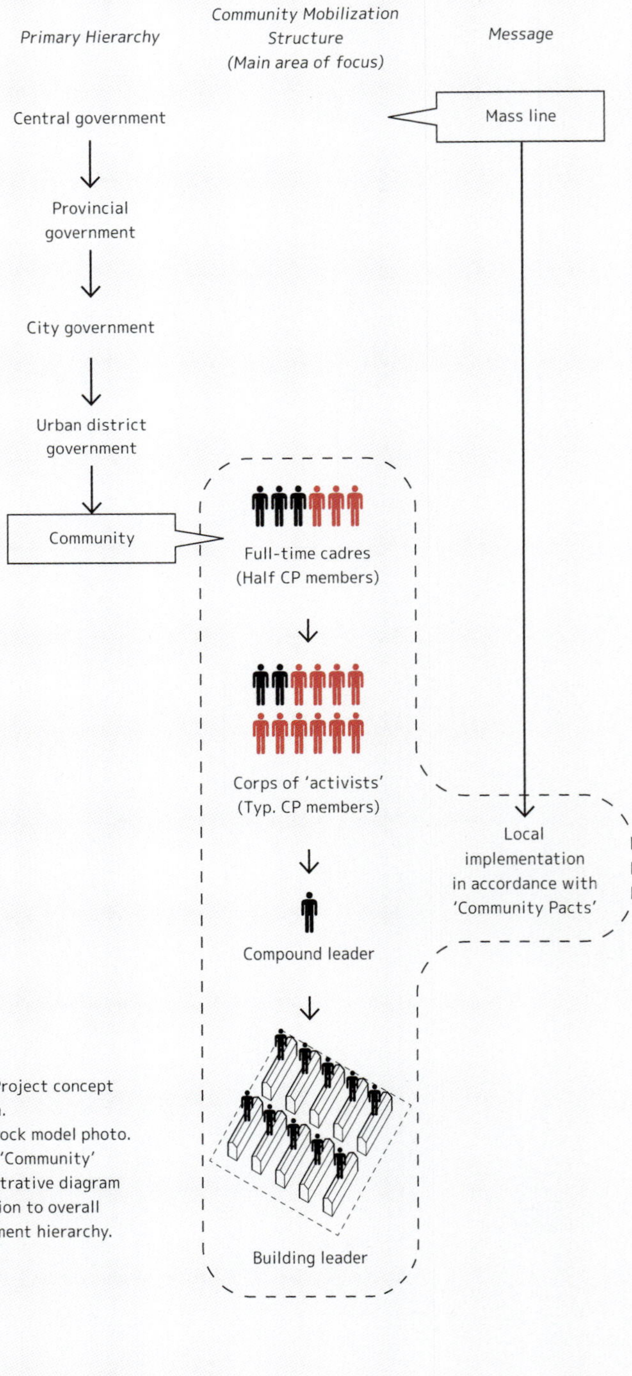

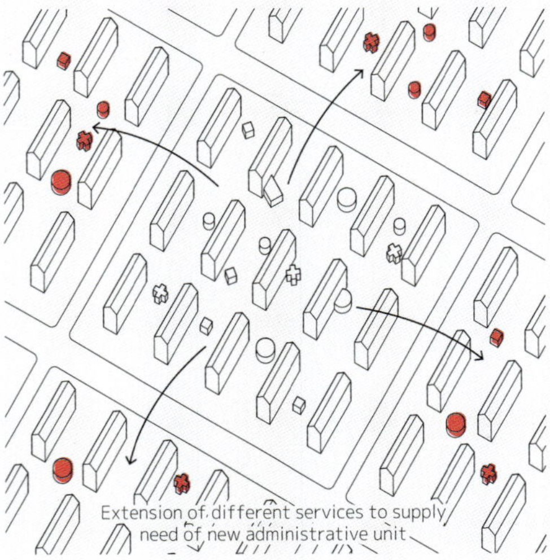

The method of aggregation would grow to fill out other portions of the community, crossing borders of the *xiaoqu* development in order to consolidate and link the larger community. The proposed method of service distribution would become a model for 'community building' in an effort to tie many (dispersed) neighborhoods together in a more effectual administrative framework (left).

(Left) Project concept diagram.
(Top) Block model photo.
(Right) 'Community' administrative diagram in relation to overall government hierarchy.

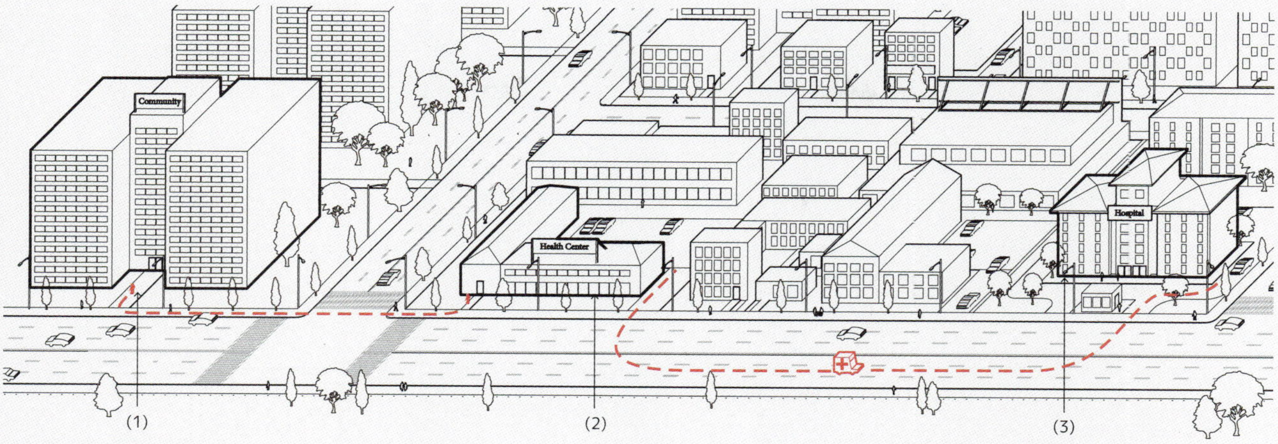

Ideal Healthcare Referral System

(1) from Local Community
If the local community block does not already have adequate health services, the local Community Health Center is located within ten minutes from every community.

(2) to Community Health Center
To deal with the local patient load adequately, the Community Health Center is the primary care unit. If specialty care is needed, the Health Center will give a referral to the resident to go to a city, county, or specialty hospital.

(3) to City or County Hospital
The large hospital units provide specialty or intensive care to those who need it, while chronic and less problematic issues are dealt with at the local level in a Community Health Center.

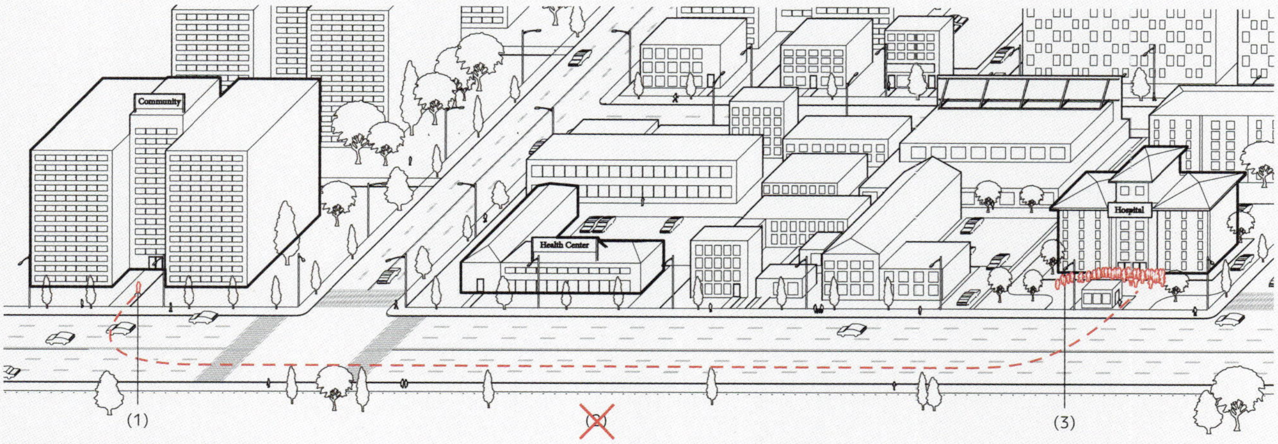

Actual Healthcare Referral System

(1) from Local Community
Instead of visiting the primary care in the local Community Health Center, residents prefer to make appointments at well-known or high-status hospitals in the region...

(2) not to Community Health Center
The local Community Health Center is usually not visited or it is bypassed as residents prefer to go to a hospital with a higher status, disrupting the referral system.

(3) to City or County Hospital
As many residents vie for an appointment, resources may be wasted and time and equipment spent on issues that may be dealt with at local Health Centers.

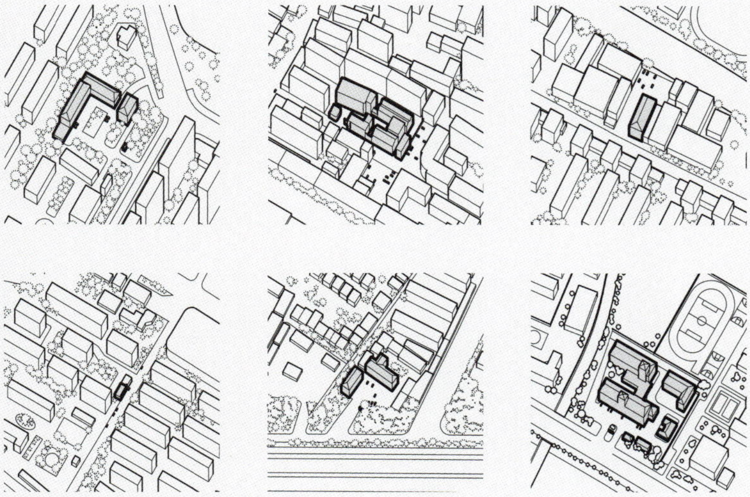

(Above) A diagram to explain the general tendencies of the healthcare referral system.

(Left) A preliminary study of various health centers and stations as they are aggregated in Songjiang. The study analyzed the positions and accessibility of the centers.

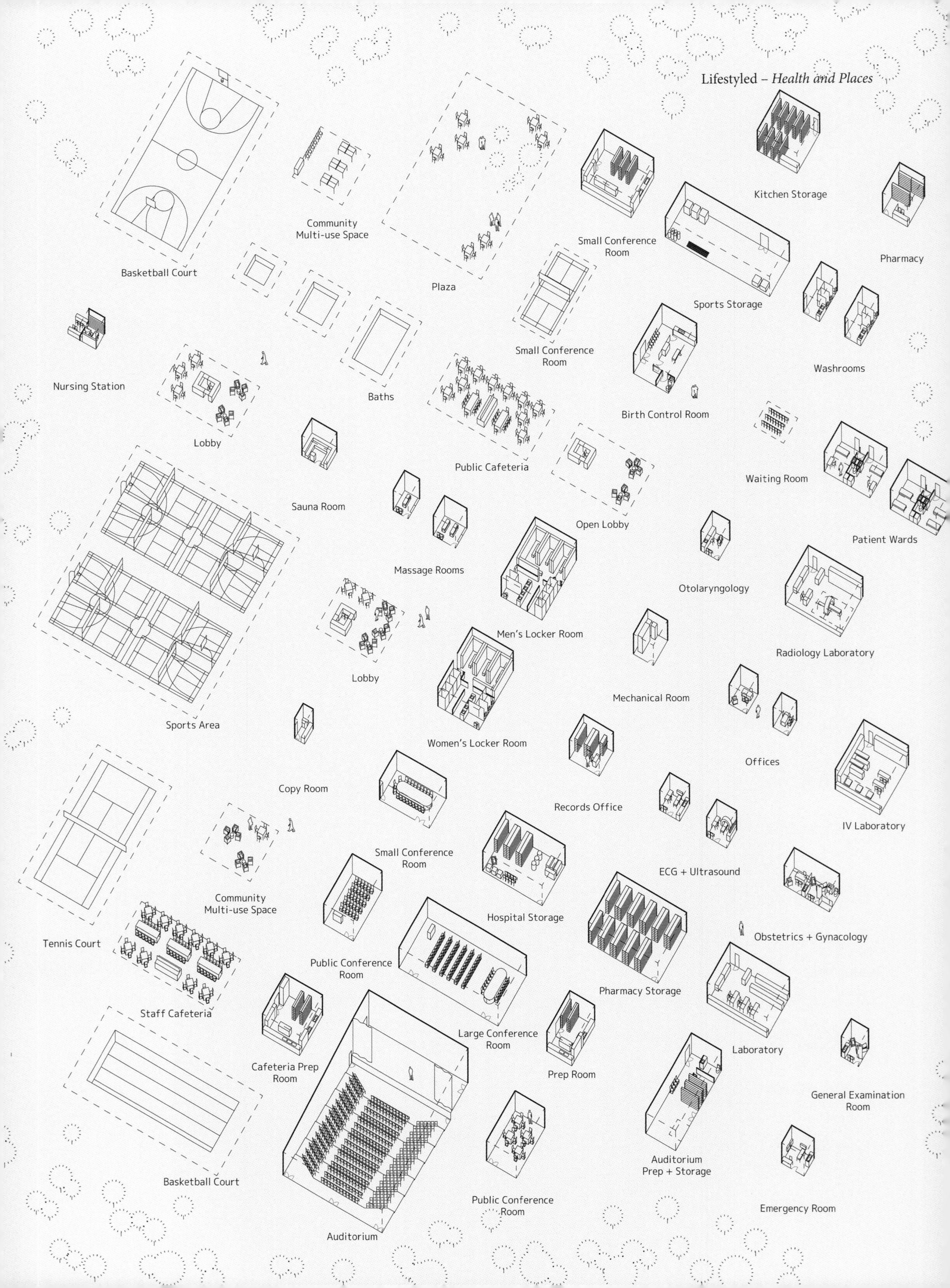
Lifestyled – *Health and Places*
Basketball Court
Community Multi-use Space
Plaza
Small Conference Room
Kitchen Storage
Pharmacy
Sports Storage
Small Conference Room
Washrooms
Nursing Station
Lobby
Baths
Birth Control Room
Public Cafeteria
Waiting Room
Sauna Room
Open Lobby
Patient Wards
Massage Rooms
Otolaryngology
Men's Locker Room
Radiology Laboratory
Lobby
Mechanical Room
Sports Area
Women's Locker Room
Offices
Copy Room
Records Office
IV Laboratory
Small Conference Room
ECG + Ultrasound
Community Multi-use Space
Hospital Storage
Obstetrics + Gynacology
Tennis Court
Public Conference Room
Pharmacy Storage
Staff Cafeteria
Large Conference Room
Laboratory
Cafeteria Prep Room
Prep Room
General Examination Room
Auditorium Prep + Storage
Basketball Court
Public Conference Room
Emergency Room
Auditorium

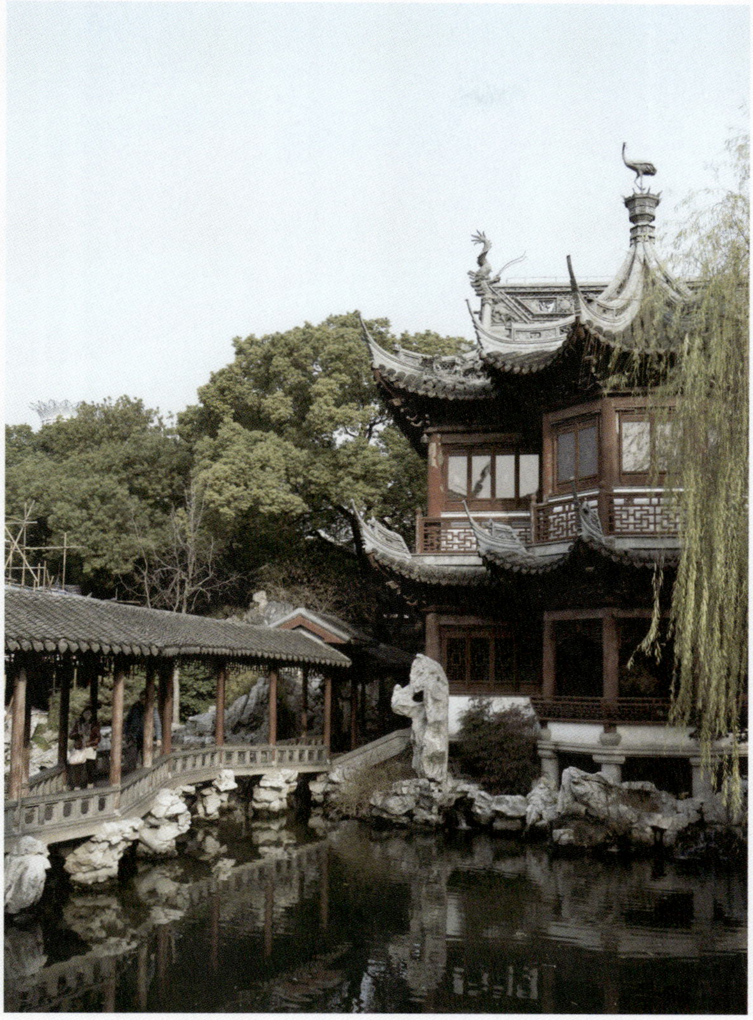

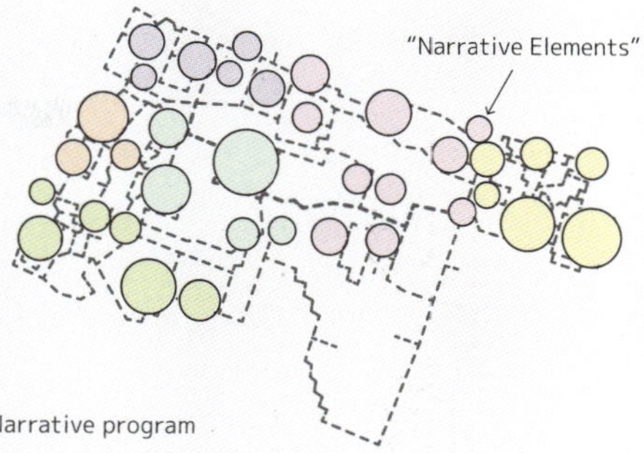

Narrative program

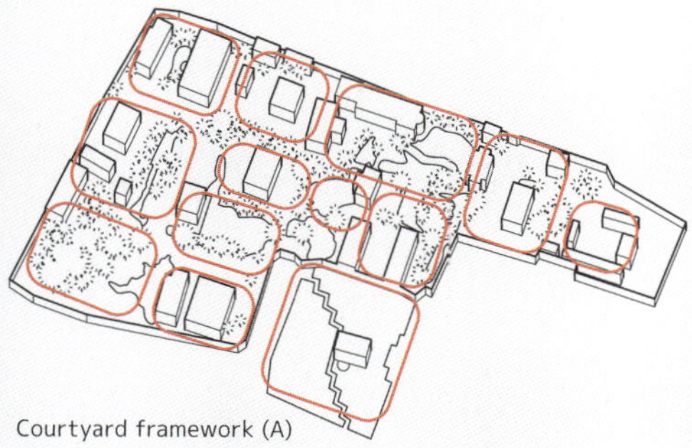

Courtyard framework (A)

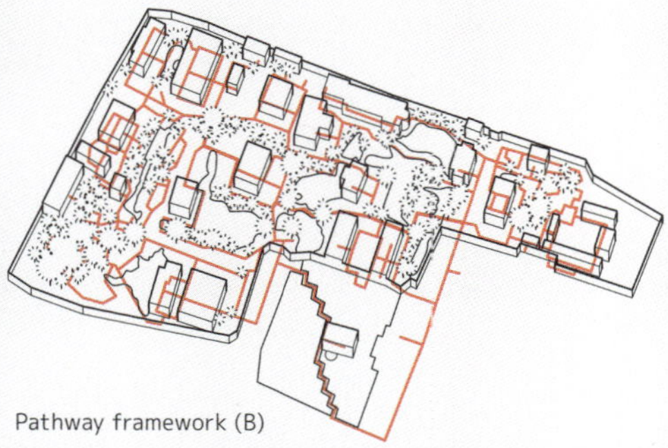

Pathway framework (B)

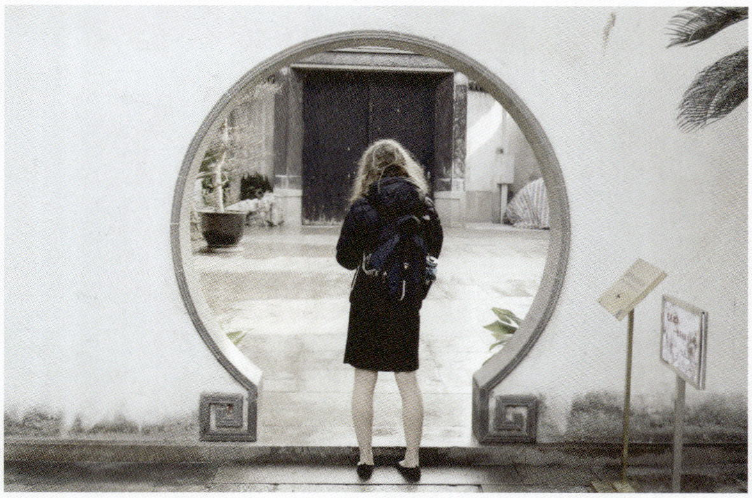

"Whoever knows how to design a park well will have no difficulty in tracing the plan for the building of a city according to its given area and situation. There must be regularity and fantasy, relationships and oppositions, and casual, unexpected elements that vary the scene; great order in the details, confusion, uproar, and tumult in the whole."

Marc Antoine Laugier 1765, Observations sur l'Architecture, Saillant, La Haye et Paris.

The Chinese garden serves as an abstract framework from which to compose the program within the block. Using a loose framework, the Chinese garden may compose a network of spaces that can serve various functions—connected, but discreet; reorganized, but flexible.

(Top Left) Yuyuan garden, Shanghai.
(Right) Yuyuan garden spatial framework diagram.

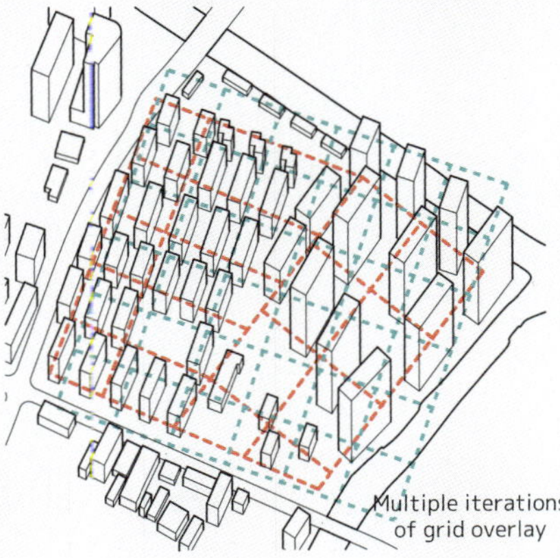

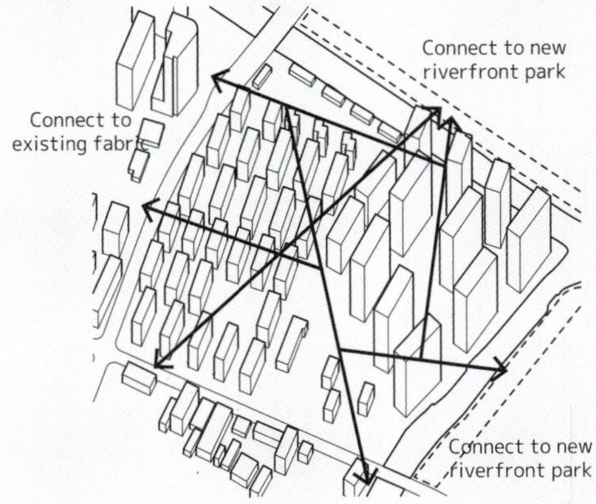

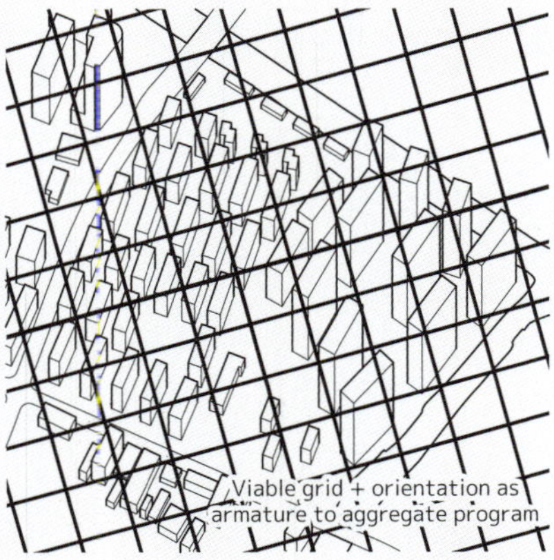

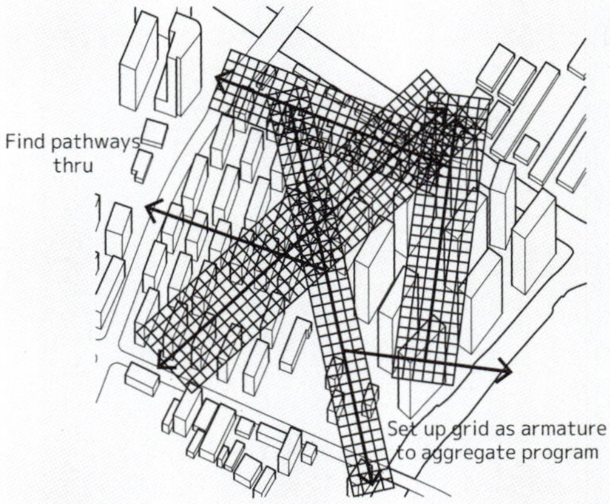

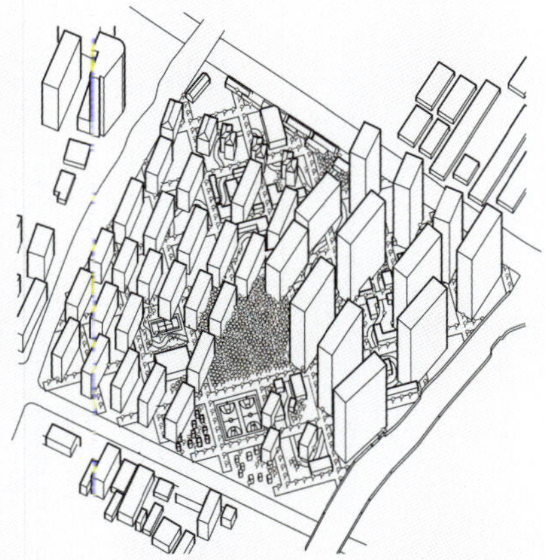

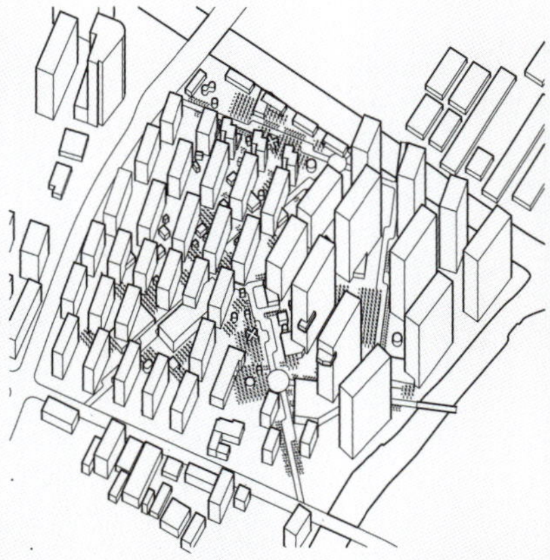

A Courtyard Scheme

This method is an application of a grid which begins to embed a new landscape of healthcare in the neighborhood. It provides a scale that is between the urban and the communal. By applying the Cartesian grid in this instance, we allow for the idiosyncrasies of the collisions, skewed alignments, and subdivisions of space that we can see in more organic contexts, while also denoting an order larger than the neighborhood itself.

B Pathway Scheme

By using the line as the primary armature from which to organize the path and program, the arrangement privileges the movement through the *xiaoqu*. Elements are directly connected and are locally articulated in response to the context. This method encourages flow and connection between each particular area. While the areas remain connected, using a secondary armature, a grid grouping similar programs can be articulated and separated.

(1) At certain instances, a program may intersect with an existing residential building. (2) The program will repurpose and take over the floor it is connected to to reappropriate existing elements. (3) The added program will allow for the existing structure to function properly. (4) Given the aggregation of other elements (trees, plantings, paths) the new interface activates the adjacent space with the program—resulting in a "courtyard"-like resulting space.

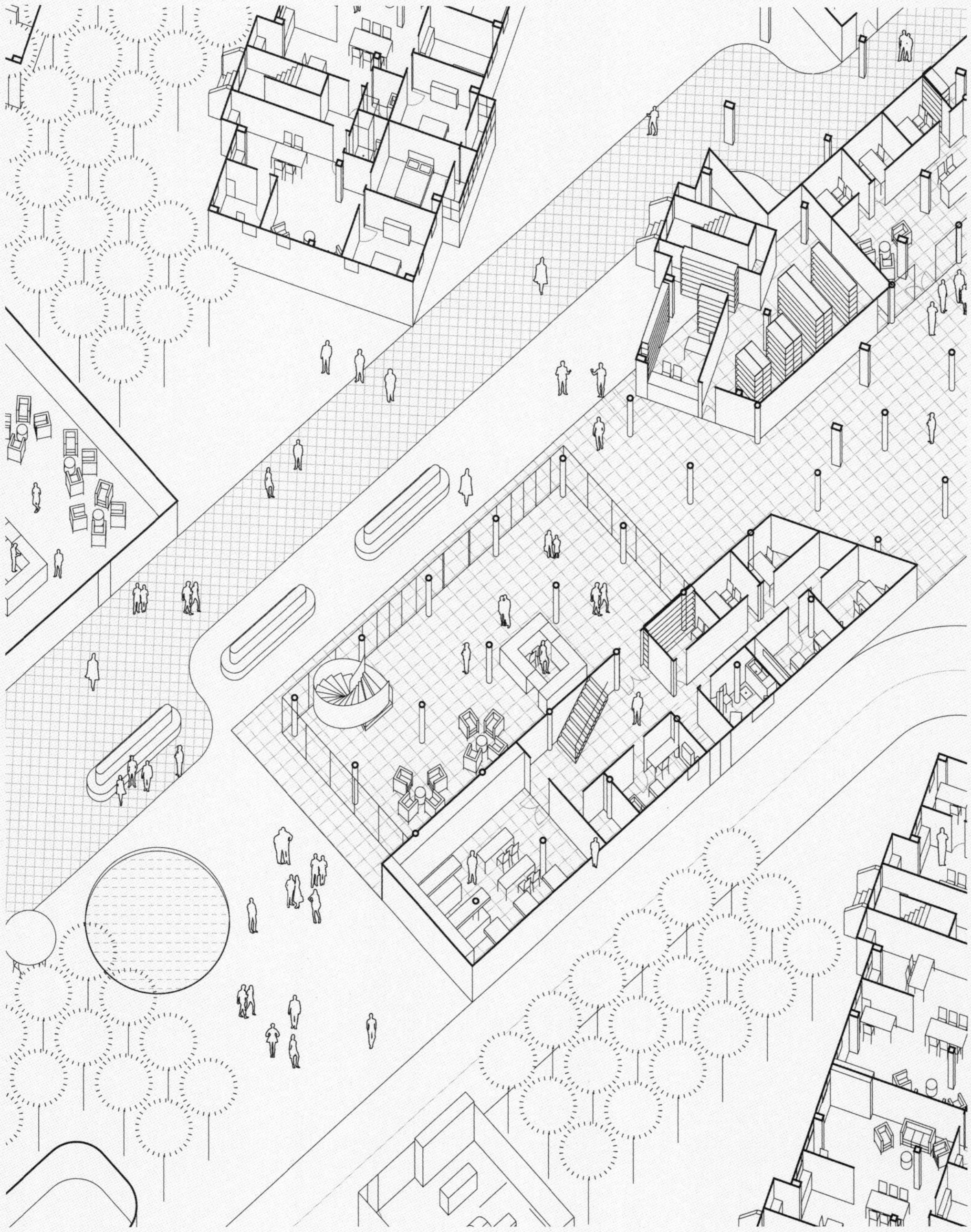

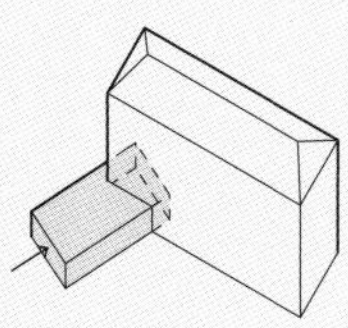

(1) Insert

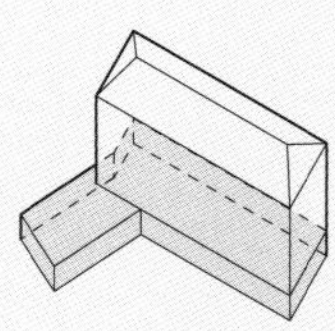

(2) Take floor

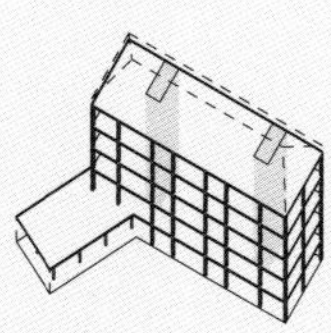

(3) Structural + circulatory negotiation

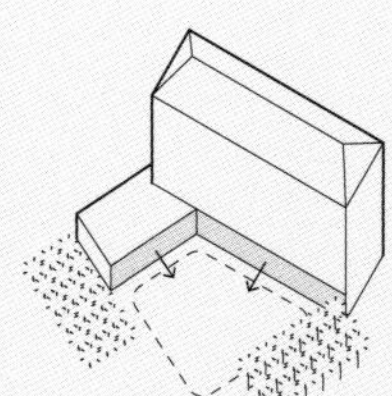

(4) Activate space

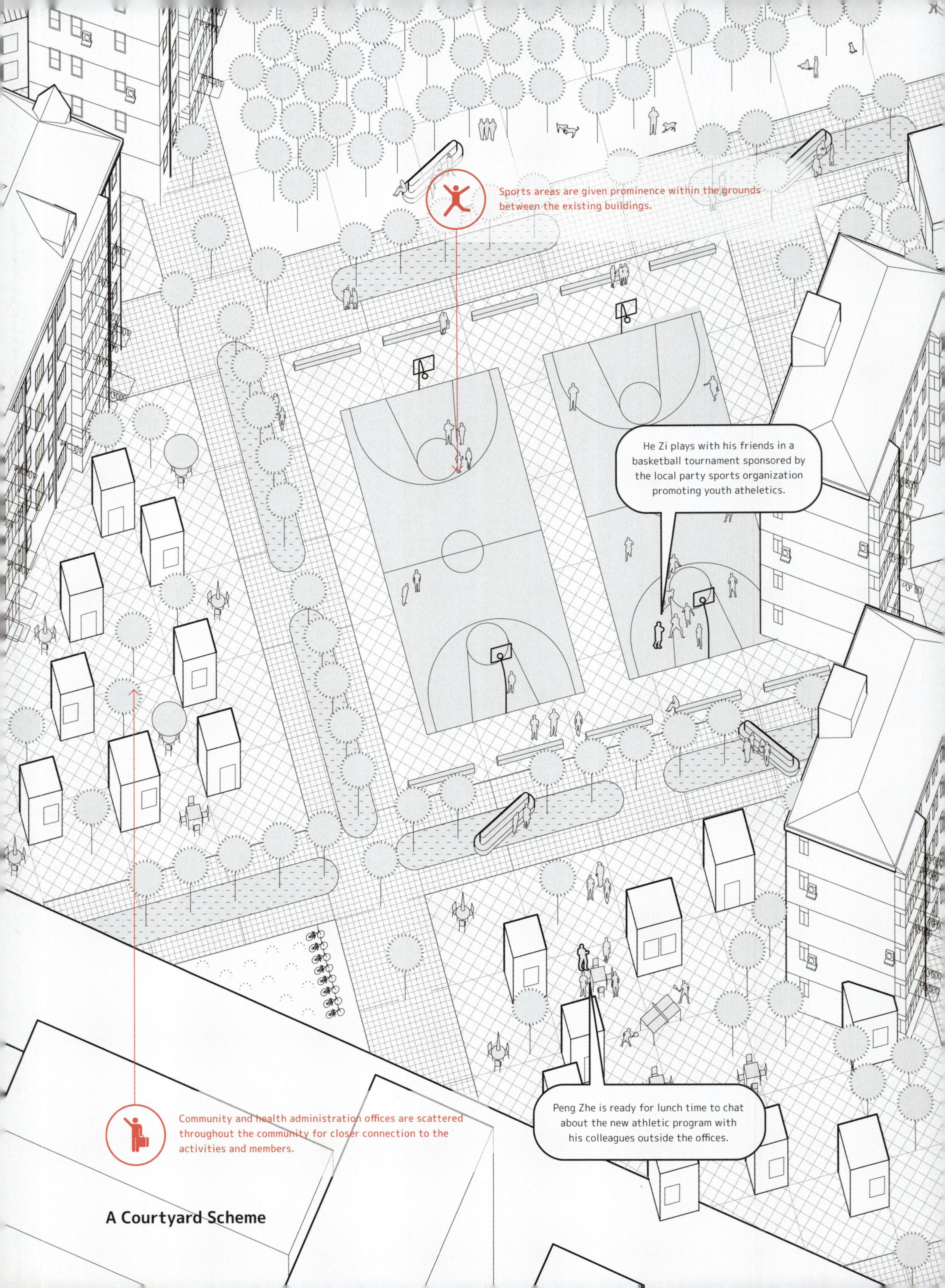

A Courtyard Scheme

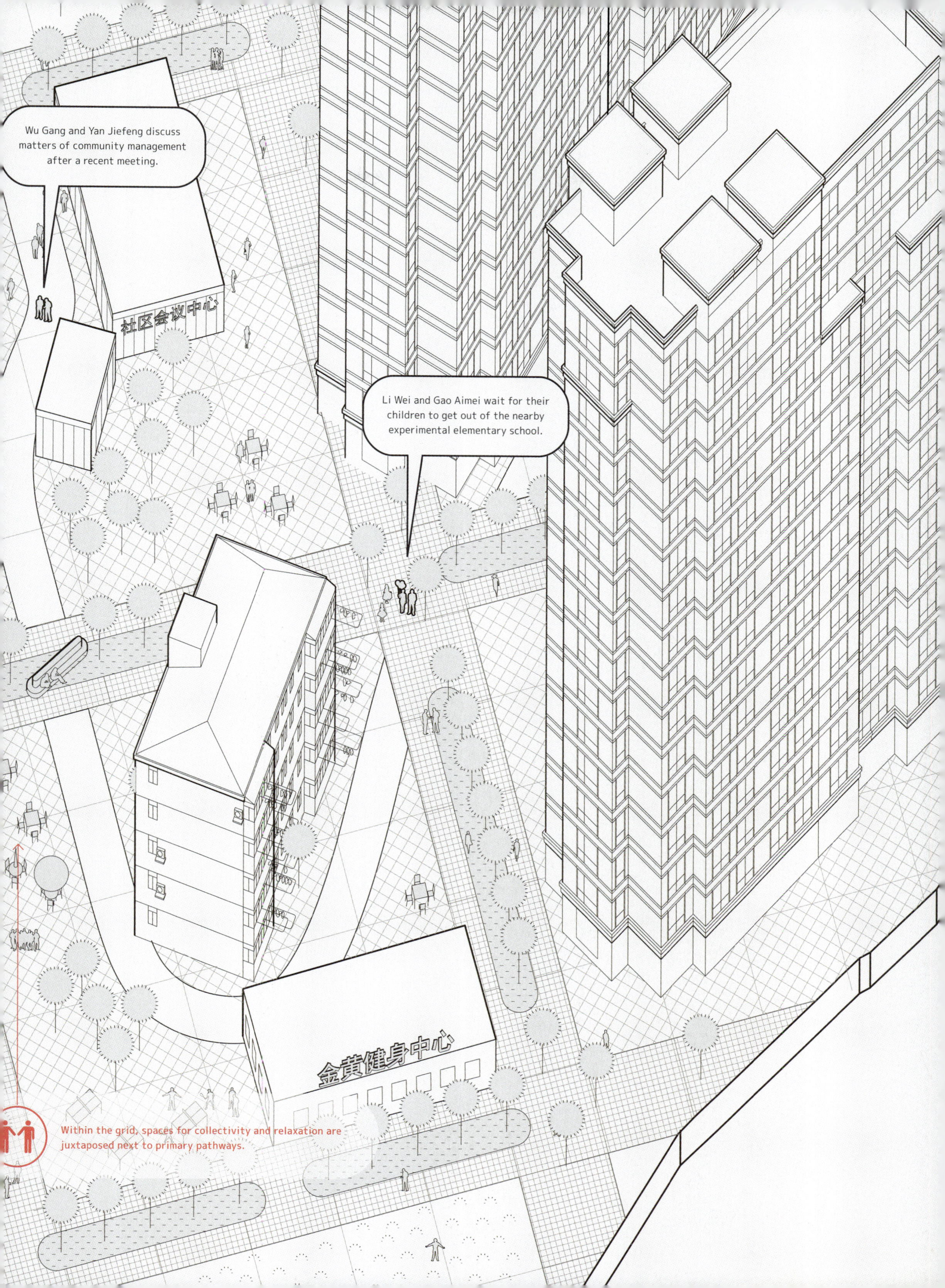
Wu Gang and Yan Jiefeng discuss matters of community management after a recent meeting.
社区会议中心
Li Wei and Gao Aimei wait for their children to get out of the nearby experimental elementary school.
金黄健身中心
Within the grid, spaces for collectivity and relaxation are juxtaposed next to primary pathways.

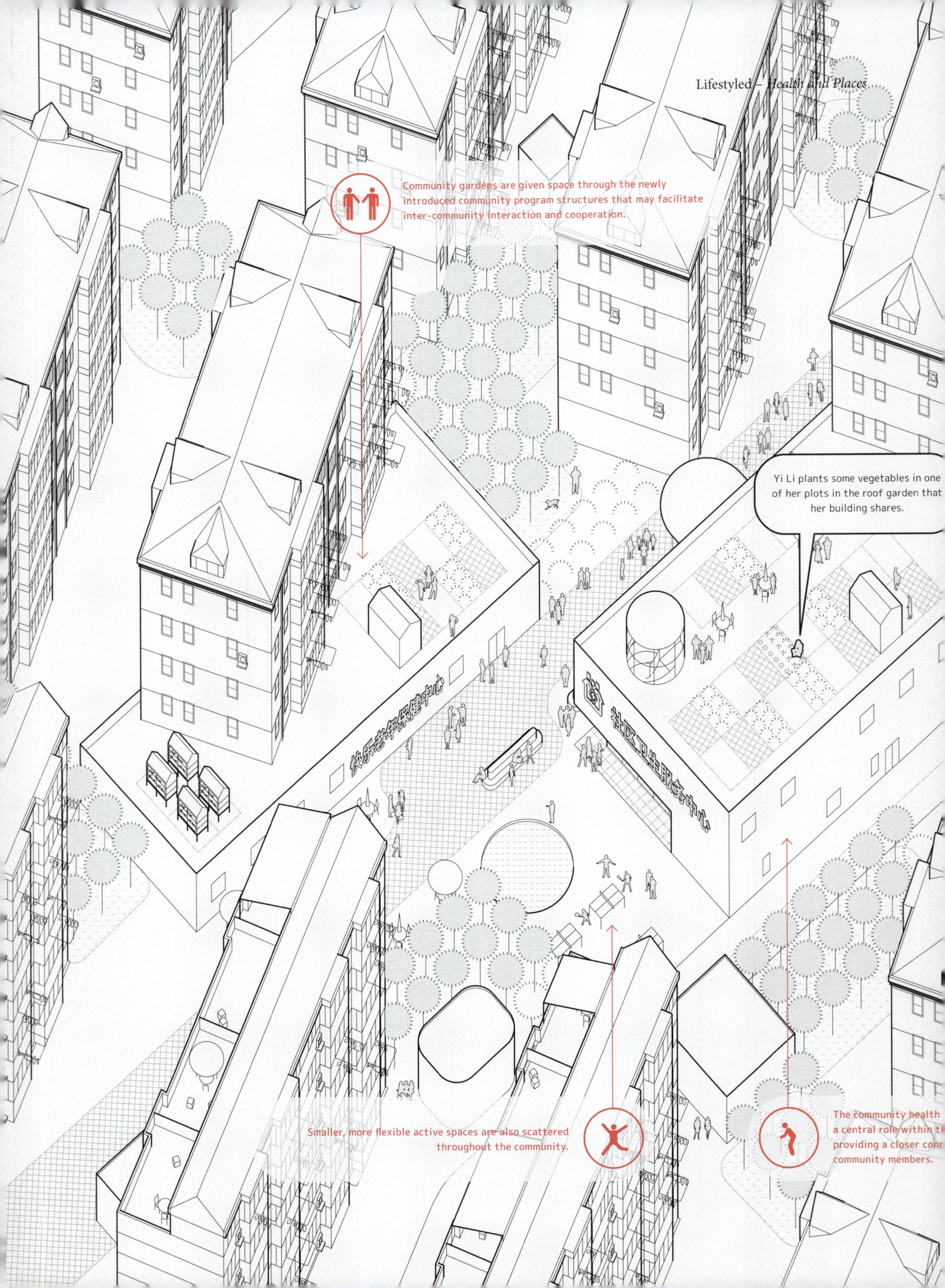
Community gardens are given space through the newly introduced community program structures that may facilitate inter-community interaction and cooperation.
Yi Li plants some vegetables in one of her plots in the roof garden that her building shares.
快乐老年保健中心
社区卫生服务中心
Smaller, more flexible active spaces are also scattered throughout the community.
The community health
a central role within
providing a closer
community members.

B Pathway Scheme

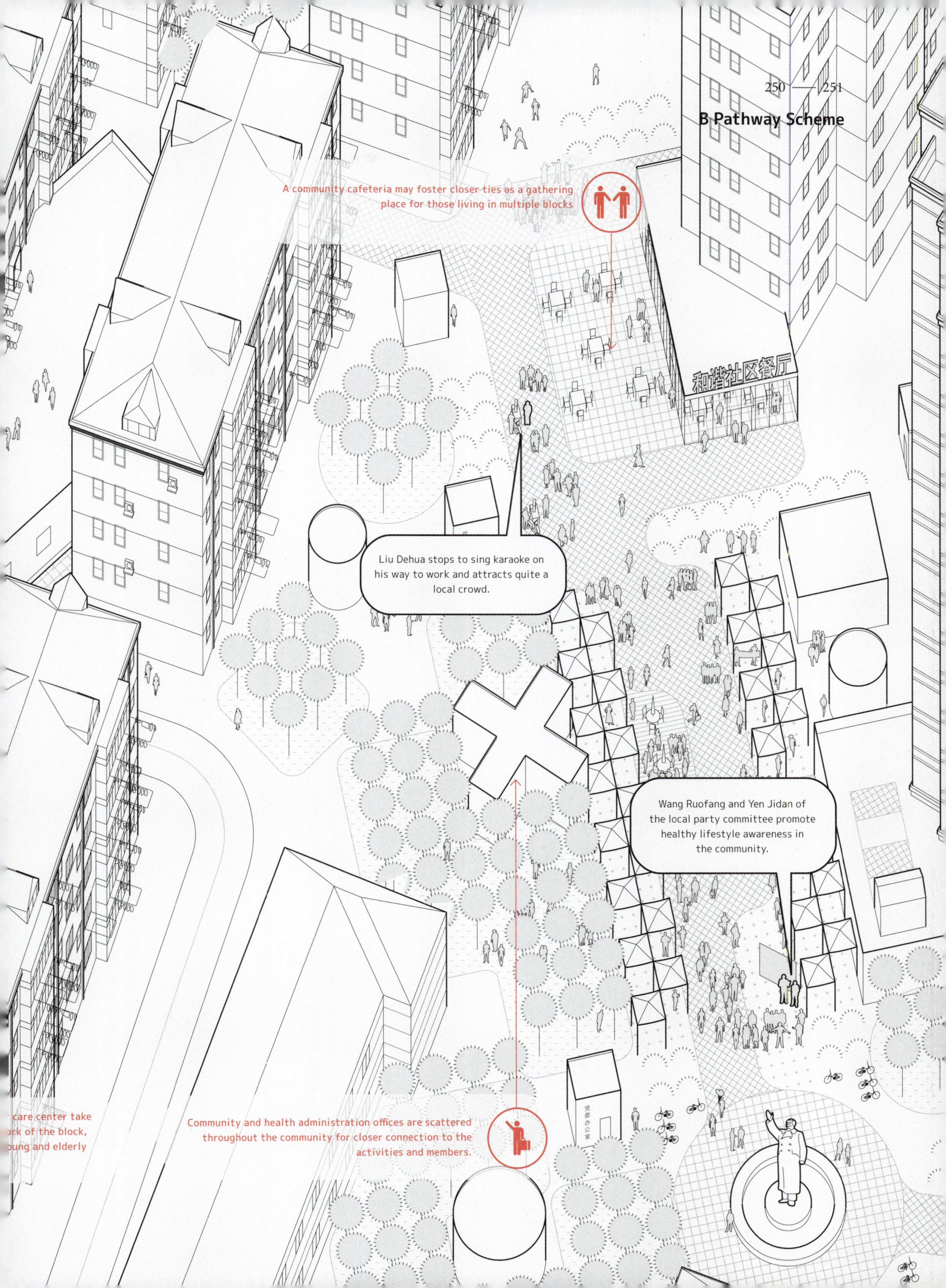

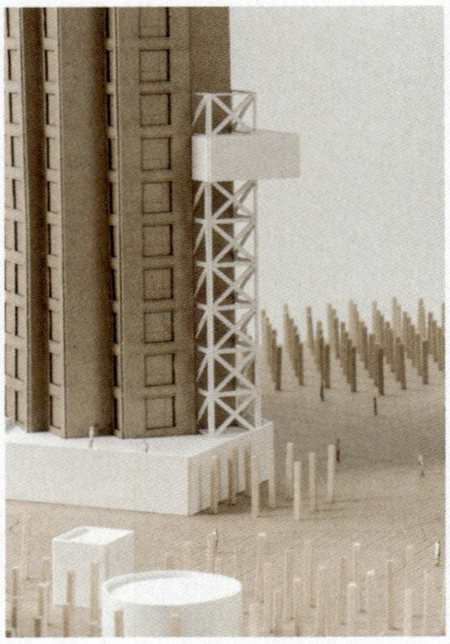

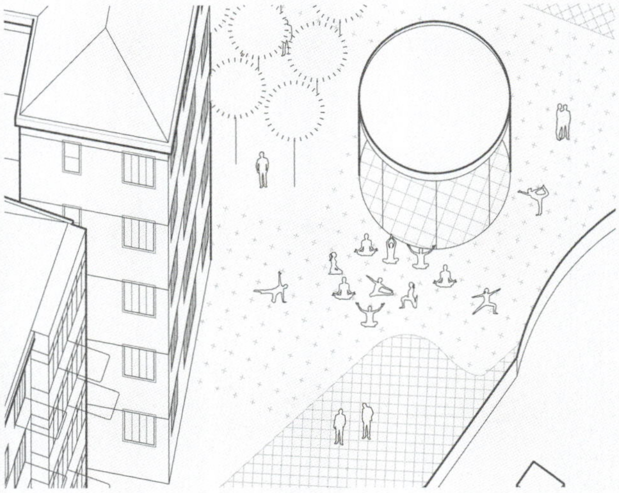

Photographs of large models. White buildings are inserted programs, attaching themselves to the exisiting (brown) residential buildings imbuing them with mixed programmatic uses. (Photographs by Anita Kan)

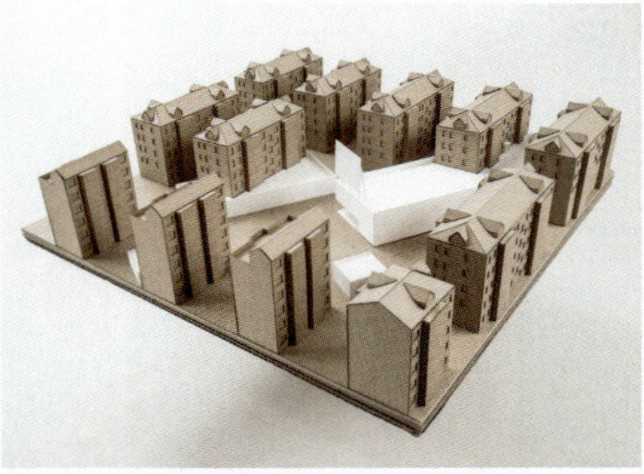

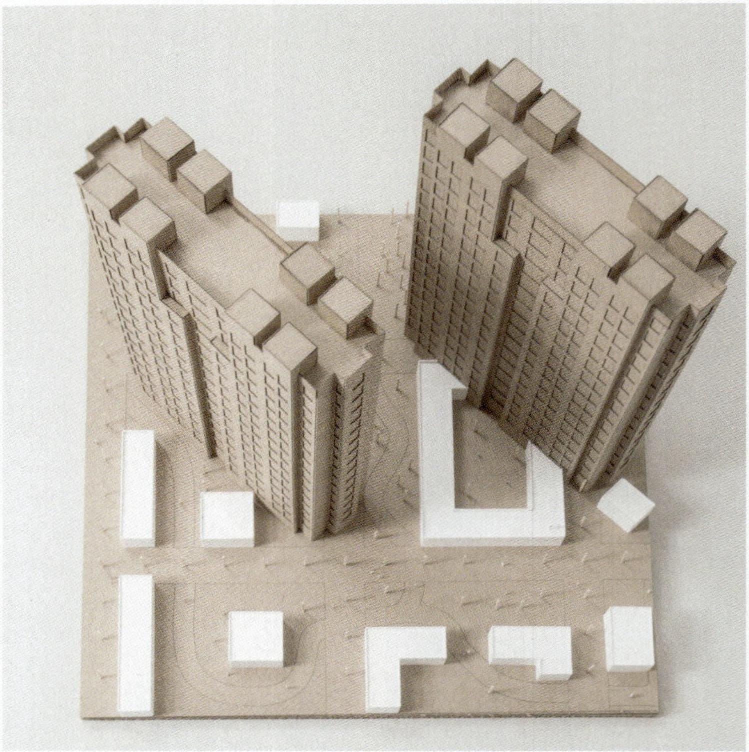

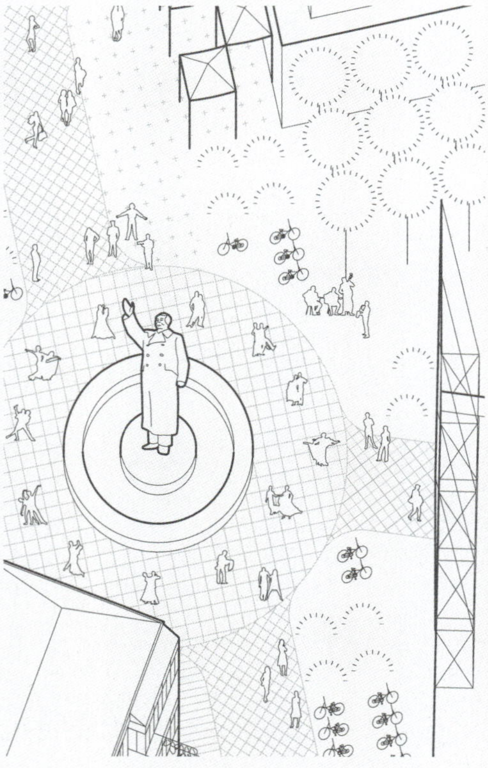

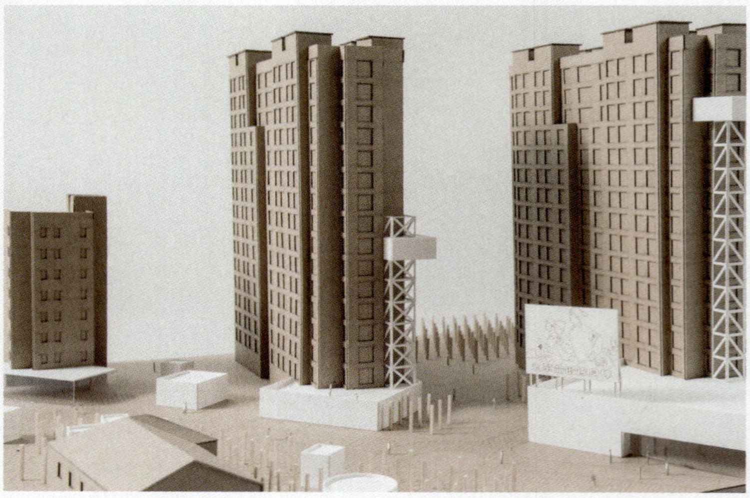

A Life Aquatic

Alejandro Lara + Dima Rachid

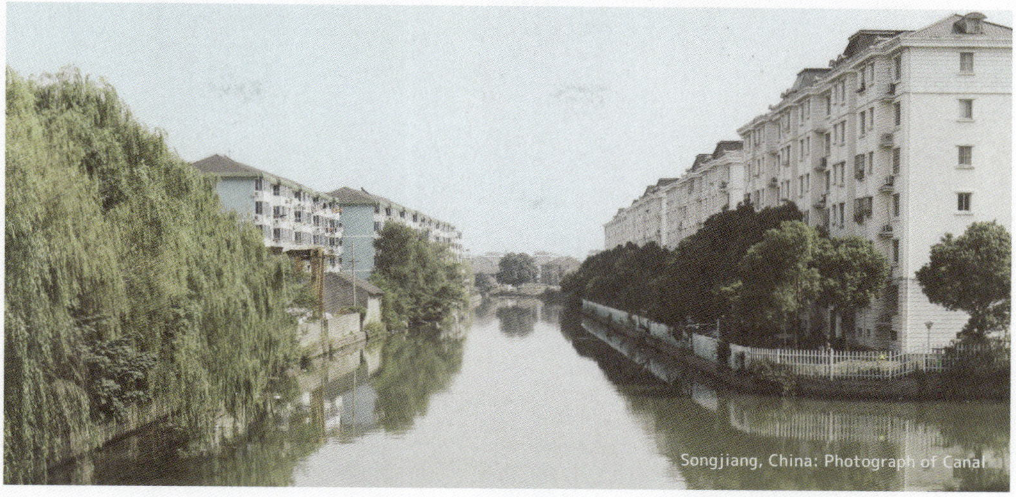

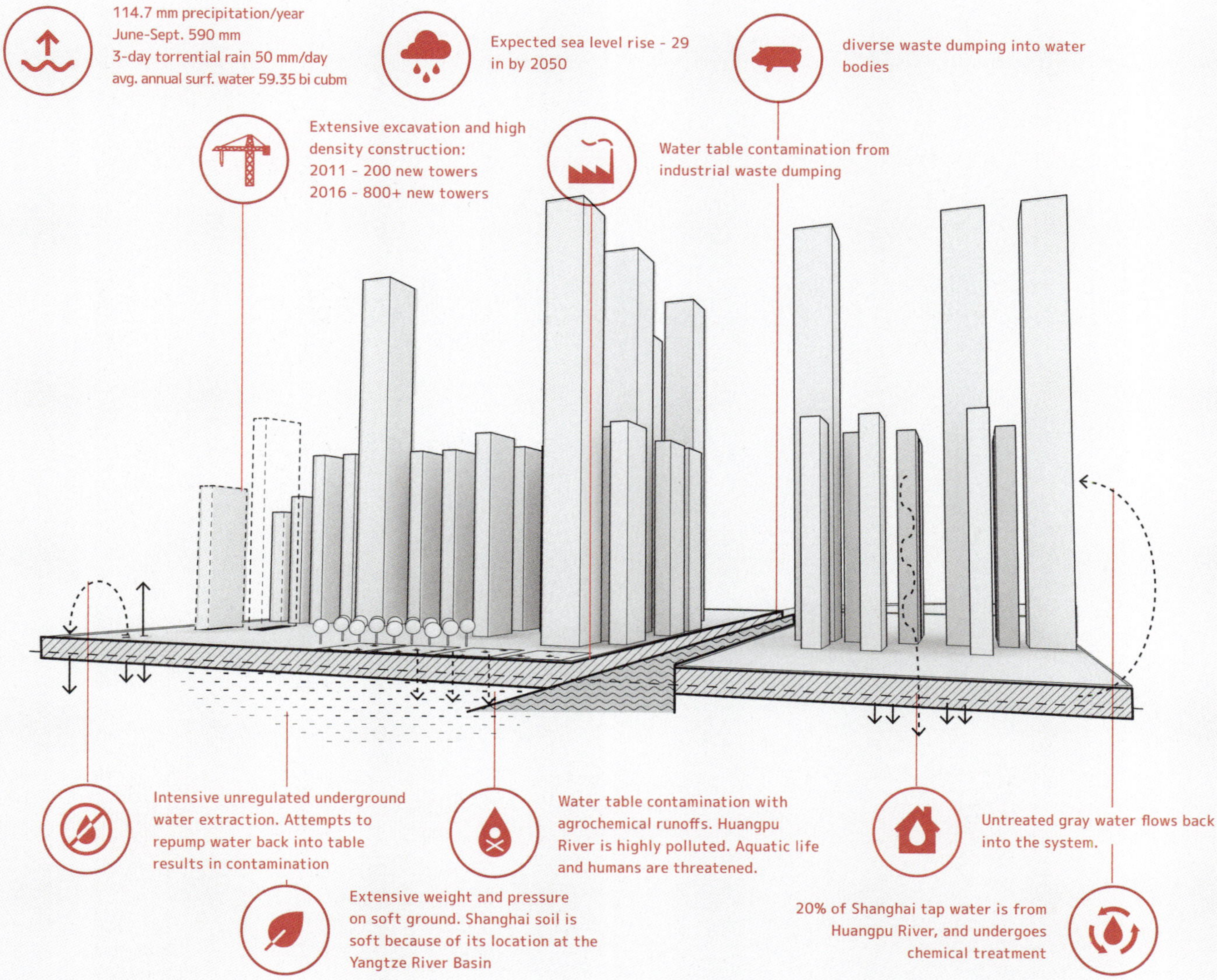

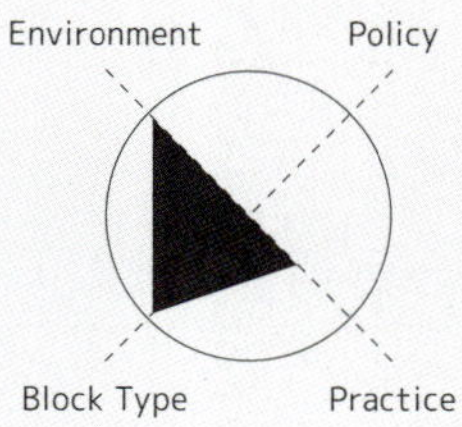

China's Water Crisis - Shanghai's Water Risks

While Shanghai enjoys an abundance of water resources, it faces a major crisis of water pollution and poor water quality. Major Chinese cities to the north face significant water shortages, while most urban areas in the country suffer from a general problem of extreme water contamination. This is often associated with spikes in cancer rates among populations, making the impulse to address the water quality issue a matter of public concern. Authorities in Shanghai say that over half of the 2,500 lakes and rivers near the city are heavily polluted.

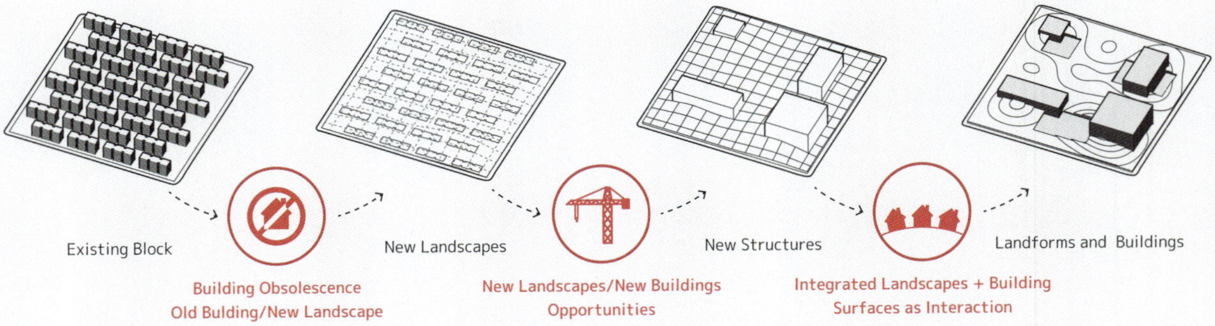

Average Chinese House
72 sqm/Unit

Average Chinese Family
3.13 People/Household

Average Chinese Family
Water Consumption
322.5 Liter/Day

Gray Water-Wetland Area
0.4 sqm/Liter

According to a 2010-2012 city water census, 53% of Shanghai's water was rated the worst category out of five levels, while only 3% of surface water was deemed as being fit for fish farms and household use.

Over the last twenty years, almost half of China's rivers have disappeared in large part due to water extraction. Furthermore, over half of the country's water sources are considered unsafe for human consumption and a quarter; unusable even for industrial purposes (according to a government report in 2010). In 2011, authorities claimed that 43% of state-monitored rivers were so polluted that they were not considered safe for human contact.

While industrial practices and bad hydrological management constitute the majority of the causes for this situation, urbanization also contributes towards the problem. Urban runoff and mismanaged storm water treatment processes can cause significant damage to the city's water sources. A model of urbanization that addresses this problem, if adopted as a prevailing model, may help improve the general problem of the city's damaged water resources.

This proposal pairs two problematic processes associated with China's current development practices in order to locate opportunities for an improved model of urbanization. The rapid rate of obsolescence of China's building fabric means that much of the city will soon be subject for renewal. By reusing the sorted debris and rubble from this renewal process, new topographies and landforms may be deployed to produce a base from which renewed neighborhoods can develop. This new engineered topography may be deployed to create a new aquatic landscape of wetlands that treat and leverage the gray water and runoff of its adjacent neighborhoods to provide both a greatly needed infrastructure and a renewed environment that can operate as a valuable social and ecological resource.

The association with older forms of neighborhoods in China such as Songjiang's old town and Suzhou, offers a neighborhood model that resonates with tradition. The remodeled landscape is used as an opportunity for enabling lifestyles that take advantage of its close relationship with water, creating a series of social and public spaces ranging from water gardens and public boardwalks to the possibility of floating amenities and markets.

Gray water from Residents

Sinks, Showers, Washing Machine

Water is considered easy to treat + safe for contact

Residents' Water is Treated on a Daily Basis

Day 1. Water Discharge

Park Space/Resilient Zone

Shallow Flow of Water Growing Grass

Fine Sand Filtration Removes Contaminants

Detoxification Zone

Metals and Toxins Removed by Sedimentation

Oxydation and Dissolution of Chemicals

Day 2-3. Water Absorption

Shallow Zone - Vegetation Filter

De-Nitrification in Anaerobic Zone

Sludge Treatment Separates Water and Waste

Coarse and Fine Gravel Bed

Water Emergent and Free Floating Vegetation

Dispersion and Difussion of Chemical Leftover

Day 4-5. Water Filtration

Deep Zone - Water Mixture

Polishing Pond

Floating Vegetation

Underwater Vegetation

Water Aeration Before Discharge

Clay and Mud Bottom Dissolve Contaminants

Day 6-7. Water Mixing

Wetland Detention Pond

Wetland Pond for Water Use

Clean Pond Safe for Fauna

Underwater Vegetation Filter Deep Water

Day 8. Clean Water

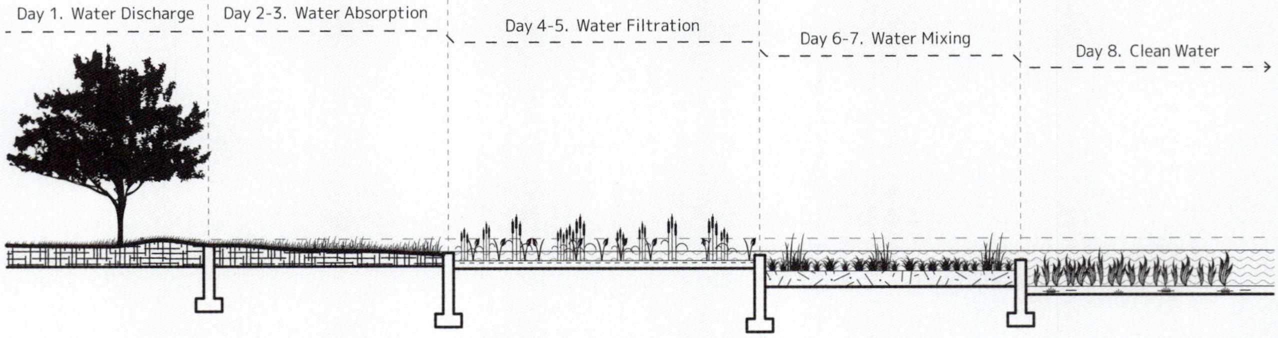

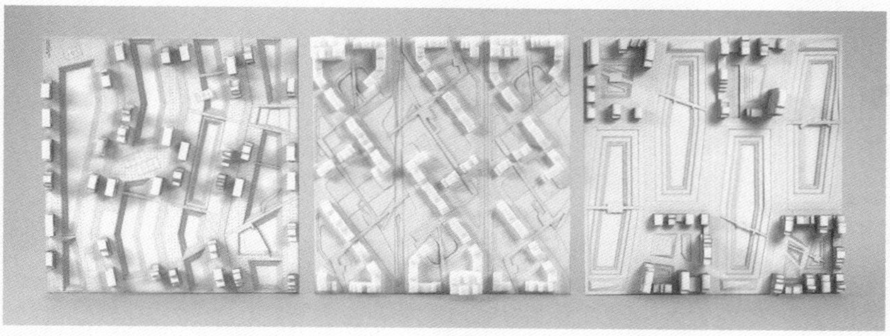

(Left) Photograph of block-scale model iterations. (Photograph by Anita Kan)

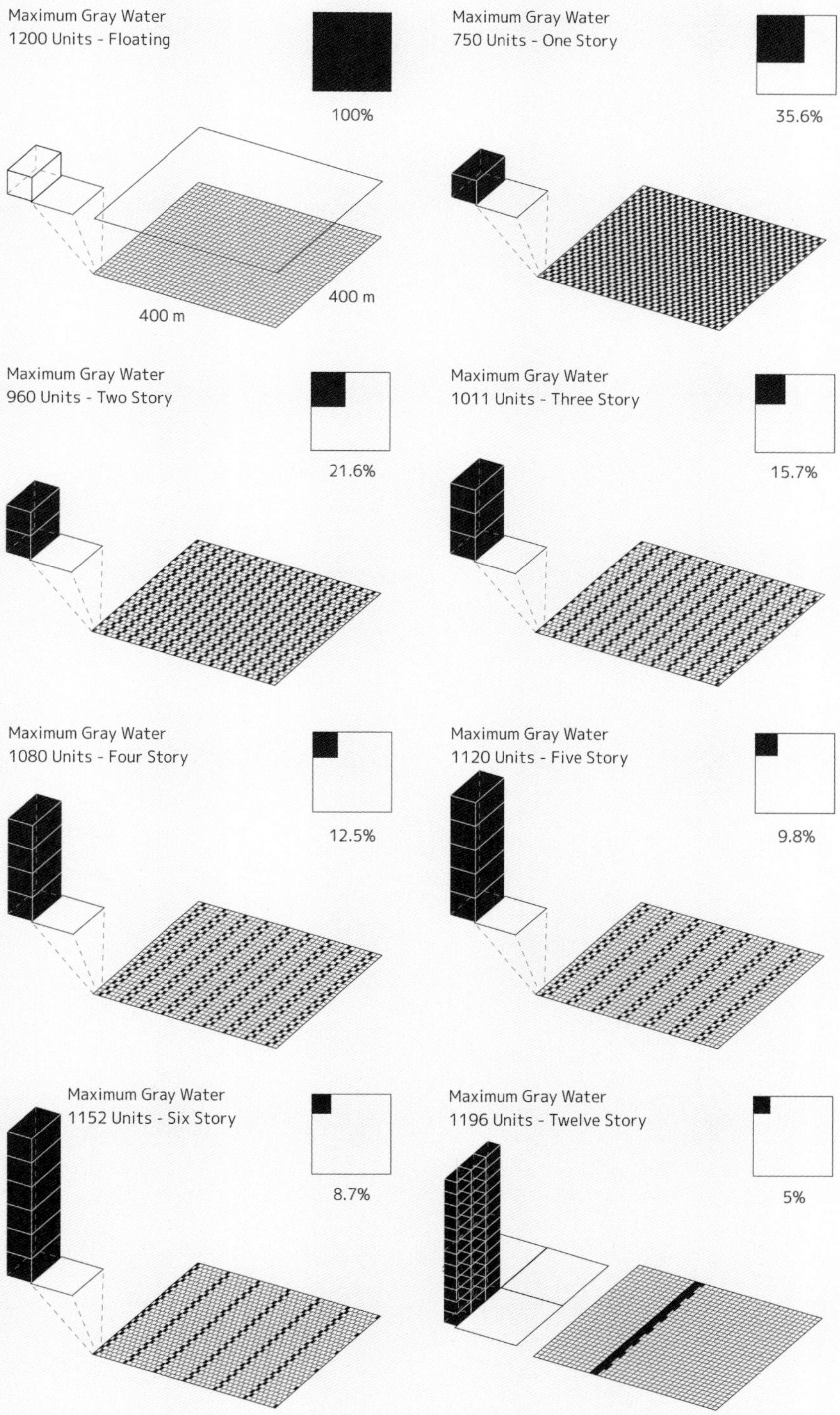

Urban Block Density Gradation

A 12-14-Storey High-Rise

B 6-Storey Mid-Rise

C 5-Storey Slabs

D 4-Storey Slabs

E 3-Storey Walk-Ups

D 2-Storey Sixpacks

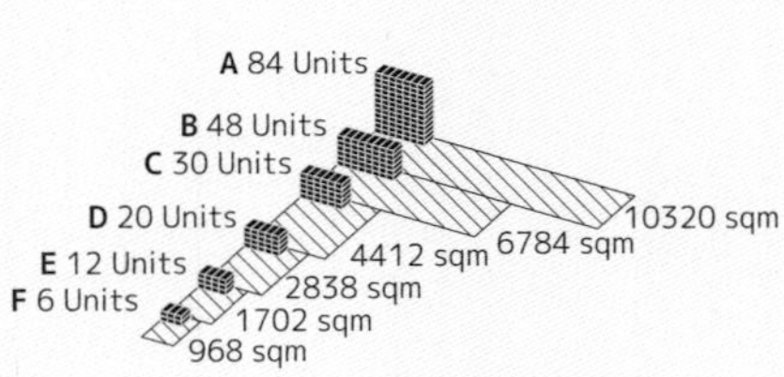

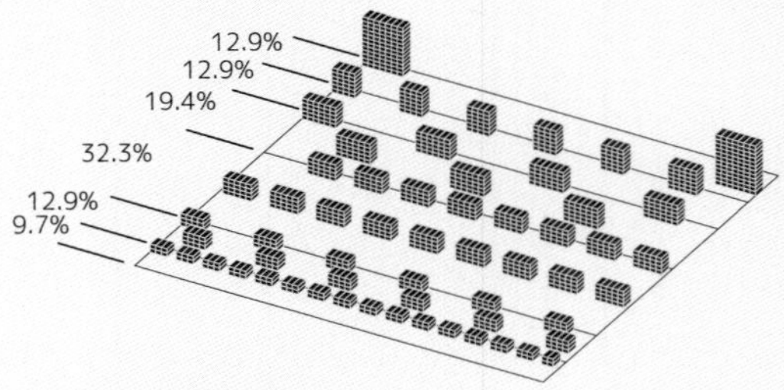

Urban Block / Water Configurations

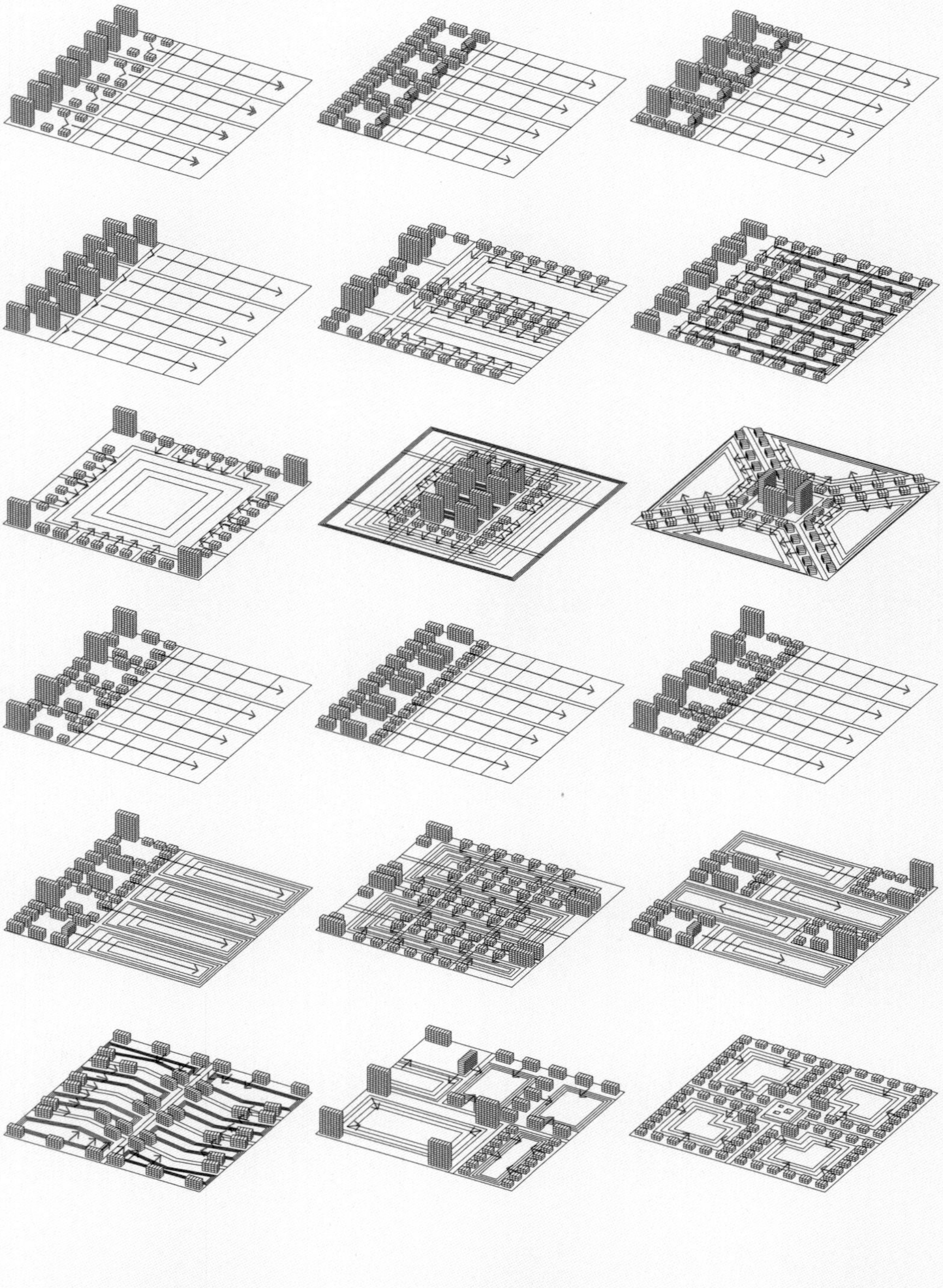

Density - Water
Density Focused on the Street Edge and Allowing the Inner Part of the Block to Respond to Context

Linear Water Ways
Density Focused on the Inner Street Edge to Create Waterways as Part of the Block

Water Isolation
Density Focused on Isolation and Maximizing the Water Bodies as Large Individual Units

Density - Water Courtyards
Density Focused on the Street Edge as Courtyards, Leavingthe Rest of the Block as a Wetland

Mixed Water Bodies
Density Alternating on the Street Edge Creating a Mixture of Density and Water Bodies

Water Mosaic
Density Focused on patterns that Maximize the Water Bodies as Repetition and Endless Possibilities

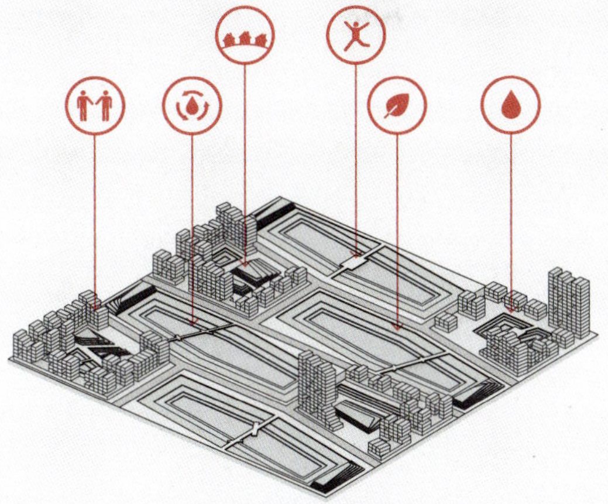

An arrangement of the block utilizing clusters of basins and buildings. These produce a series of courtyards or discrete, framed water gardens as well as the larger open basins. The resulting urban form is also discrete and scattered, producing smaller complexes or enclaves rather than a consistent fabric. This block arrangement cultivates a more private environment for the residential developments, with clearly demarcated spaces related to each complex while also offering the larger open spaces of the basins.

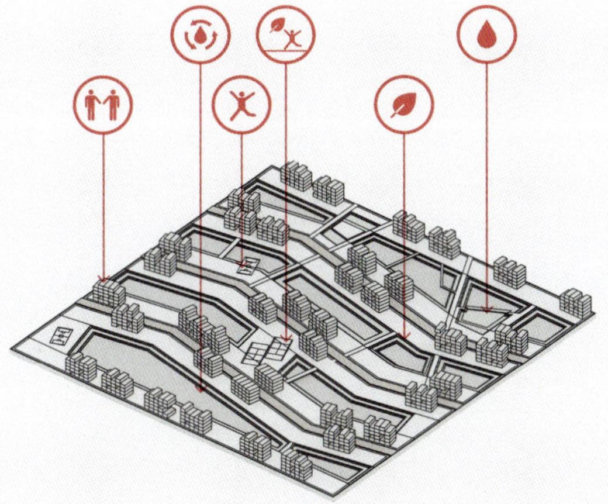

A striated arrangement of linear waterways and buildings produces a neighborhood configuration that allows for buildings with water adjacencies on both sides. A linear configuration of the building fabric mirrors row house block types such as Shanghai's *linong* districts and London's nineteenth century terrace houses. This fabric is more open, having a more immediate relationship between the continuous communal landscape and the buildings.

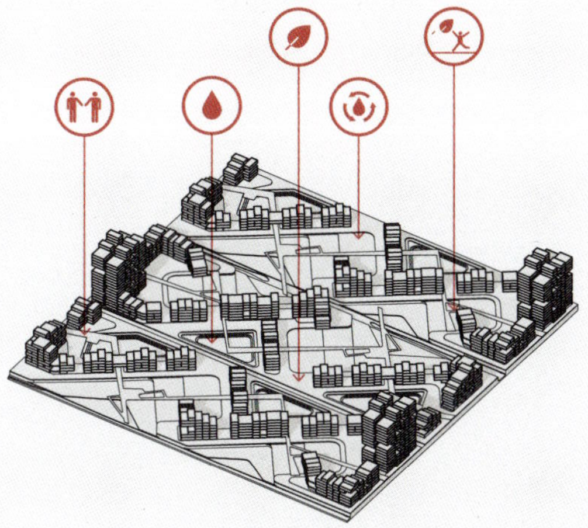

A hybrid between the two previous arrangements allows for a range of different kinds of spaces and relationships between buildings and the landscape. Framed, more intimate courtyards are continuous with more open bay-like configurations, offering a gradient transition between different types of open spaces. Differentiated building types are also deployed in this arrangement with courtyard arrangements as well as the more linear fabrics. High-rise and row house types are integrated within the block together with smaller, discrete pavilion buildings, offering a diversity of housing types.

Detailed Landscape Treatments

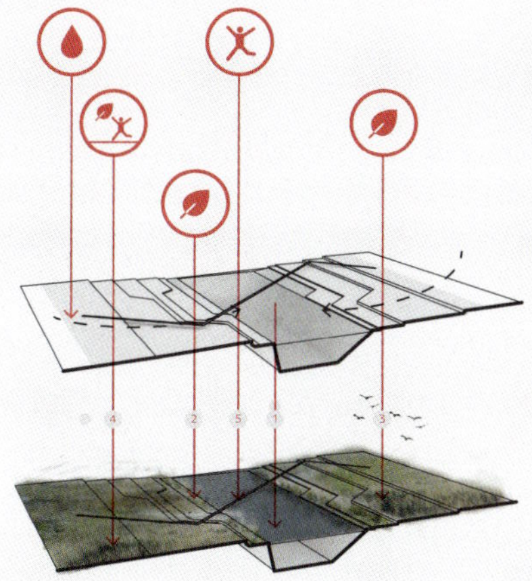

(Left) Constructed wetlands 3-phase at River Edge
(1) Existing Water Canal
(2) Overflow Zone
(3) Infiltration Trays
(4) Landform Top Platform
(5) Pedestrian Walkway/Bridge

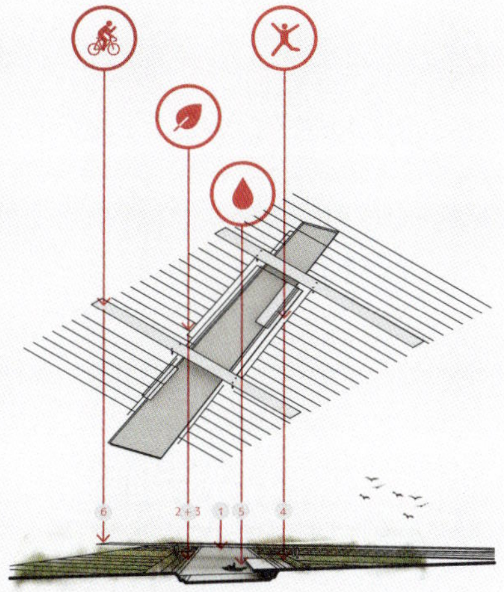

(Right) Constructed wetlands at Canal Edge
(1) Existing Water Canal
(2) Overflow Zone
(3) Infiltration Trays
(4) Cantilevered Platform
(5) Boat Marina
(6) Existing Bridge

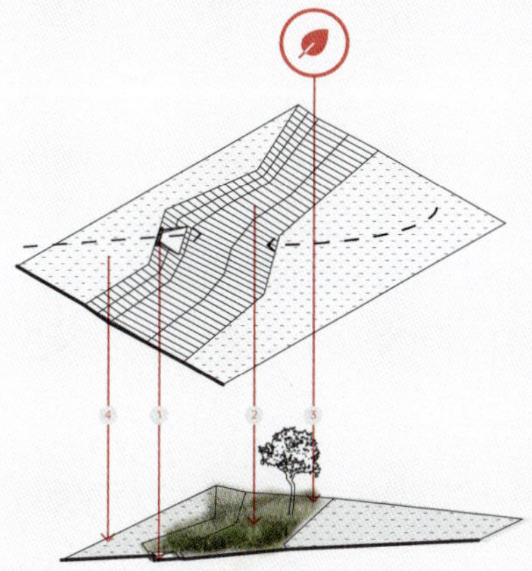

(Left) Surface Runo Filter at Urban Edge
(1) Water Conduit Discharge
(2) Trench
(3) Softscape (Remediated/Ornamental)
(4) Urban Surface/Hardscape

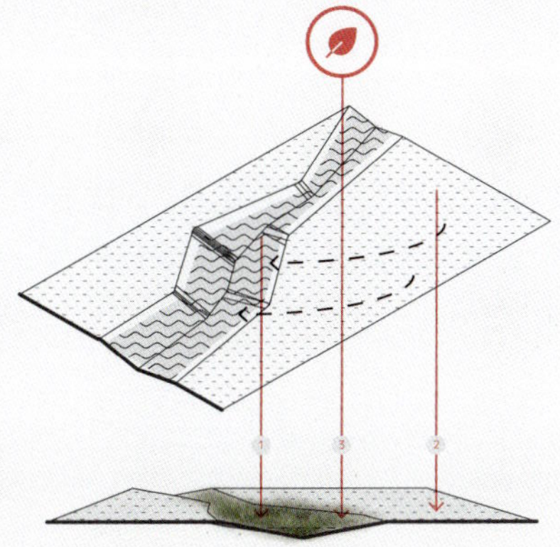

(Right) Surface Runo Bioswale No-Channel at Urban Edge
(1) Shallow Trench
(2) Sloped Surface
(3) Softscape

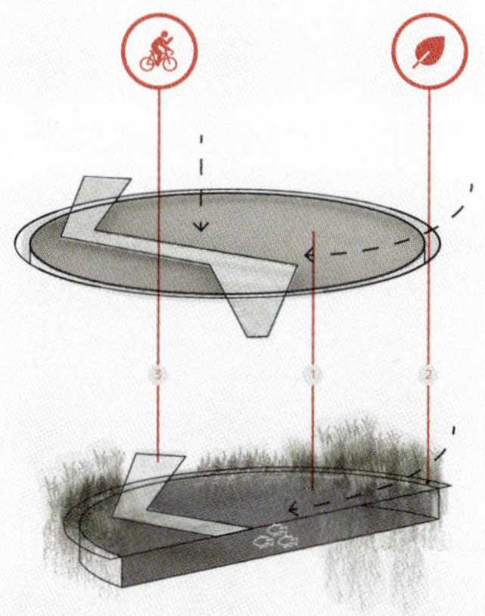

(Left) Water Collection Pod at Inland/Existing Body
(1) Water Collection Pod
(2) Buffer/Remediation Tray
(3) Platform/Connector

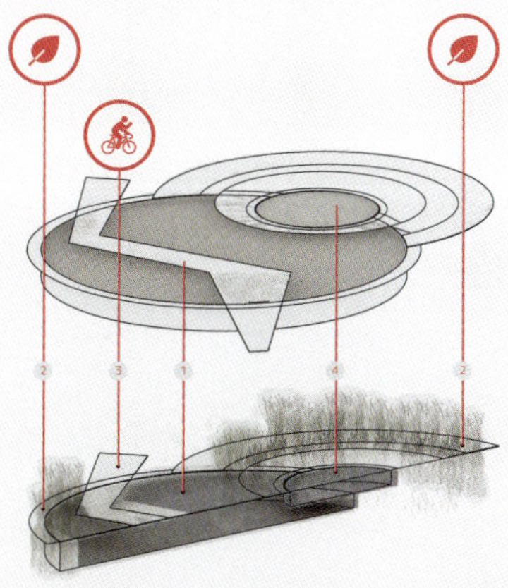

(Right) Surface Runo Bioswale No-Channel at Urban Edge
(1) Shallow Trench
(2) Sloped Surface
(3) Softscape

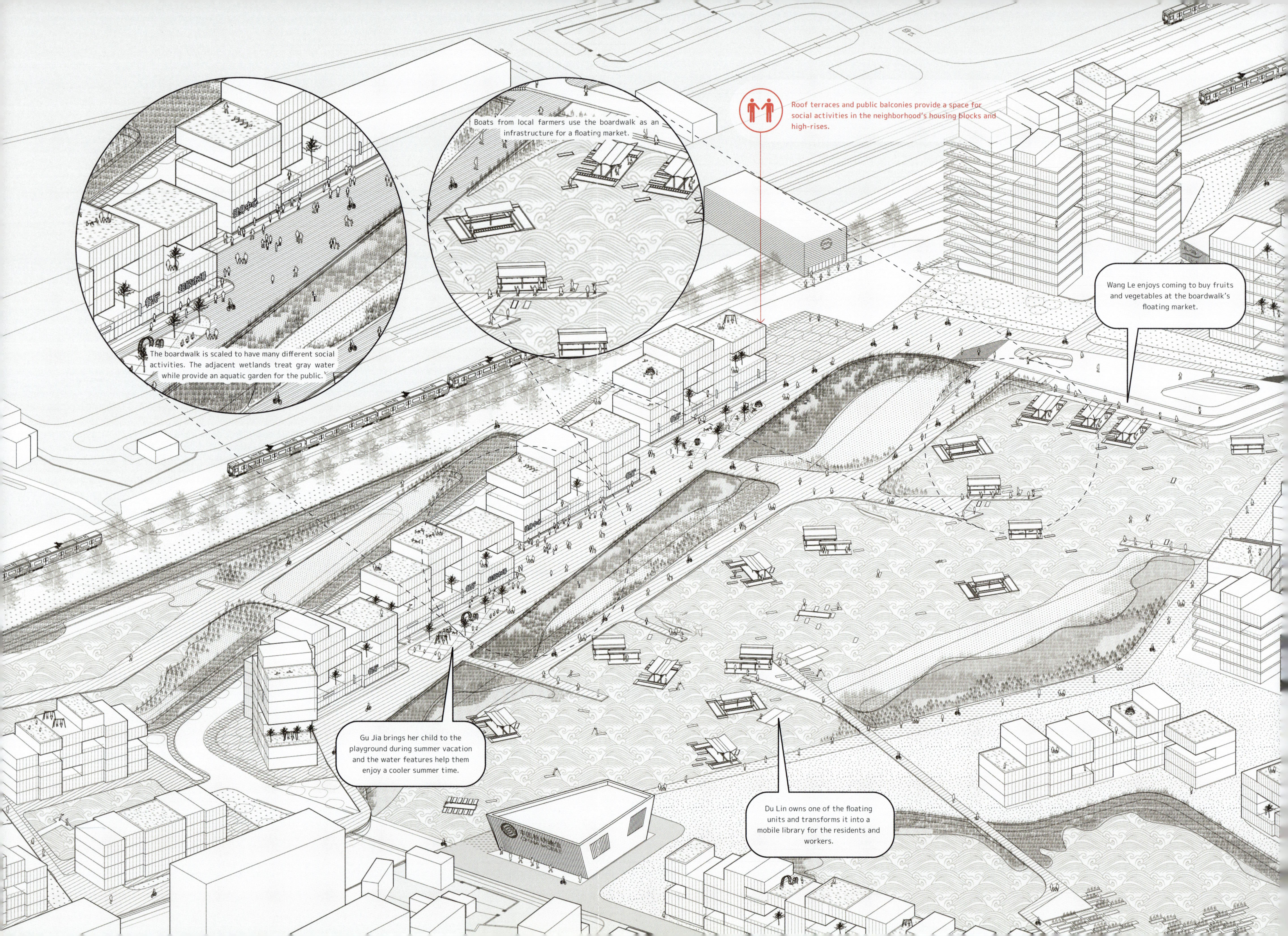
The boardwalk is scaled to have many different social activities. The adjacent wetlands treat gray water while provide an aquatic garden for the public.
Boats from local farmers use the boardwalk as an infrastructure for a floating market.
Roof terraces and public balconies provide a space for social activities in the neighborhood's housing blocks and high-rises.
Wang Le enjoys coming to buy fruits and vegetables at the boardwalk's floating market.
Gu Jia brings her child to the playground during summer vacation and the water features help them enjoy a cooler summer time.
Du Lin owns one of the floating units and transforms it into a mobile library for the residents and workers.

Implementation Scenario - Songjiang Old Town

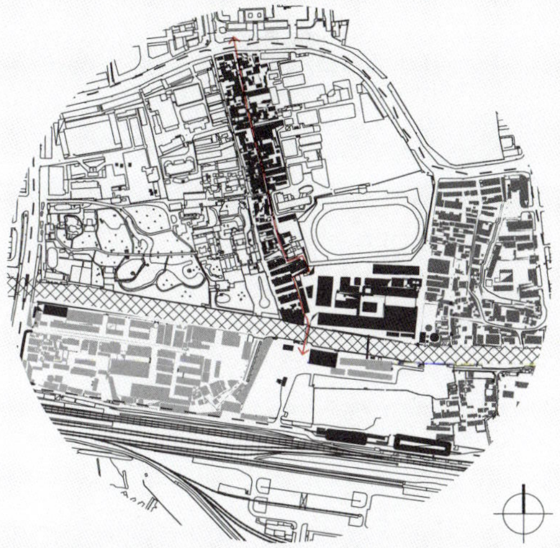

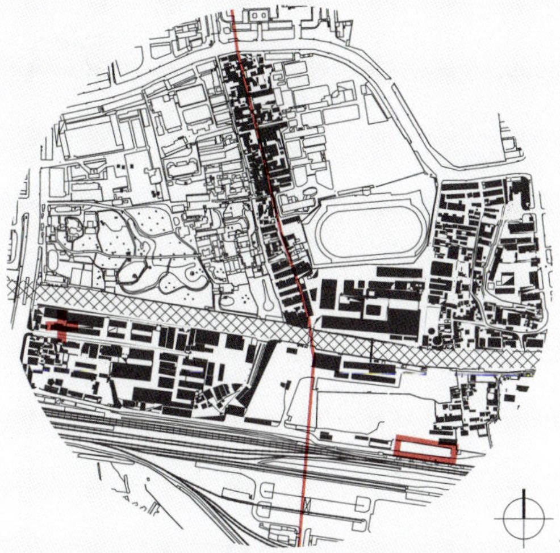

Existing Condition / Land Use and Circulation

- Low-income/ Low-rise Housing
- Brownfields
- High End Housing Under Construction
- Footpath

Planned Condition / Urban Planning Department Plan

- Main Circulation
- Proposed New Main Road
- Proposed Civic Center
- Metro Station

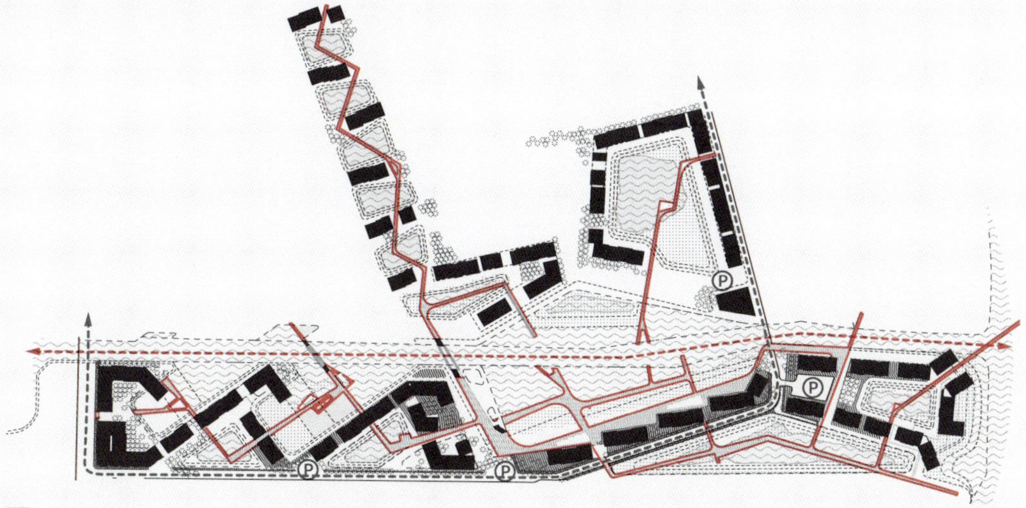

- Housing
- Main Circulation
- Main Vehicular Access
- Parking

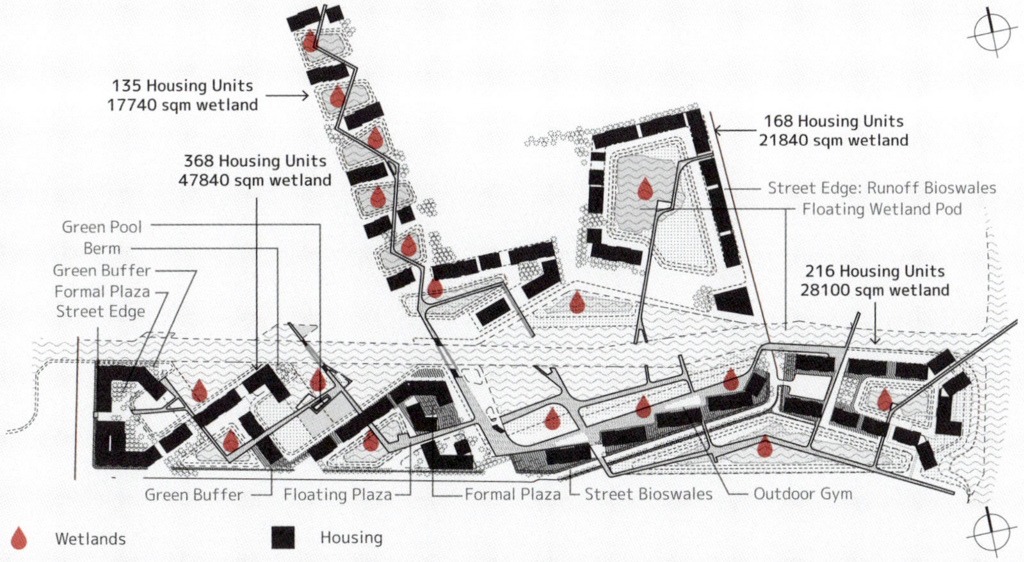

- Wetlands
- Housing

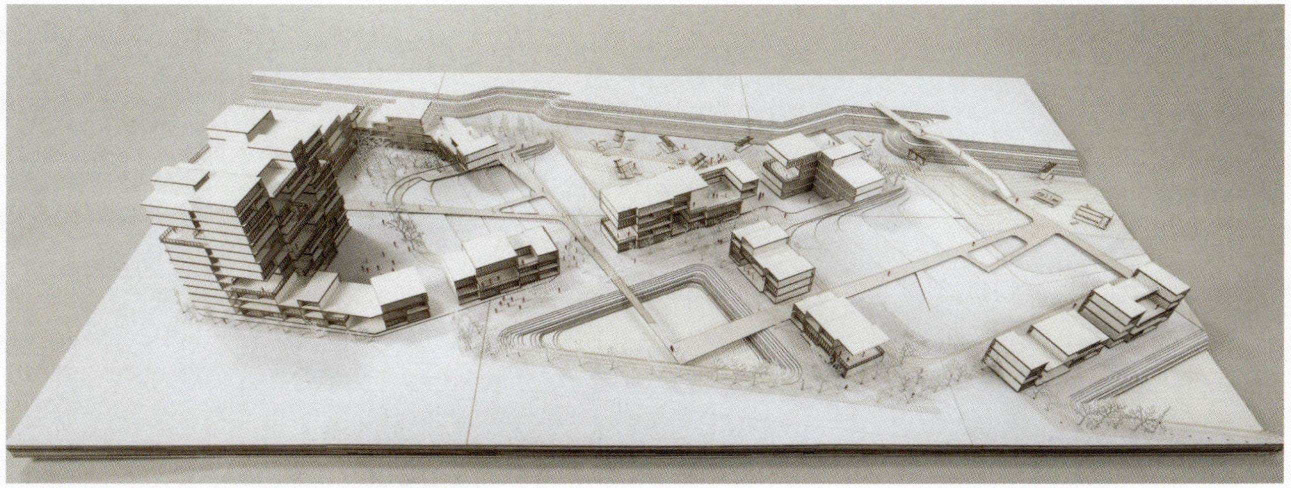

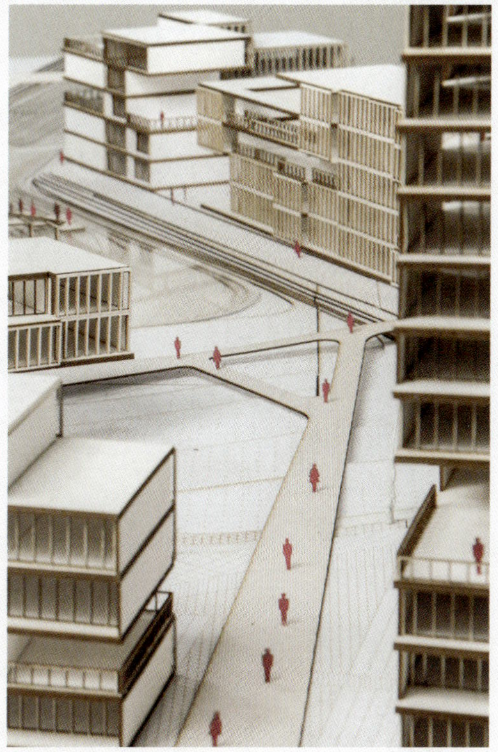

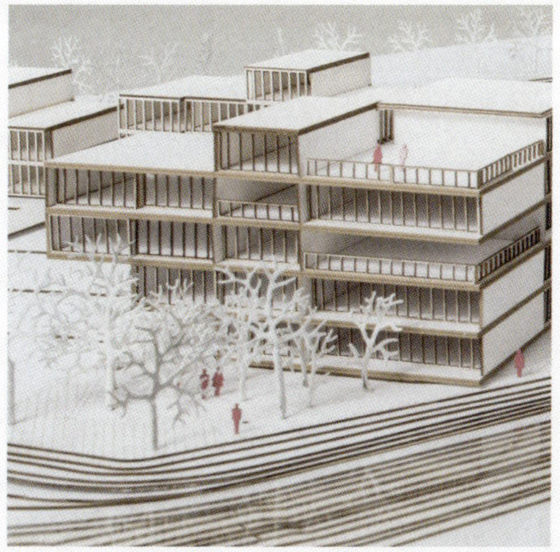

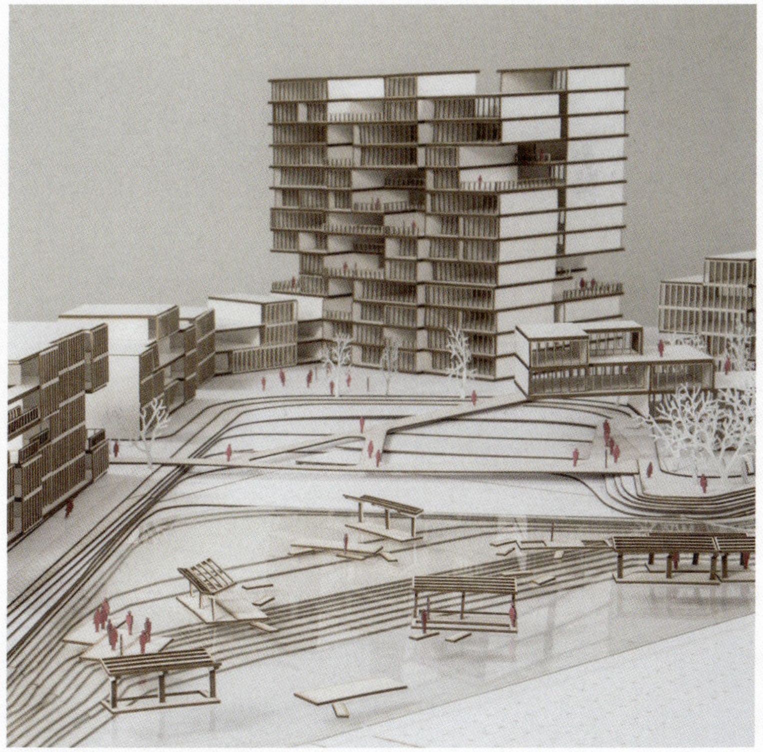

(Top) Overall photograph of large-scale model
(Left + Right Middle, Bottom) Photographs of large-scale model in detail. (Photographs by Anita Kan)

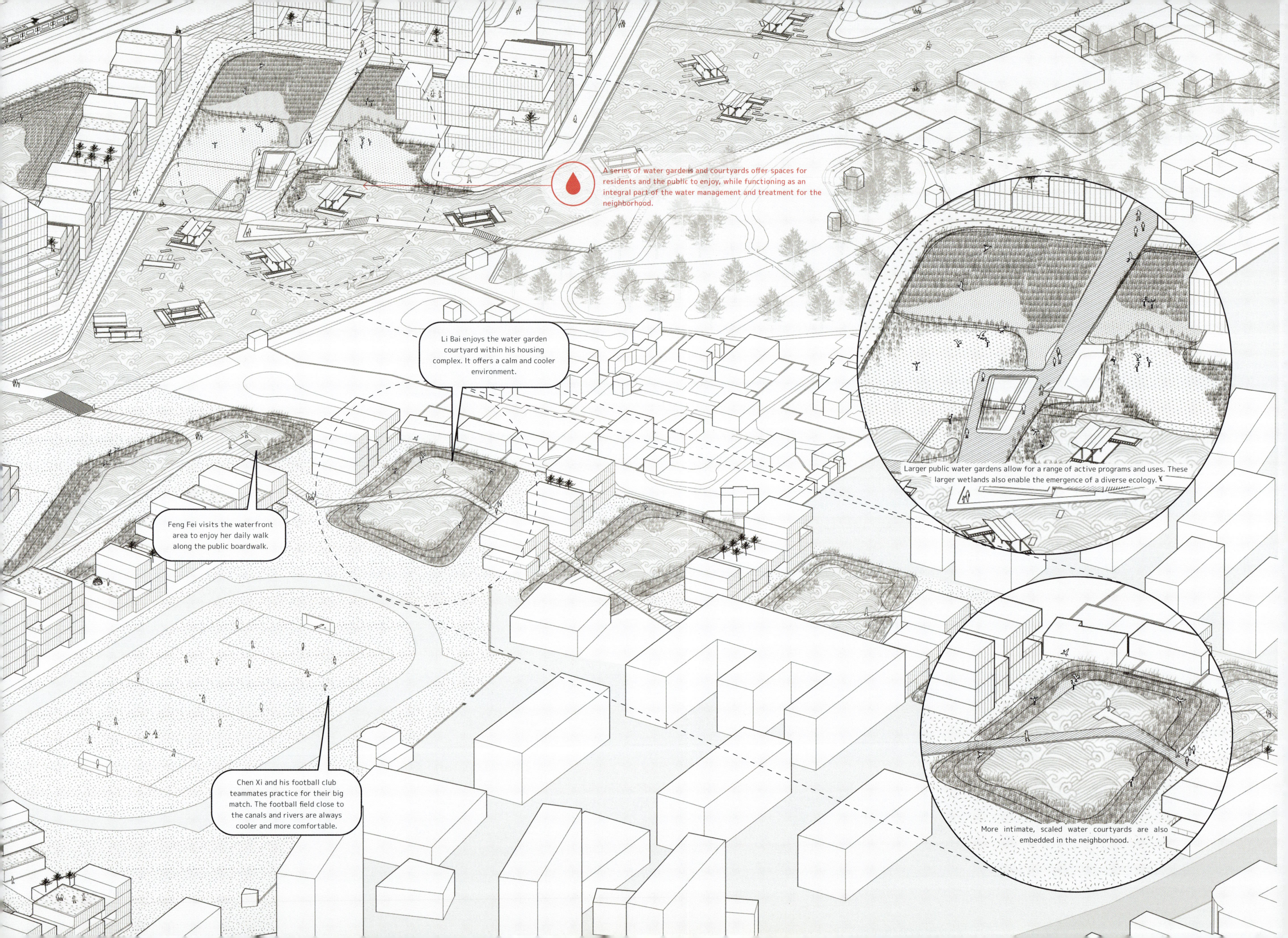
A series of water gardens and courtyards offer spaces for residents and the public to enjoy, while functioning as an integral part of the water management and treatment for the neighborhood.
Li Bai enjoys the water garden courtyard within his housing complex. It offers a calm and cooler environment.
Feng Fei visits the waterfront area to enjoy her daily walk along the public boardwalk.
Chen Xi and his football club teammates practice for their big match. The football field close to the canals and rivers are always cooler and more comfortable.
Larger public water gardens allow for a range of active programs and uses. These larger wetlands also enable the emergence of a diverse ecology.
More intimate, scaled water courtyards are also embedded in the neighborhood.

Seeing the Forest for the Trees

Wen Wen +Joon Won

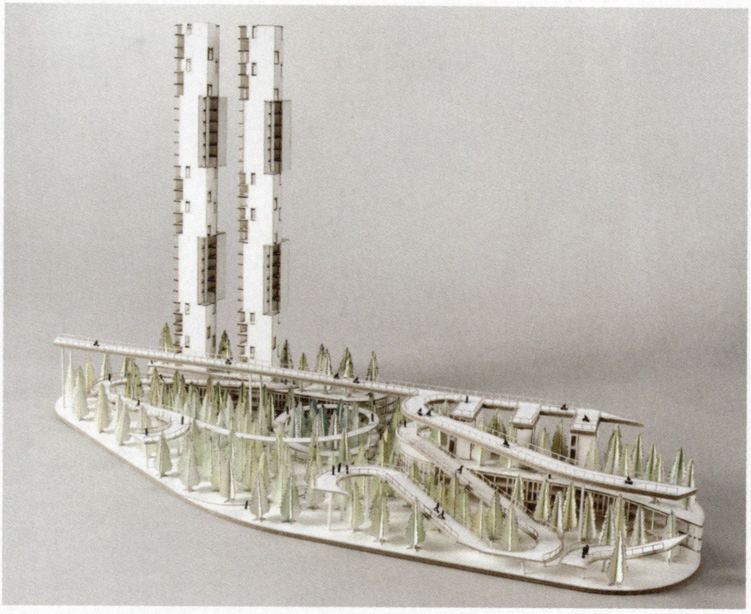

(Photograph by Anita Kan)

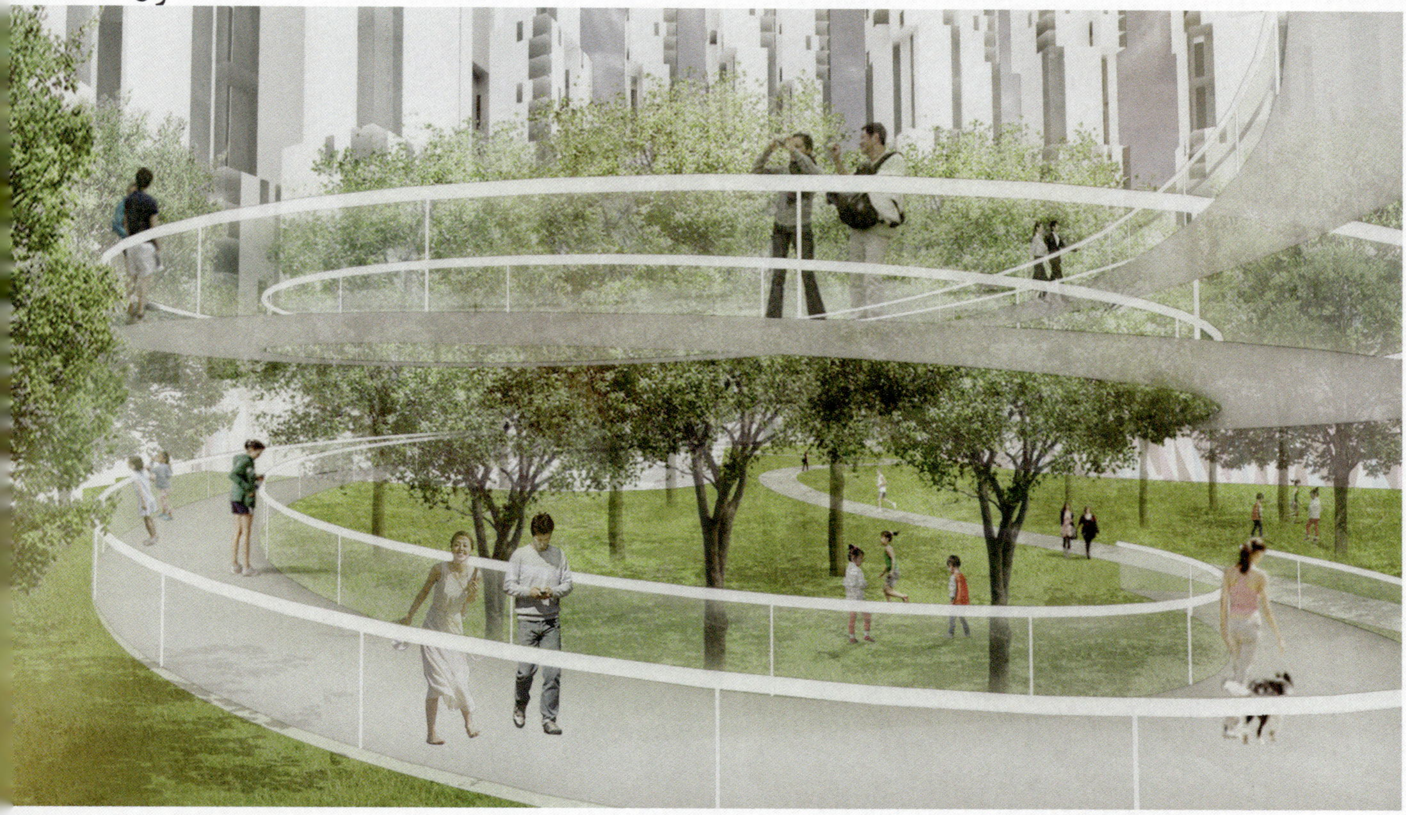

Taking three specific factors related to human health as a guide, Wen Wen, Won Joon Seol and Whitney Hansley identified a range of associations or relationships between aspects of the built environment and its capacity to support healthy life practices. These factors were identified as physical activity, diet, and sustainable environments. These three factors were extrapolated into a series of quantifiable parameters that could be used to determine significant aspects of the block's organization and design features.

The ambition of the projects developed by Wen Wen and Won Joon Seol as well as Whitney Hansley, offers a view of the consequences of quantified health related parameters driving the arrangement of our built environment in a largely singular manner. Almost myopic in its dedicated attempt to accommodate these concerns within a block, the projects locate opportunities in ratios that impose difficult constraints.

The projects also propose a model of neighborhoods that make explicit and tangible the typically abstract ideas of human and environmental health by making the consequences of their lifestyle choices physical and immediately evident to its residents and users. The result are neighborhoods that achieve some didactic value in communicating these issues while also offering a vision of novel living environments that creates a potentially desirable quality of life based on quantitative data.

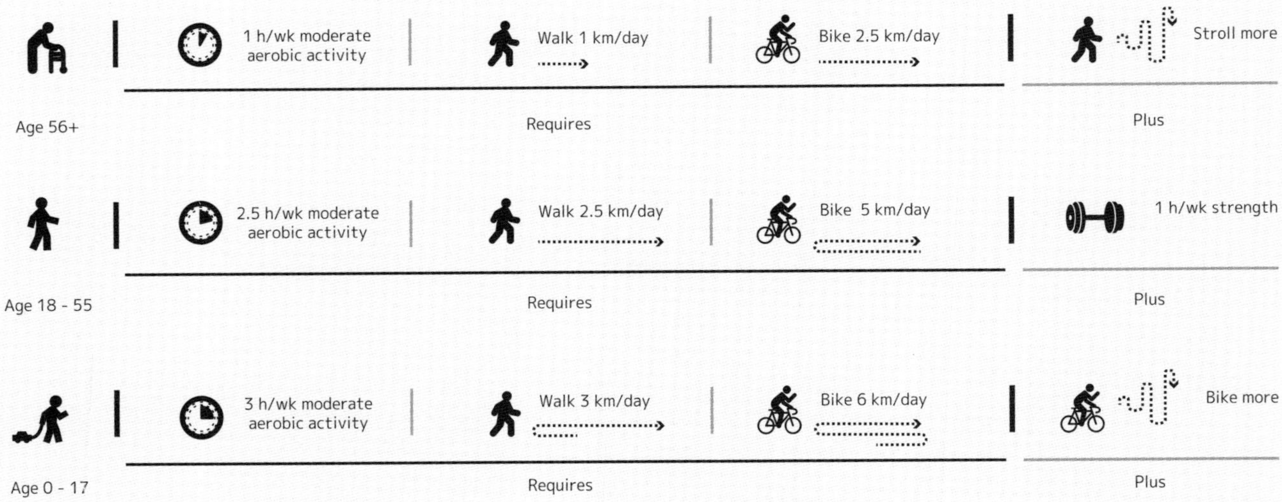

Physical activity was formulated into a series of metrics for the appropriate level of exercise each age range is expected to partake in on a daily basis in order to maintain a healthy lifestyle. These were then translated into daily walking distances and actual linear meters of track or paths that would be needed to facilitate this. The intention would be to embed this requirement within the block itself.

Source: Health and Places Initiative, 2014

"METs" means "metabolic equivalents."
One Met is the amount of energy a person would expend while sitting quietly. The amount of energy a person uses depends on the intensity of the activity, and the person's body mass. To find out how many calories you have burned, use the following formula: Energy expenditure (in calories per minute) = 0.0175 cals/kg/min x MET x Body mass (kg) x time (minutes).

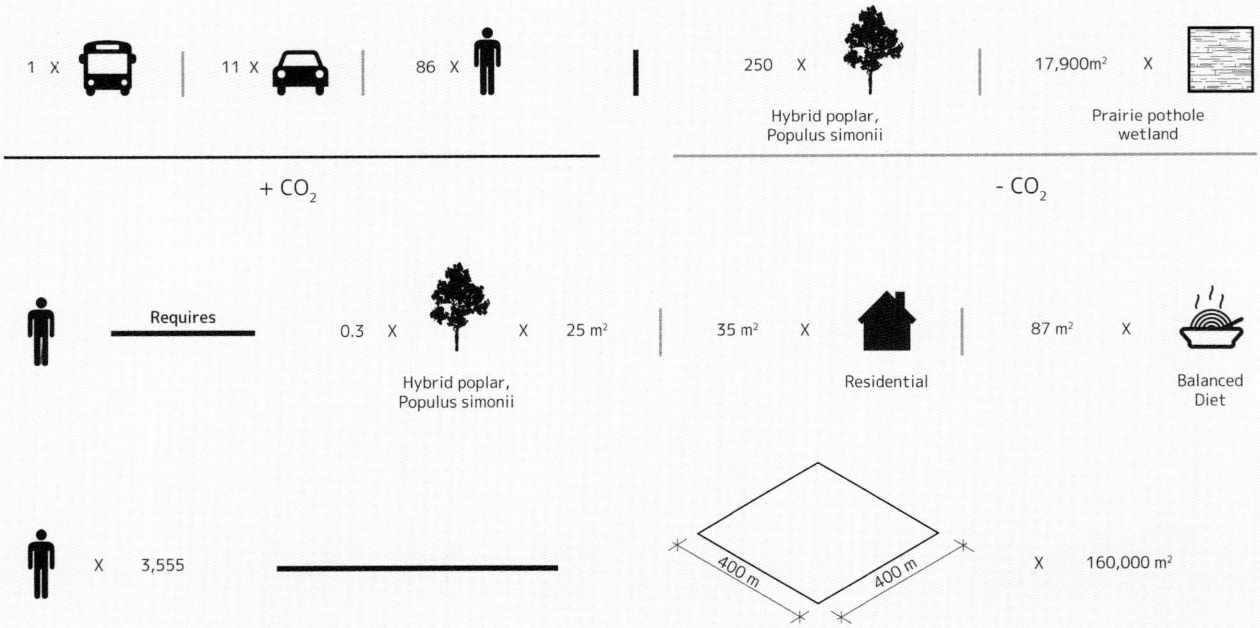

Making the block support the health of the environment was structured as a relationship between carbon sequestration and car ownership. An assumed level of car ownership and its use was translated into levels of carbon production. To make the consequence of this life choice visible and also as a means to mediate this potentially damaging practice (for the environment as well as human health), trees and wetland areas were studied for their capacity for carbon sequestration. A one-to-one relationship between car ownership and the amount of trees or wetland area that would need to be cultivated in the block to counter or offset the carbon produced was identified. This would simultaneously be a punitive measure (the higher the car ownership, the more of the block area you will need to retain for trees) and perhaps a positive quality for the neighborhood (the more the trees, the more "nature" or recreational forest it would have).

Source: Health and Places Initiative, 2014

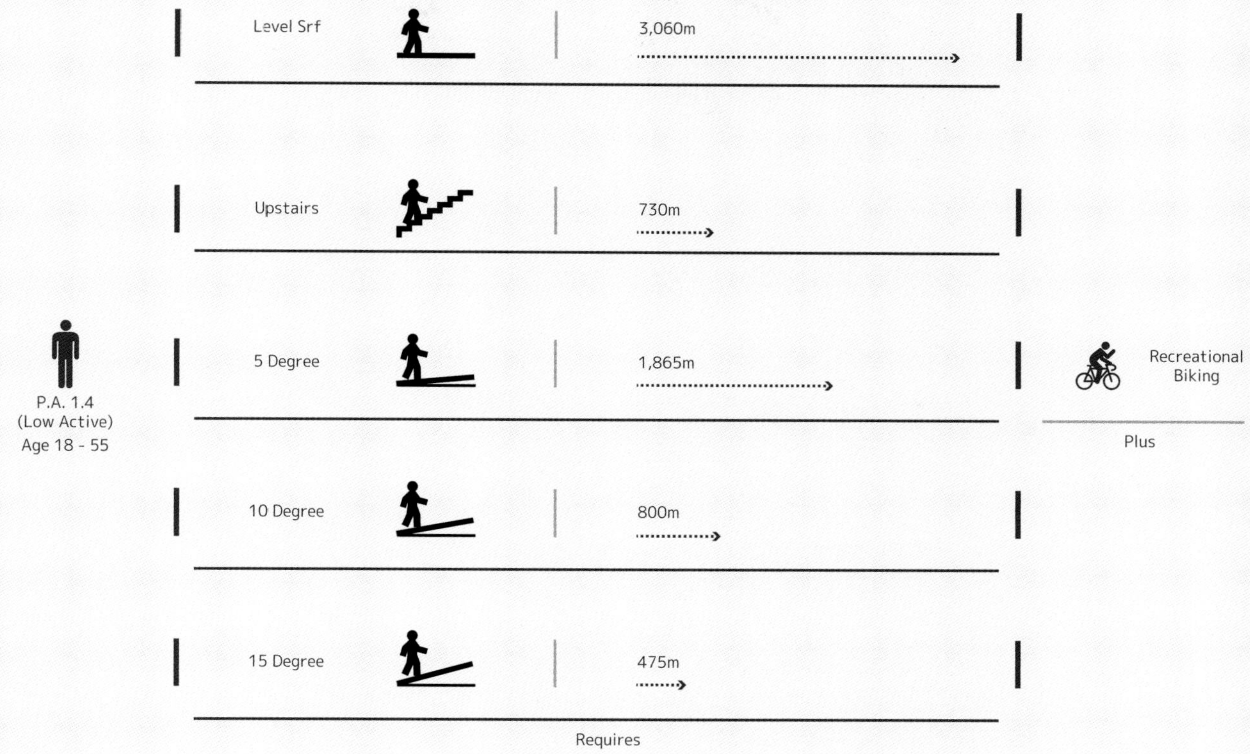

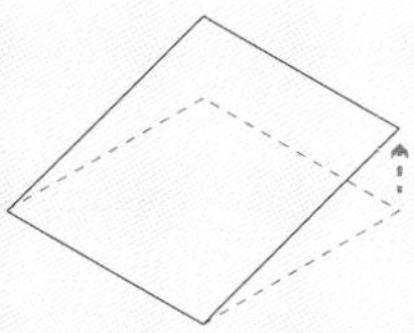

Another way to accommodate the recommended physical activity of its residents is through the introduction of slopes and gradients to the walking and cycling tracks. These can help alleviate the necessary linear meters of circulation paths as more METs are expended when the level of difficulty of walking is increased by a steep incline. The pedestrian and cycling network for the block were considered both as a means for commuting and circulation as well as a form of exercise or gym equipment.

Source: Health and Places Initiative, 2014

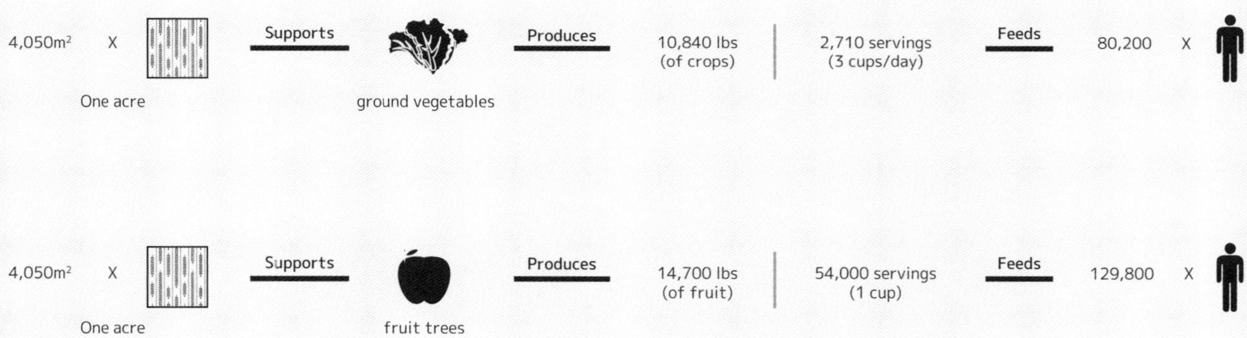

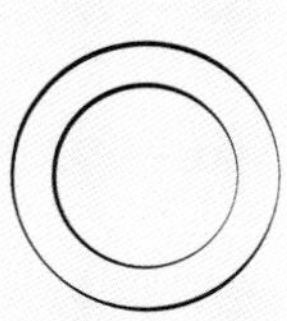

Dietary habits and nutrition were considered in relationship to the amount of area required to cultivate fruits and vegetables to support a healthy eating habit for its residents. One of the problems with China's food security can be identified in the broken cold chain. It was decided by the team that cultivating many of the perishables needed for a healthy diet close to the residents would provide many benefits such as preventing waste, and potentially ensuring quality while, again; making the consequences of the resident's healthy life choices tangible.

Source: World Health Organization, 2015

Schematic Visualizations

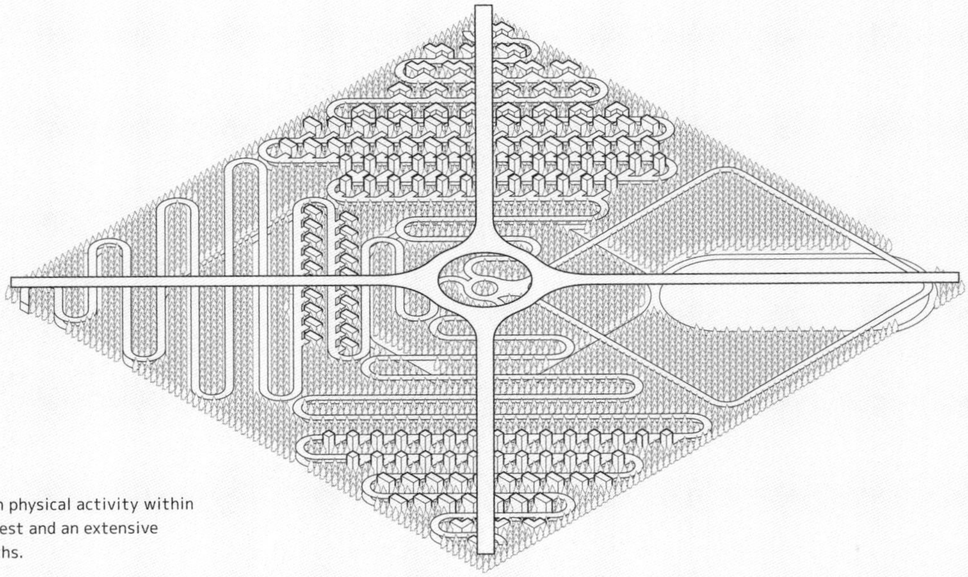

Scenario 1
Balancing carbon sequestration with physical activity within the block. This results in a large forest and an extensive network of pedestrian and cycle paths.

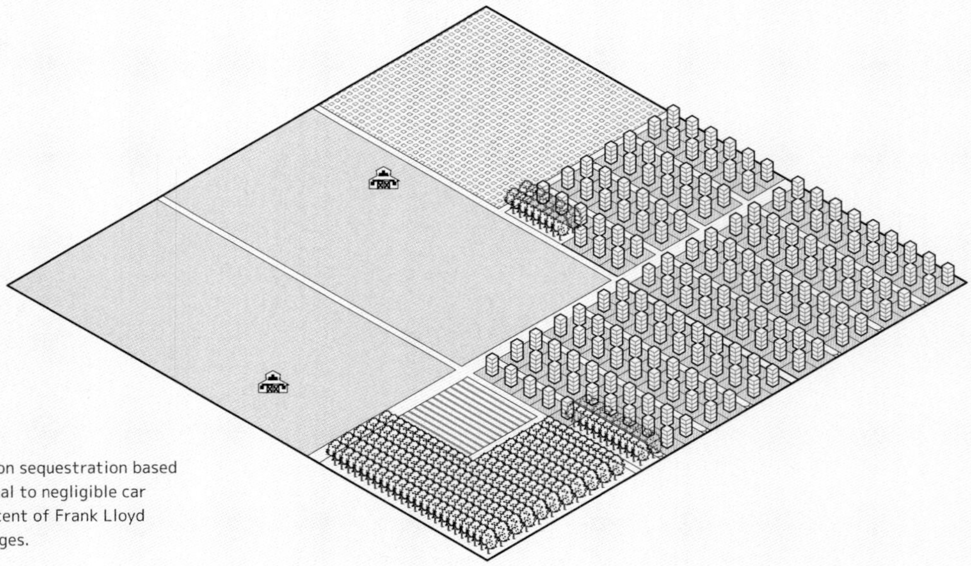

Scenario 2
Balancing food production and carbon sequestration based on a resident population with minimal to negligible car ownership. An organization reminiscent of Frank Lloyd Wright's Broadacre City model emerges.

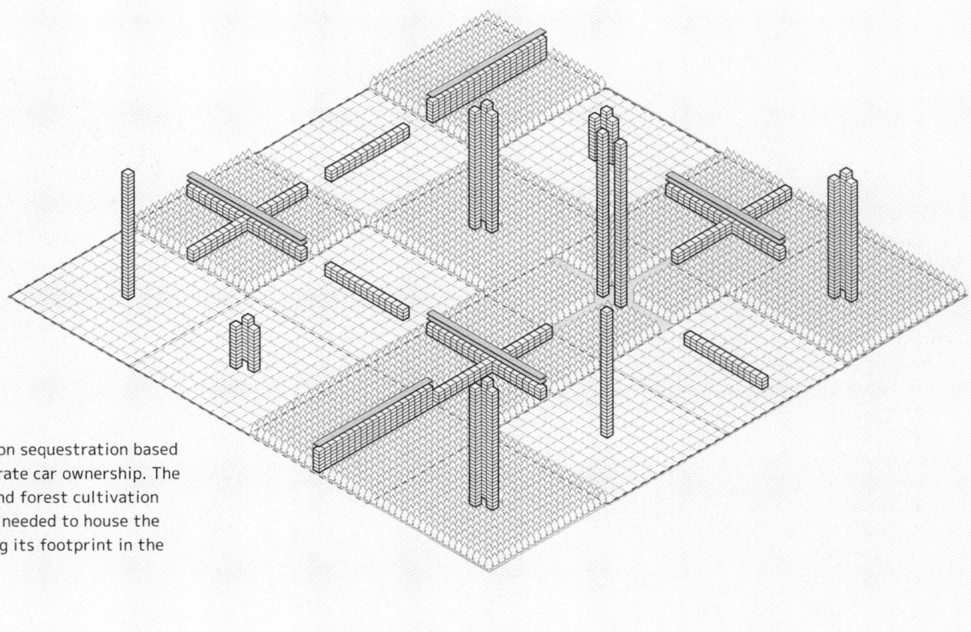

Scenario 3
Balancing food production and carbon sequestration based on a resident population with moderate car ownership. The amount of area dedicated to food and forest cultivation impacts the kinds of building types needed to house the resident population while minimizing its footprint in the block.

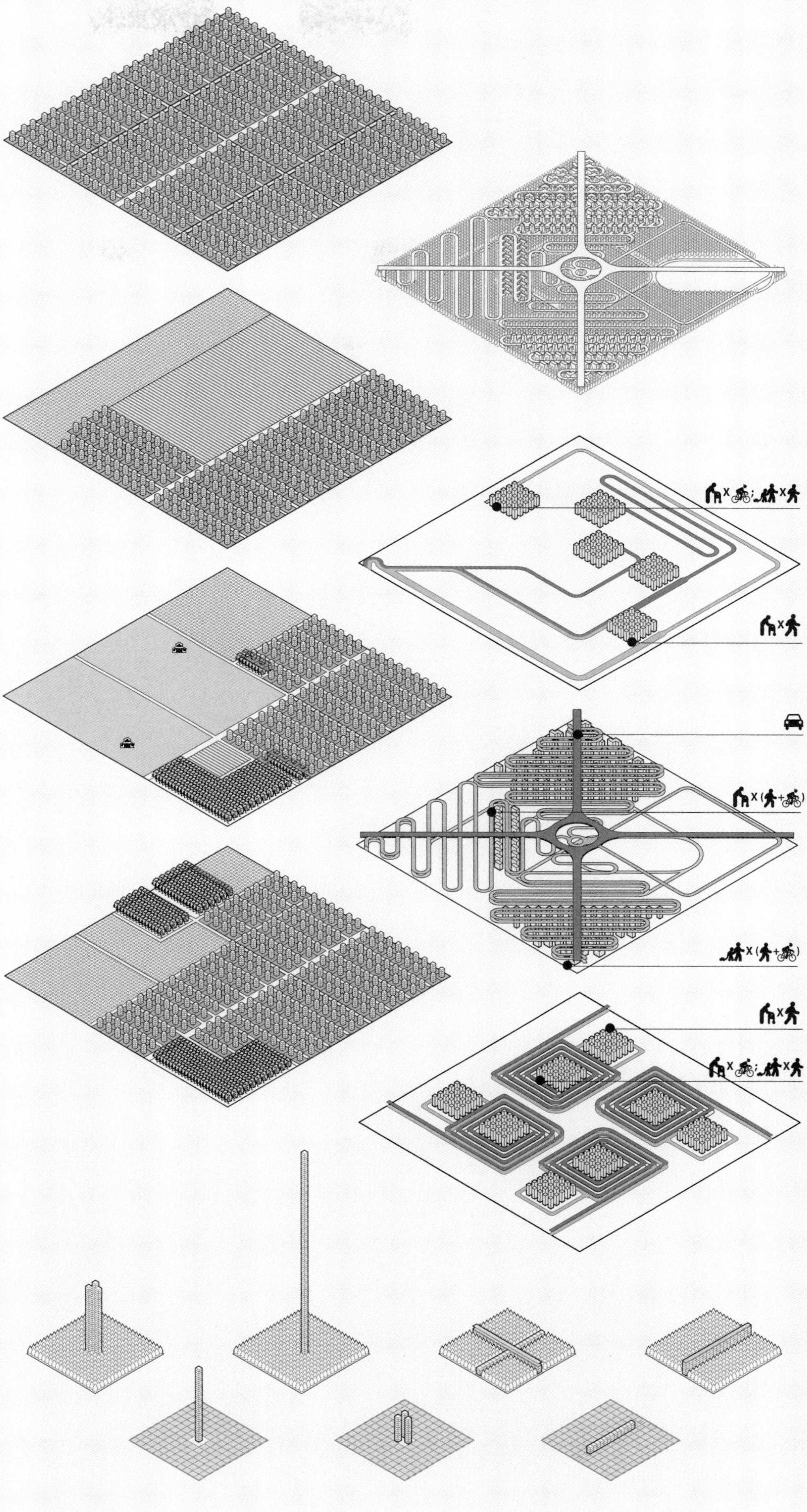

Varying iterations and scenarios generated by multiple negotiations between the health-related parameters and projected residential populations. The wide range of possible scenarios motivated the decision to propose two separate detail design proposals based on different iterations / scenarios: one developed by Wen Wen and Joon Won, the other by Whitney Hansley.

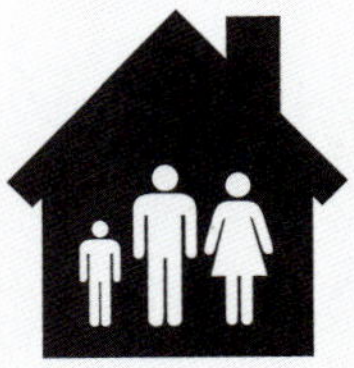

Unit and building types are informed by a series of projected lifestyle scenarios centered on a number of assumed subjects / actors. Design and organization features were guided by a strategy to encourage physical activity even within buildings.

"Villa" Type

The "villa type" features a three-bedroom unit that is distributed over three floors. Vertical circulation on opposite ends of the floor plate promotes physical activity within the residential portion (staircases).

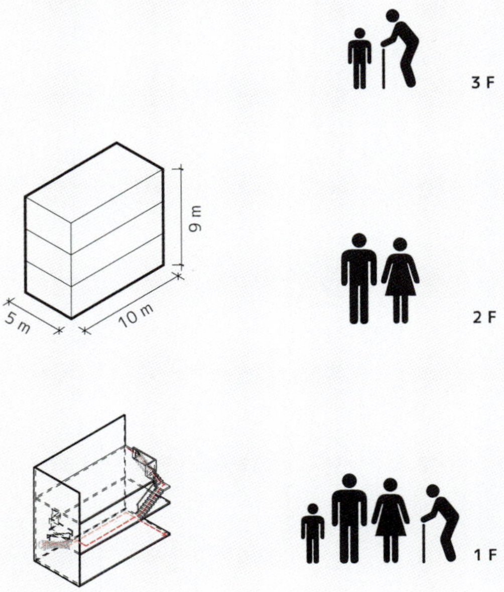

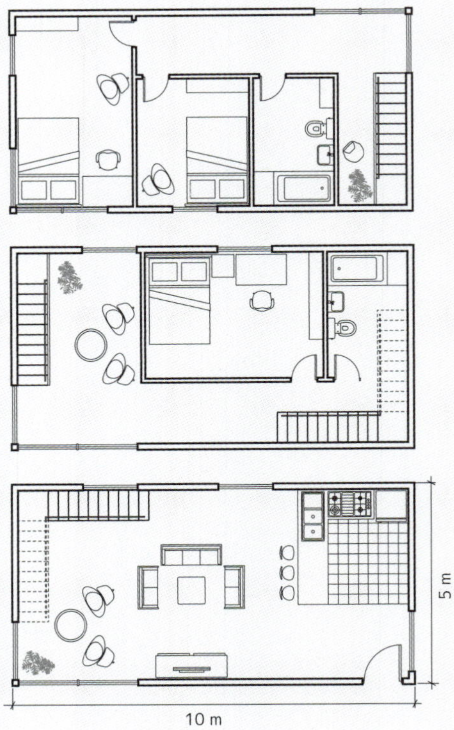

"Studio" Type

The "studio type" features a studio unit that occupies one entire floor. Three studios make up one module, and are connected by staircases on the exterior. These units can be accessed by foot on the ground level, and by bike on the roof level.

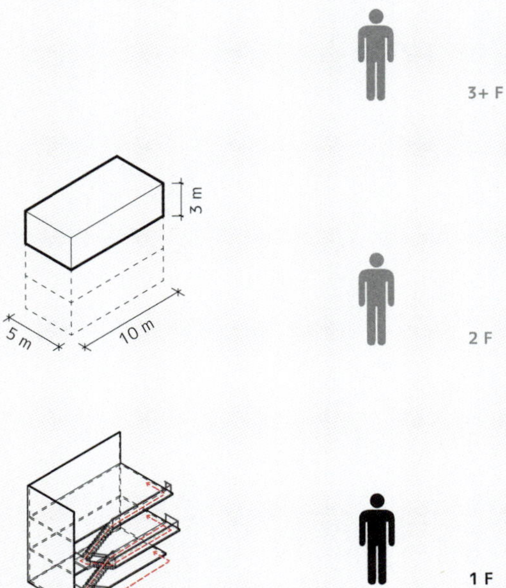

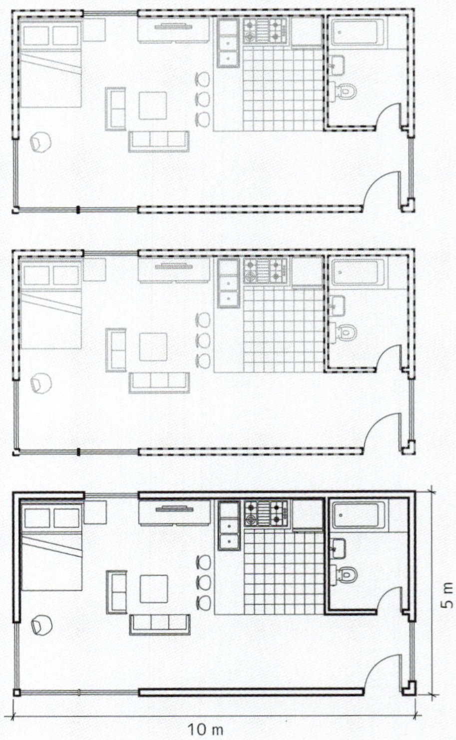

In Wen Wen and Joon Won's final block proposal, the team chose to focus on balancing physical activity and carbon sequestration concerns.

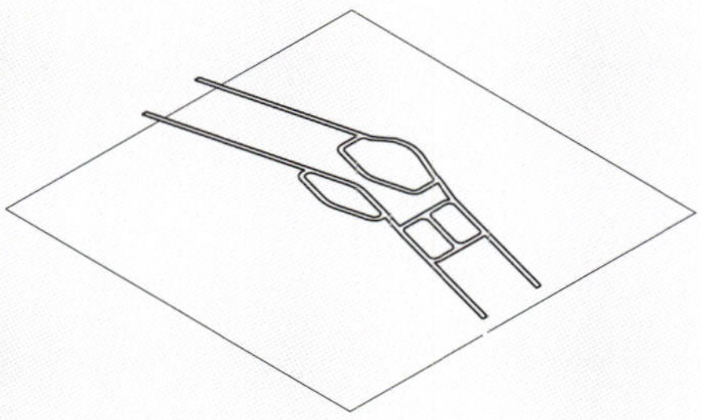

Elevated cycle network

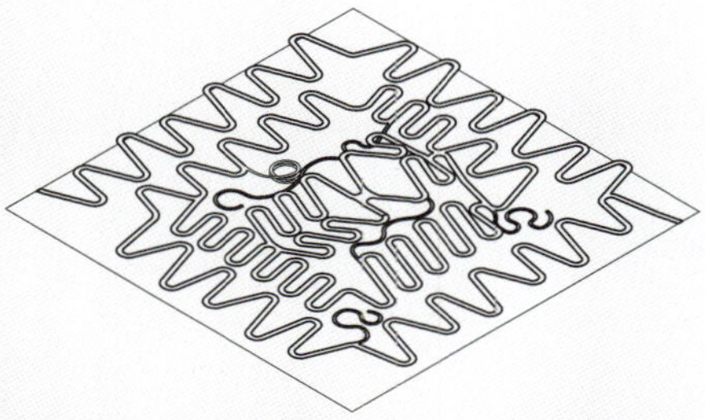

Elevated pedestrian network

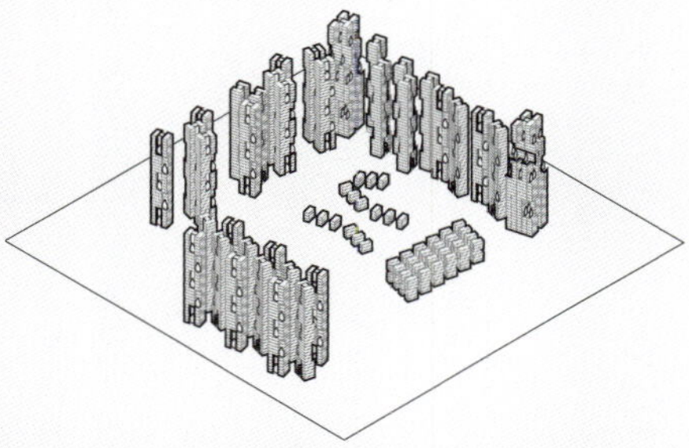

Residential buildings (including live / work units)

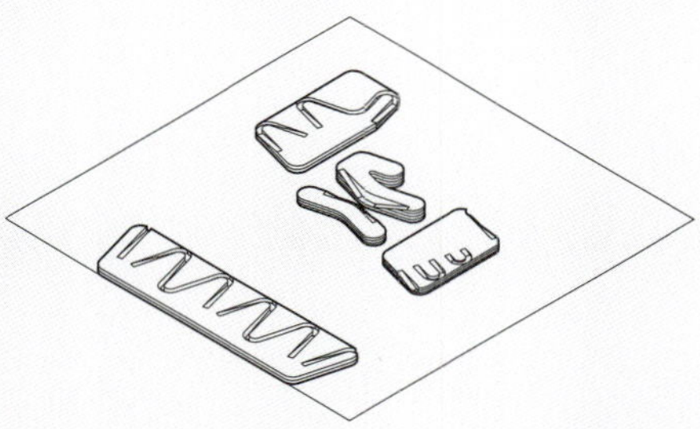

Amenities, retail and large offices

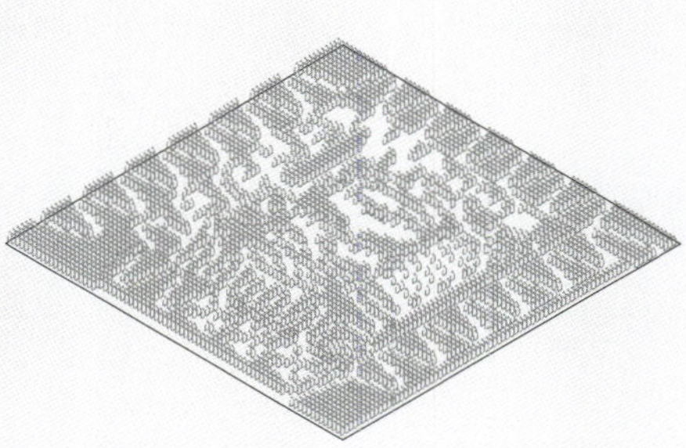

Forest

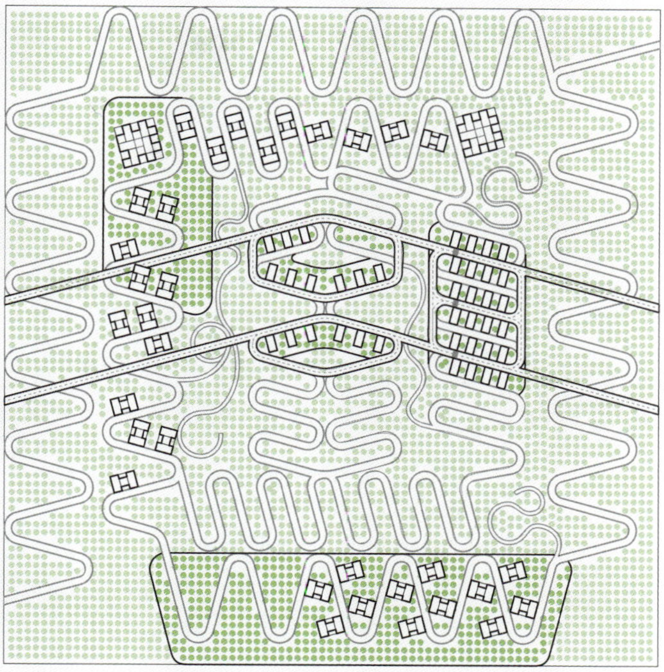

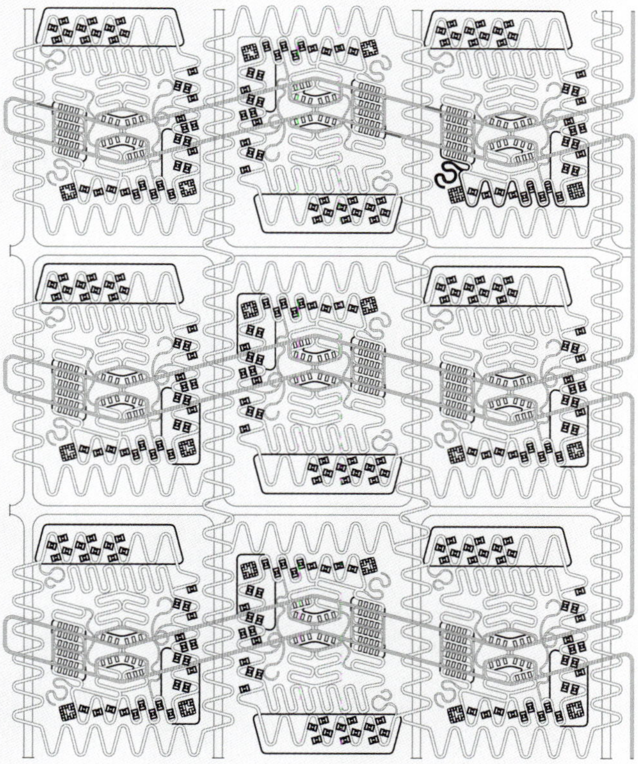

Schematic Plan of Larger Neighborhood (composed of nine blocks)

When aggregated at larger scales, the proposal transforms a wider area into a large forest / park criss-crossed by an extensive commuting / recreational exercise network of cycle, running and pedestrian tracks / trails.

The distribution of unit and housing types is determined by the appropriate physical activity quota for different age groups.

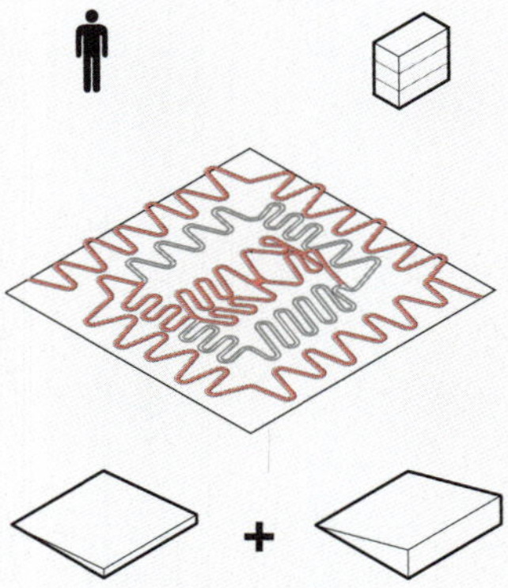

Youth/able-bodied network (access to studio units includes steepest sloped walkways)

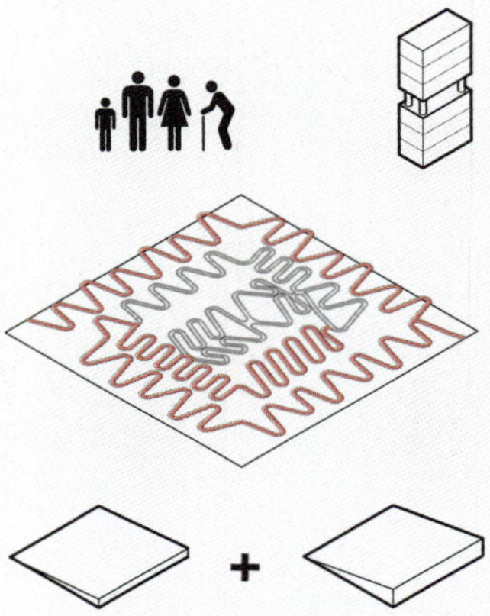

Family / elderly network (access to medium-rise and villa-type housing)

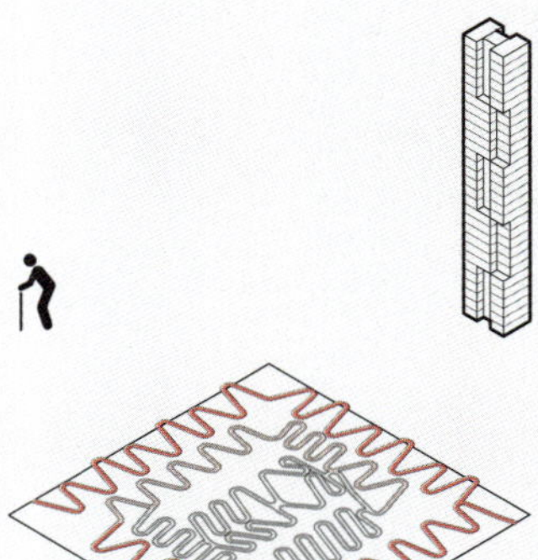

Elderly network (access to high-rises with elevators)

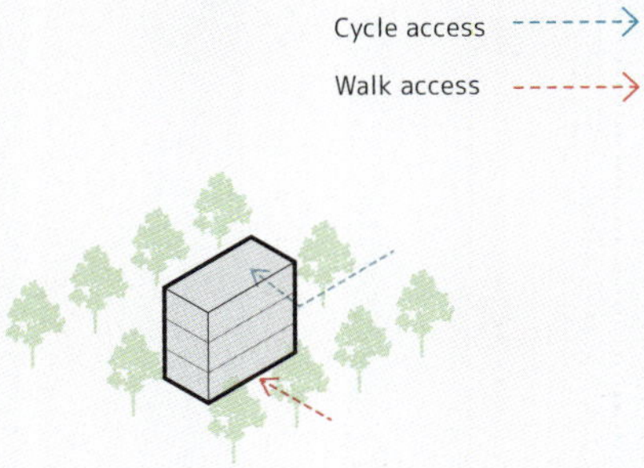

Studio units are distributed as pavilion type structures in the deepest part of the block. It's a long walk but you enjoy the most immersive experience of living in "nature".

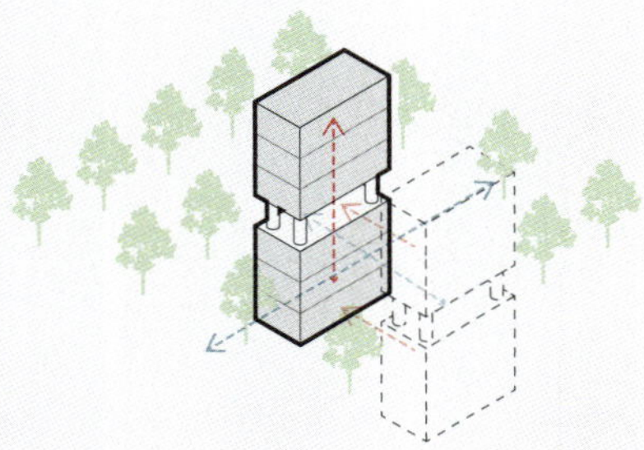

Villa units allow cycle and pedestrian access from the middle floors of the building, encouraging walking up and down to your units.

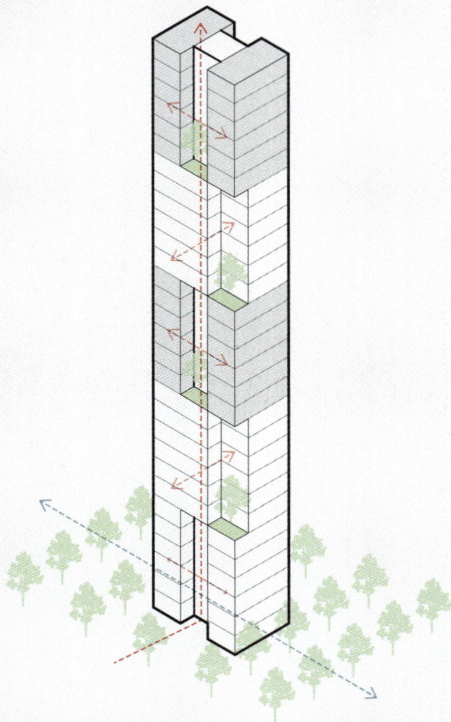

High-rise units are the only building types that require elevators. These are most suitable for the very elderly and people who require assistance for walking. Social spaces are scattered throughout the height of the building to encourage short walks from the resident's respective units.

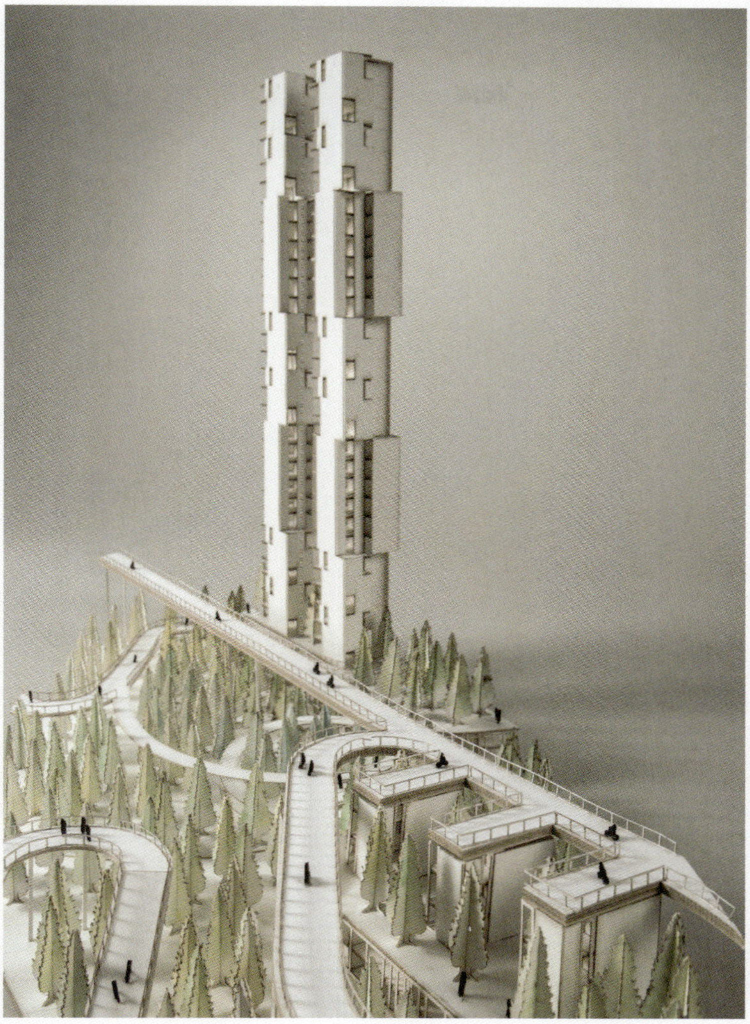

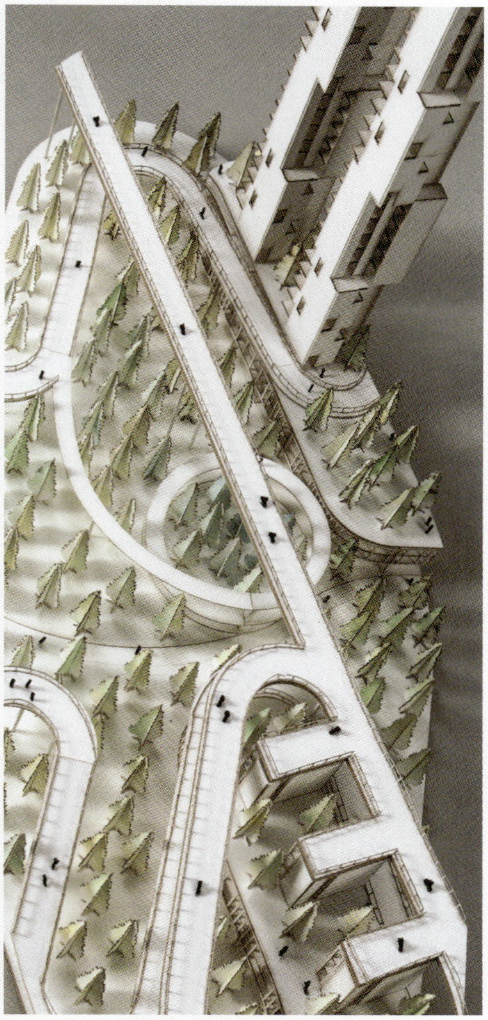

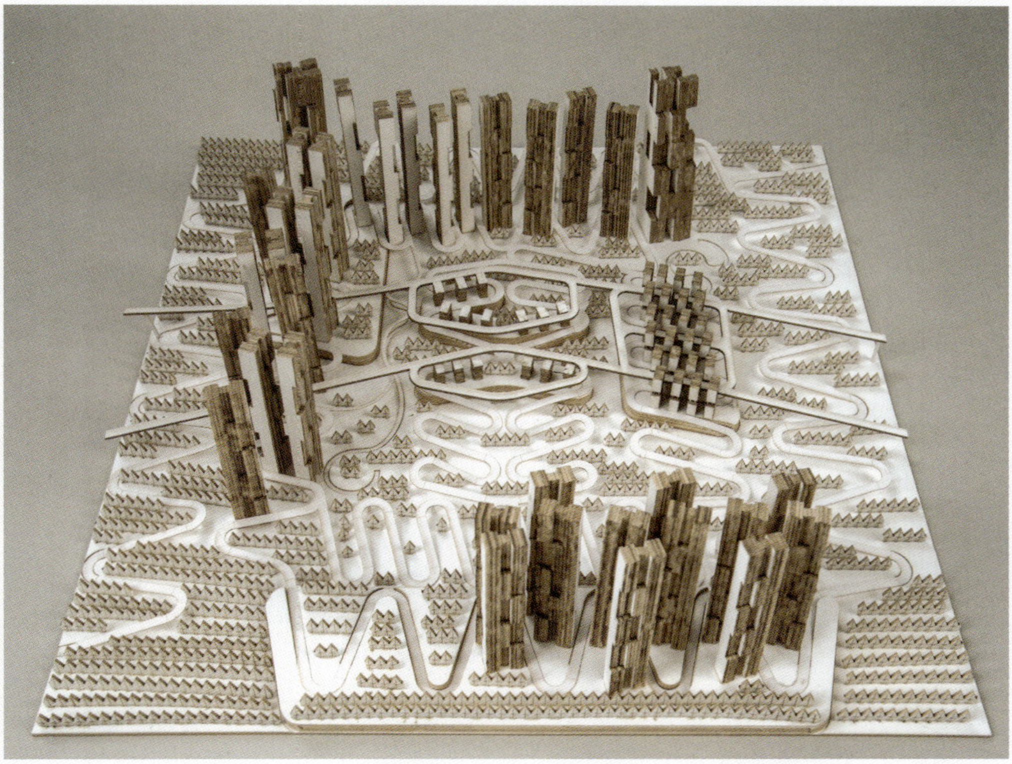

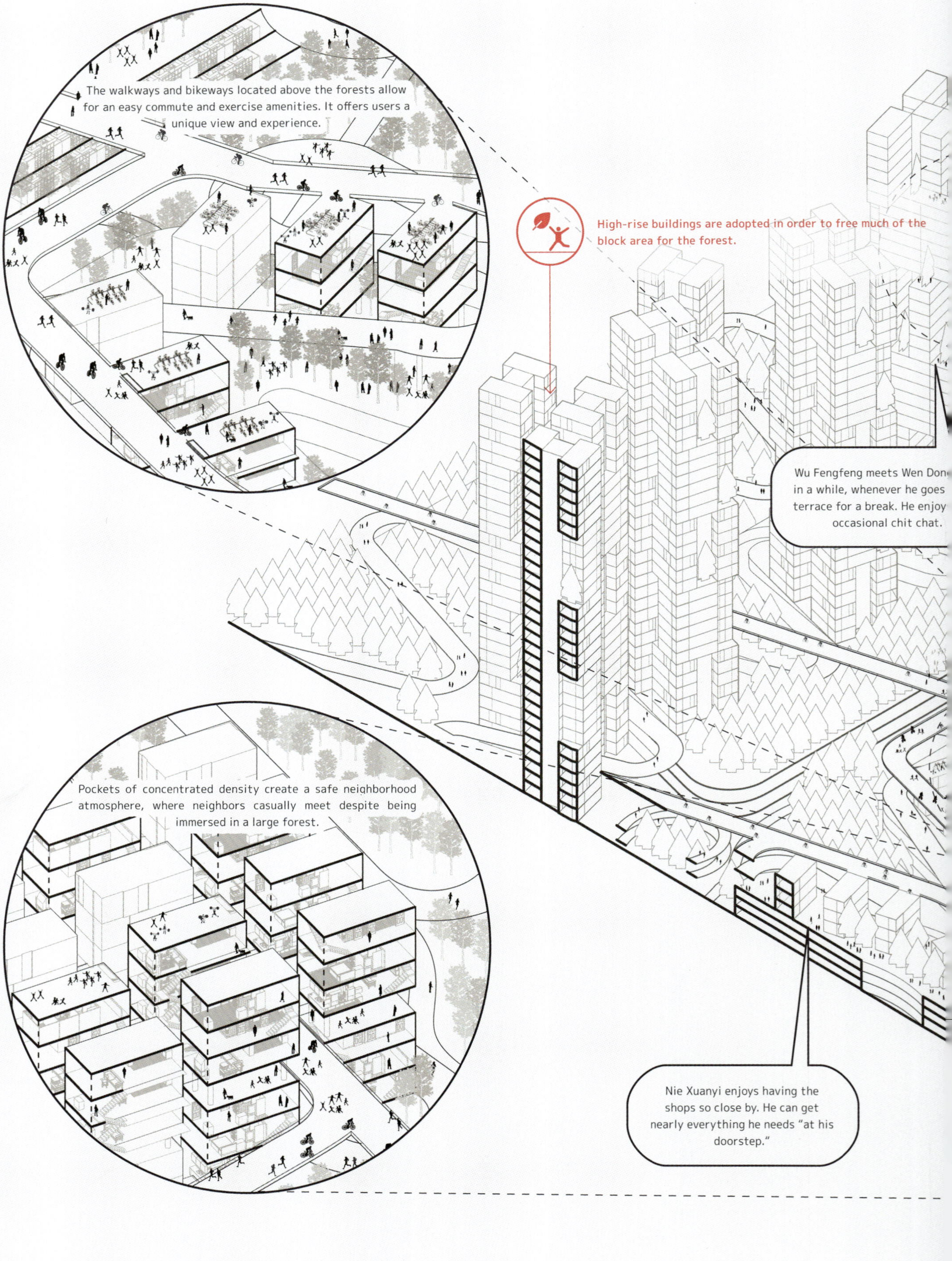
The walkways and bikeways located above the forests allow for an easy commute and exercise amenities. It offers users a unique view and experience.
High-rise buildings are adopted in order to free much of the block area for the forest.
Wu Fengfeng meets Wen Don
in a while, whenever he goes
terrace for a break. He enjoy
occasional chit chat.
Pockets of concentrated density create a safe neighborhood atmosphere, where neighbors casually meet despite being immersed in a large forest.
Nie Xuanyi enjoys having the shops so close by. He can get nearly everything he needs "at his doorstep."

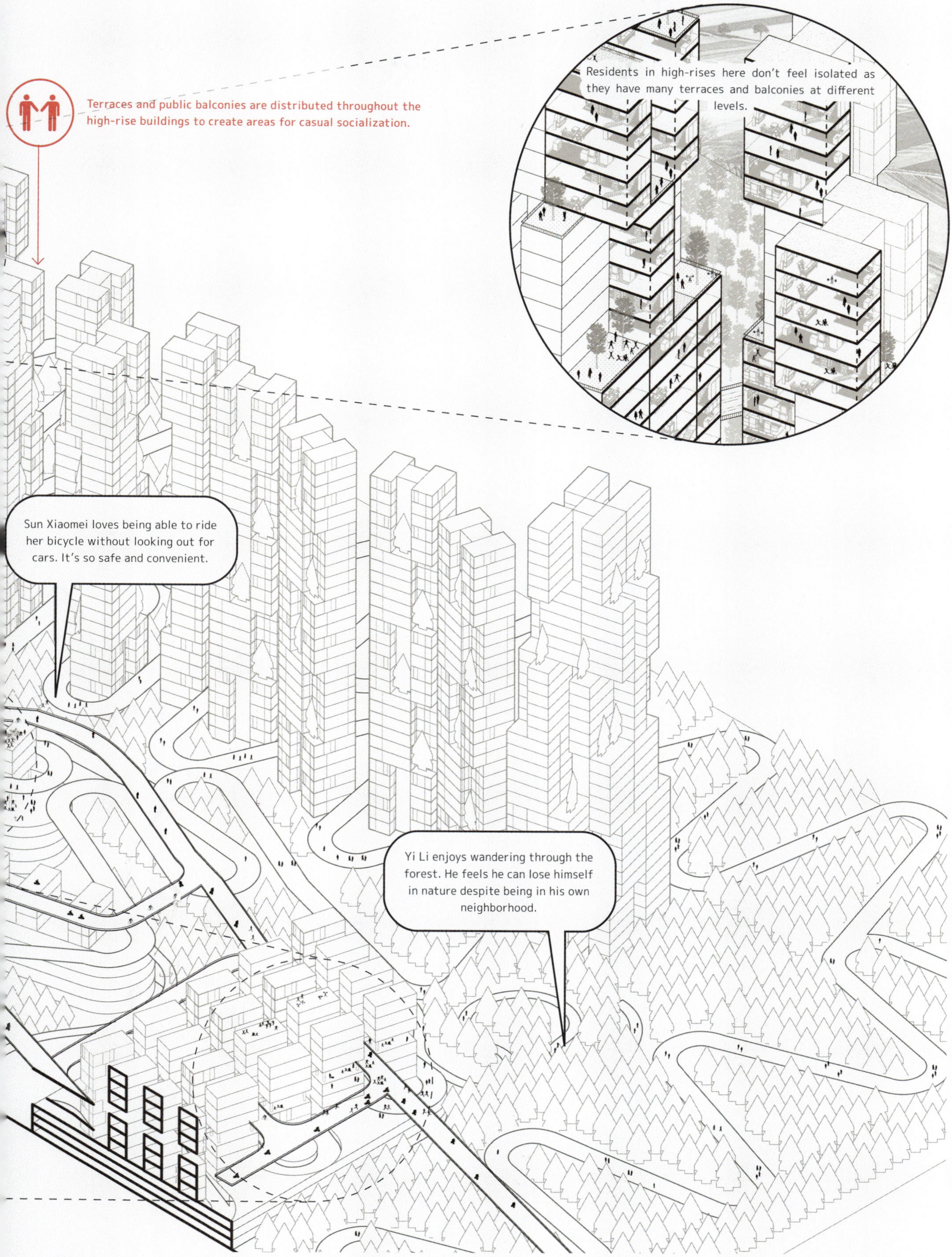
Terraces and public balconies are distributed throughout the high-rise buildings to create areas for casual socialization.
Residents in high-rises here don't feel isolated as they have many terraces and balconies at different levels.
Sun Xiaomei loves being able to ride her bicycle without looking out for cars. It's so safe and convenient.
Yi Li enjoys wandering through the forest. He feels he can lose himself in nature despite being in his own neighborhood.

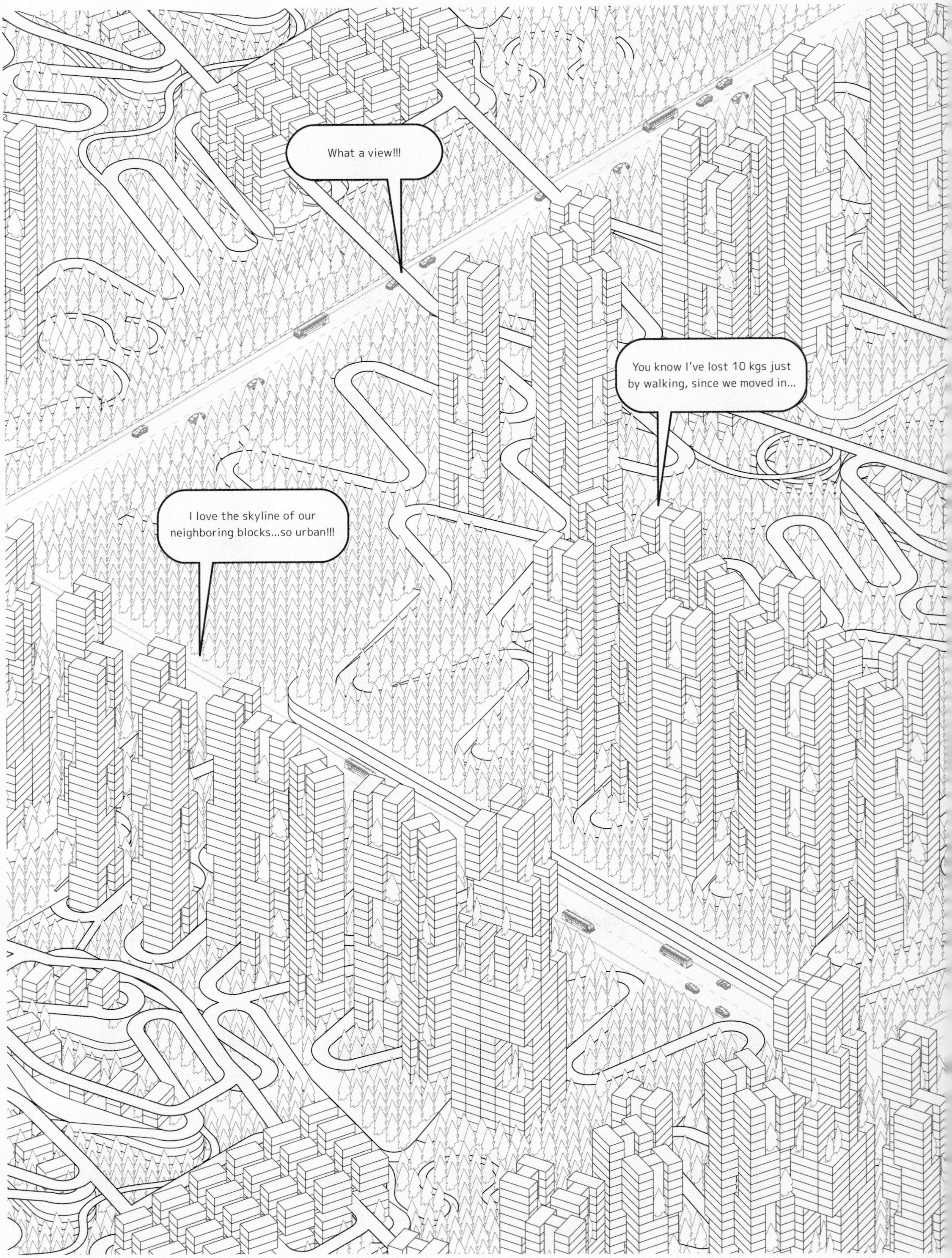
What a view!!!
You know I've lost 10 kgs just by walking, since we moved in...
I love the skyline of our neighboring blocks...so urban!!!

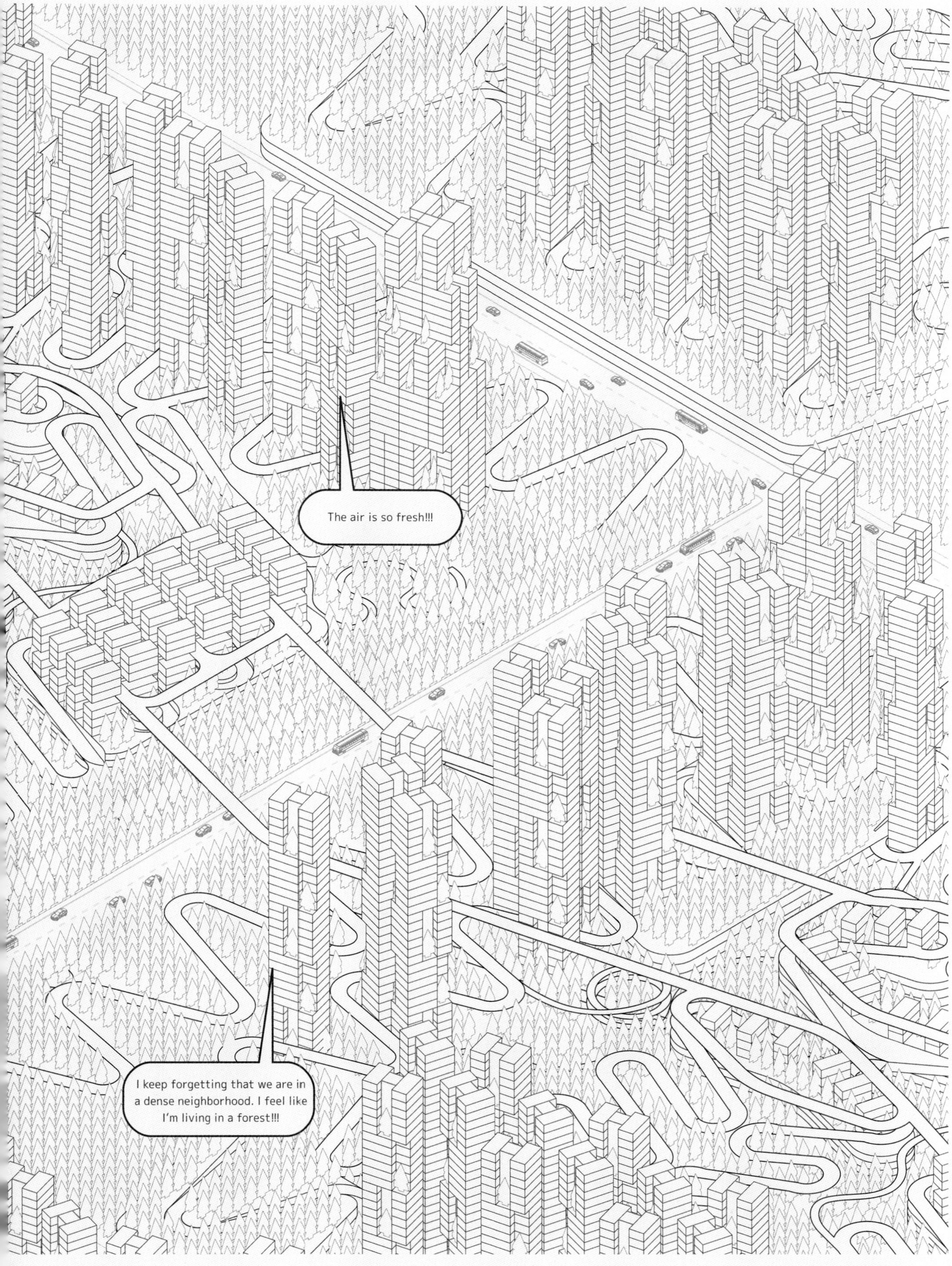
The air is so fresh!!!
I keep forgetting that we are in a dense neighborhood. I feel like I'm living in a forest!!!

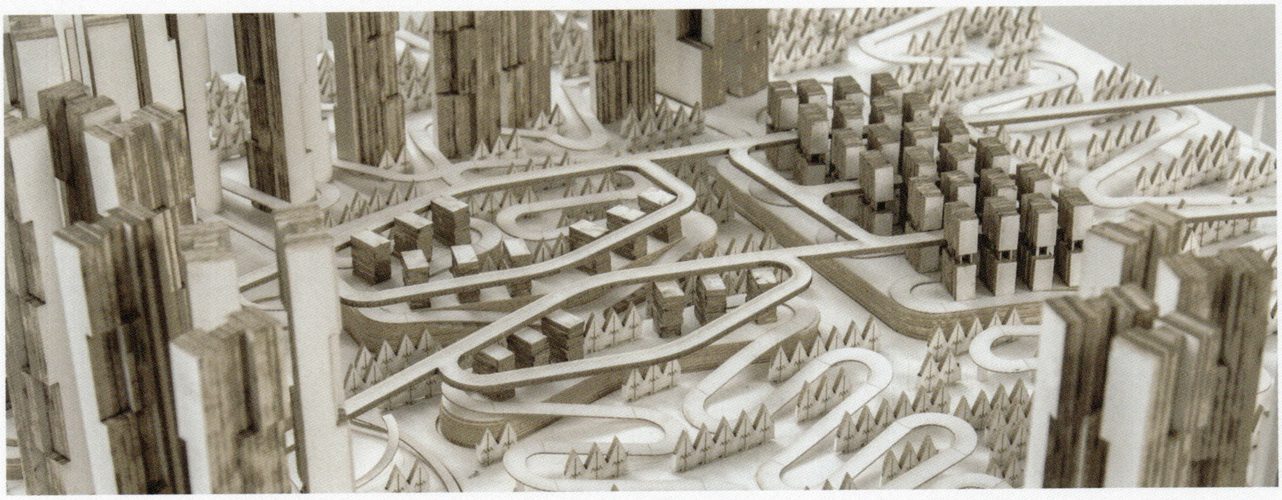

(Page 257) Views of detail and overall massing models (This Page, Top) Detail view of overall massing model (This Page, Bottom) Detail view of the elevated pedestrian and cycle network. (Photographs by Anita Kan)

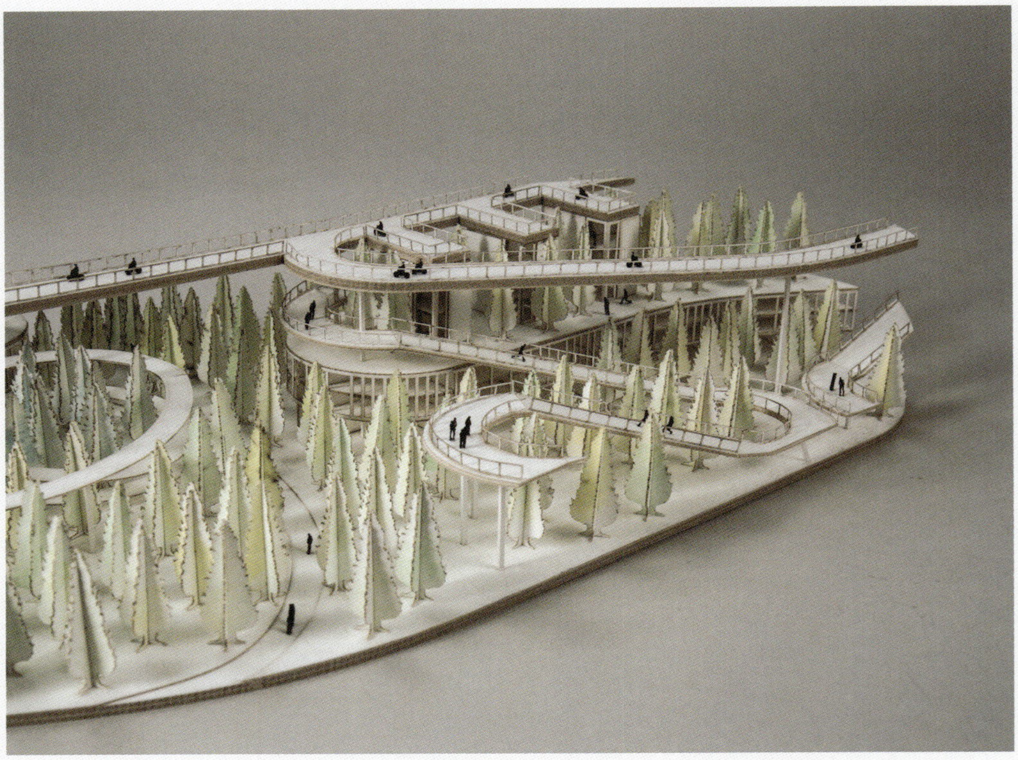

References

Health and Places Initiative, 2014, "Physiology and Psychology of Aging, Health, and Place. A Research Brief." http://research.gsd.harvard.edu/hapi/files/2014/10/HAPI_ReserachBrief-Aging-PhyPsy-102814-FINAL.pdf.

Health and Places Initiative, 2014, "Physical Activity, Health, and Place. A Research Brief." Version 1.0. http://research.gsd.harvard.edu/hapi/.

World Health Organization, 2015, "Physical Activity and Young People." Accessed May 29, 2015. http://www.who.int/dietphysicalactivity/factsheet_young_people/en/.

Farms, Forks, and the METs Between

Whitney Hansley

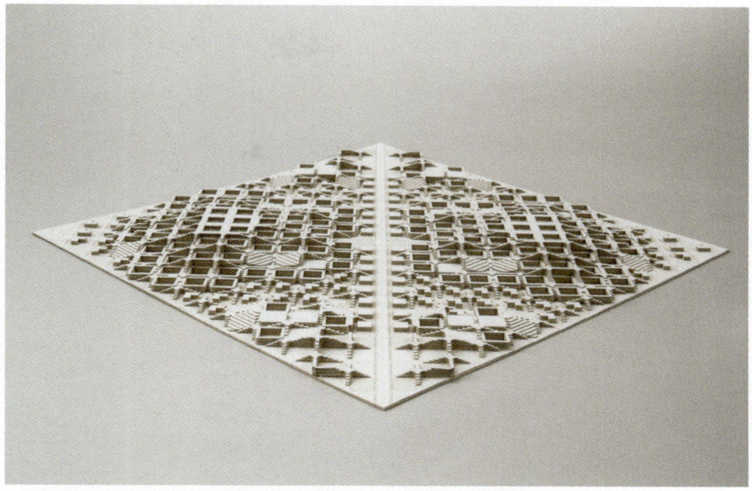

Massing model overall view. (Photograph by Anita Kan)

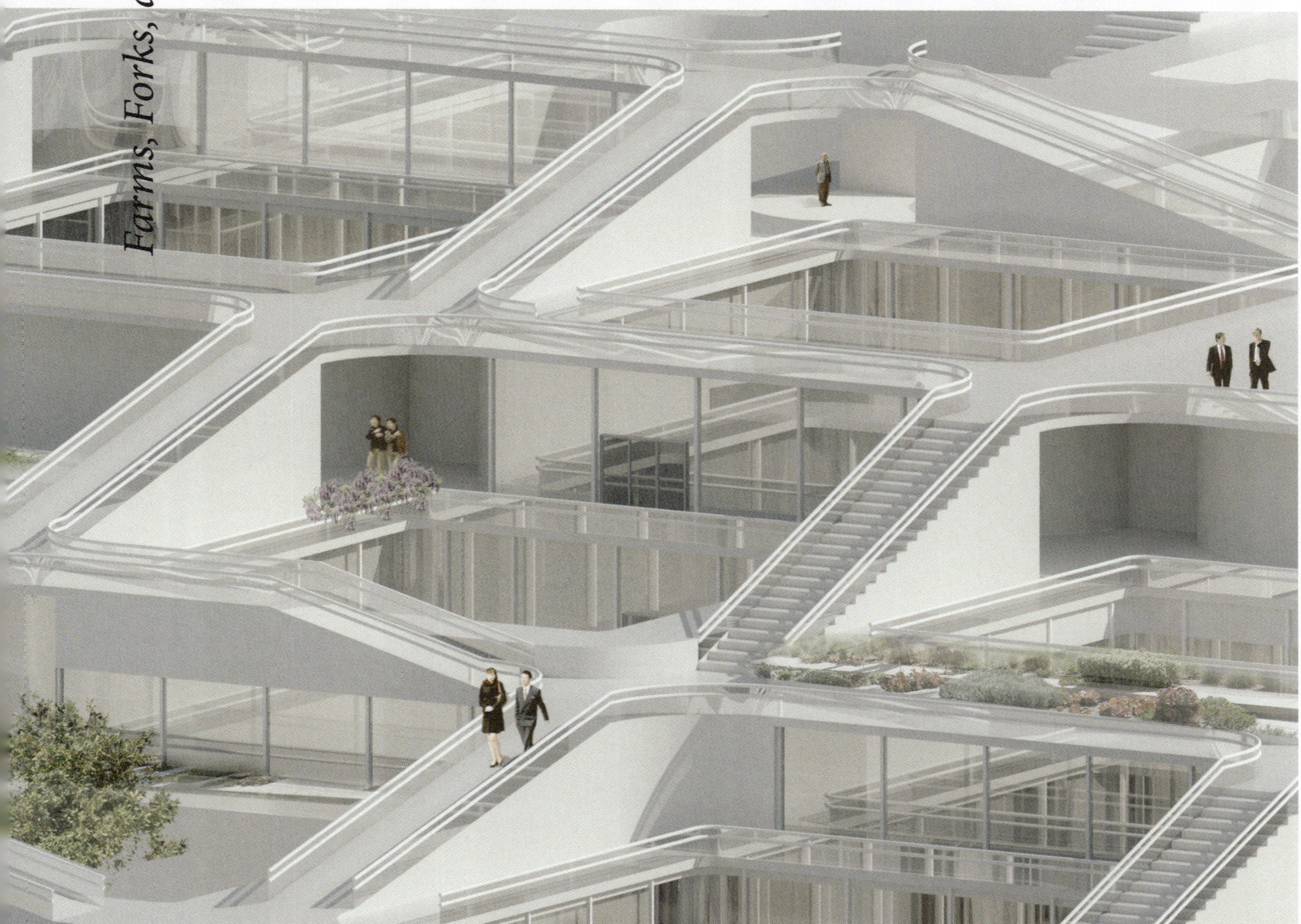

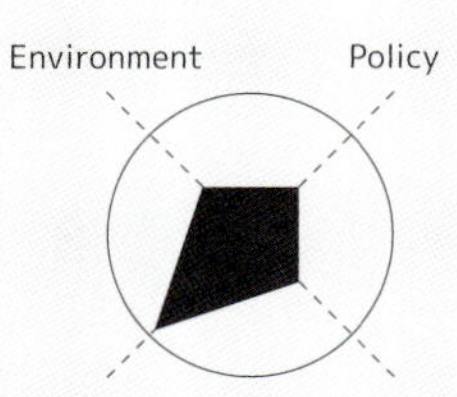

The Cold Chain in China is severely fragmented. Approximately twenty-five percent of all fruits and vegetables and twelve to fifteen percent of meat spoil due to improper refrigeration during the journey from fork to table. This project aims to tackle this problem through an architectural lens. Structured as a continuation of an earlier exploration, the project holds a desire to maintain immediate proximity to foods within the cold chain with the intention of increasing physical activity and offsetting carbon emissions. Recognizing that people will ultimately choose the course of actions they prefer, the intent is to offer a matrix of endless possible routes and destinations so that they are able to both increase physical activity and constantly surround themselves with healthy food choices.

A Table of Area Requirements for Cultivating Food and its Capacity to Feed Residents

One animal	Needs	Produces	Feeds
	8,100m²	96 servings of milk/day (1 cup)	768 X
	0.36m²	8 servings/ whole chicken (3 oz) 1 serving/ day (1 egg)	3.2 or 0.4 X
	1,350m²	50 servings/ whole pig (3 oz)	20 X

One acre	Supports	Produces		Feeds
4,050m²	ground vegetables	10,840 lbs (of crop)	2,710 servings (3 cups/day)	80,200 X
4,050m²	fruit trees	14,700 lbs (of fruit)	54,000 servings (1 cup)	129,800 X
4,050m²	rice / wheat	6,500 lbs (of crop)	52,000 servings (1/4 cup)	2,054,320 X

Overall Schematic Block Organization

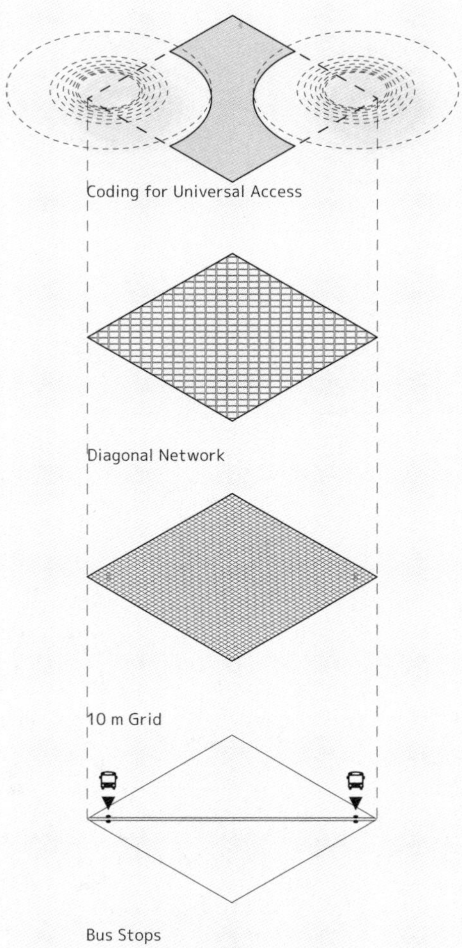

Schematic Block Organizations Based on Scenario of DifferentRatios Between Food Cultivation and Populations

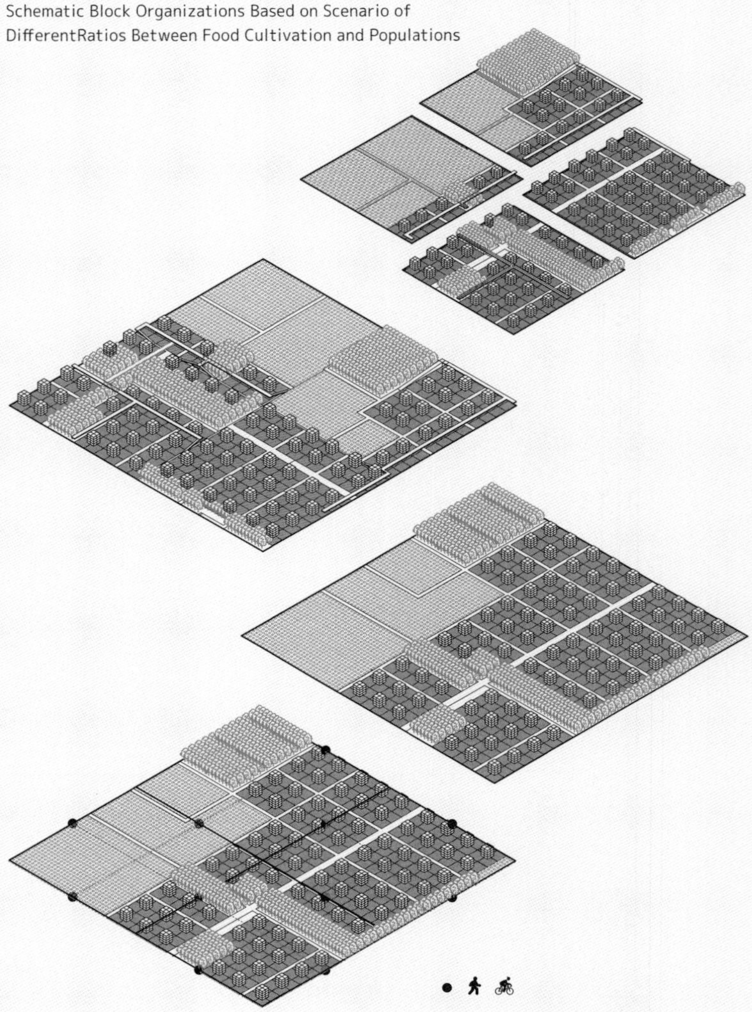

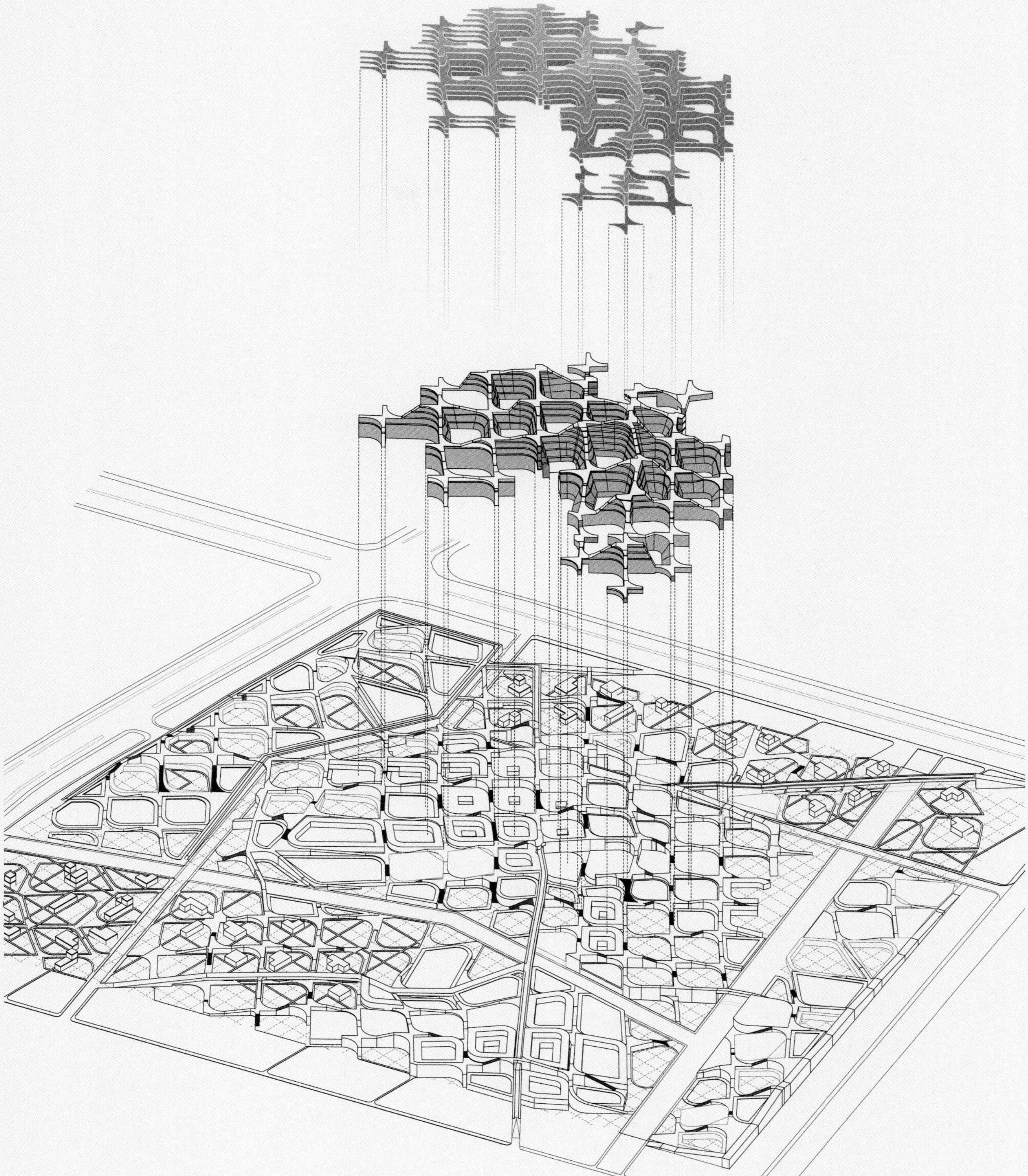

(Above) Exploded axonometric of the block's "topography." The block develops a new ground over, within, and under which its residents live.

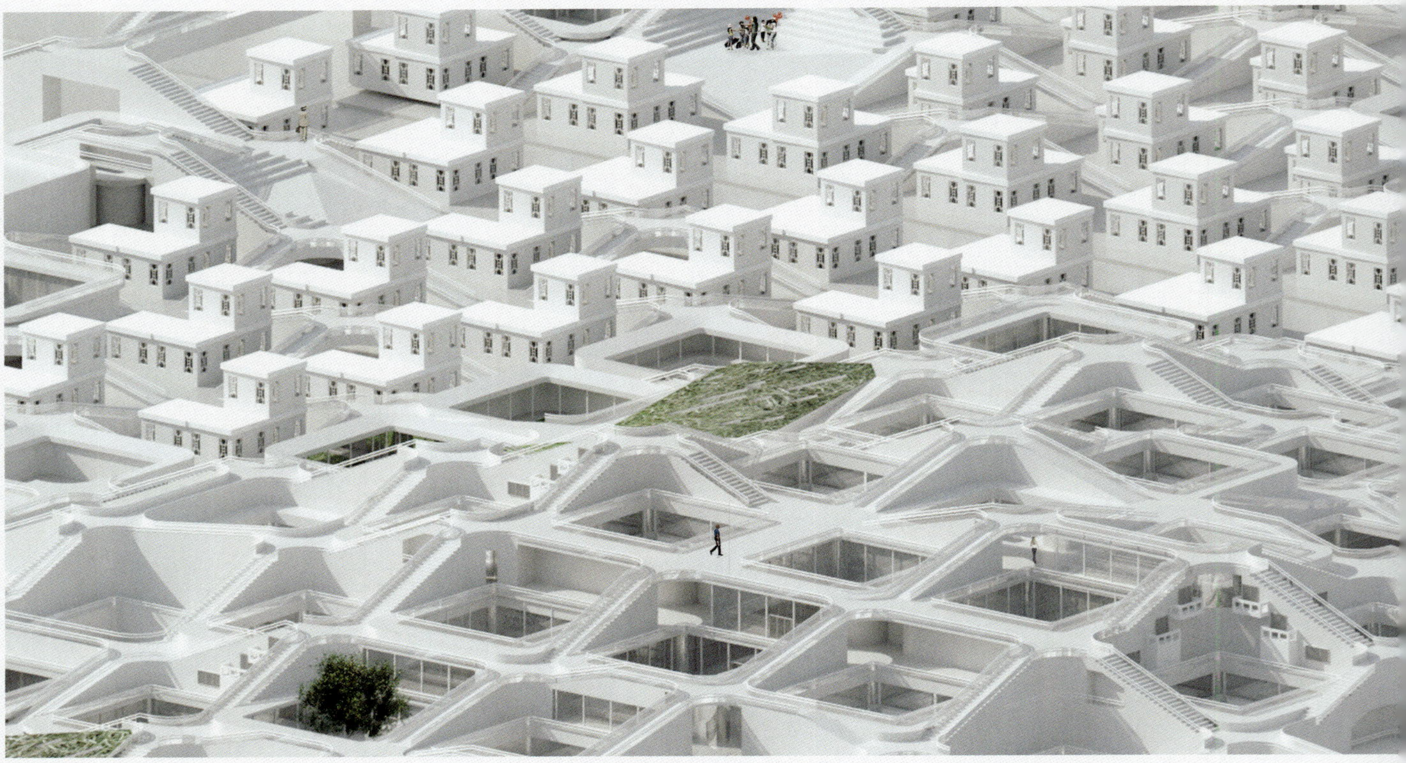

(Above) Detail of neighborhood block.
(Below) Section through topographic complex.

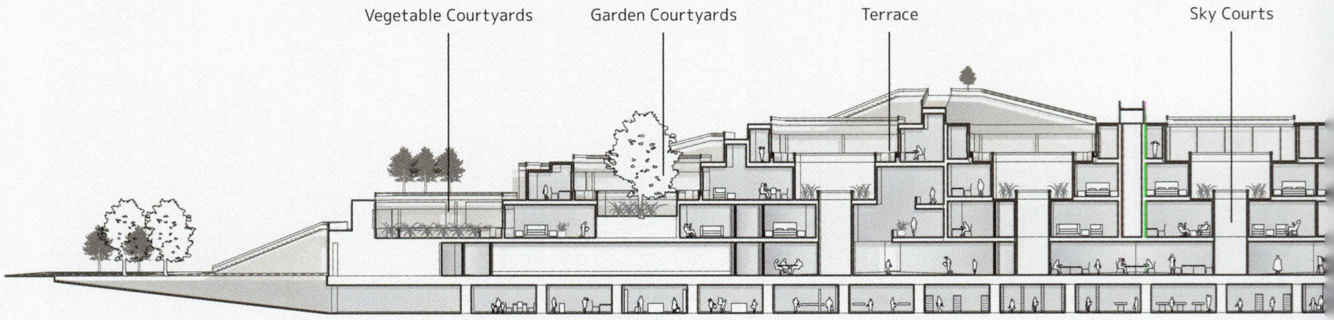

To accommodate the programs and ground area required for the cultivation, "topographic" building complexes are proposed that embed a "crust" of ground for physical excercise as well as smaller orchards and vegetable gardens.

Plan Diagram of the Distribution of the Block's Programs

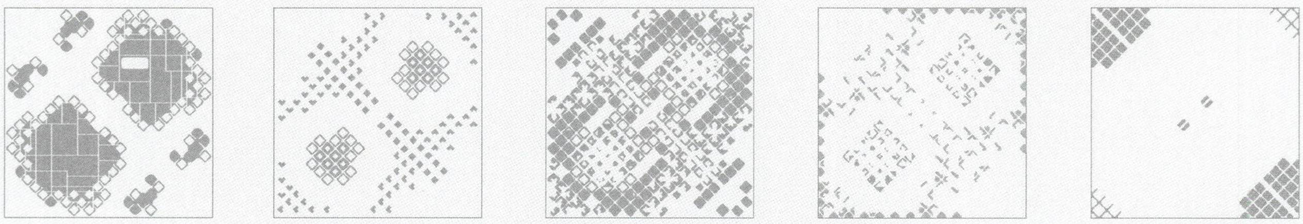

Commercial GSF
53,465m²

Residential GSF
14,970m²

Vegetable Land Area
67,750m²

Fruit Land Area
21,355m²

Hybrid Poplar Land Area
21,355m²

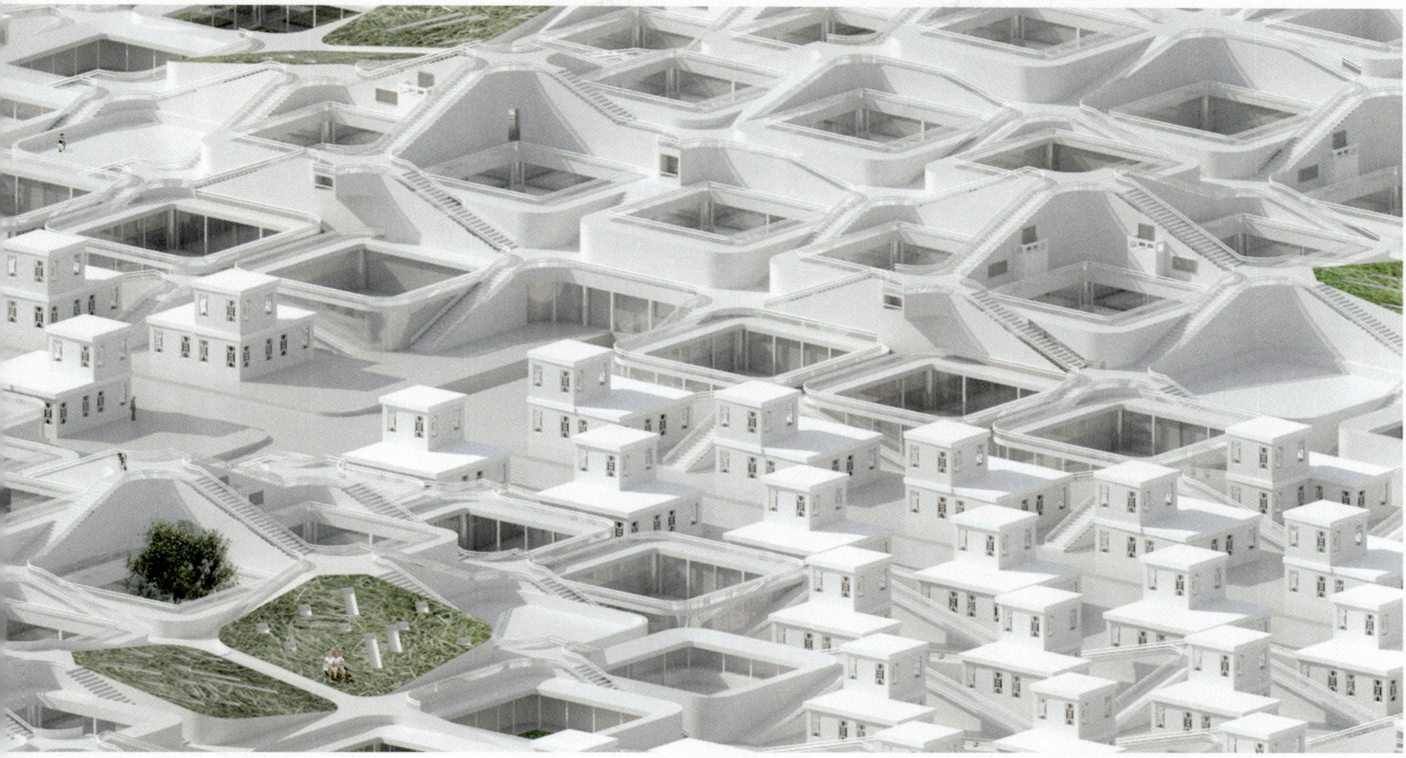

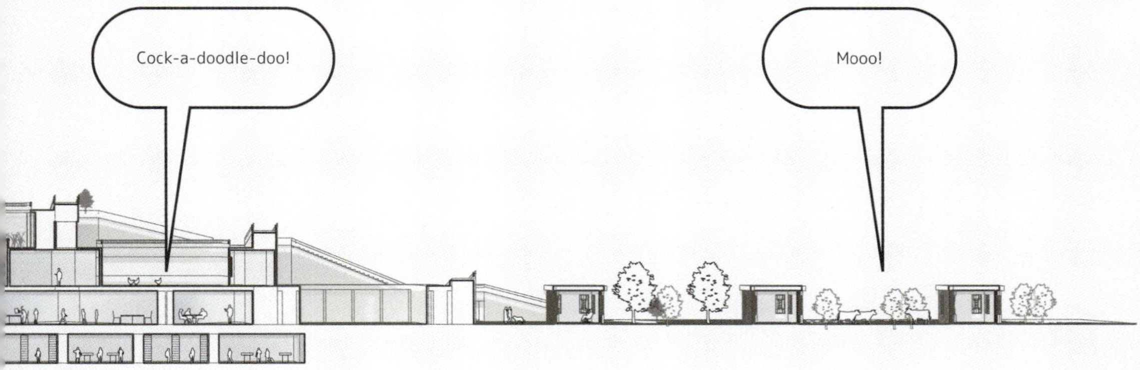

Massing model overall view. (Photograph by Anita Kan)

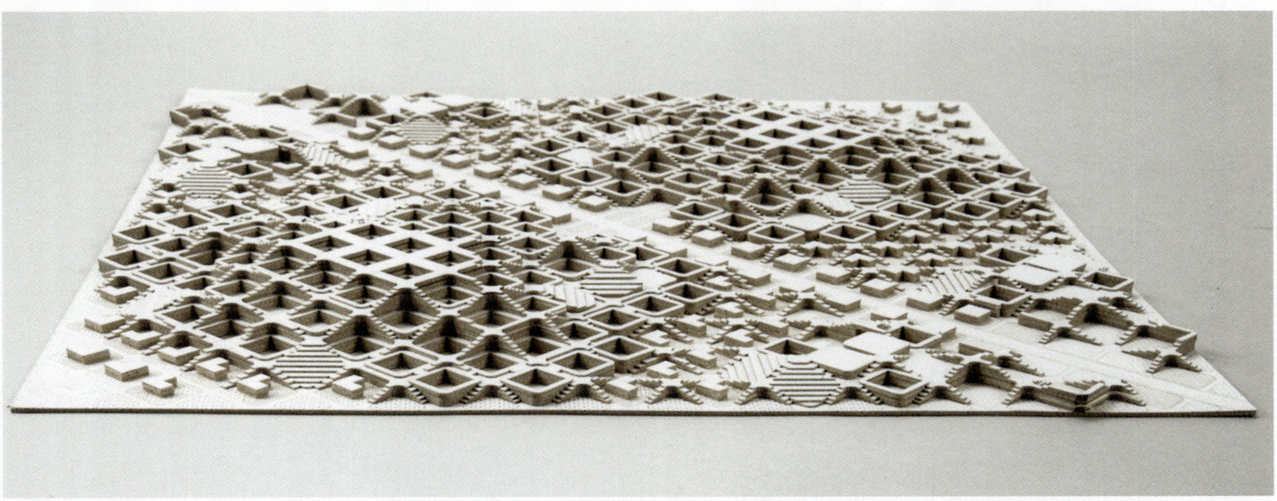

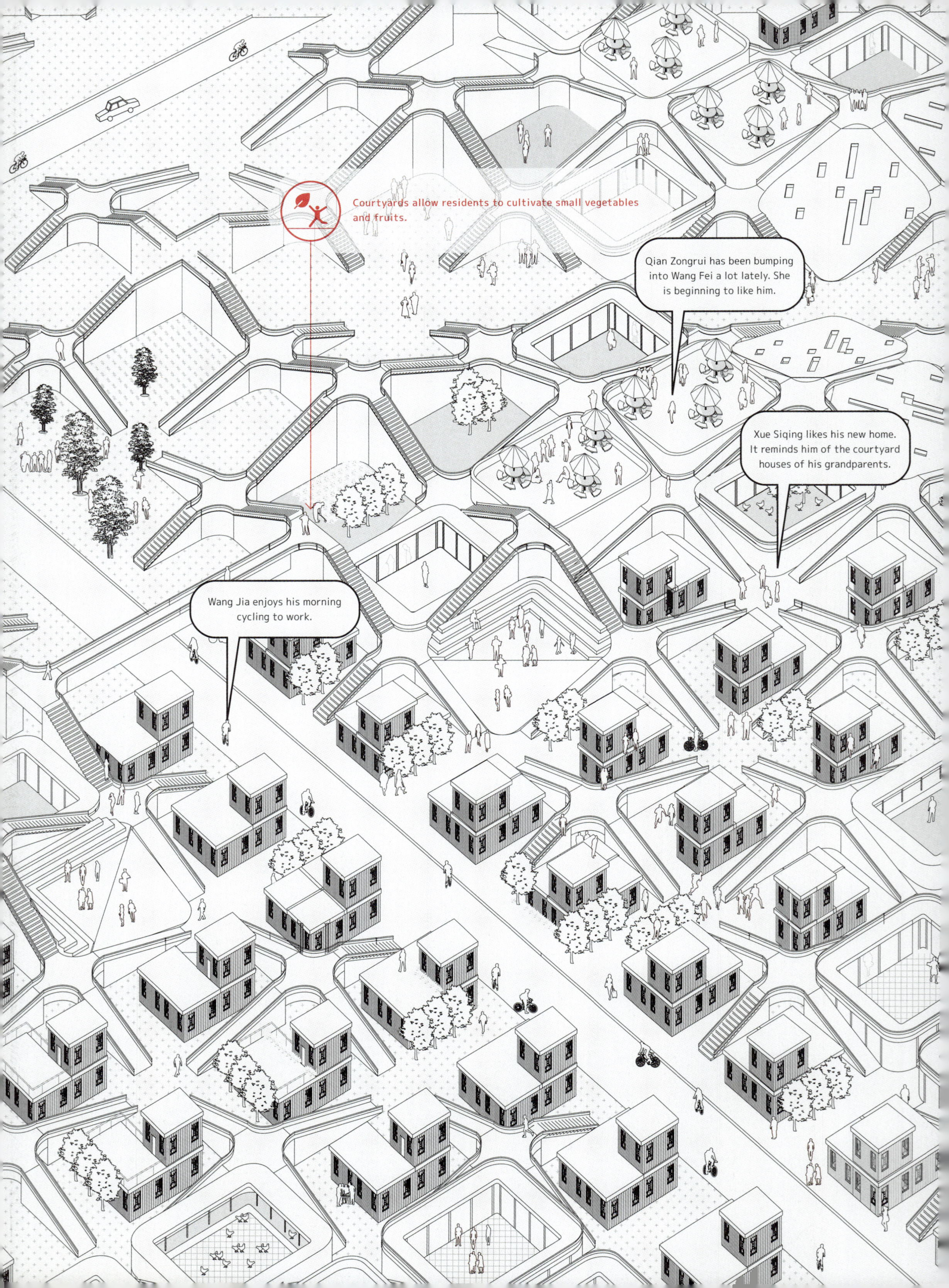

Courtyards allow residents to cultivate small vegetables and fruits.
Qian Zongrui has been bumping into Wang Fei a lot lately. She is beginning to like him.
Xue Siqing likes his new home. It reminds him of the courtyard houses of his grandparents.
Wang Jia enjoys his morning cycling to work.

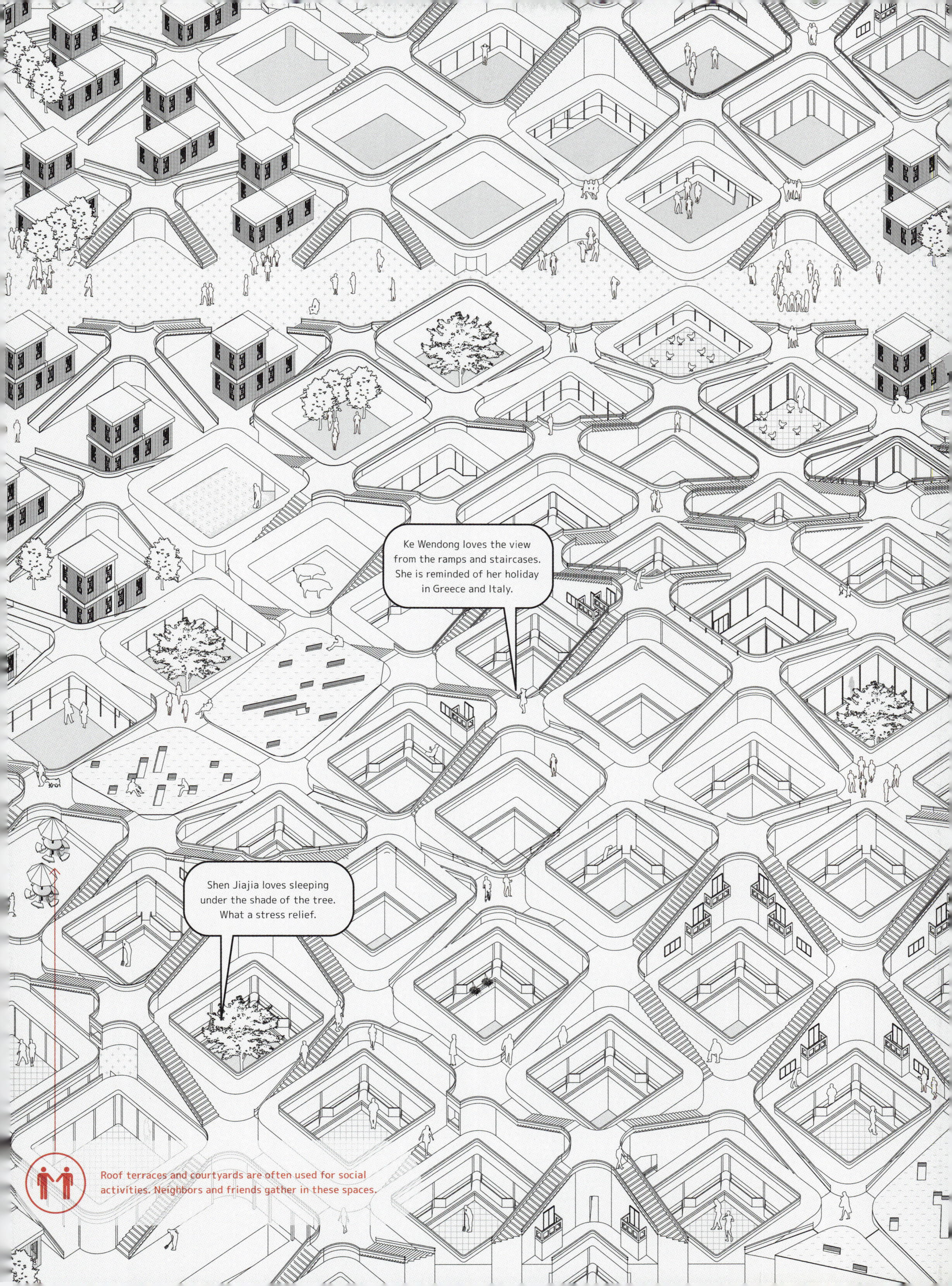
Ke Wendong loves the view from the ramps and staircases. She is reminded of her holiday in Greece and Italy.
Shen Jiajia loves sleeping under the shade of the tree. What a stress relief.
Roof terraces and courtyards are often used for social activities. Neighbors and friends gather in these spaces.

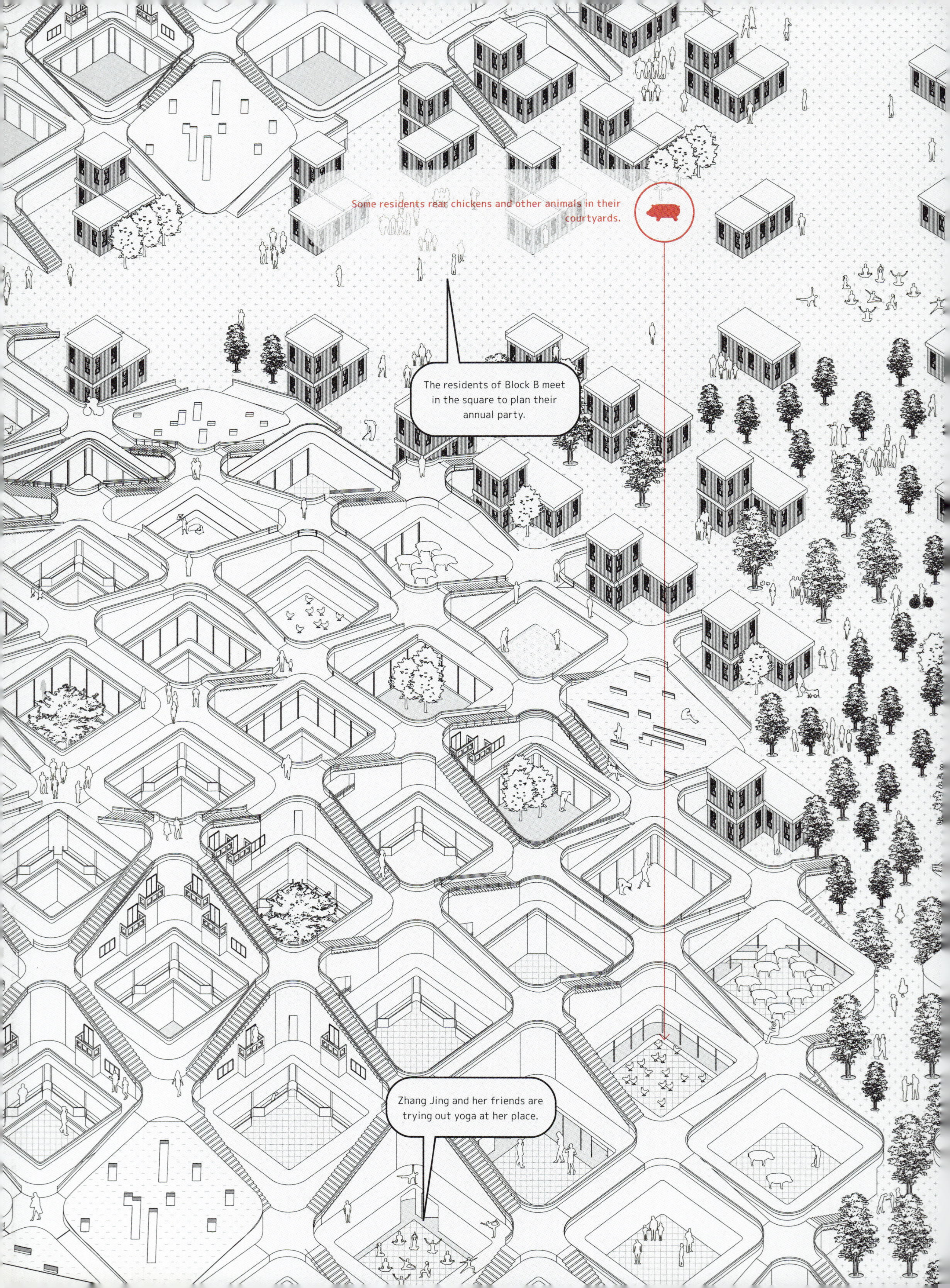
Some residents rear chickens and other animals in their courtyards.
The residents of Block B meet in the square to plan their annual party.
Zhang Jing and her friends are trying out yoga at her place.

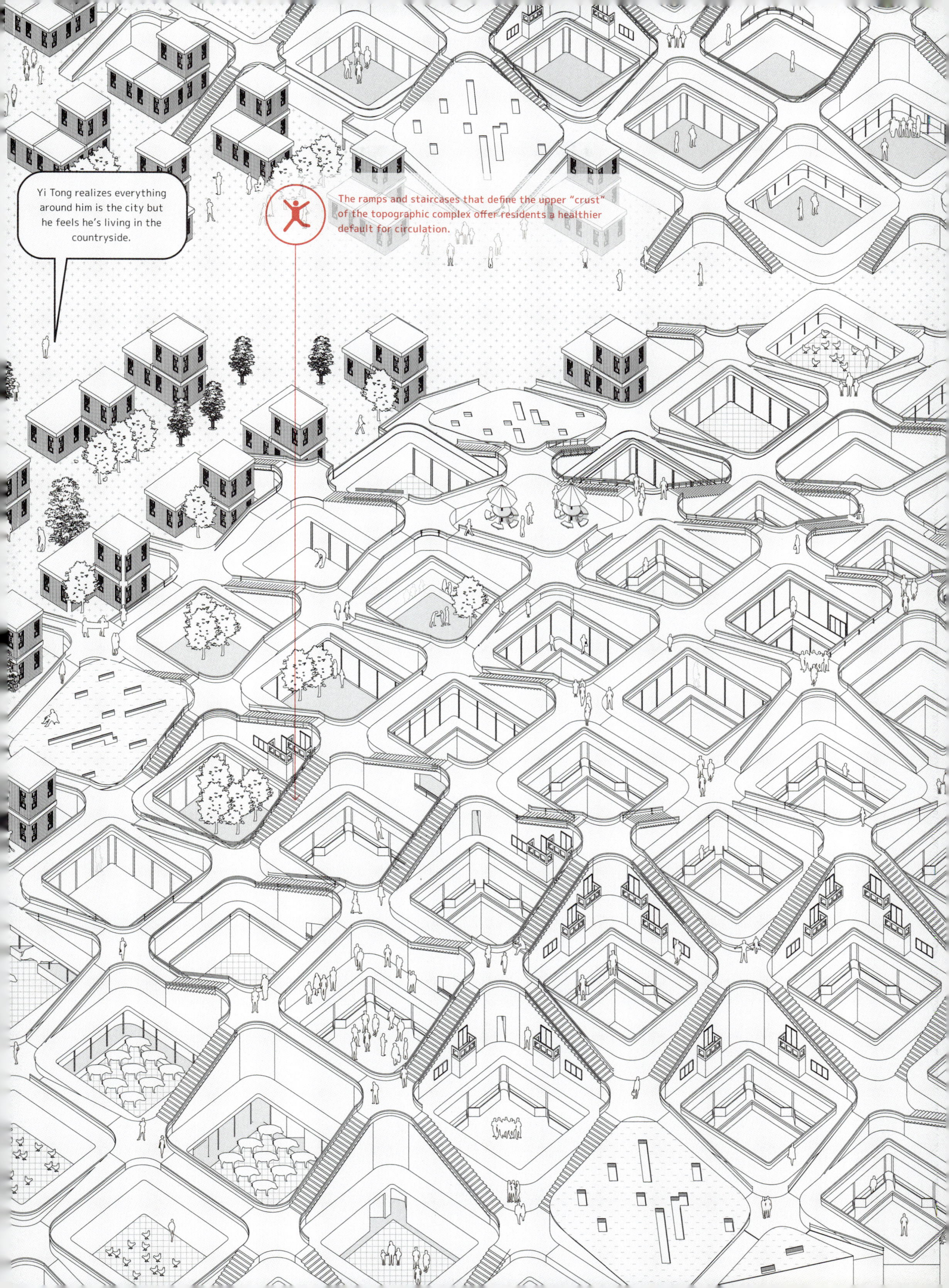
Yi Tong realizes everything around him is the city but he feels he's living in the countryside.
The ramps and staircases that define the upper "crust" of the topographic complex offer residents a healthier default for circulation.

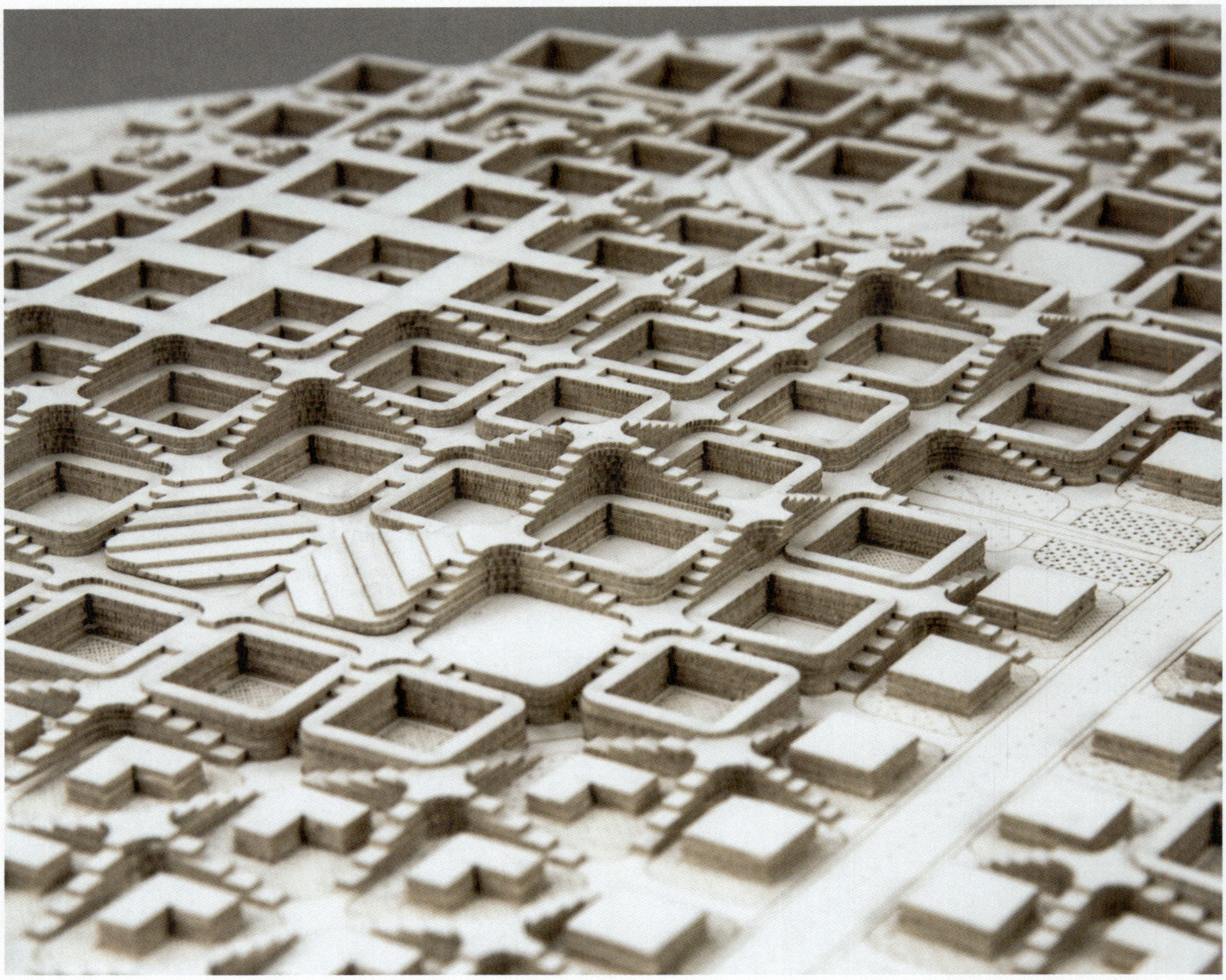

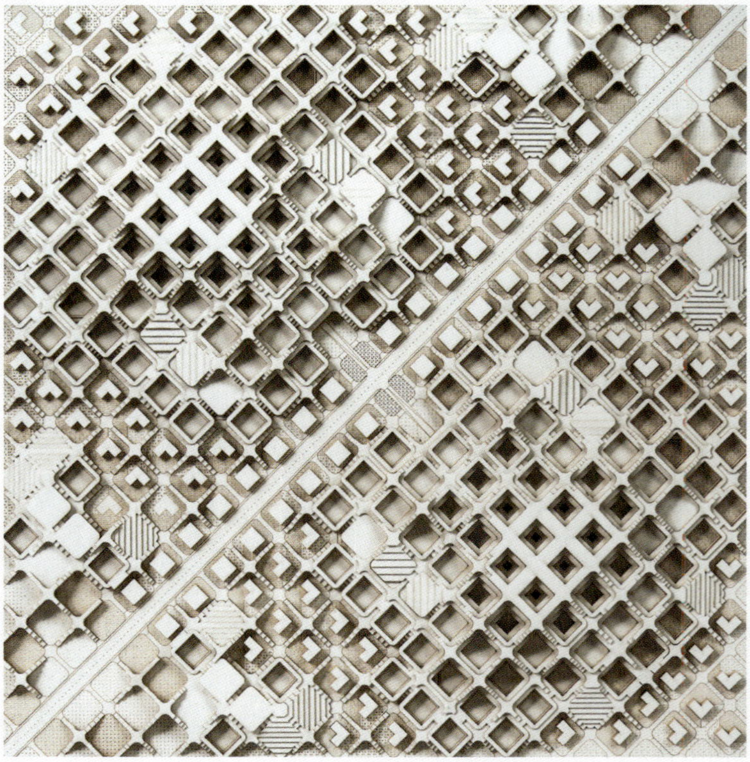

(Above + Right) Detail and plan view of overall massing model.
(Photographs by Anita Kan)

Linong Evolution

Rituparna Simlai + Wei Lin

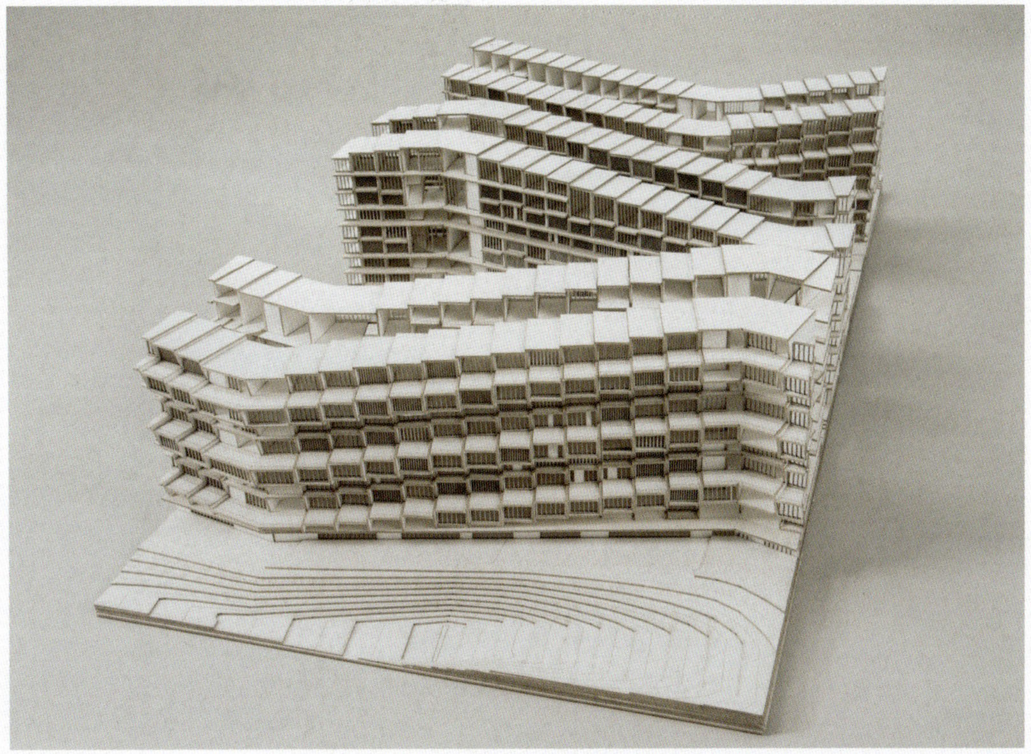

(Photograph by Anita Kan)

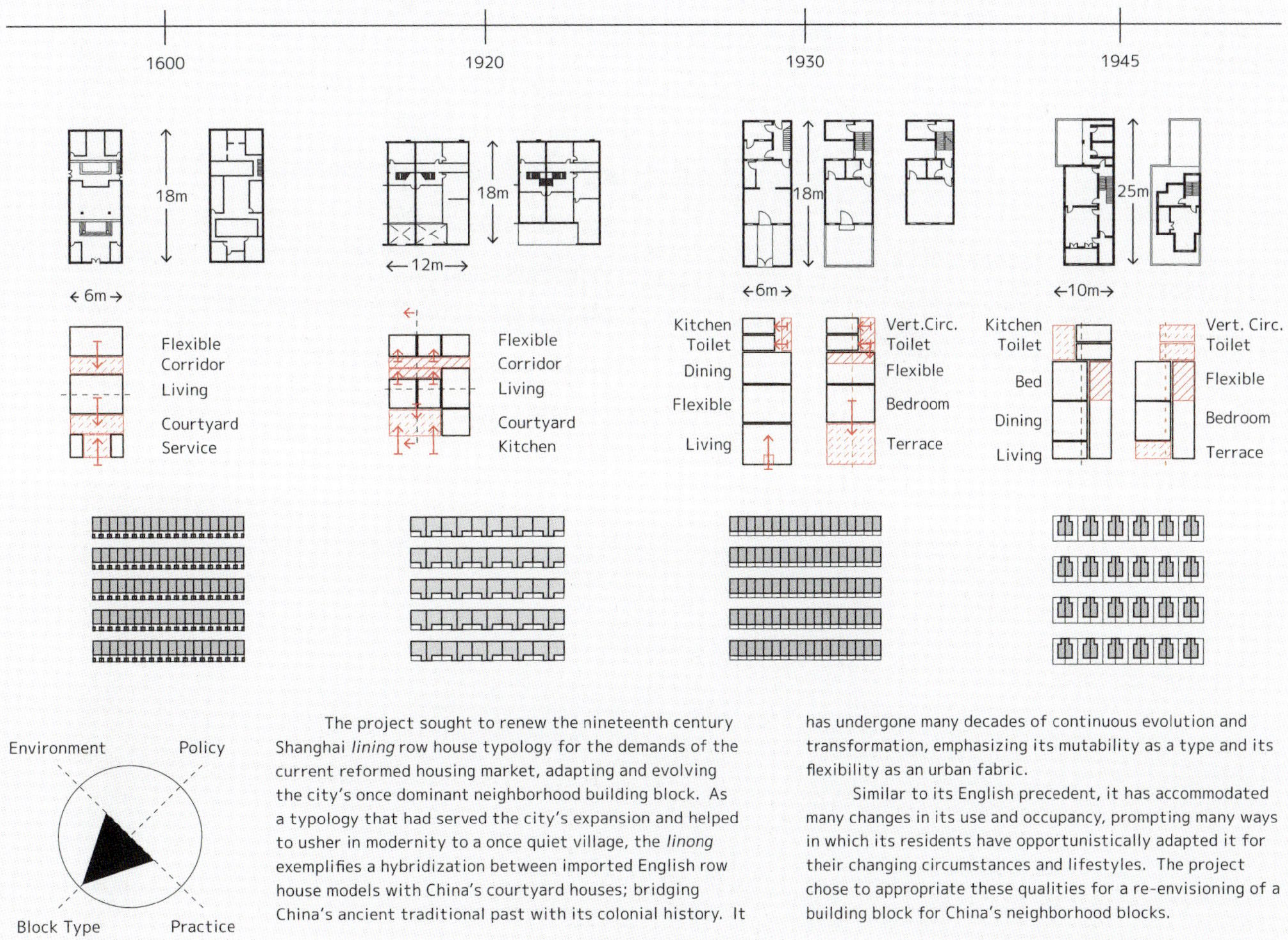

The project sought to renew the nineteenth century Shanghai *lining* row house typology for the demands of the current reformed housing market, adapting and evolving the city's once dominant neighborhood building block. As a typology that had served the city's expansion and helped to usher in modernity to a once quiet village, the *linong* exemplifies a hybridization between imported English row house models with China's courtyard houses; bridging China's ancient traditional past with its colonial history. It has undergone many decades of continuous evolution and transformation, emphasizing its mutability as a type and its flexibility as an urban fabric.

Similar to its English precedent, it has accommodated many changes in its use and occupancy, prompting many ways in which its residents have opportunistically adapted it for their changing circumstances and lifestyles. The project chose to appropriate these qualities for a re-envisioning of a building block for China's neighborhood blocks.

(Below) A Sample of Possible Unit Configurations

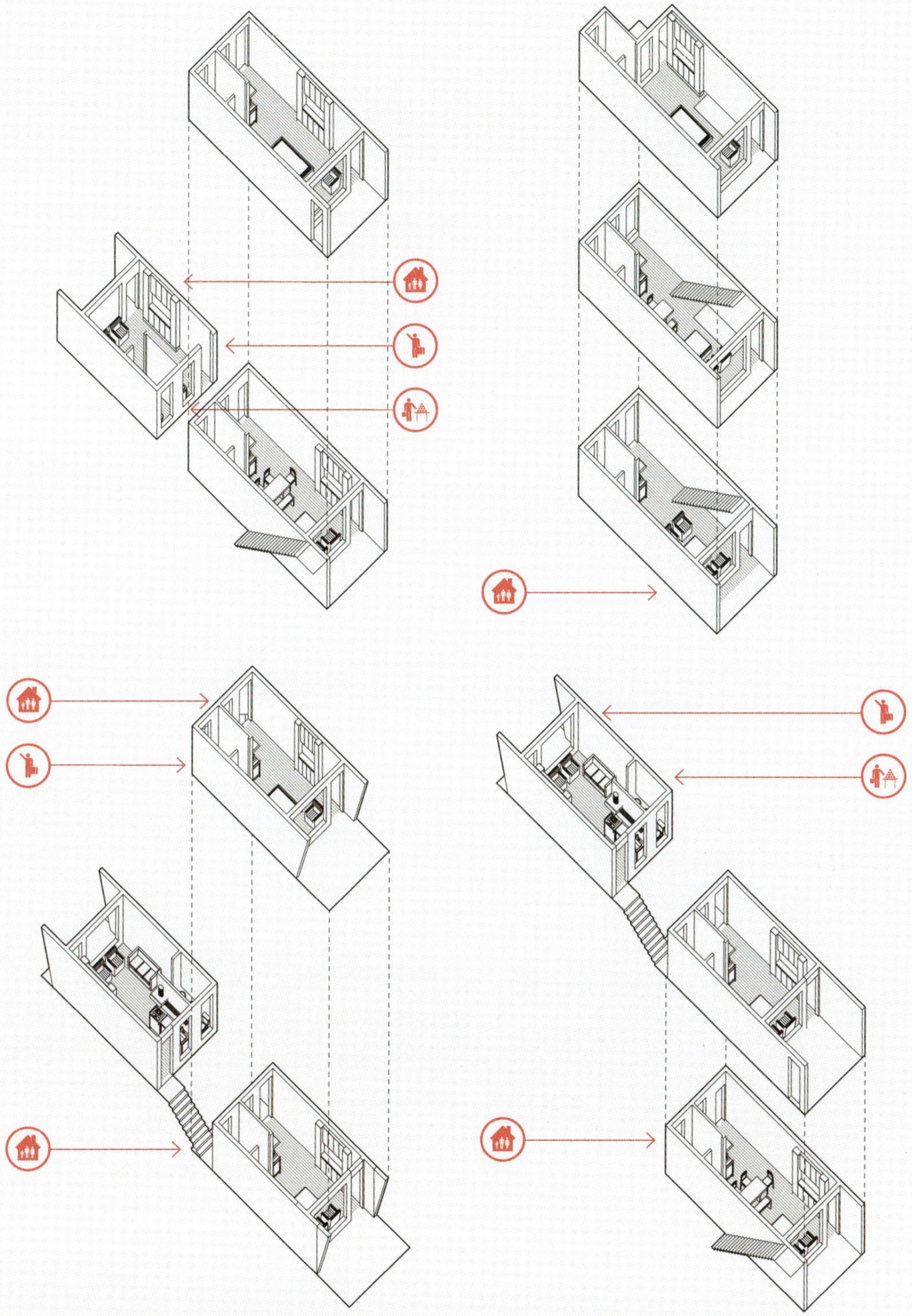

Unit configurations may be flexibly accommodated within the buildings, where anything from single units to aggregations of multiple units are possible arrangements. Learning from the flexibility of the London row house precedents and the *linongs*, the proposed buildings allow for the accommodation of a range of living arrangements as well as programs. In London, we see the typology house a panoply of housing unit arrangements, educational institutions (the Architectural Association), museums (Sir John Soane's Museum), offices, stores and many other different uses.

The two sides of the building are arranged as split levels, allowing for a more gradual transition vertically through the building and retaining visual relationships across the floors while also encouraging physical activity. The central vertical circulation is celebrated with daylighting from above and provides a healthier default for circulation through the building while the ramping building variations also allow for movement vertically through the building on its outside façade. These design features are intended as sites of social bridges as well as "nudges" towards healthier, physically active life practices.

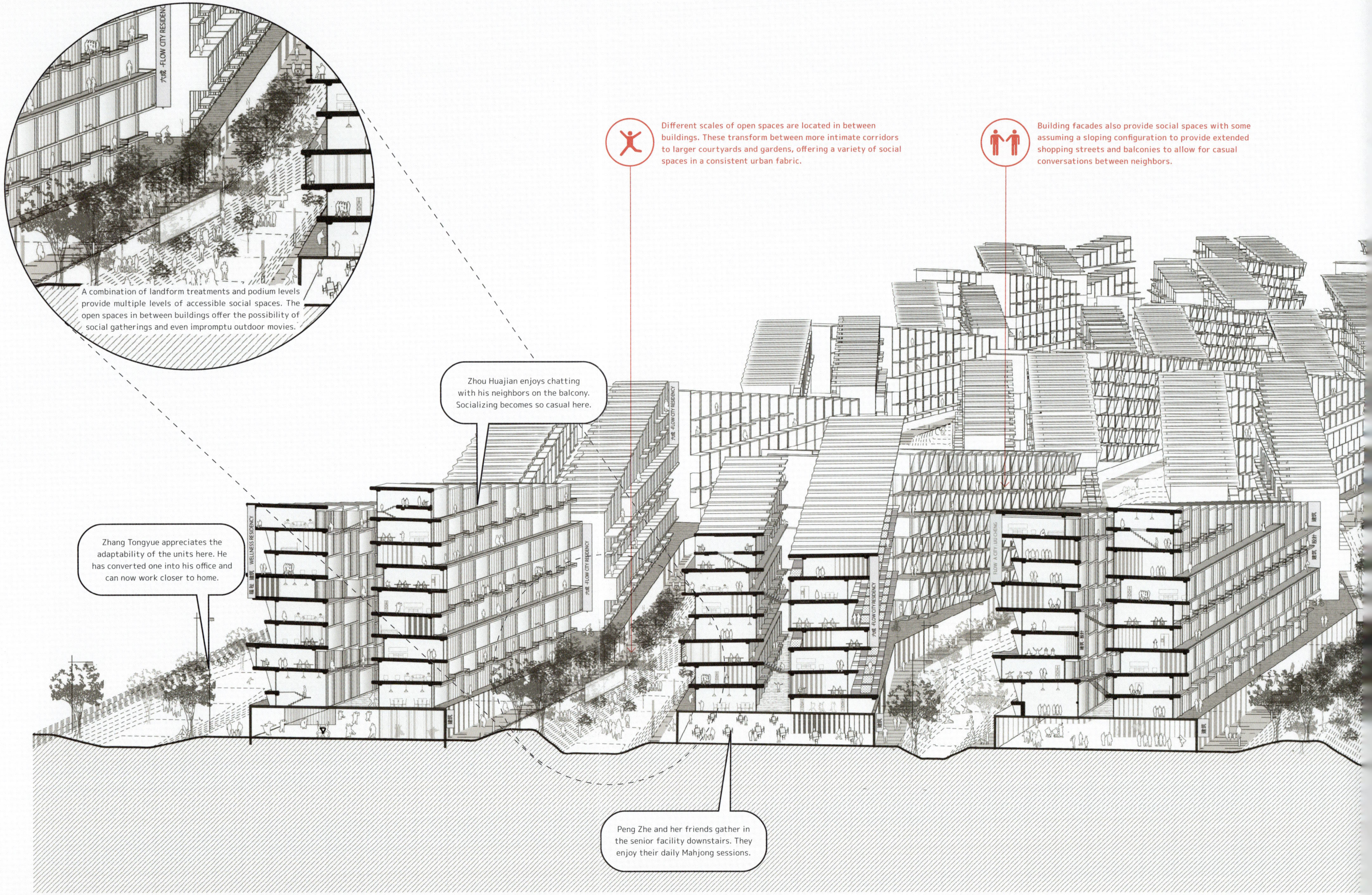

A combination of landform treatments and podium levels provide multiple levels of accessible social spaces. The open spaces in between buildings offer the possibility of social gatherings and even impromptu outdoor movies.
Different scales of open spaces are located in between buildings. These transform between more intimate corridors to larger courtyards and gardens, offering a variety of social spaces in a consistent urban fabric.
Building facades also provide social spaces with some assuming a sloping configuration to provide extended shopping streets and balconies to allow for casual conversations between neighbors.
Zhou Huajian enjoys chatting with his neighbors on the balcony. Socializing becomes so casual here.
Zhang Tongyue appreciates the adaptability of the units here. He has converted one into his office and can now work closer to home.
Peng Zhe and her friends gather in the senior facility downstairs. They enjoy their daily Mahjong sessions.

Implementation Scenario - Songjiang New Town

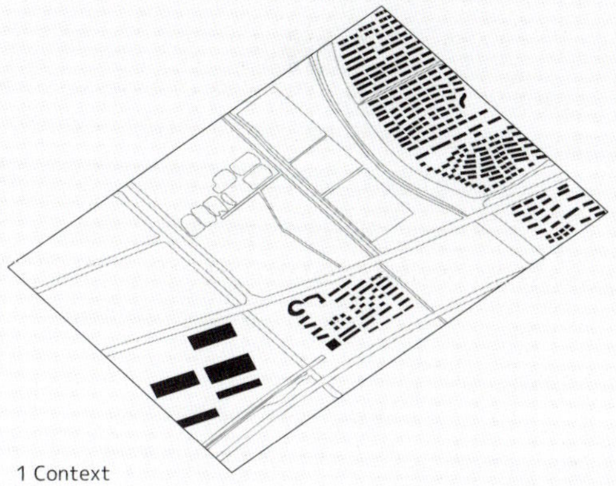
1 Context

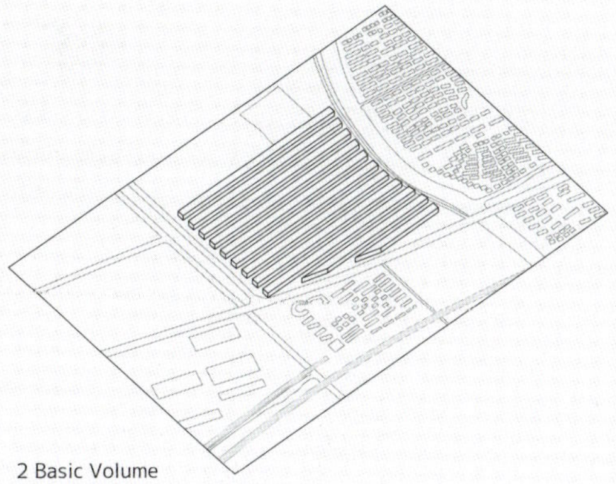
2 Basic Volume

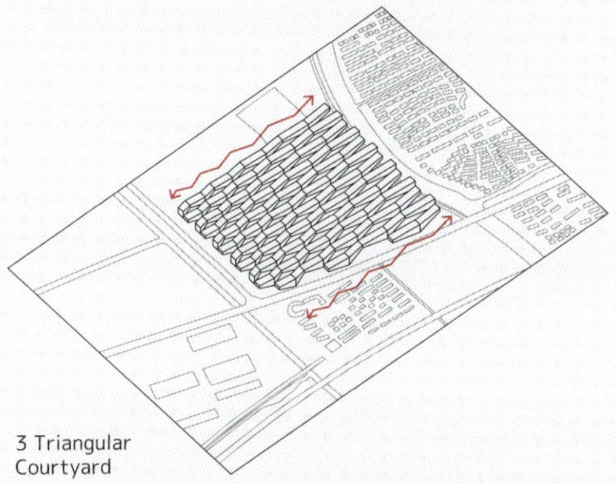
3 Triangular Courtyard

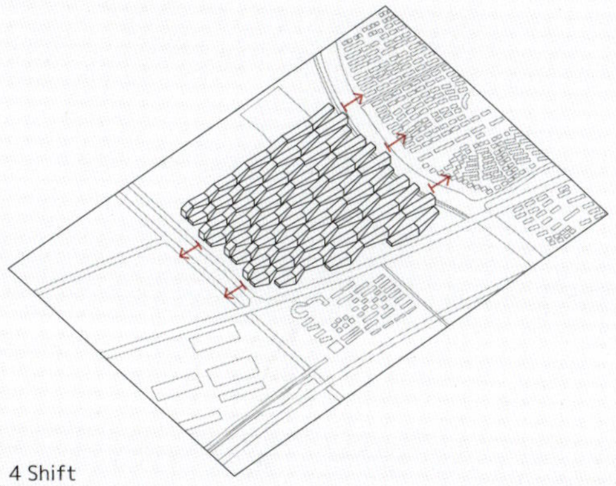
4 Shift

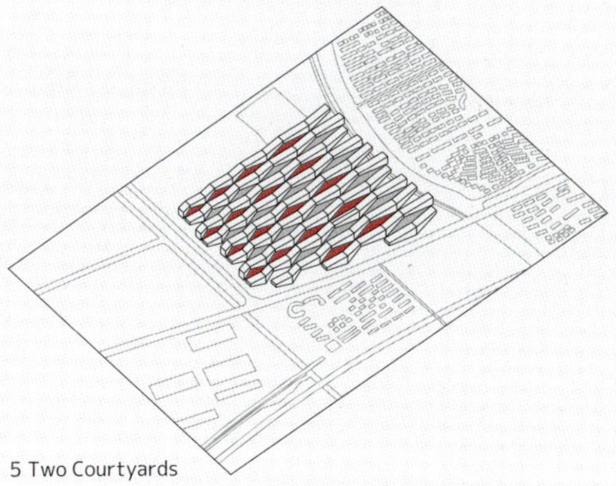
5 Two Courtyards

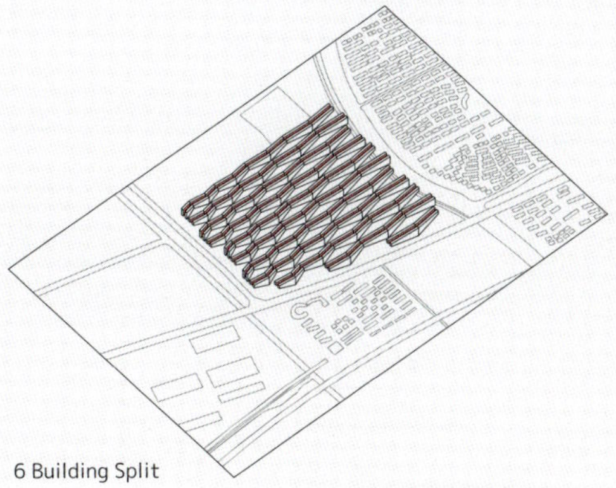
6 Building Split

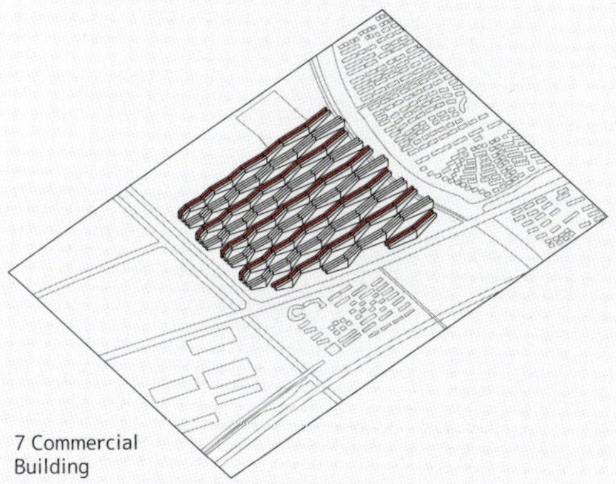
7 Commercial Building

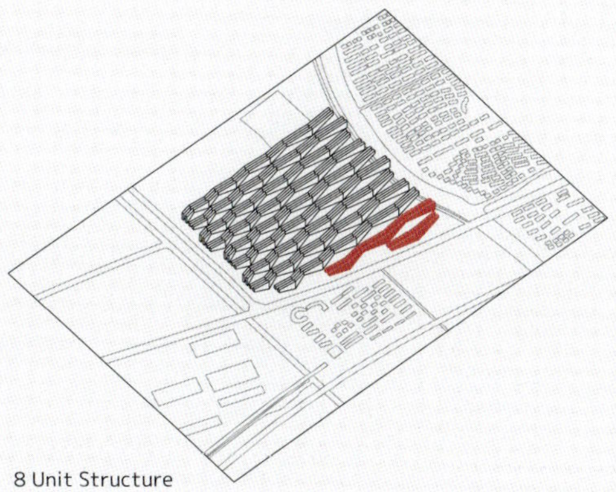
8 Unit Structure

(Right) Diagram of light restrictions on form.
(Below) Formal variations based on sunlight studies.

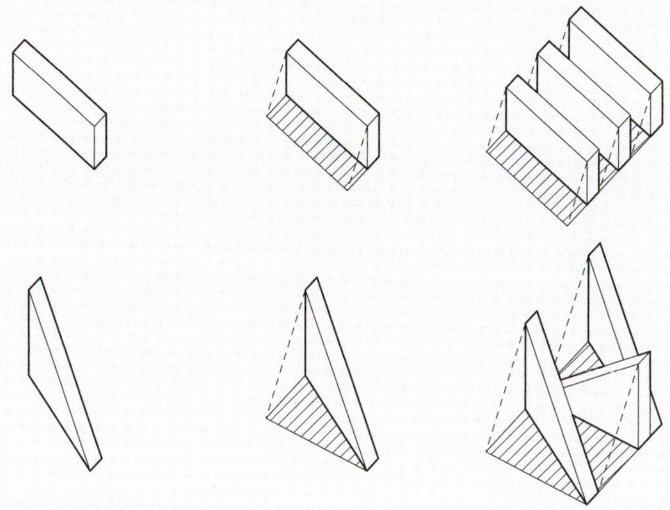

The row house type was reconsidered to be able to accommodate higher densities as well as a greater diversity of spaces through the introduction of a capacity for fabric differentiation. By allowing for vertical transformation as well as a shift to diagonal orientations, the original *linong* configuration could be evolved into one that would embed a gradient of different scales of spaces and building heights within a consistent fabric. Courtyards and alleys or lanes blend into each other as the urban elevation shifts back and forth with an undulating roofline. Using the sunshine law as a guide for this differentiation, the different distances between rows affect the allowable heights of adjacent buildings, resulting in the possibility of an alternating rhythm of peaks and valleys.

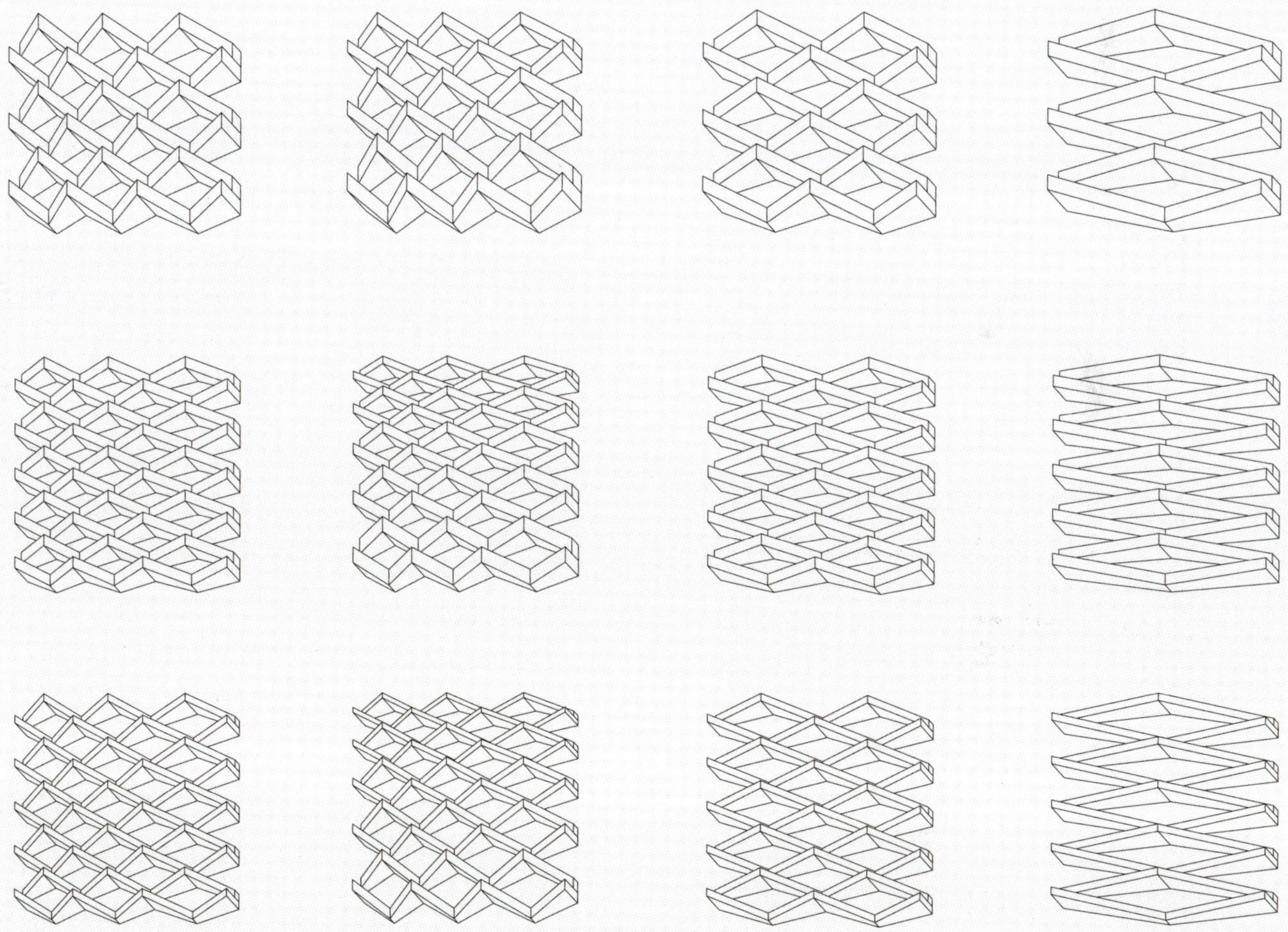

By using this association between building distance and height, based on the sunshine law, a range of possible fabric configurations may be generated to produce different urban grains as well as a diversity of open space patterns.

The capacity to provide anything from smaller yet regular framed courts to single, large central fields is dependent on the specific rhythms of the shifting orientations of the building fabric.

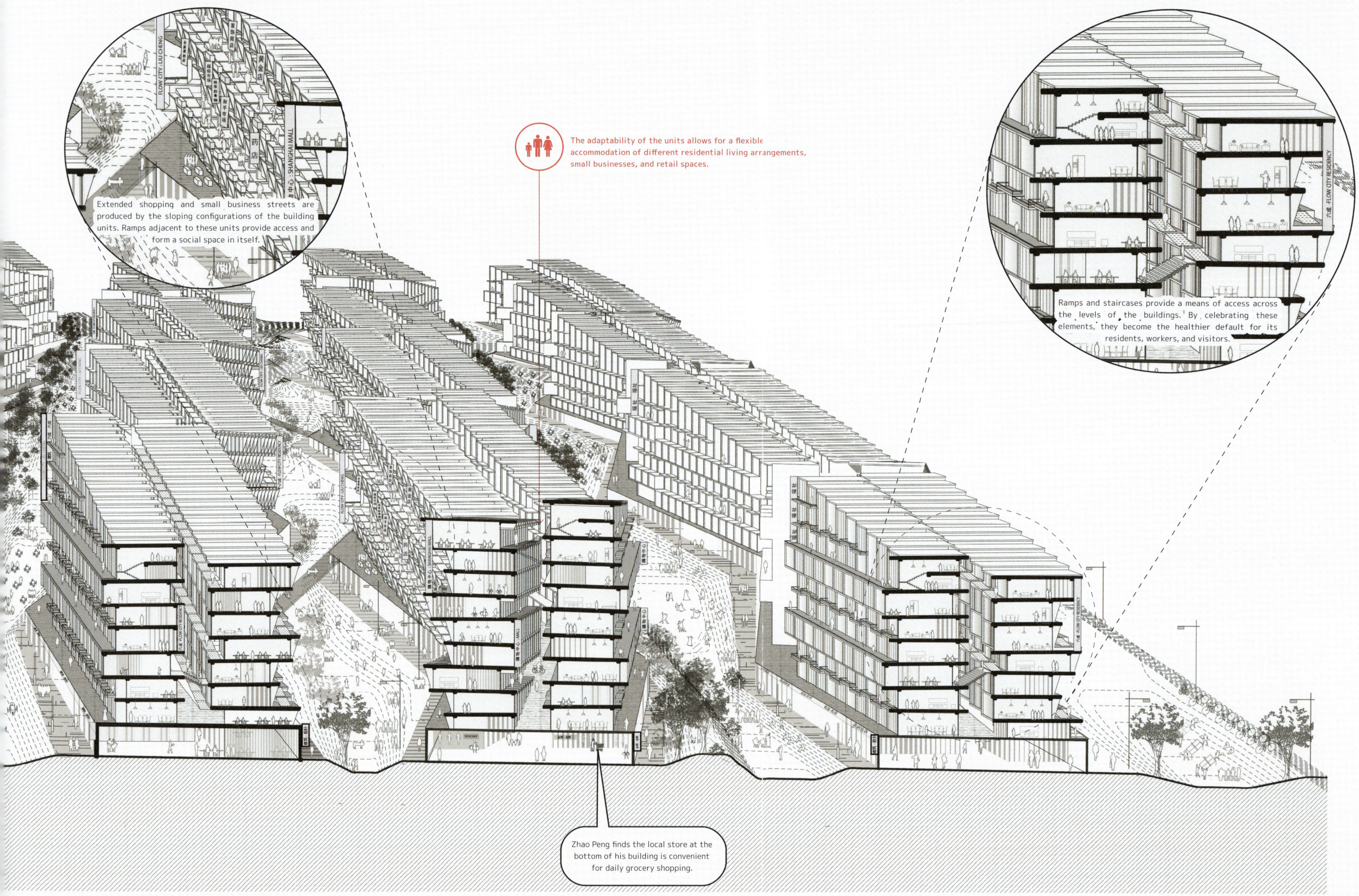

Extended shopping and small business streets are produced by the sloping configurations of the building units. Ramps adjacent to these units provide access and form a social space in itself.
FLOW CITY : LIU CHENG
SHANGHAI MALL
The adaptability of the units allows for a flexible accommodation of different residential living arrangements, small businesses, and retail spaces.
Ramps and staircases provide a means of access across the levels of the buildings.[1] By celebrating these elements, they become the healthier default for its residents, workers, and visitors.
FLOW CITY RESIDENCY
Zhao Peng finds the local store at the bottom of his building is convenient for daily grocery shopping.

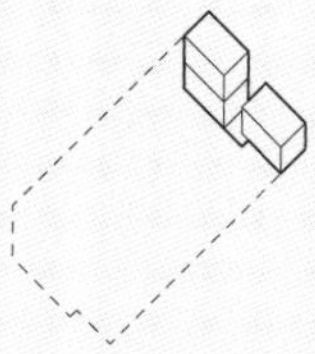

Unit Variations

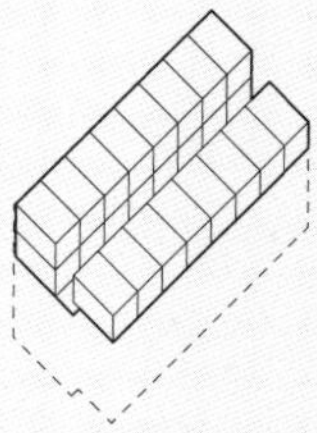

Linear Arrangement

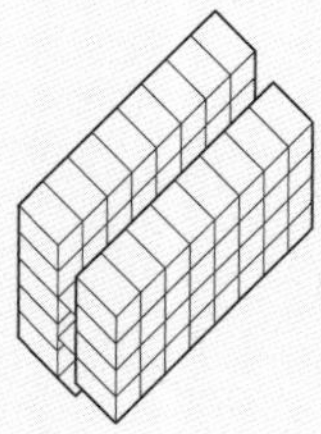

1 Linear

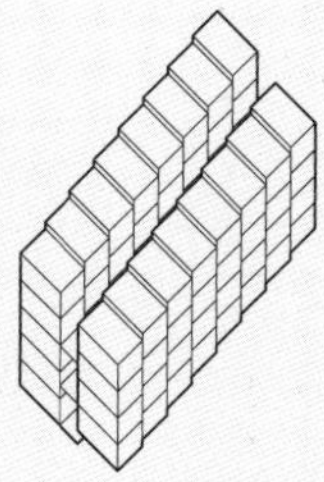

2 Ramping

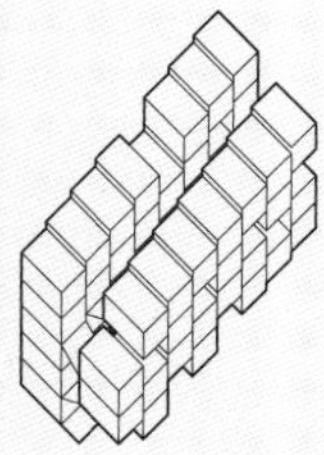

3 Void

At the smaller scale, the project utilized an adjusted variation of a *linong* type as the basic organizational unit that is multiplied to form the urban fabric. Variations in the ways in which these units may be combined allow for larger scale organizational differences such as linear or ramping aggregations. The double loaded arrangement allows for even more variations.

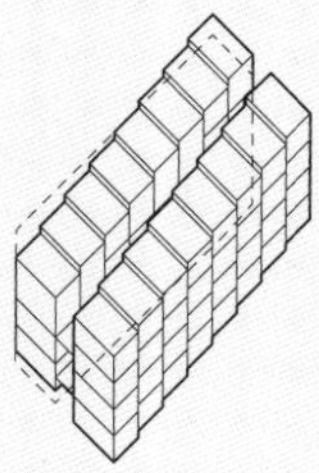

1+2 Combination

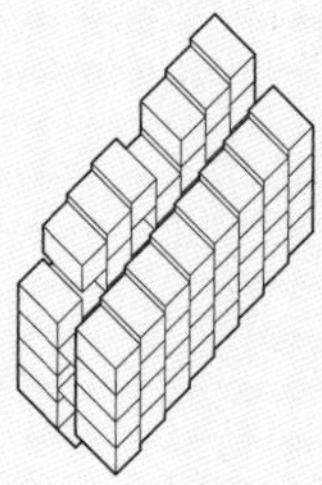

2+3 Combination

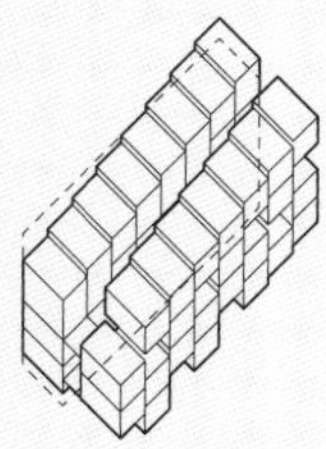

1+3 Combination

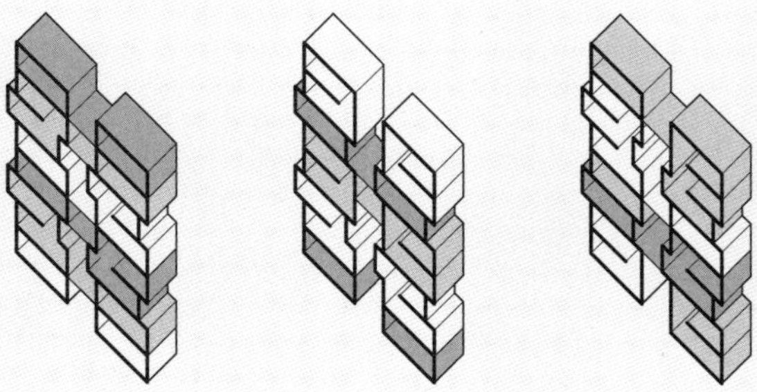

Possible Aligned Combinations

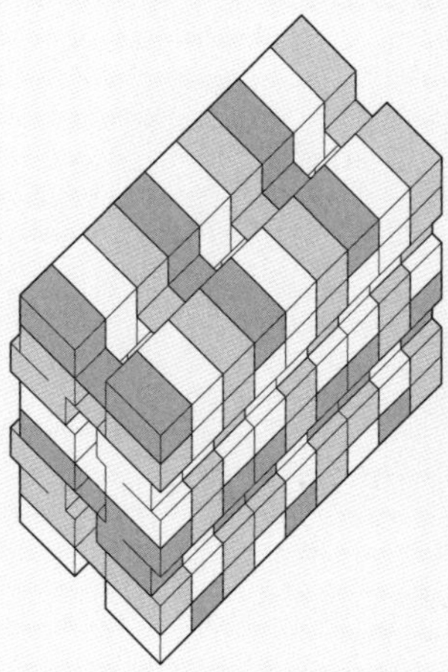

Aligned + Linear Aggregation

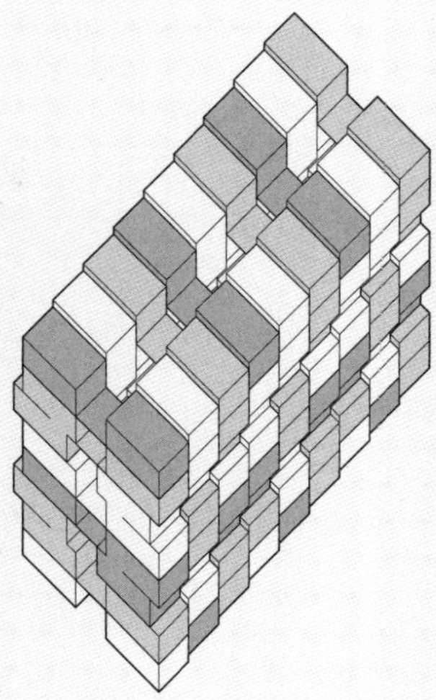

Aligned + Sloped Aggregation

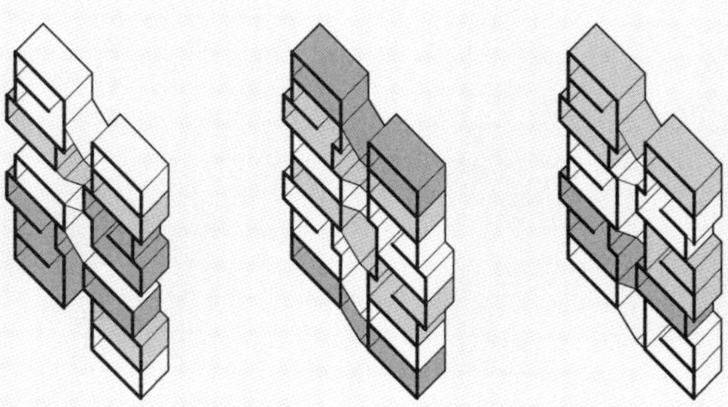

Possible Offset Combinations

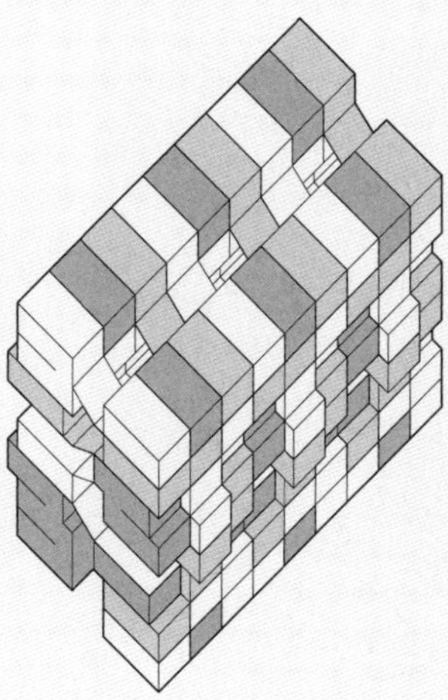

Offset + Linear Aggregation

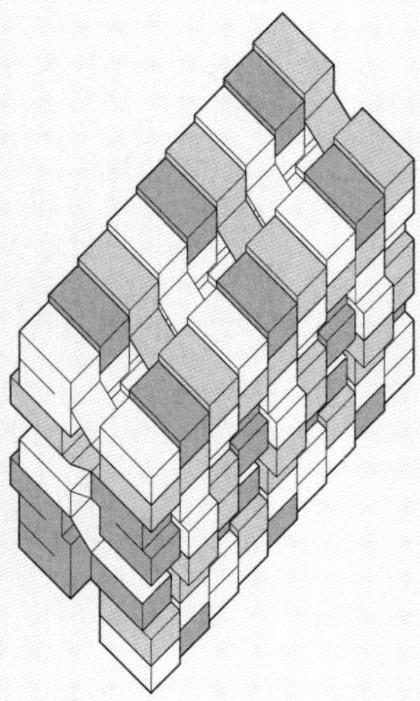

Offset + Sloped Aggregation

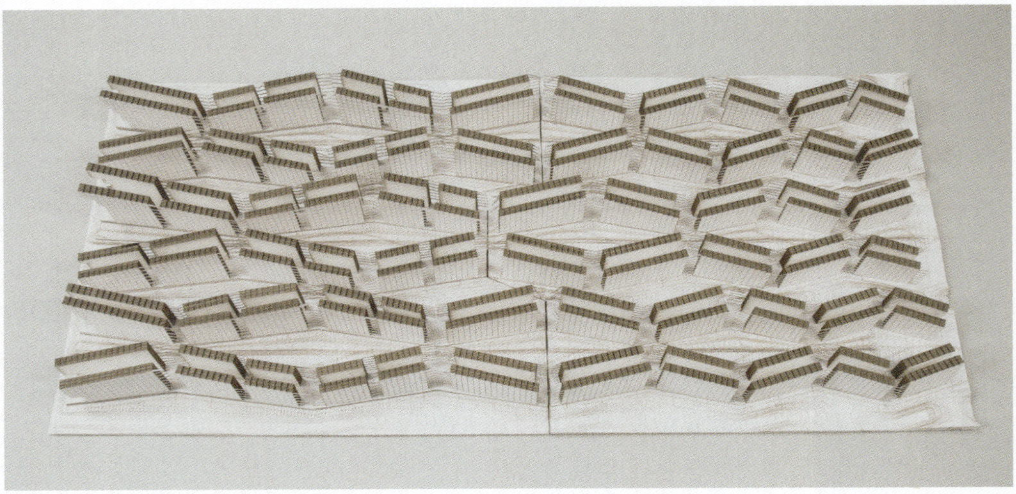

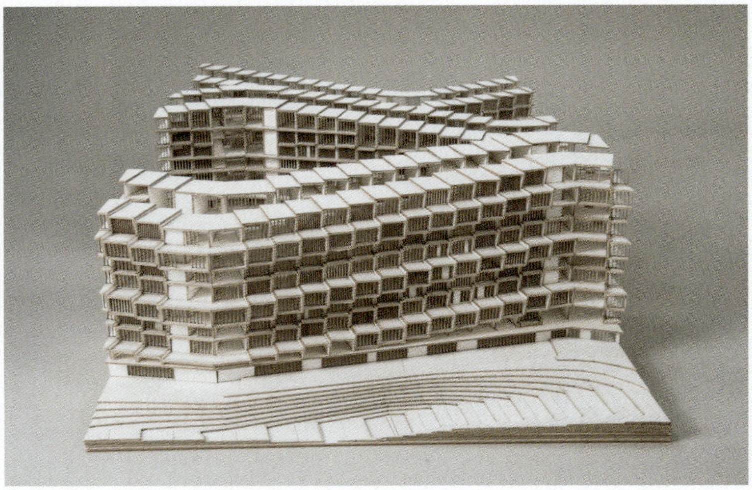

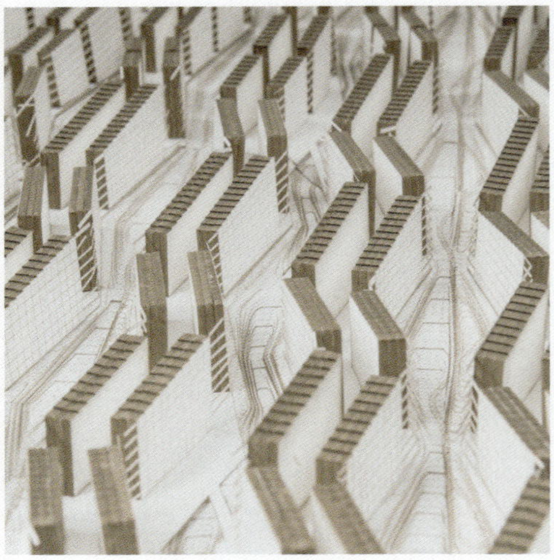

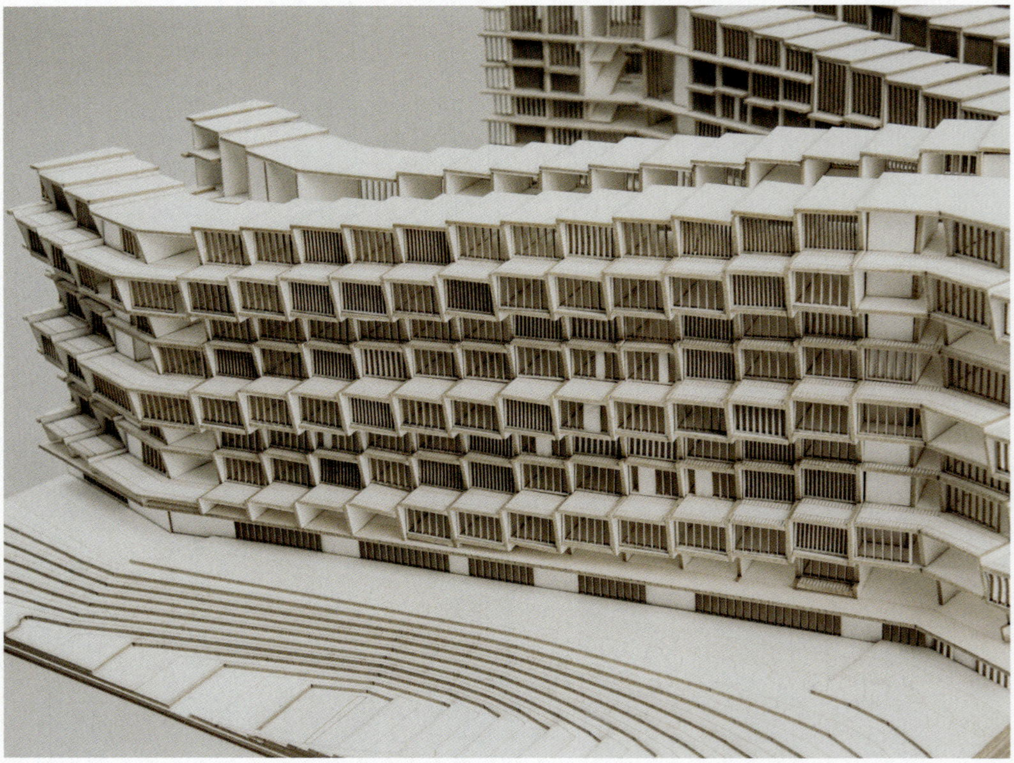

(Top, Middle Right) Photographs of overall block-scale model. (Middle Left, Bottom Right) Photographs of large-scale model. (Photograhs by Anita Kan)

A Variegated Framework for Social Life

Yi Li + Clayton Strange-Lee

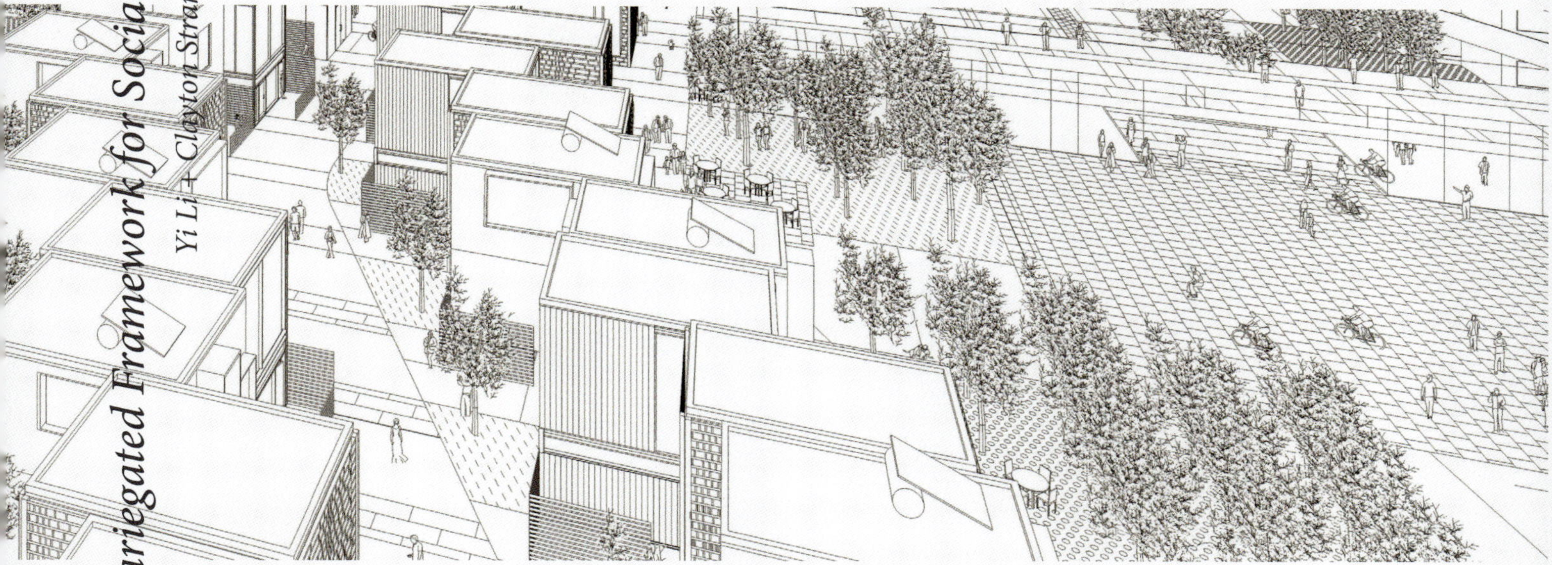

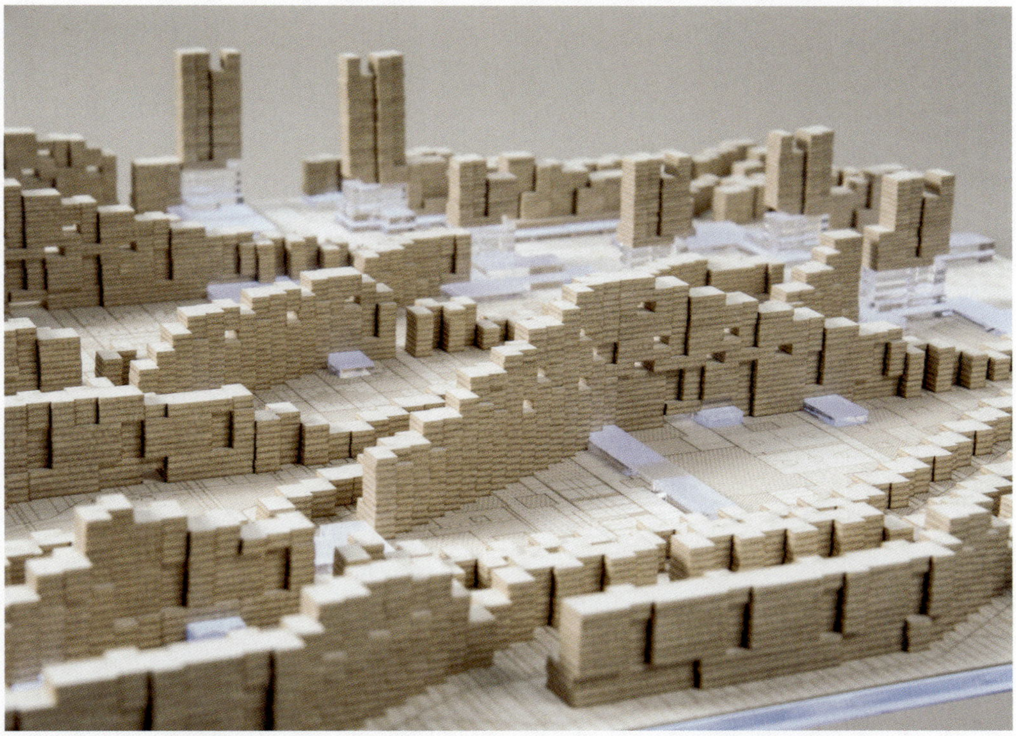

(Photograph by Anita Kan)

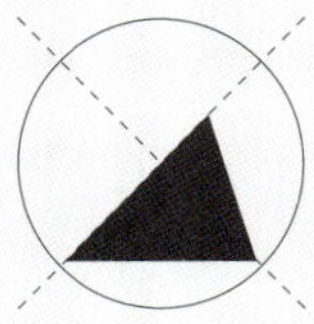

Social Capital and the Built Environment

Social engagement and community involvement are seen as having positive health consequences, where studies have shown that those who have active social lives tend to live longer and be healthier both physically and mentally. Many factors contribute to the ways in which a neighborhood may enjoy a socially engaged community but it is the physical fabric of the environment that forms the site of this activity. While active social communities can exist in many types of physical environments, the project was invested in proposing a model neighborhood environment that would be organized with this consideration as a main influence on the design.

The project began with a number of questions. How do we build resilient environments that can help buffer the population from a huge demographic and economic change? How can we bridge between older forms of social practice with the emerging lifestyles that come with China's changing society? Can the physical environment provide a vital social infrastructure?

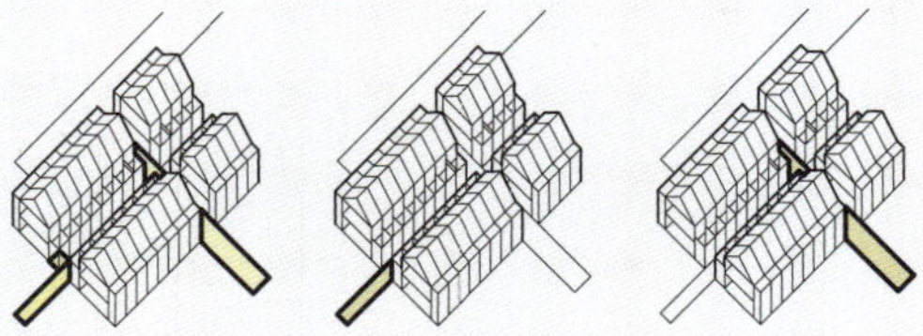

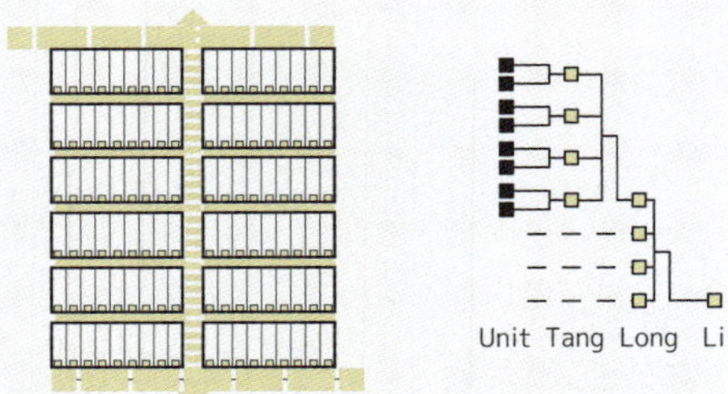

Lilong Membership
1:10:40

(legend)	Jie (街)	*City 1.6 M*	
(legend)	Li (里)	69 units	207 people
(legend)	Long (弄)	23 units	68 people
(legend)	Tang (堂)	2-4 units	6-24 people

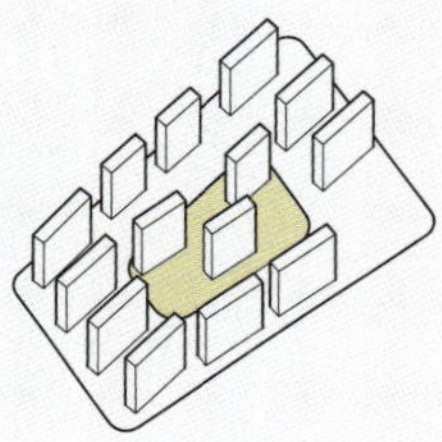

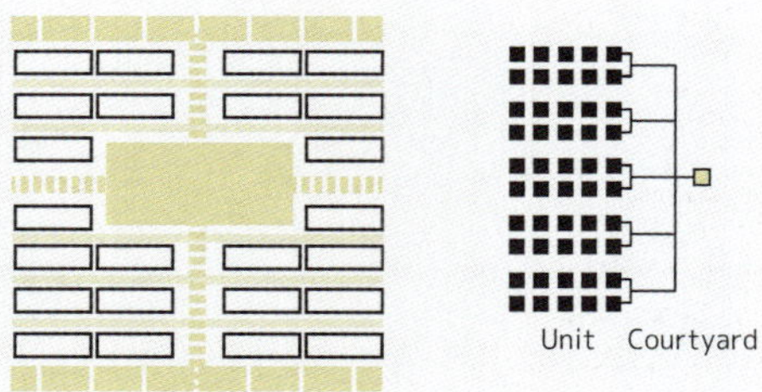

Xiaoqu Membership
1:680

(legend)	External Street	*City 1.6 M*	
(legend)	Inner Street	Block 680 units	
(legend)	Alley	Adj. Bldg.	136 units
(legend)	Central Plaza	Block 2000 people	

Events	Unit Structure	m^2 per Unit	m^2 per Person
1840-1911 Late-Feudalism	2-9	200 m^2	16 m^2
1911-1949 Republican Era	7	150 m^2	10 m^2
1949-1983 Communist PRC, Free Market Opening	5	42 m^2	7 m^2
1984-1991 "Xiaokang" Standard of Living Raised 1 Family, 1 Unit	3	100 m^2	20 m^2
1992-1997 Functional Compartmentalization Increased Unit Sizes	3	180-200 m^2	38 m^2
1998-2005 Style, Comfort, Unique	5/3/1	90-100, 60-70, 45-55 m^2	20 m^2
2005-present Economic, Compact, Transformable	3	70-80 m^2	23 m^2

Type	%	Household Structure	Unit Sizes	Bedrooms
Single	17		S	1br
Couple (Nuclear Family)	23		S, M	2br, 1br
Standard Nuclear Family	31		M, L	2br, 3br
3 Linear Family	12	or	L	3br, 4br, 5br
Complex Family	3	or	L	3br, 4br, 5br

By studying a range of neighborhood types found in Shanghai throughout history, we can recognize the streamlined and "efficient" structure of contemporary *xiaoqu* housing developments. These standard forms of contemporary development offer a very clear differentiation and compartmentalization of a range of neighborhood activities (necessary or everyday essential, voluntary and social activities). In the *xiaoqu*, nearly all the spaces for necessary activities are embedded within the private realm of the housing unit, while specific areas that may allow voluntary and social activities are greatly reduced. When studying an older emblematic neighborhood type; the *linong*, a more gradated transition between the private housing units and the public world of the *li* (the major alleys) is clear. The distribution of activities in the *linong* neighborhood is more dispersed with many opportunities for casual social engagement, where many activities overlap in the finer grain fabric of houses, *li* (major alley), *long* (minor alley) and *tang* (interior courtyard).

The linong spatial hierarchy itself is distributed in very fine grains when compared to the *xiaoqu* models, matching the spatial arrangements of various activities. Public spaces are divided into numerous more intimate scales, allowing various groups to develop a better sense of membership to the community and neighborhood by having specific spaces that they can identify a sense of belonging to. The responsibilities for managing and maintaining the internal public spaces are typically divided amongst the

(Top Left) Lilong membership diagram. (Middle Left) *Xiaoqu* membership diagram. (Top Right) Structure of chinese housing history. (Middle Right) Chinese household structure. (Right Page) Sunlight/form diagram.

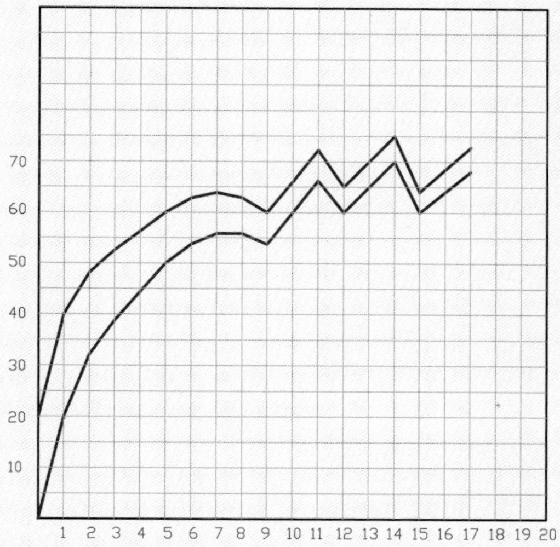

Based on the Sunshine Law in China, every room in China must receive at least one hour of direct sunlight. From this we derived a graph which illustrates the connection between building heights and building spacing.

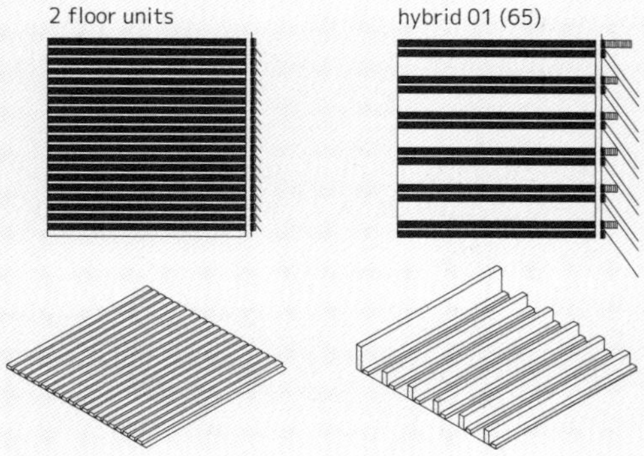

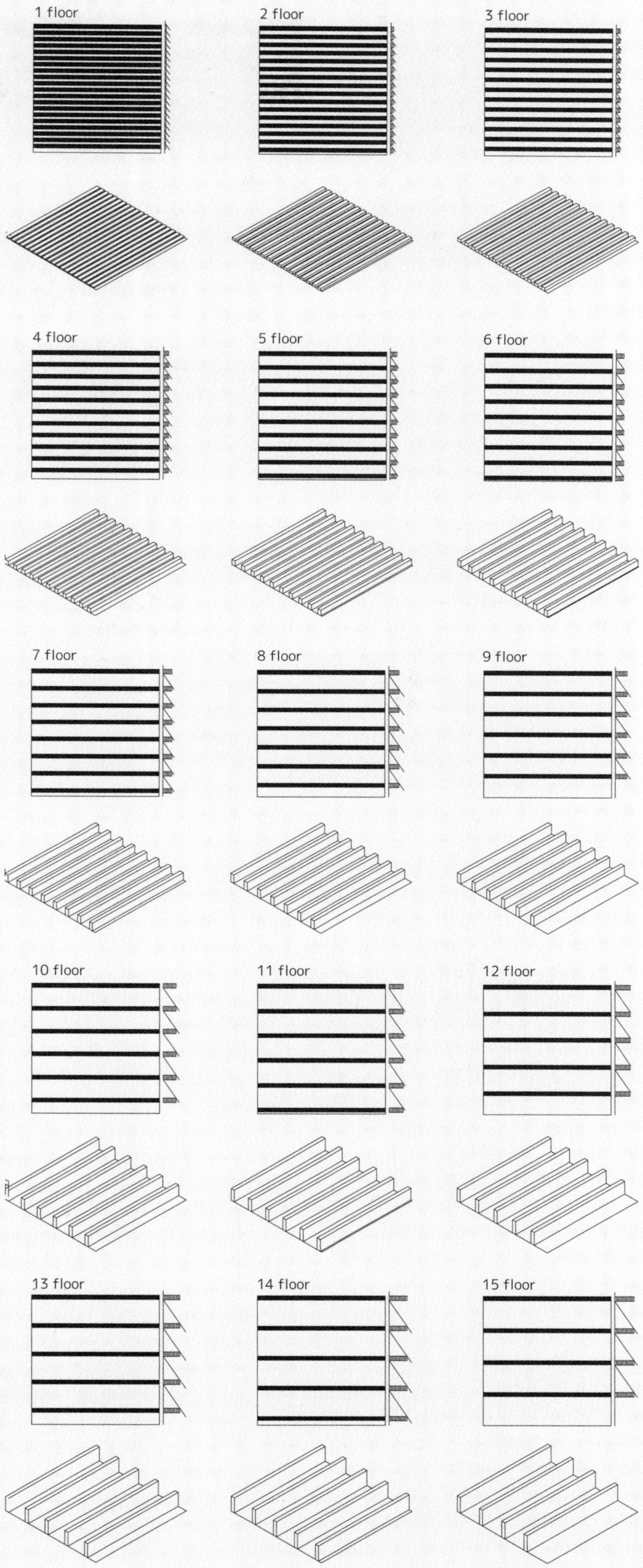

residents of the adjacent units fostering even further a sense of collective ownership. The *xiaoqu* spatial hierarchy is typically less nuanced and is often organized with its main public spaces consolidated in a central space within the block. Residents of the *xiaoqu* have membership to the central plaza but the huge scale often dilutes a direct sense of attachment. The management and maintenance of these spaces are also often reliant on a third party maintenance company.

The study of the sunshine laws effect on urban grain or building density and the resulting open space pattern also suggests the great variety of fabric types that may be generated from this simple association alone. The objective for the project was to embed difference within the urban grain, learning from the finer differentiated grain of older Chinese urban fabrics. We chose to utilize this law that was established to ensure healthier living environments as the mechanism to deliver this. From one association aimed at delivering healthier living environments, we hoped to generate a series of physical fabrics that allow for the emergence of a setting within which another factor that contributes to health may thrive; social life.

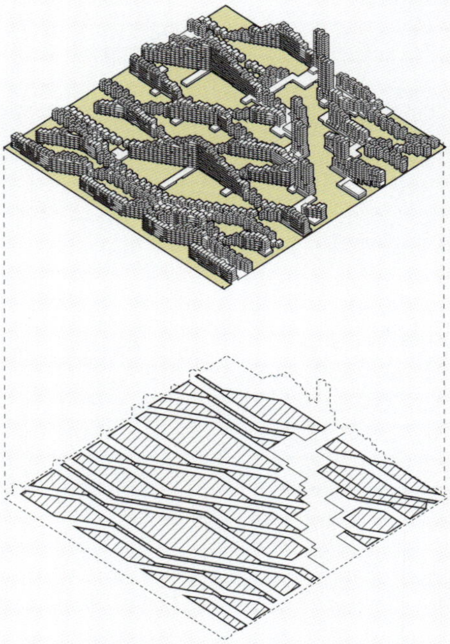

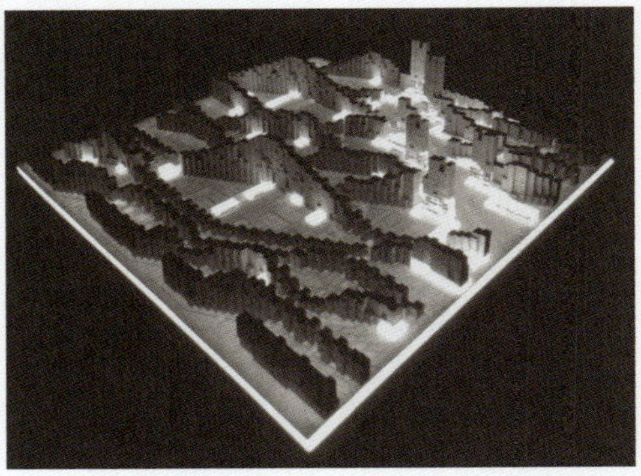

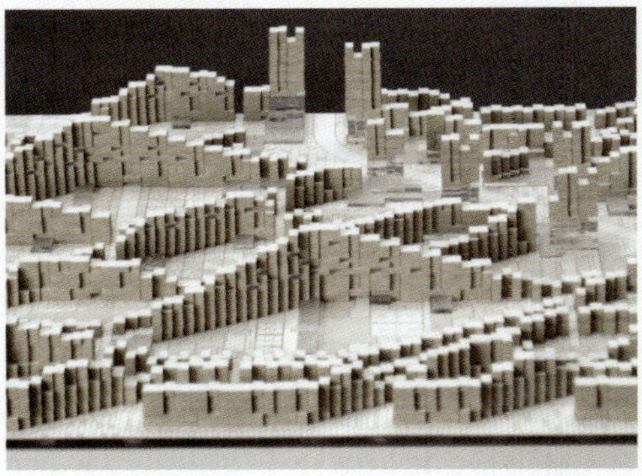

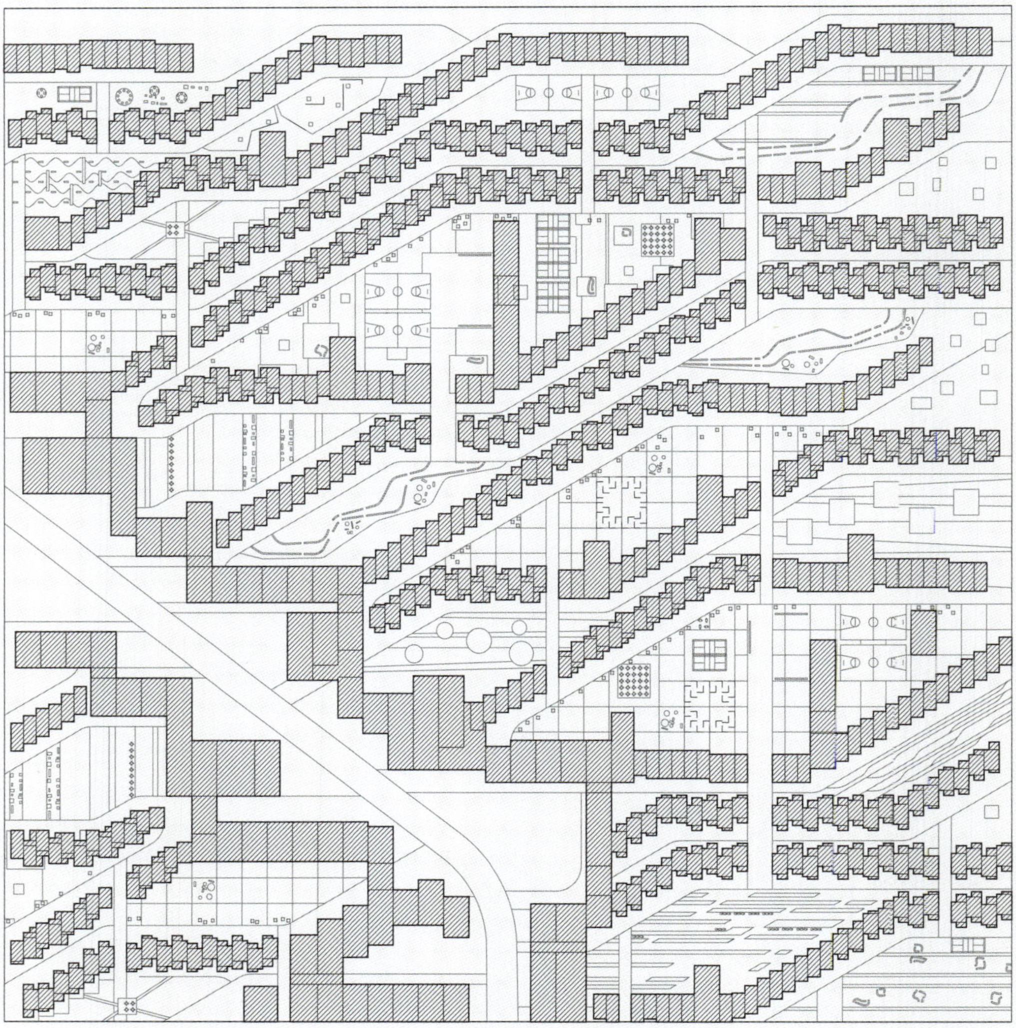

(Top Left) Courtyard/alley distribution
(Top Middle) Model photographs. (Photographs by Anita Kan)
(Left Bottom) Prototypical site plan.

Instead of creating a system of evenly distributed courtyards and laneways, or a purely concentrated system, we propose to build a system with varied scale and different levels of space sharing.

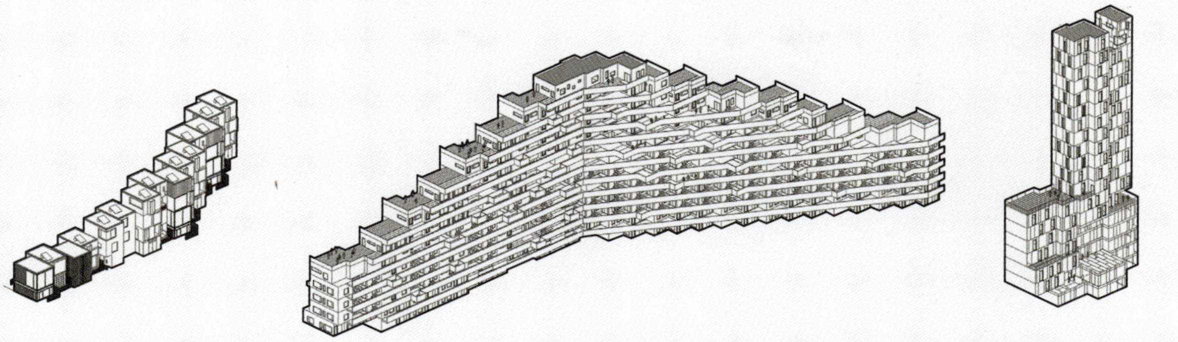

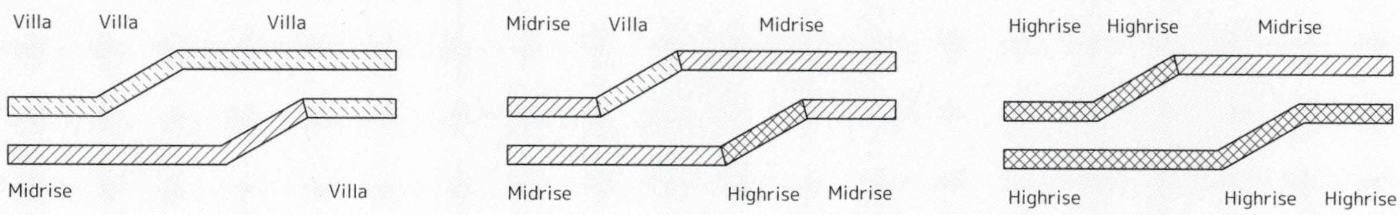

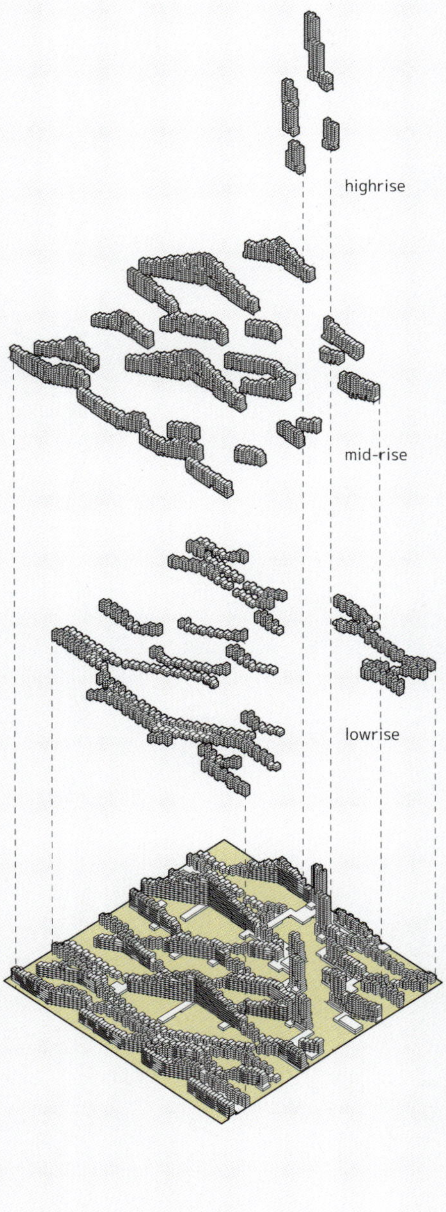

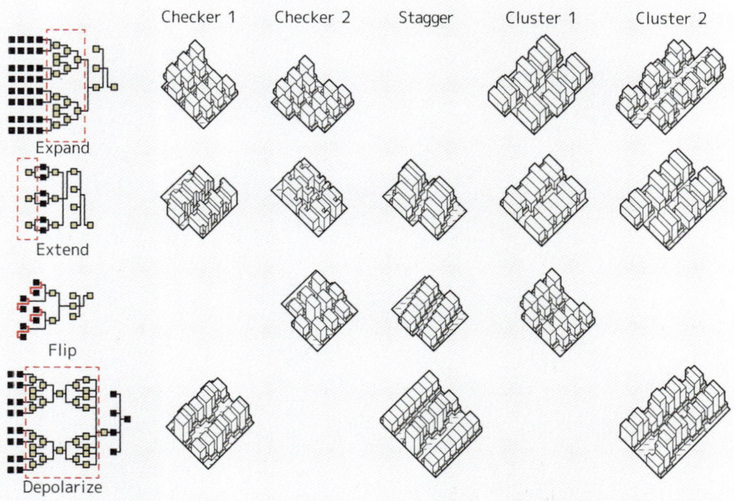

In the nineteenth century, older public health reform campaigns in the west sought to improve the living conditions of urban populations by imposing clear order and standardization. The *xiaoqu* is a result of this impulse inherited from the hygiene movement. We propose that a return to a more ambiguous and gradated series of spaces offering models for neighborhood environments that invite chance encounters, overlapping itineraries, and even occasional congestion. The project was invested in the notion that spatial diversity and a finer grain is a valuable quality for the neighborhood, while understanding that China's contemporary urbanization demand higher densities than the older models can deliver. Through a series of graph diagrams, we were able to describe organizational structures that support a more nuanced and graduated distribution of a neighborhood's activities throughout its physical fabric. These were translated into a number of design strategies and various organizational design features that supported (1) the expansion of the zone of shared spaces, (2) the extension of the interior private spaces by adding additional buffer zones, (3) flipping orientations and front-to-back relationships to create the possibility of chance encounters and contiguities, (4) and depolarizing the linear transition in the hierarchy of spaces into a more intricate and gradated zone.

(Top) Density types.
(Top-Middle) Arrangement of density.
(Left) Aggregation diagram.
(Bottom) Configuration diagram.

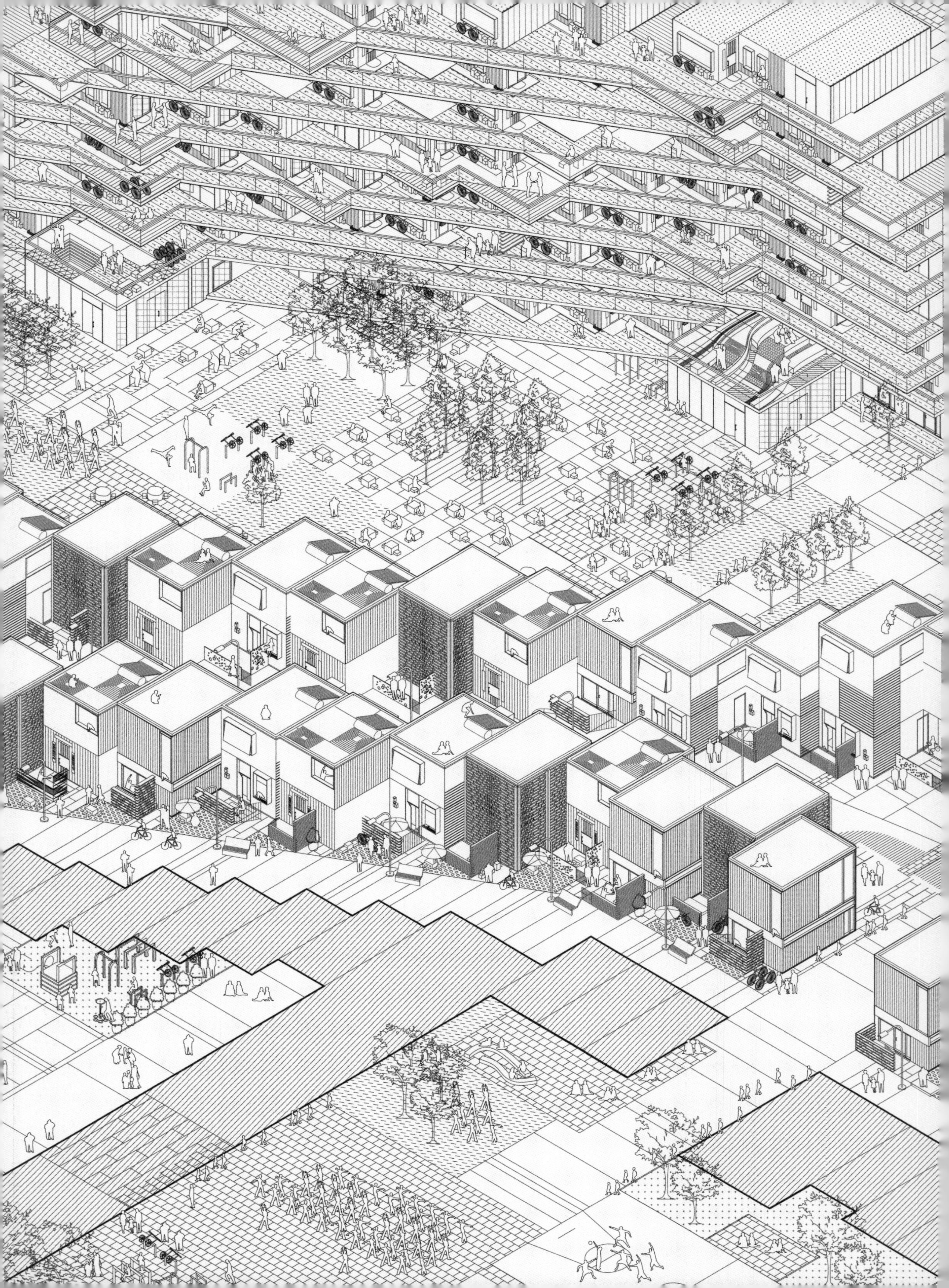

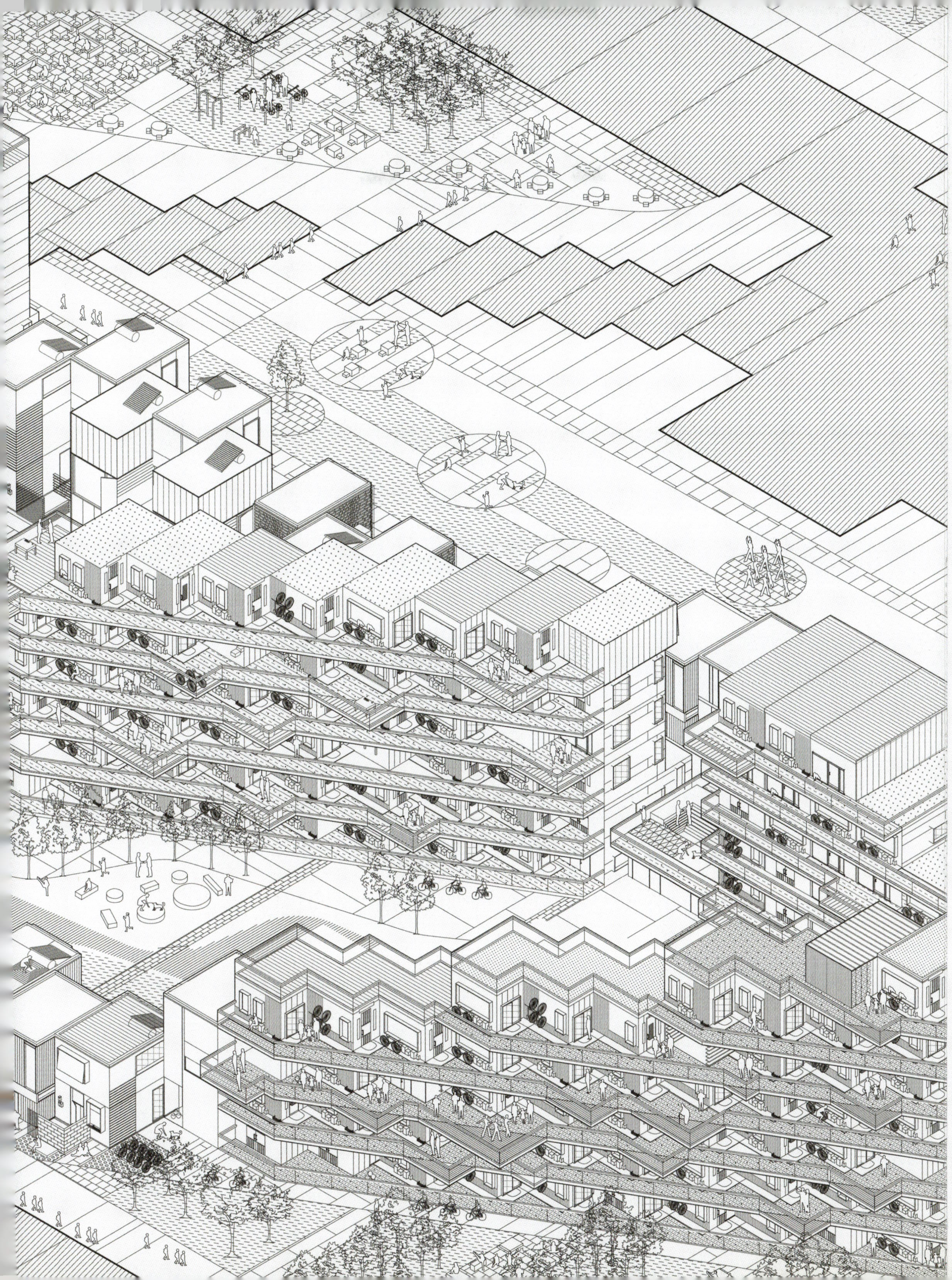

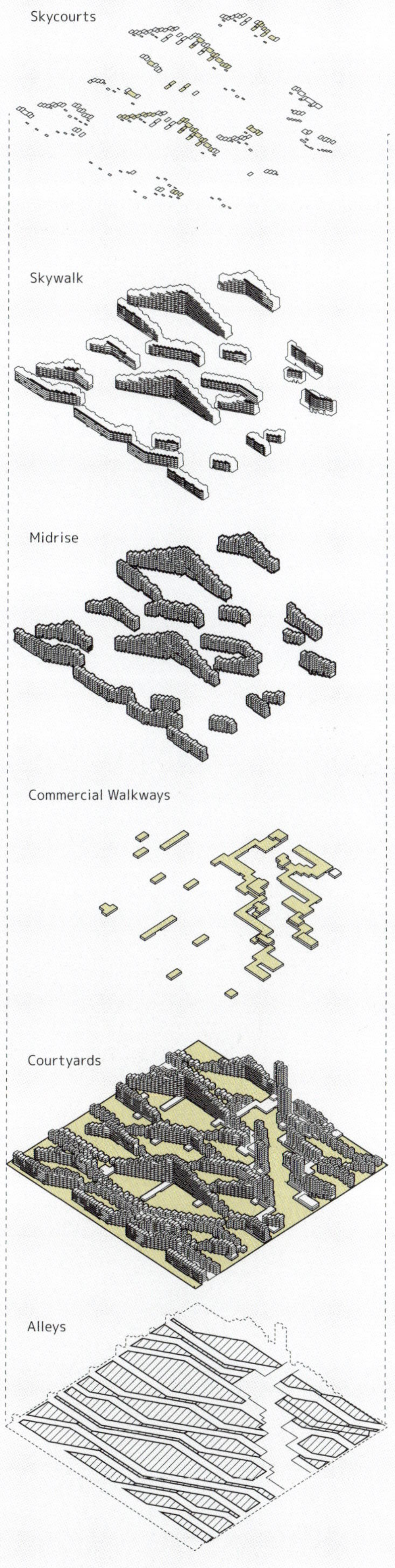

The overlapping of multiple layers of "ground" levels allows for the capacity to introduce the finer grain of social spaces found in models like the *linong* within a high density and sometimes high-rise typology. Roof terraces, expanded balconies, and differing scales of forecourts and backyards are scattered throughout the neighborhood. The diverse physical fabric offers a kaleidoscopic array of different housing types, social spaces, and landscape experiences as well as the possibility of embedding amenities, services, and community facilities within the block.

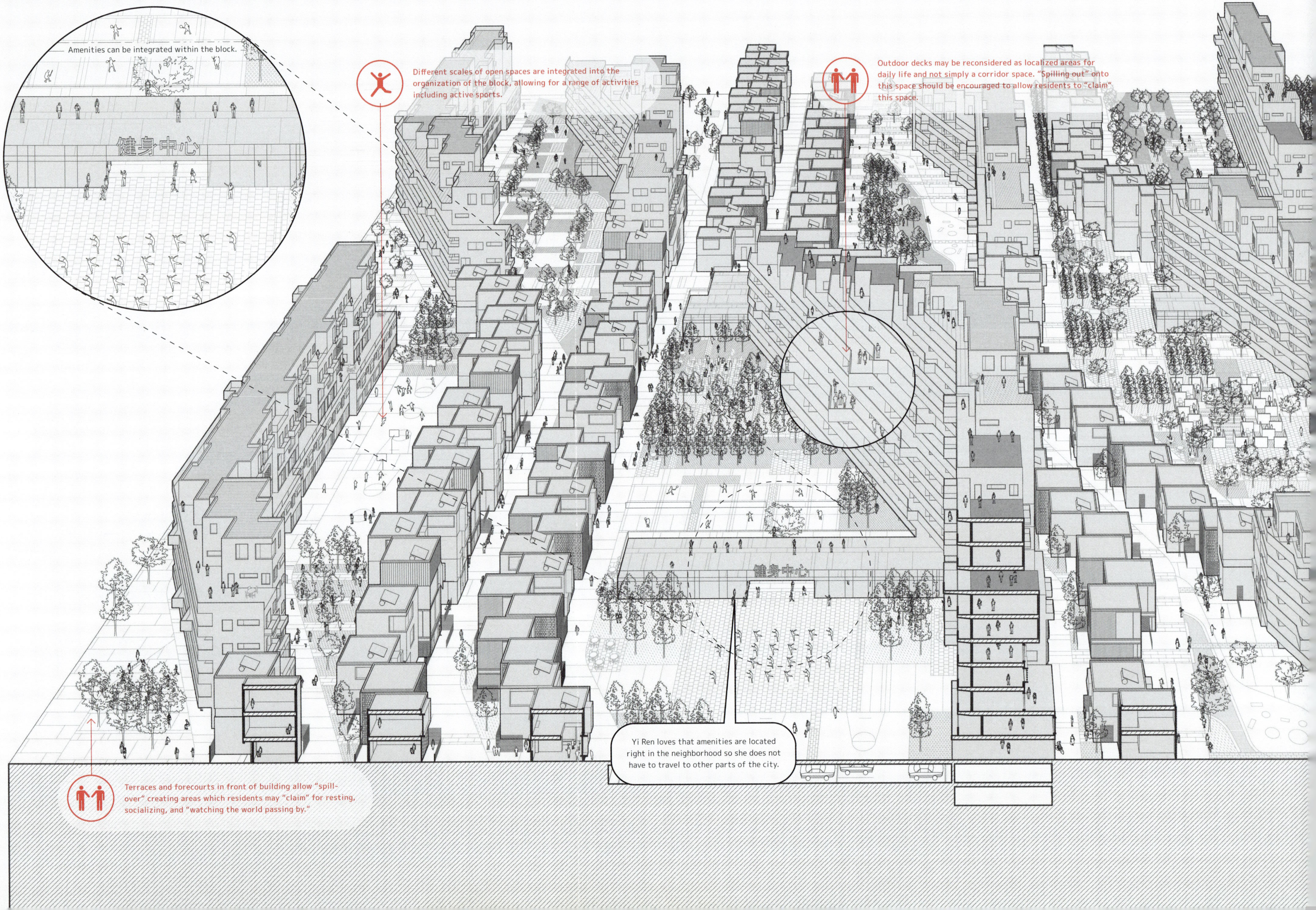
Amenities can be integrated within the block.
健身中心
Different scales of open spaces are integrated into the organization of the block, allowing for a range of activities including active sports.
Outdoor decks may be reconsidered as localized areas for daily life and not simply a corridor space. "Spilling out" onto this space should be encouraged to allow residents to "claim" this space.
Yi Ren loves that amenities are located right in the neighborhood so she does not have to travel to other parts of the city.
Terraces and forecourts in front of building allow "spill-over" creating areas which residents may "claim" for resting, socializing, and "watching the world passing by."

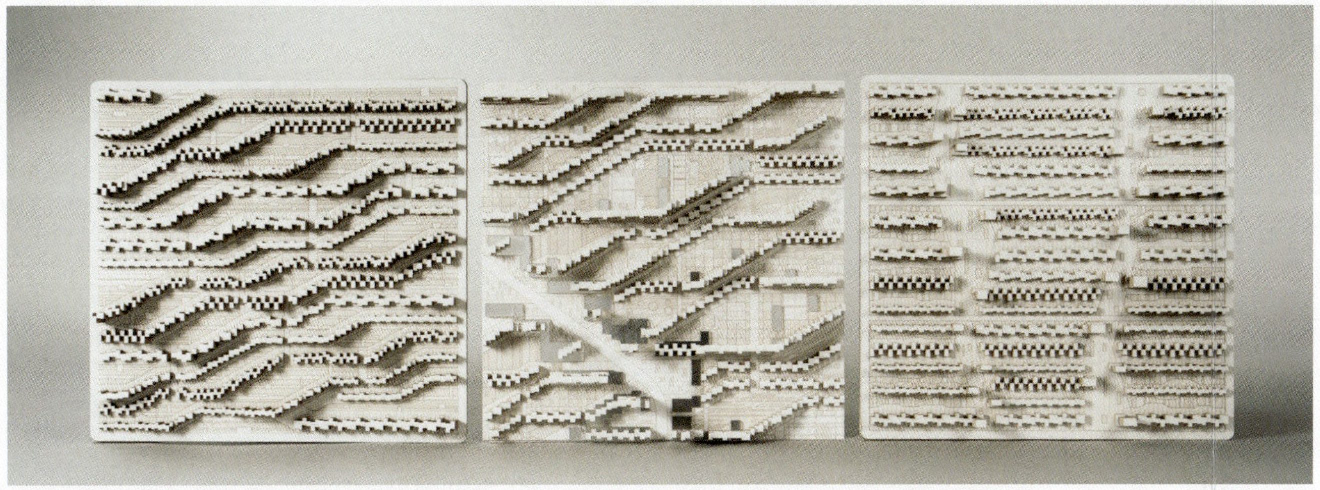

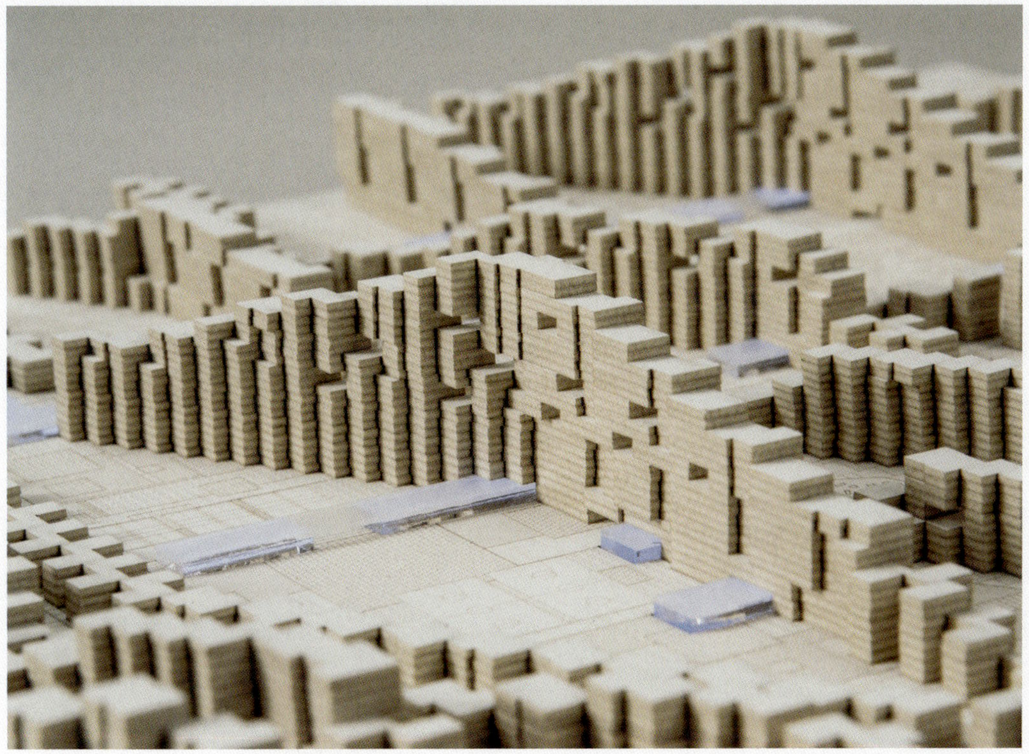

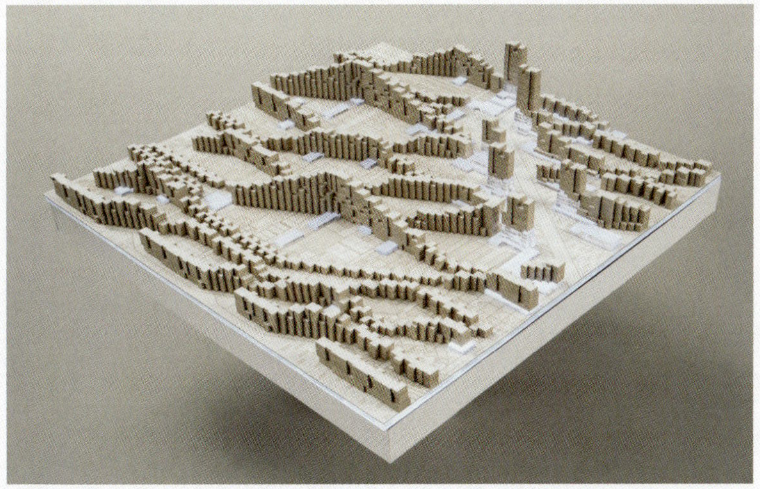

(Top) Photograph of model iterations/typologies.
(Middle) Photograph of model, close up.
(Bottom) Photograph of overall final model.

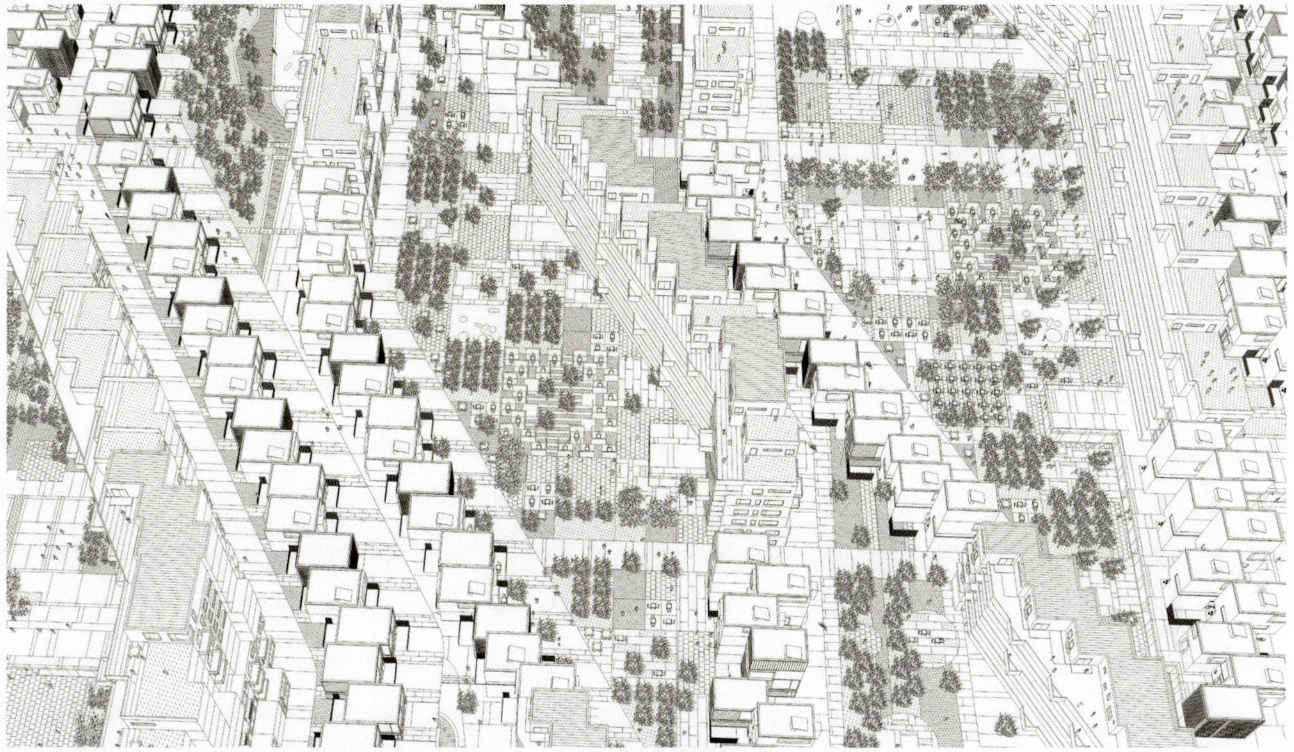

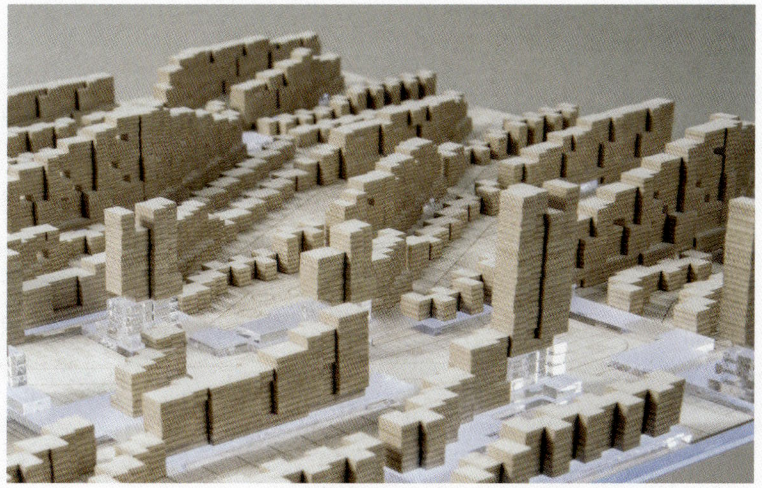

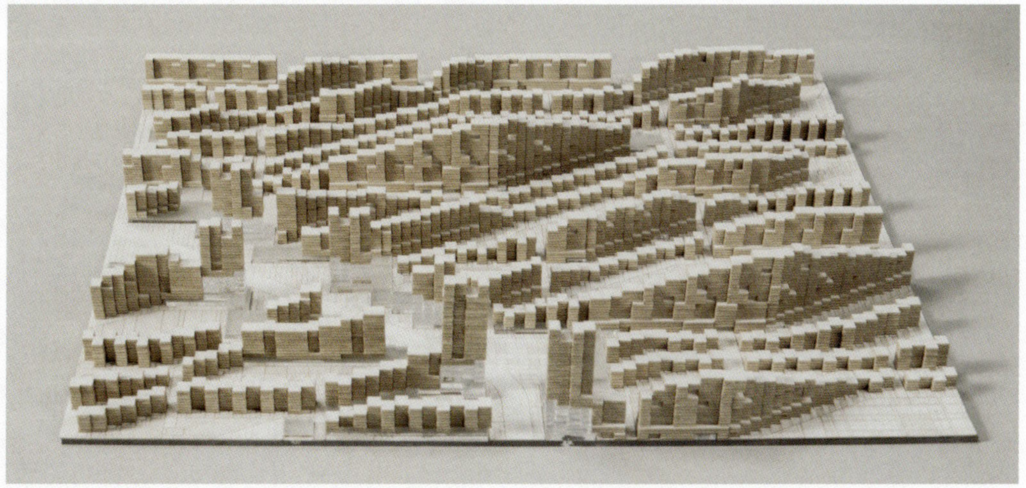

(Top) Perspective line drawing of alleys and housing.
(Middle) Photograph of model, close up.
(Bottom) Photograph of model side.
(Photographs by Anita Kan)

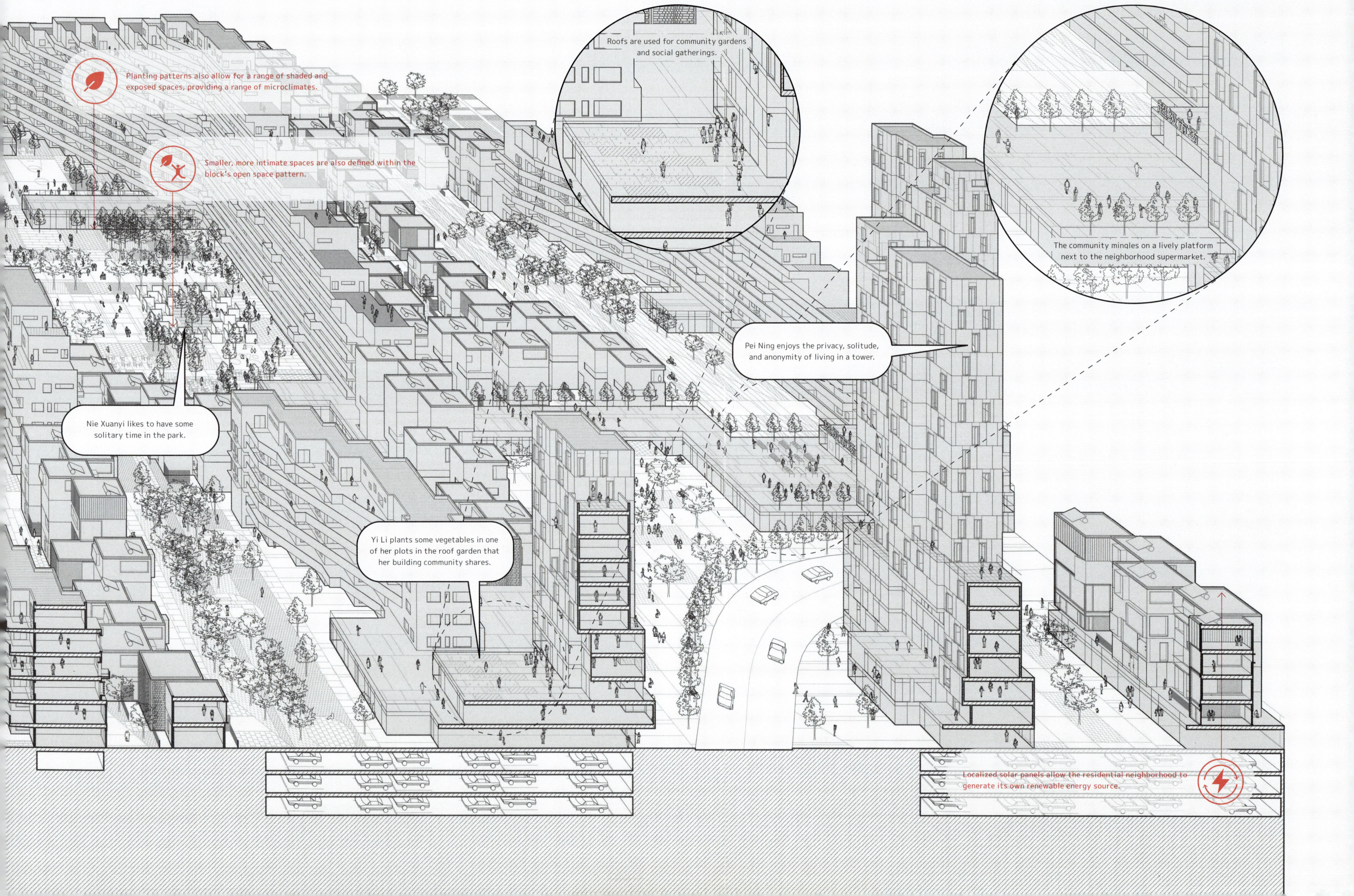
Planting patterns also allow for a range of shaded and exposed spaces, providing a range of microclimates.
Smaller, more intimate spaces are also defined within the block's open space pattern.
Roofs are used for community gardens and social gatherings.
The community mingles on a lively platform next to the neighborhood supermarket.
Pei Ning enjoys the privacy, solitude, and anonymity of living in a tower.
Nie Xuanyi likes to have some solitary time in the park.
Yi Li plants some vegetables in one of her plots in the roof garden that her building community shares.
Localized solar panels allow the residential neighborhood to generate its own renewable energy source.

Community for the Multitude

Yujun Yin + Zhe Peng

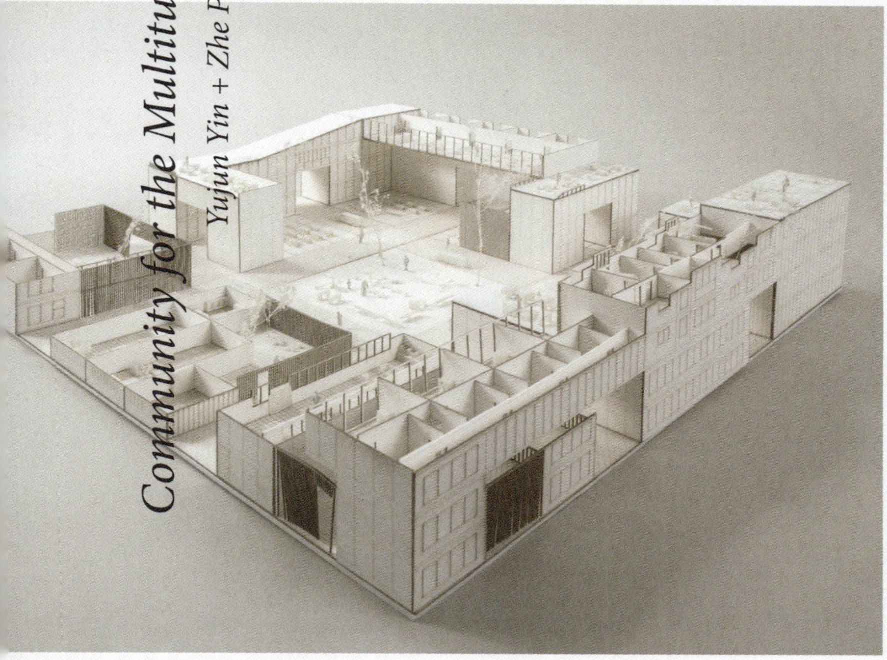

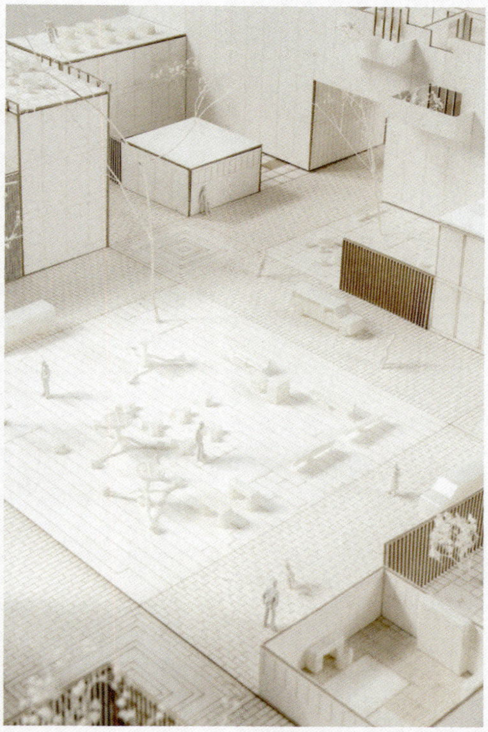

(Top Right) Close up photograph of prototype model
(Top Left) Overall photograph of prototype model
(Photographs by Anita Kan)

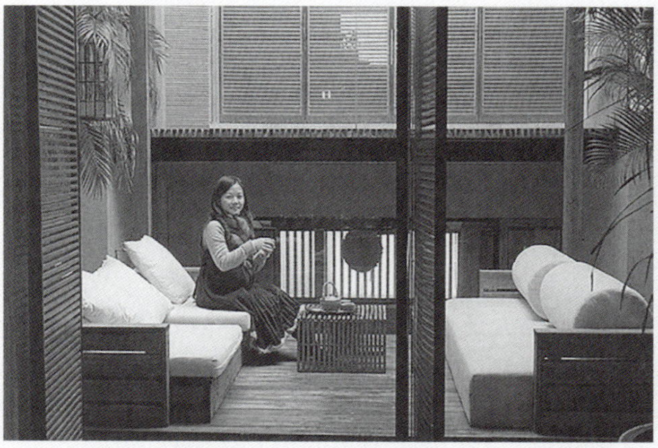

Liu Dan-Chengdu, Luxury Villas (Photograph by Xiaoci Bai)

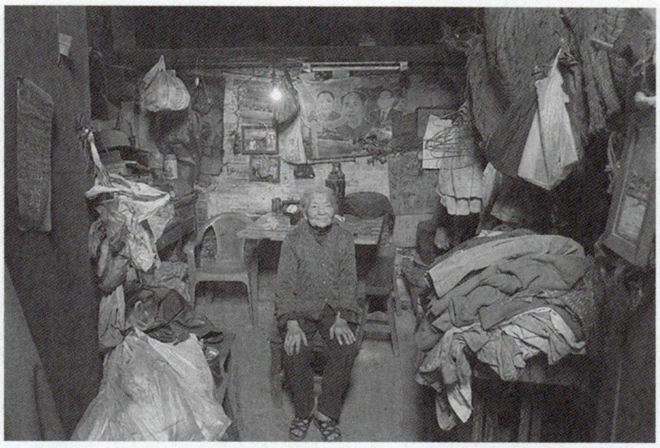

Xipu Yu-Shenzhen, "Urban Villages" Multi-family Courtyard Housing
(Photograph by Xiaoci Bai)

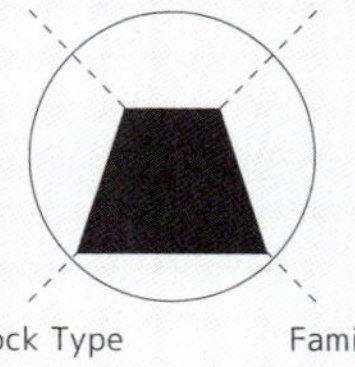

"My own view can be stated simply: the quality of life in a city is good when its inhabitants are capable of dealing with complexity. Conversely, the quality of life in cities is bad when its inhabitants are capable only of dealing with people like themselves. Put another way, a healthy city can embrace and make productive use of the differences of class, ethnicity, and lifestyles it contains, while a sick city cannot; the sick city isolates and segregates difference, drawing no collective strength from its mixture of different people."[1]

China's ongoing economic and social change has transformed the lives of many of its citizens, multiplying the number of different subjects that constitute the wide continuum of its polity. The shift towards a more capitalist economic model has brought with it an acute differentiation and inequality amongst its citizens, producing a dramatic difference in lifestyles and life chances. The gulf between urban and rural life has become even more pronounced since the emergence of what has been called a "floating population" of unregistered rural migrants living within China's urban conurbations has further contrasted the growing urban middle classes with an impoverished countryside.

The country's current urbanization has, until recently, been largely driven by a real estate boom with property developers constituting the major homebuilders nationwide. This has resulted in a residential landscape which largely caters to a market abstraction of the urban middle and upper classes, with very little concern for the urban and rural poor. Gated community models and neighborhoods marketed to, and therefore segregated in, distinct social classes have spatialized the growing inequalities by constructing enclaves.

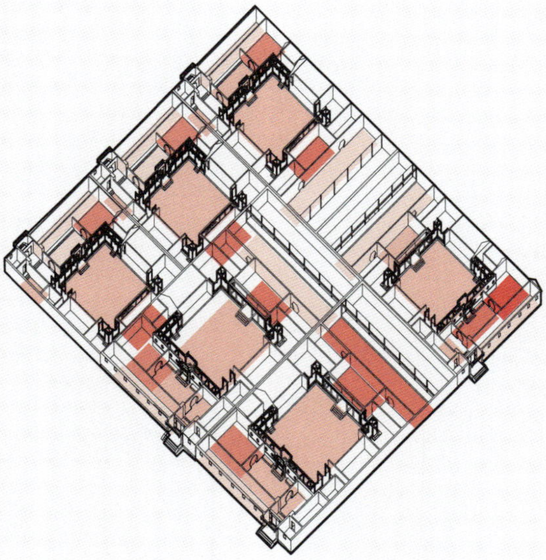

Courtyard House

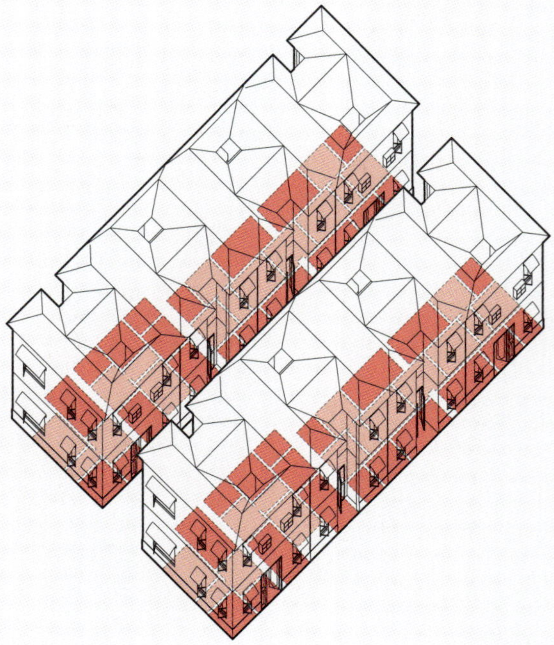

Linong Housing

Can the complexity described by Richard Sennett be reflected in or enabled by the physical fabric of China's neighborhoods? Two of China's historically significant housing types; the *Siheyuan* courtyard and *Linong* row house types formed the basic unit for its urbanization in different periods of its past. China's urbanization can be described as having often been determined by the adoption and subsequent deployment of prevailing types or models over large extensions. Despite their repetitive and standardized nature, these types have been found to be open to adaptation, accommodating a range of different lifestyles over time and can be seen to have a more intricate spatial and programmatic relationship between private and social spaces.

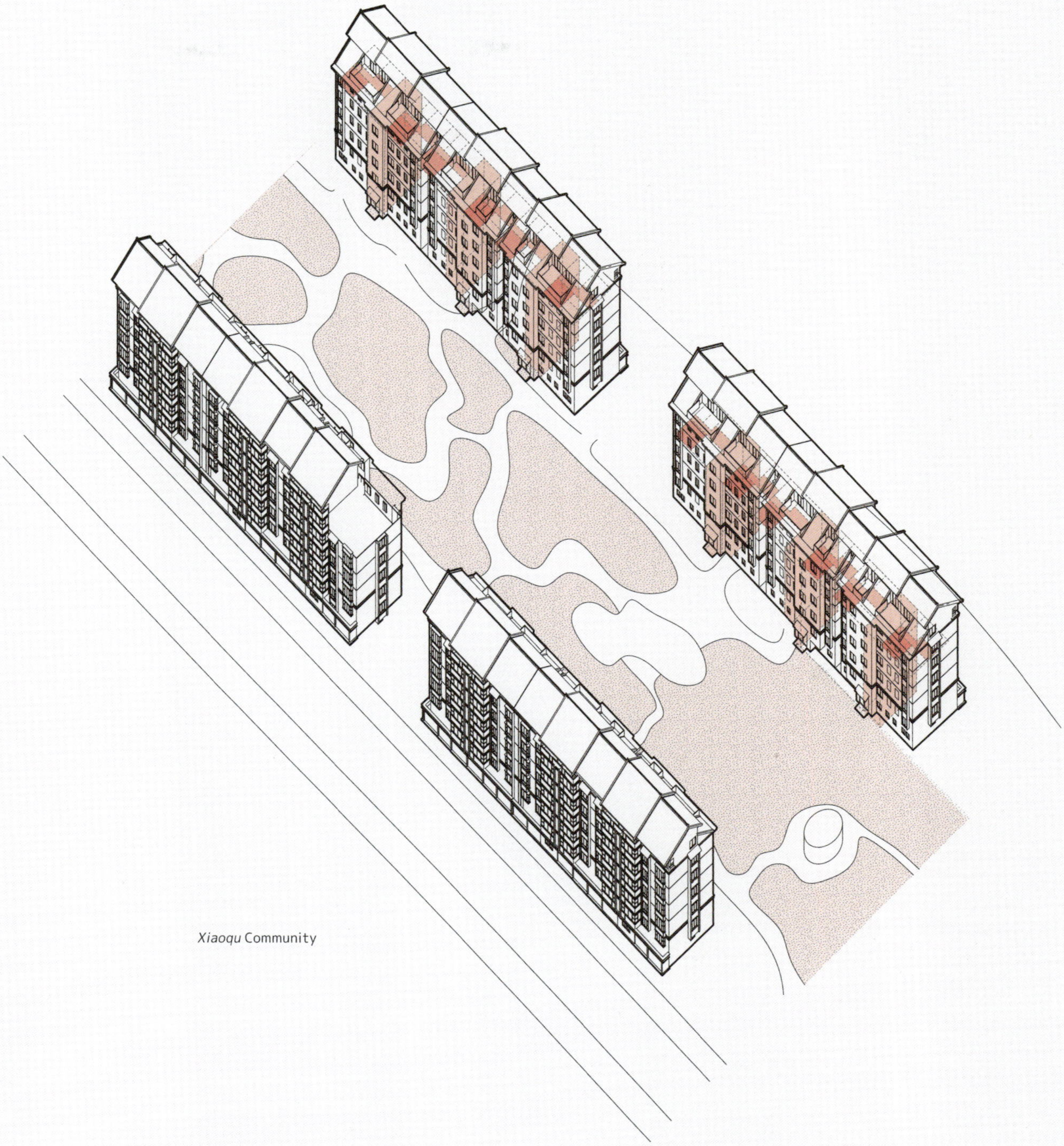

Xiaoqu Community

The contemporary housing developments offered by the market (the *xiaoqu*) offer a greatly improved built environment in terms of hygiene and its associated modern conveniences. They have, however, also adopted a model of housing that has, in many ways, failed to recognize the value of complexity. Many new residents, including those relocated from appropriated rural land, lament the lack of appropriate social spaces as well as the inflexibility of the spatial structure of these developments to accommodate different living arrangements. Many have suffered a sense of isolation and an inability to adapt to this new spatial structure. The underlying market assumptions and standard development practices that shape these places are often predicated on a narrow view of housing as a commodity. What is needed is a community for the multitude that allows for complexity and for the possibility of its residents to determine their own living spaces.

Units, Models and Aggregations

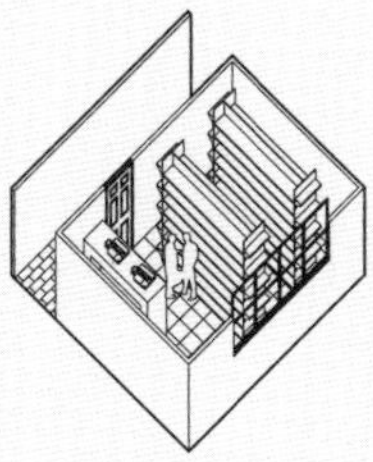

Grocery Store

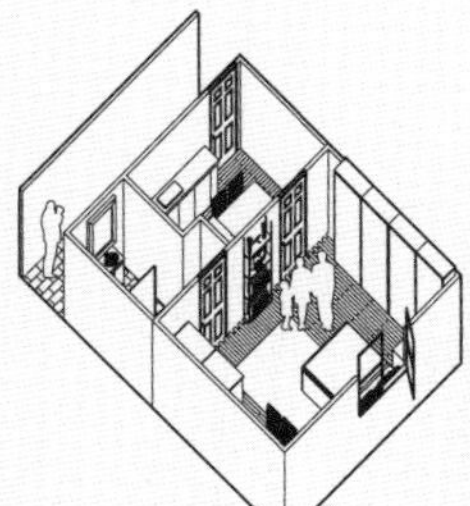

Studio type

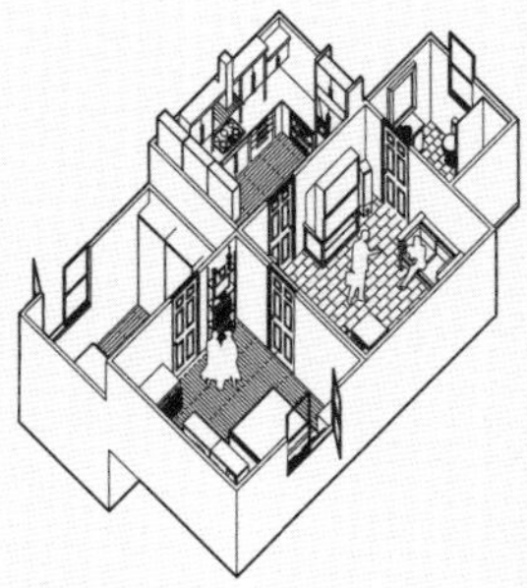

Two-Family Type

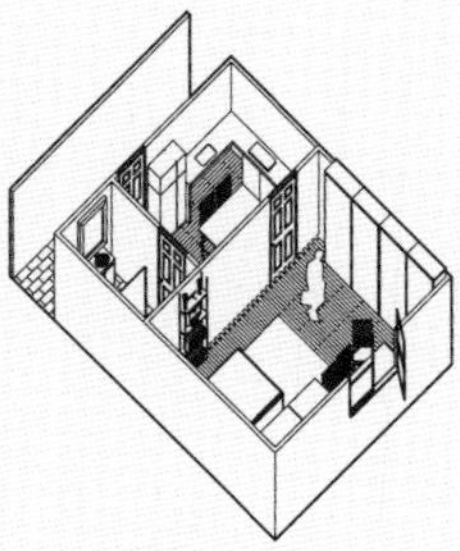

Studio Type

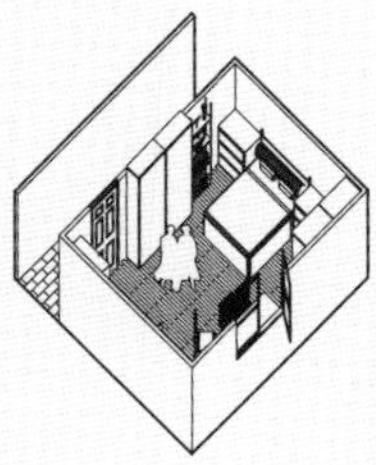

Studio Type

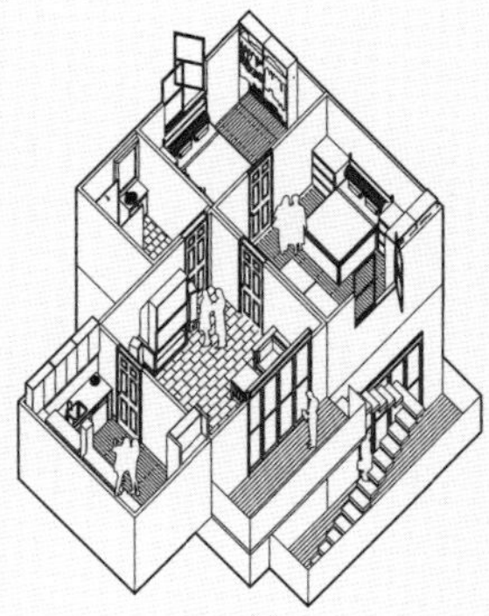

Two-Family Type

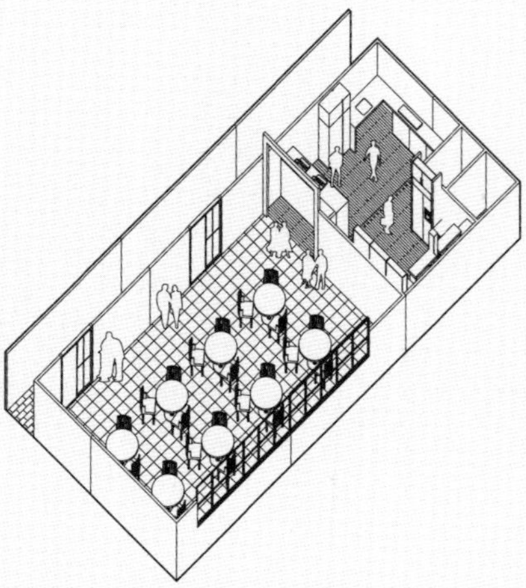

Restaurant

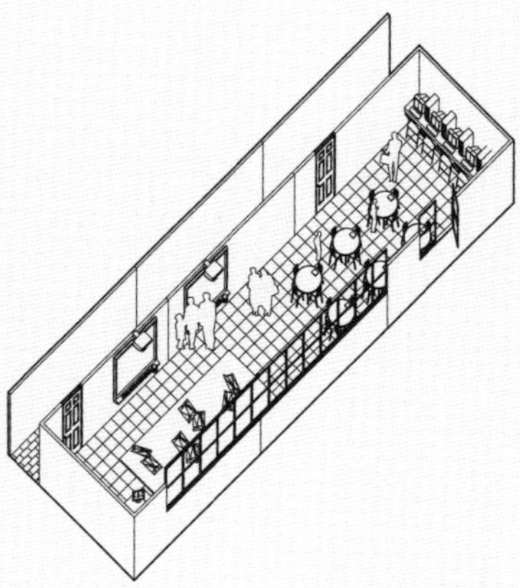

Studio Type

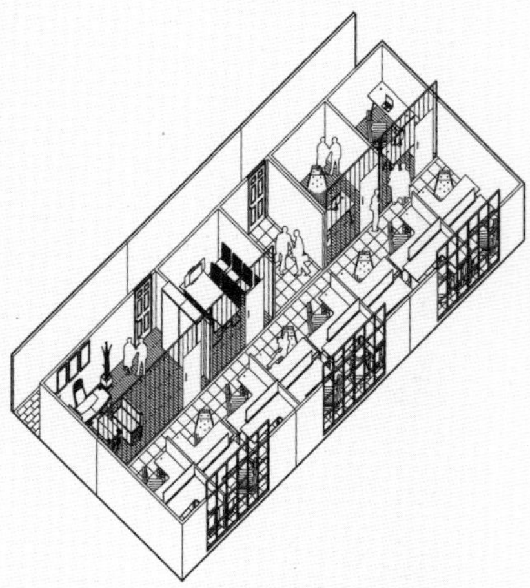

Two-Famliy Type

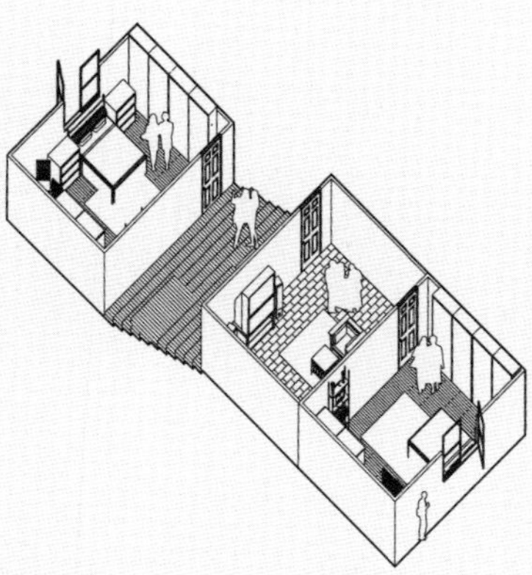

House for Single or Young Couple

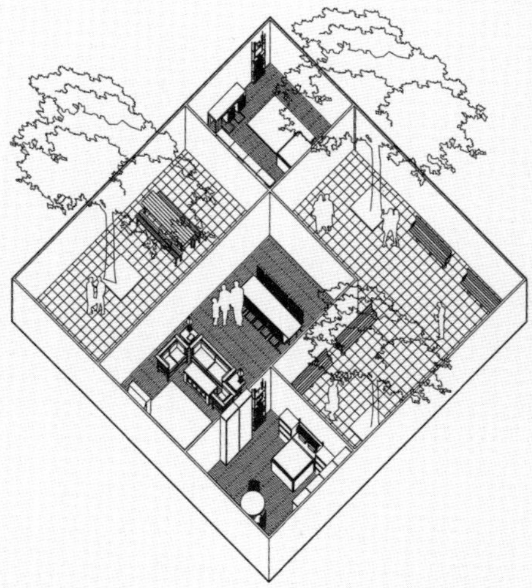

Courtyard

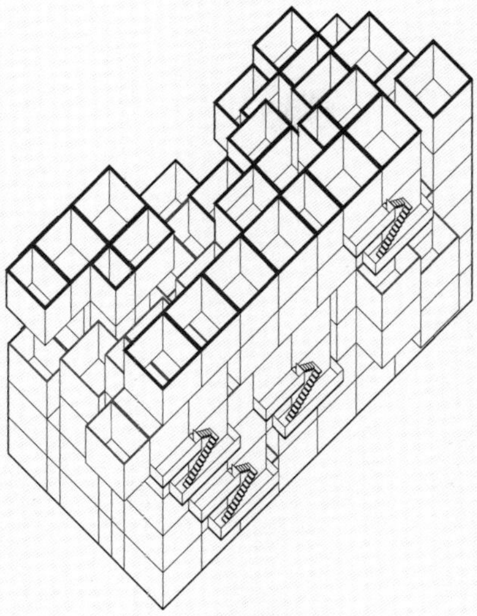
Aggregation 1

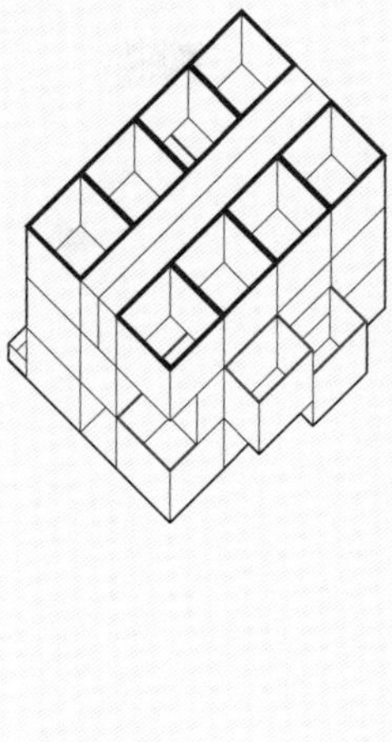
Aggregation 2

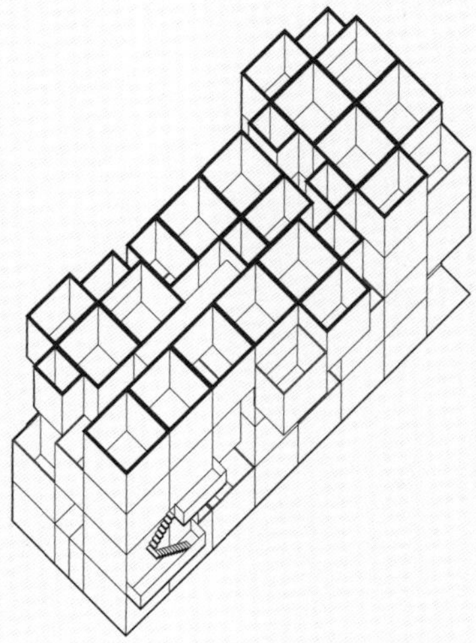
Aggregation 3

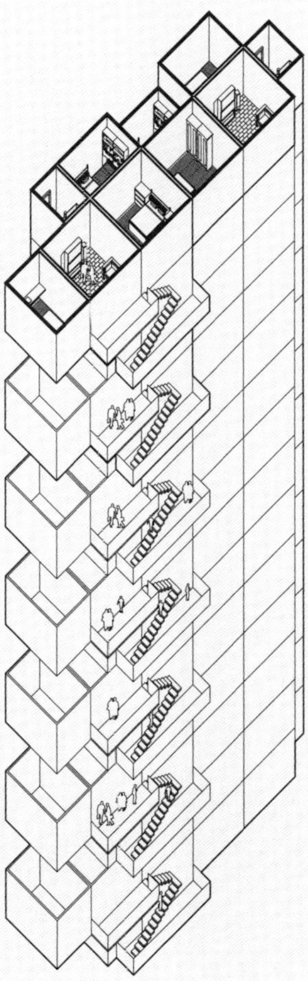
Aggregation 4

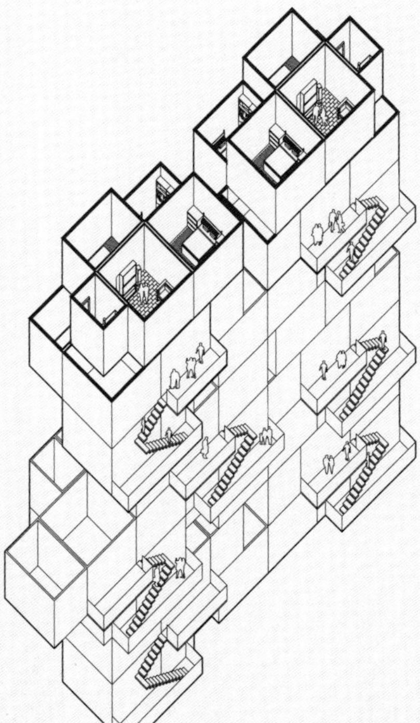
Aggregation 5

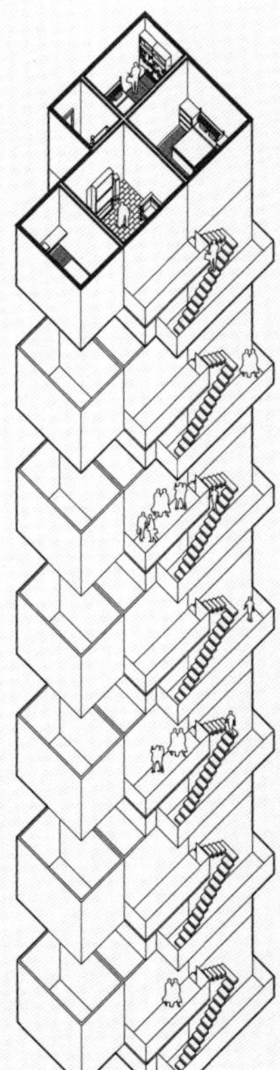
Aggregation 6

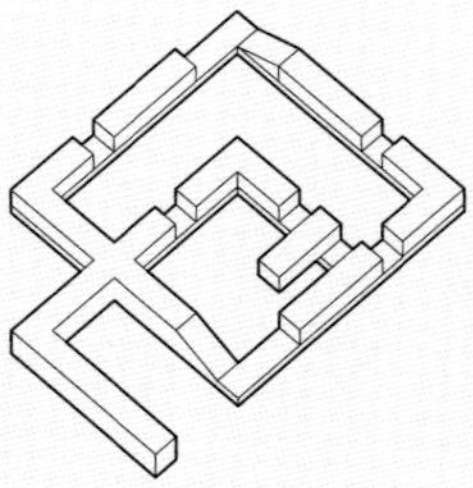

Composition 1

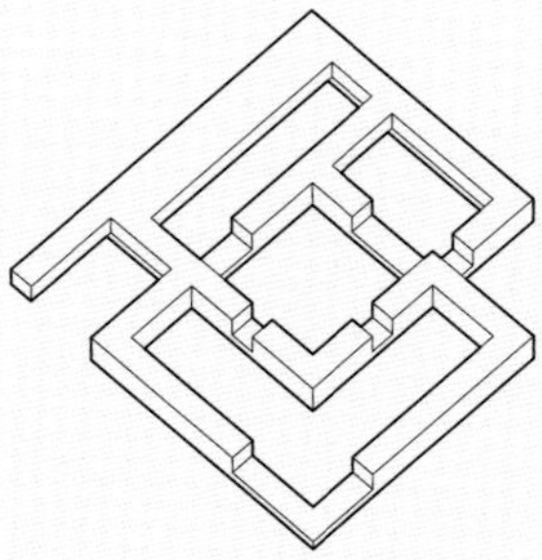

Composition 2

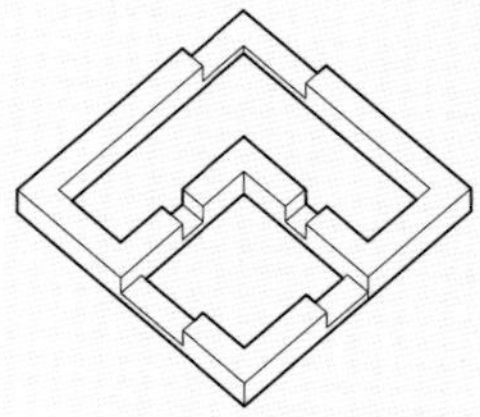

Composition 3

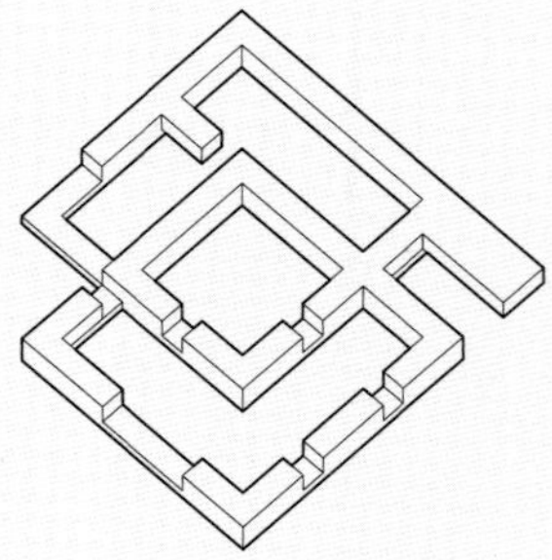

Composition 4

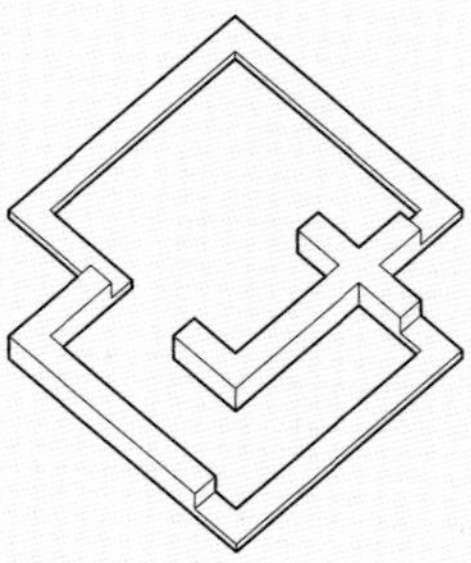

Composition 1

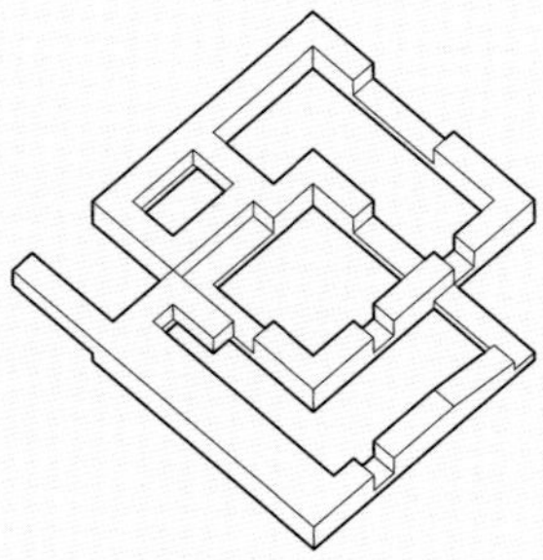

Composition 2

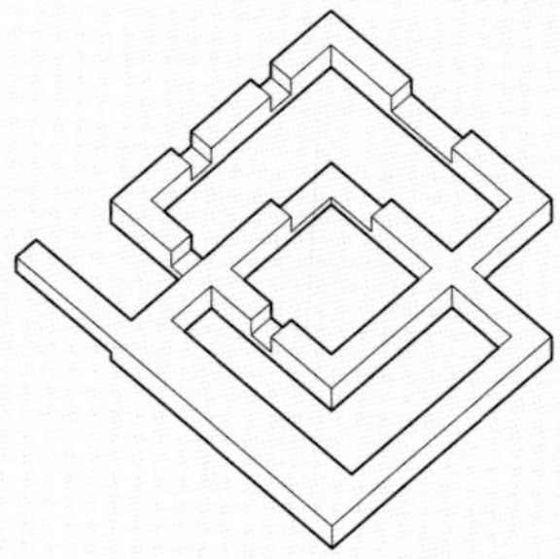

Composition 3

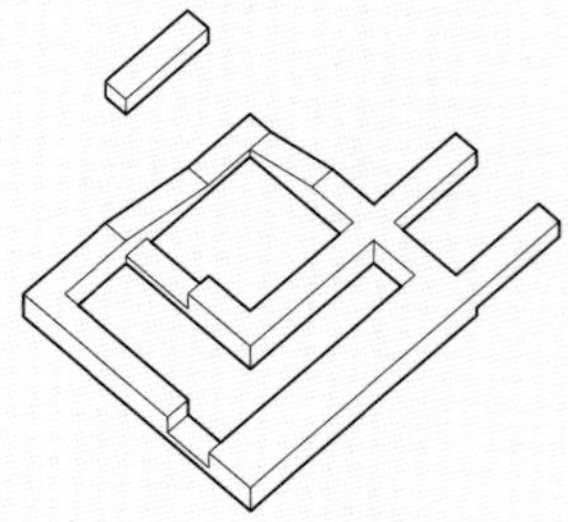

Composition 4

The neighborhood block is proposed as an aggregation of different modules across a range of scales. At the lower scales, a basic spatial unit allows for a rudimentary living space, while any number of aggregations of these units may offer residents the possibility for many different spatial configurations and possible uses. Because of their modularity, these spaces also allow for the negotiation and transformation of uses and residencies over time, opening it up to the possibility of adaptation. These can form a range of units at the next order of scale that, when aggregated in different ways, begin to form a variety of urban textures. Various compositions may be arranged at various heights throughout the block to define a varying order of large courtyards and urban fabrics. The resulting spatial intricacy is intentional both in organizational and expressive terms; it acts as the environment in which a complex array of China's citizens may come to claim a space for themselves within a larger aggregation.

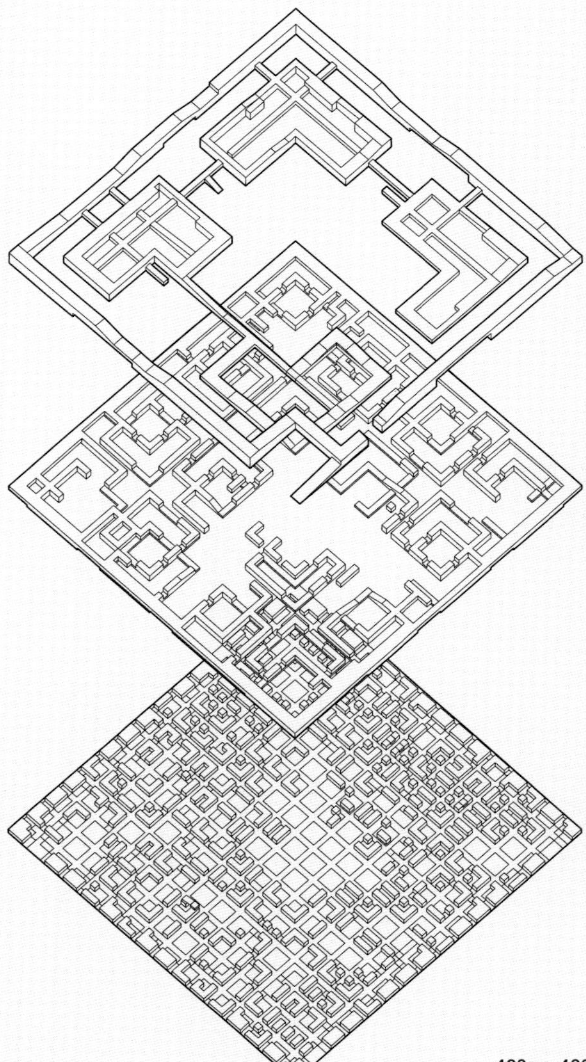

400m x 400m Prototype

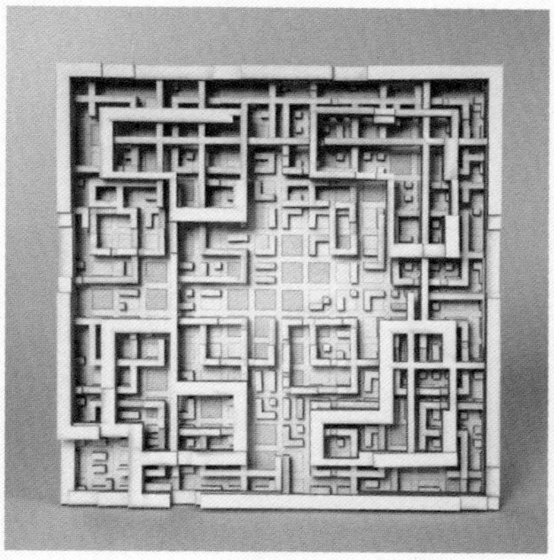

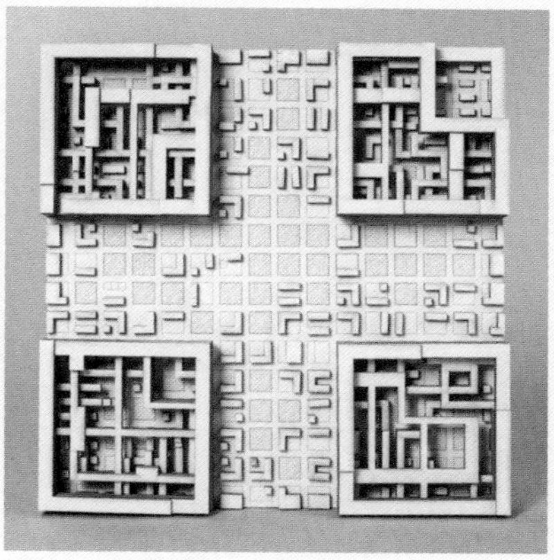

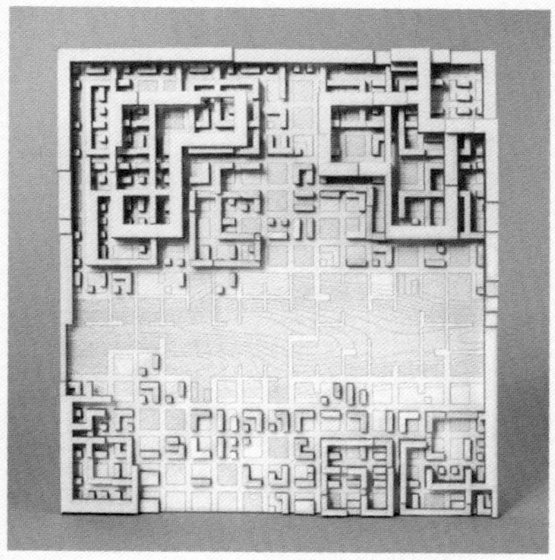

(Above) Site models
(Photographs by Anita Kan)

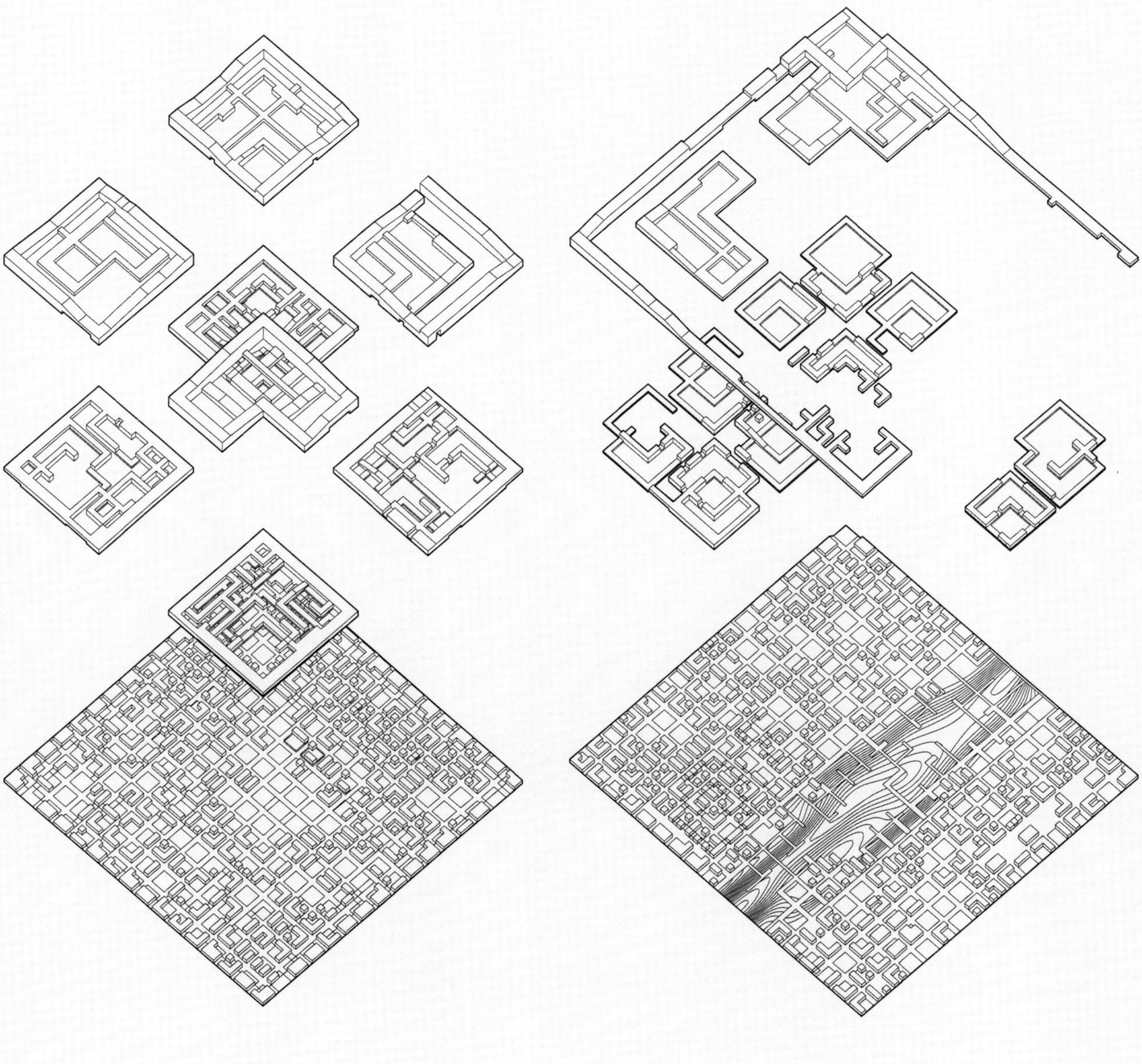

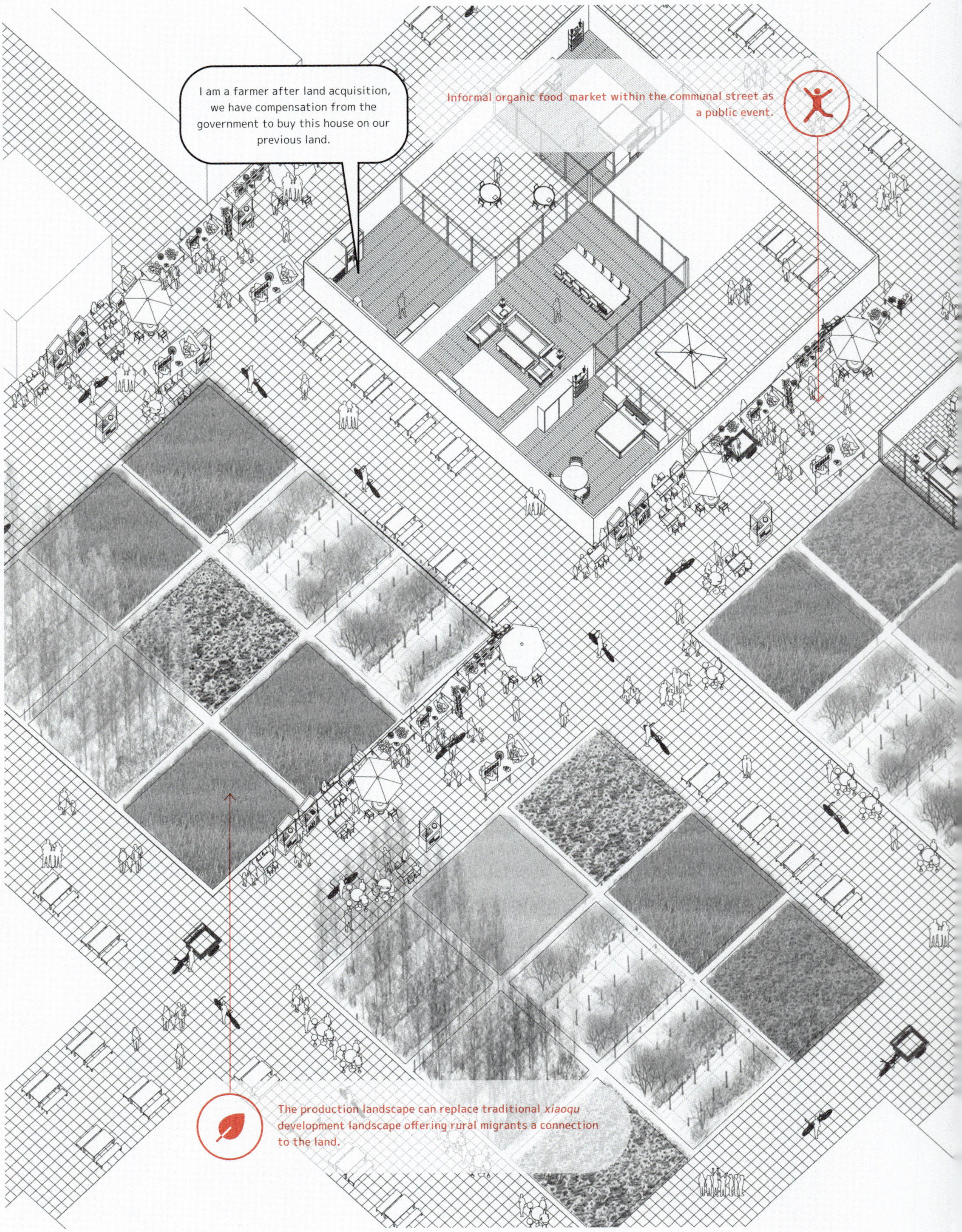
I am a farmer after land acquisition, we have compensation from the government to buy this house on our previous land.
Informal organic food market within the communal street as a public event.
The production landscape can replace traditional *xiaoqu* development landscape offering rural migrants a connection to the land.

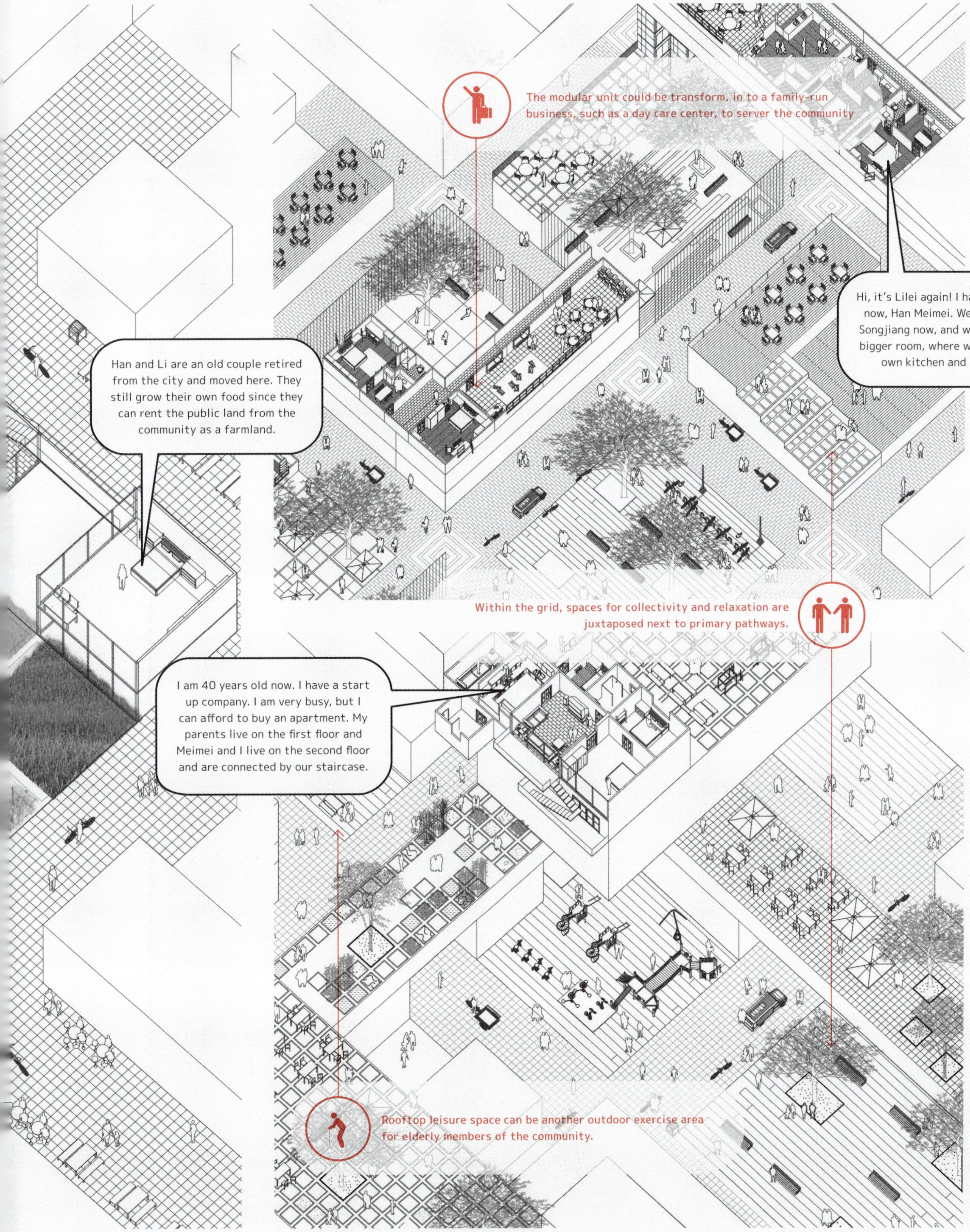
The modular unit could be transform, in to a family-run business, such as a day care center, to server the community
Hi, it's Lilei again! I have a girlfriend now, Han Meimei. We both work in Songjiang now, and we moved into a bigger room, where we can have our own kitchen and bathroom.
Han and Li are an old couple retired from the city and moved here. They still grow their own food since they can rent the public land from the community as a farmland.
Within the grid, spaces for collectivity and relaxation are juxtaposed next to primary pathways.
I am 40 years old now. I have a start up company. I am very busy, but I can afford to buy an apartment. My parents live on the first floor and Meimei and I live on the second floor and are connected by our staircase.
Rooftop leisure space can be another outdoor exercise area for elderly members of the community.

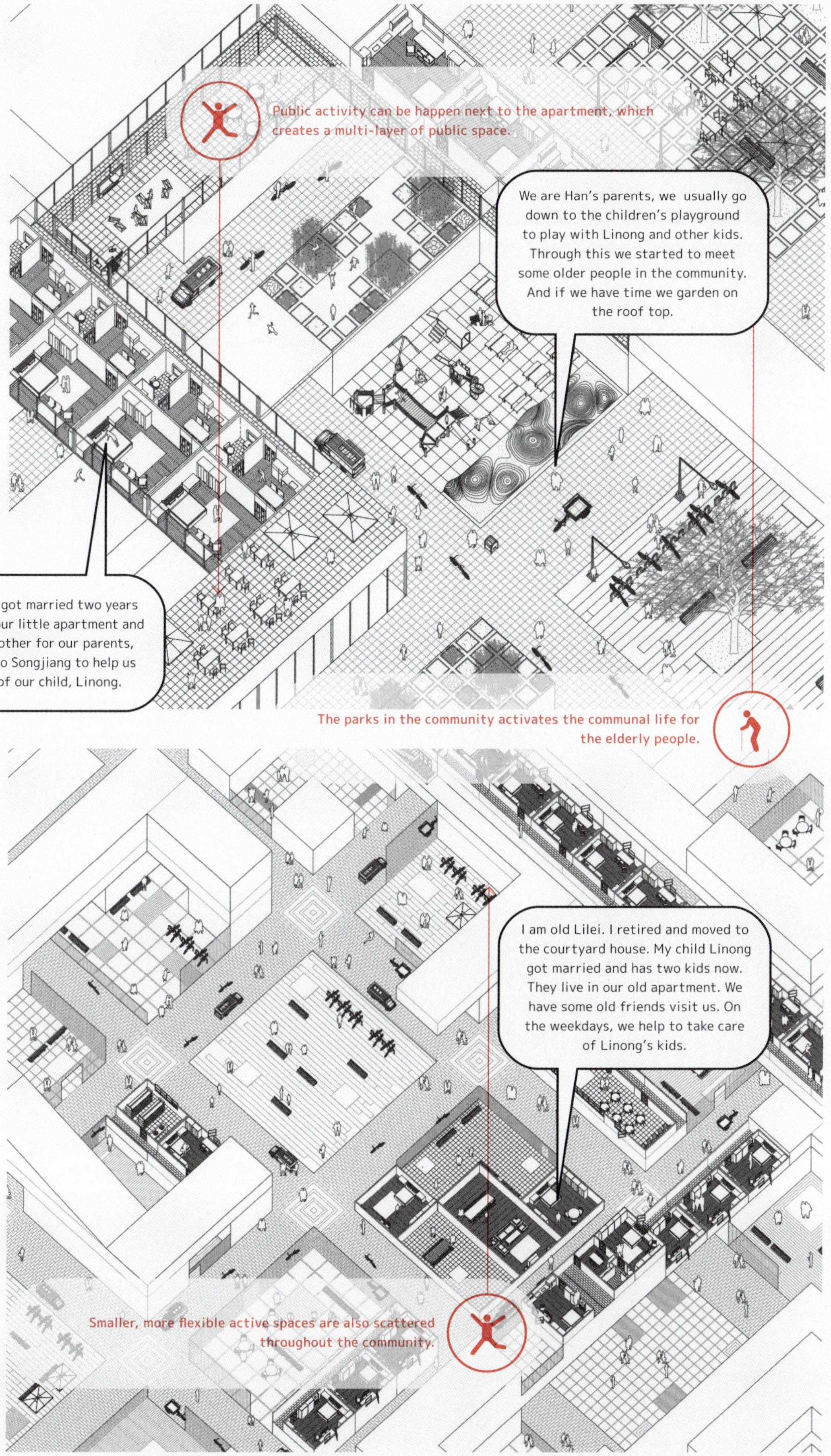
Public activity can be happen next to the apartment, which creates a multi-layer of public space.
We are Han's parents, we usually go down to the children's playground to play with Linong and other kids. Through this we started to meet some older people in the community. And if we have time we garden on the roof top.
Meimei and I got married two years ago. We own our little apartment and also rent another for our parents, who moved to Songjiang to help us take care of our child, Linong.
The parks in the community activates the communal life for the elderly people.
I am old Lilei. I retired and moved to the courtyard house. My child Linong got married and has two kids now. They live in our old apartment. We have some old friends visit us. On the weekdays, we help to take care of Linong's kids.
Smaller, more flexible active spaces are also scattered throughout the community.

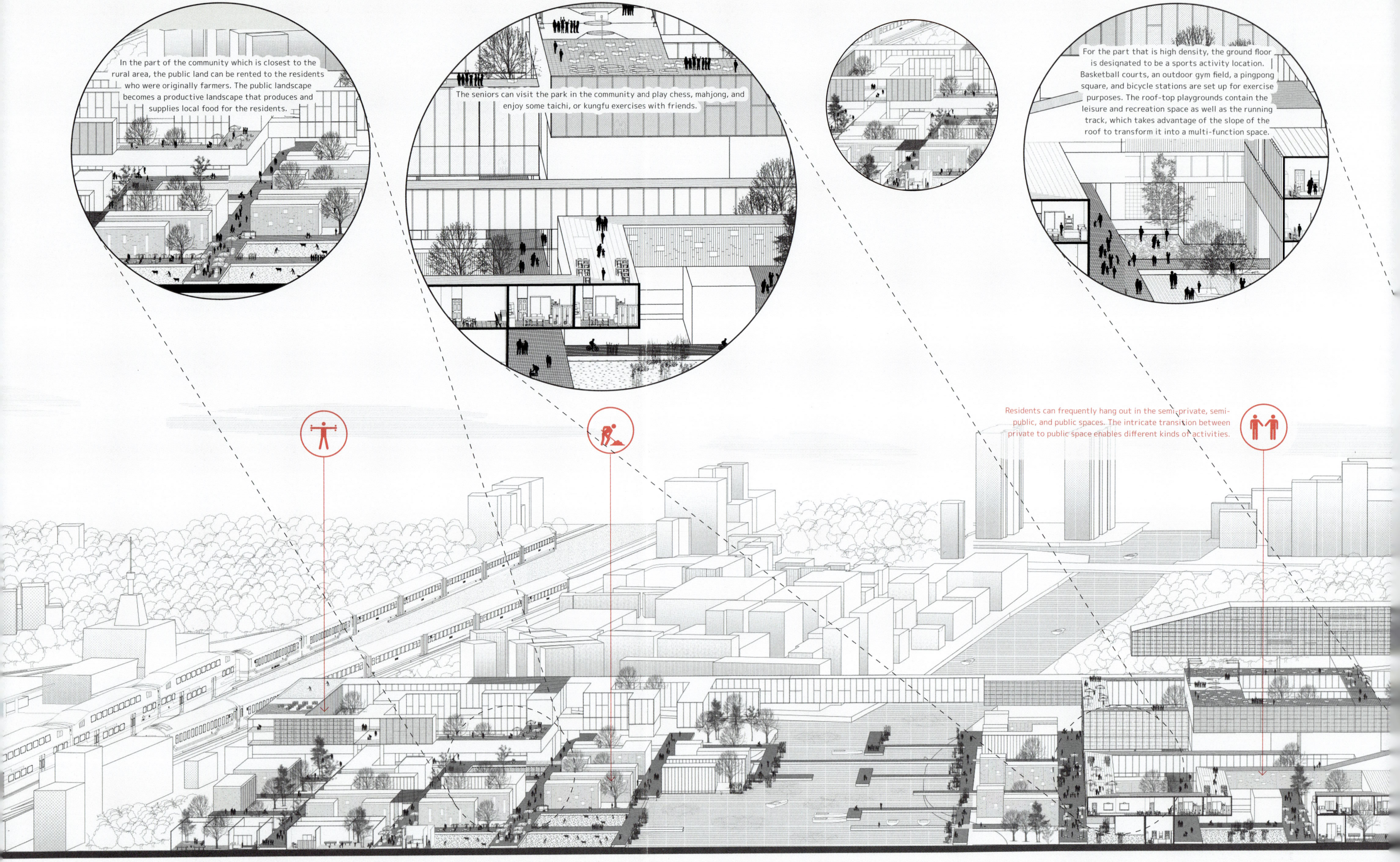
In the part of the community which is closest to the rural area, the public land can be rented to the residents who were originally farmers. The public landscape becomes a productive landscape that produces and supplies local food for the residents.
The seniors can visit the park in the community and play chess, mahjong, and enjoy some taichi, or kungfu exercises with friends.
For the part that is high density, the ground floor is designated to be a sports activity location. Basketball courts, an outdoor gym field, a pingpong square, and bicycle stations are set up for exercise purposes. The roof-top playgrounds contain the leisure and recreation space as well as the running track, which takes advantage of the slope of the roof to transform it into a multi-function space.
Residents can frequently hang out in the semi-private, semi-public, and public spaces. The intricate transition between private to public space enables different kinds of activities.

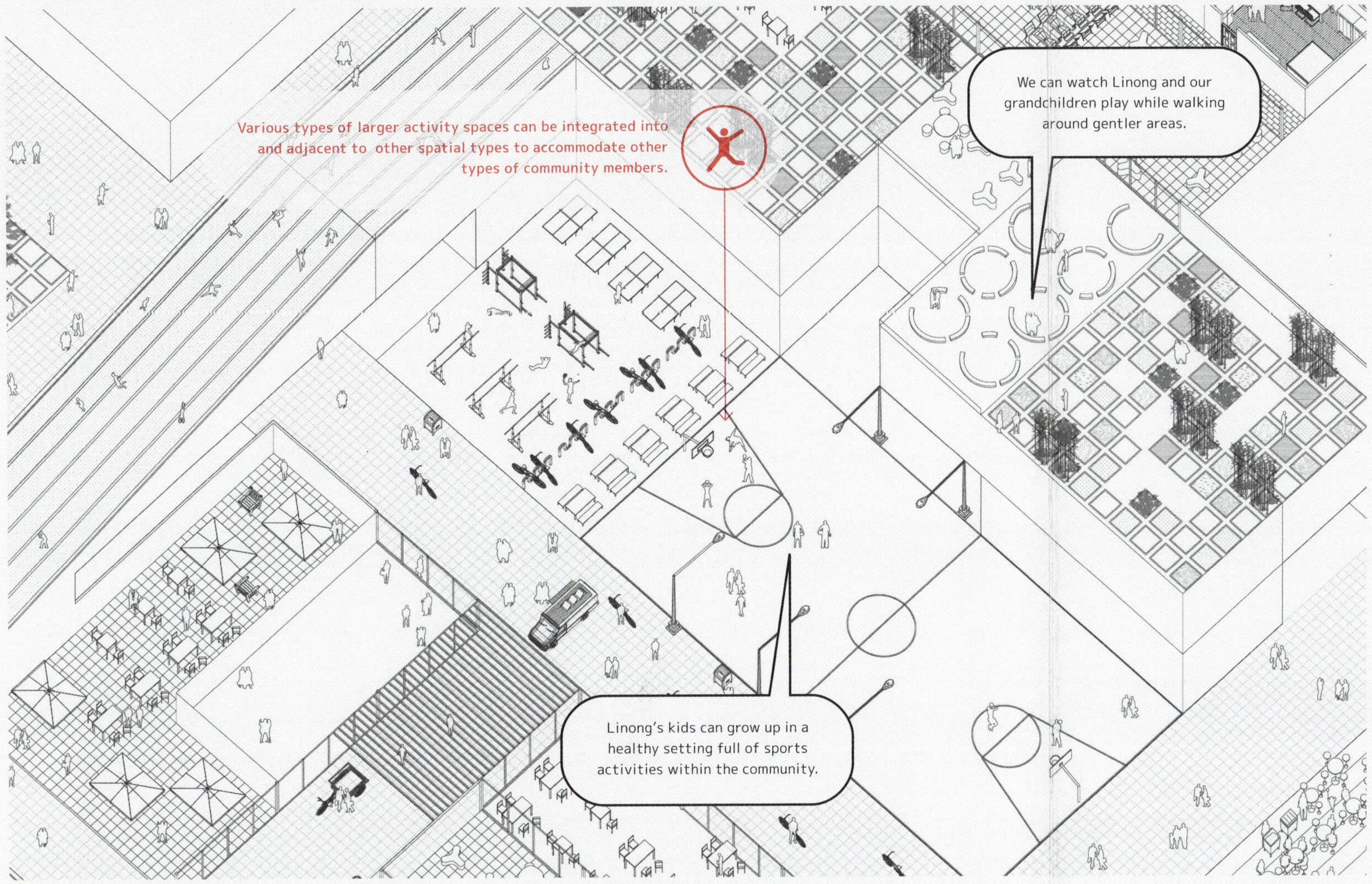

(Left) Axonometric Drawing
(Right Top-Bottom) Photographs of scale model
(Photographs by Anita Kan)

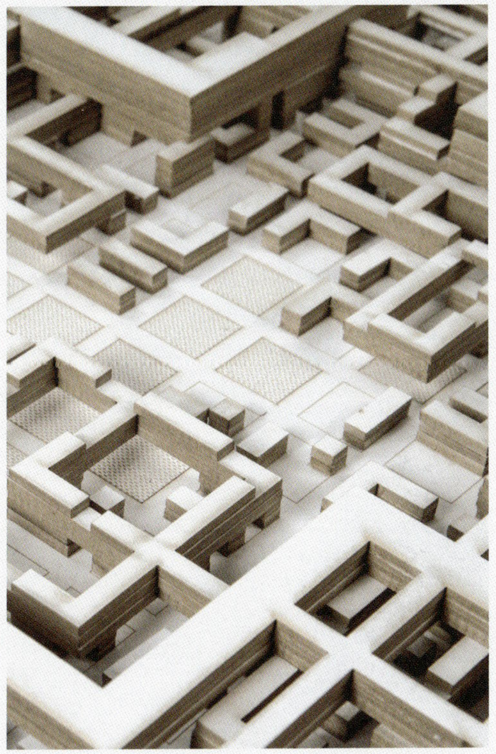

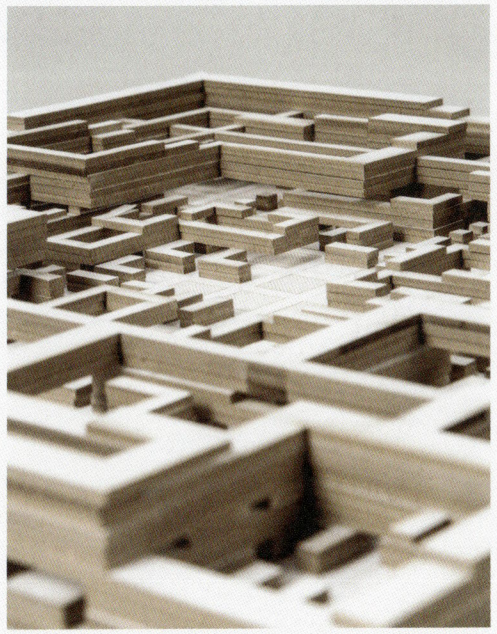

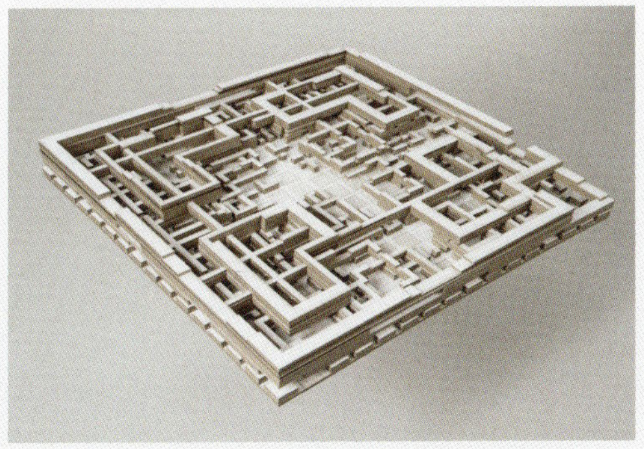

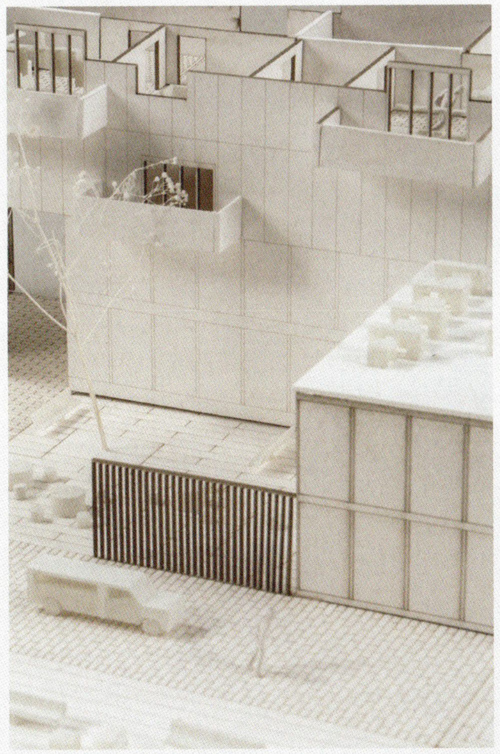

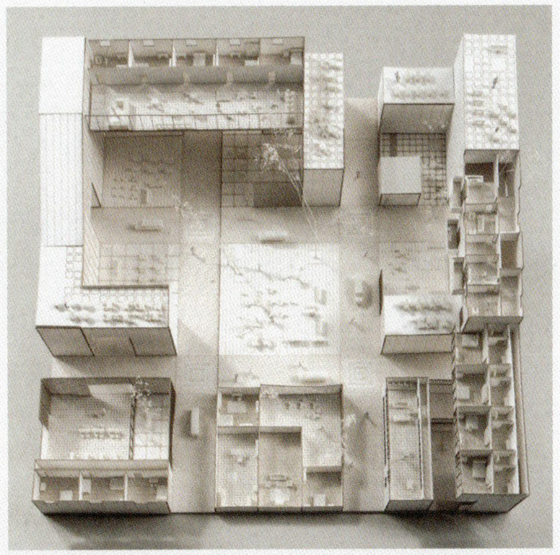

(Bottom Left) Close-up photograph of prototype model showing various boundary conditions between private and community spaces.
(Bottom Right) Overall photograph of prototype model.
(Photographs by Anita Kan)

The motivation for the proposed block's design is centered on the desire to offer a model of a neighborhood that better reflects and houses a more authentic cross section of China's citizens. A more diverse series of narratives and personal itineraries should be able to be associated with such a place, allowing for the possibility of a healthy city that resonates with the characteristics offered by Richard Senett. Through a series of scenarios and narratives, the project sought to shape and give definition to the neighborhoods spaces at the detailed level, letting a projection of multiple subjects guide our design.

Notes

1 Richard Sennett, 2011, Why complexity improves the quality of city life, LSE Cities conference; Hong Kong; Cities, Health and Wellbeing. https://lsecities.net/media/objects/articles/why-complexity-improves-the-quality-of-city-life/en-gb/.

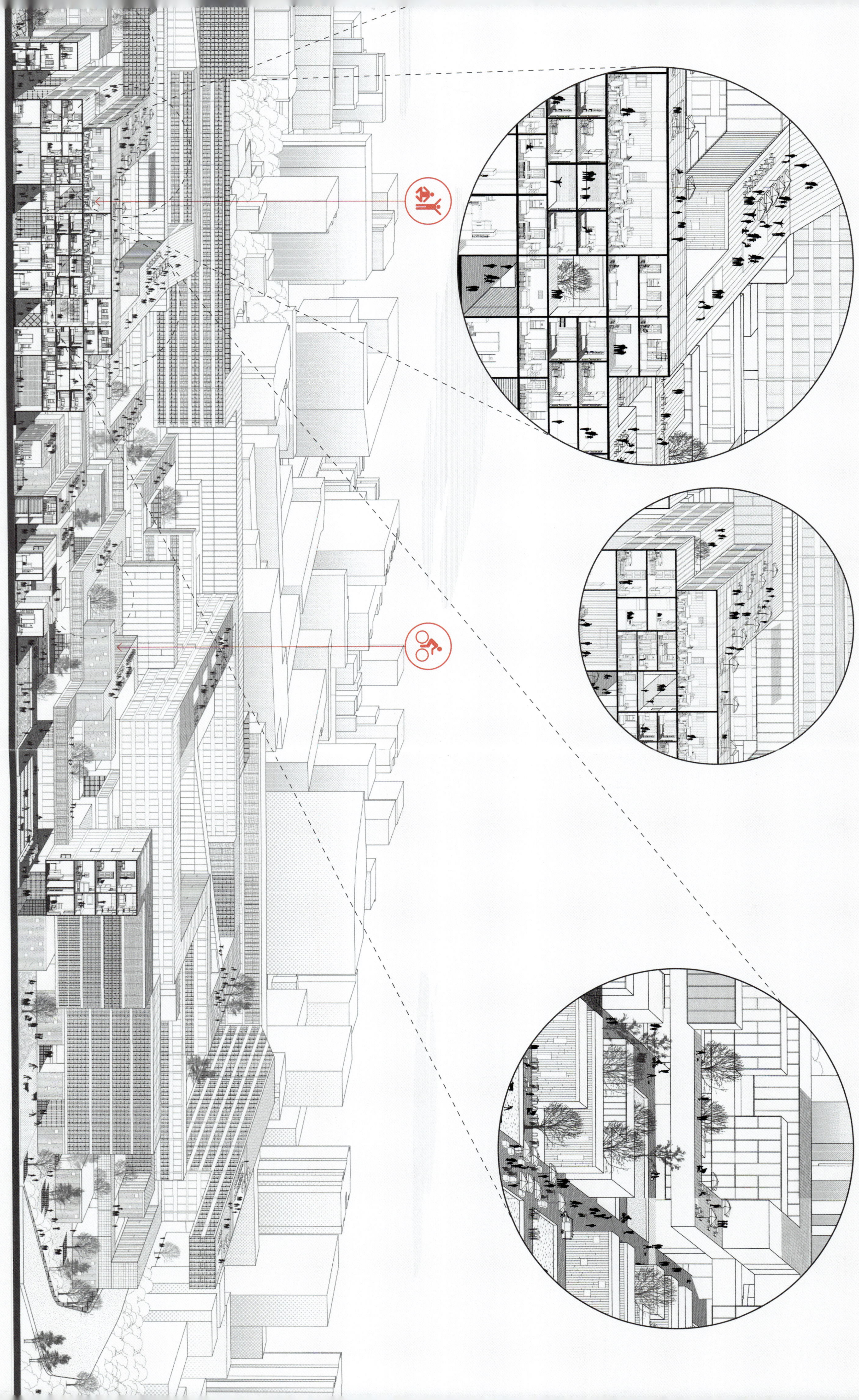

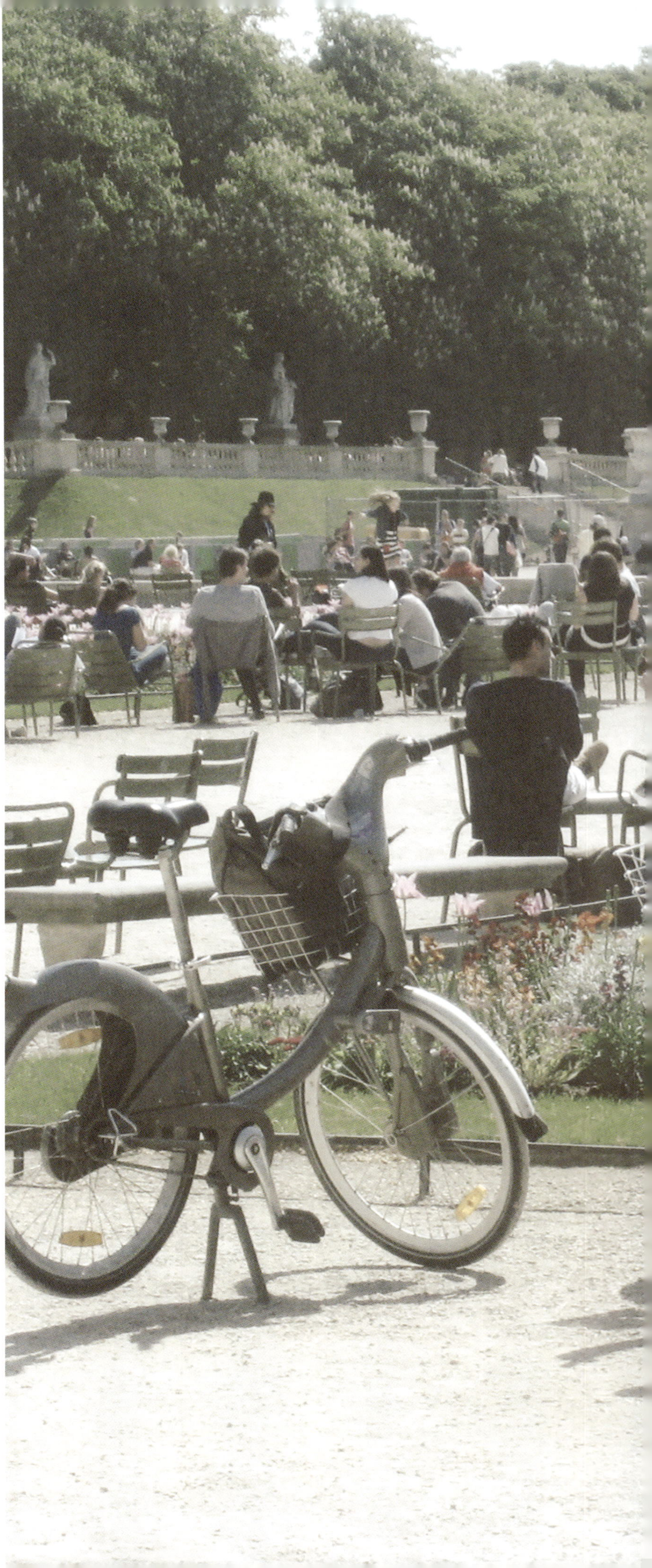

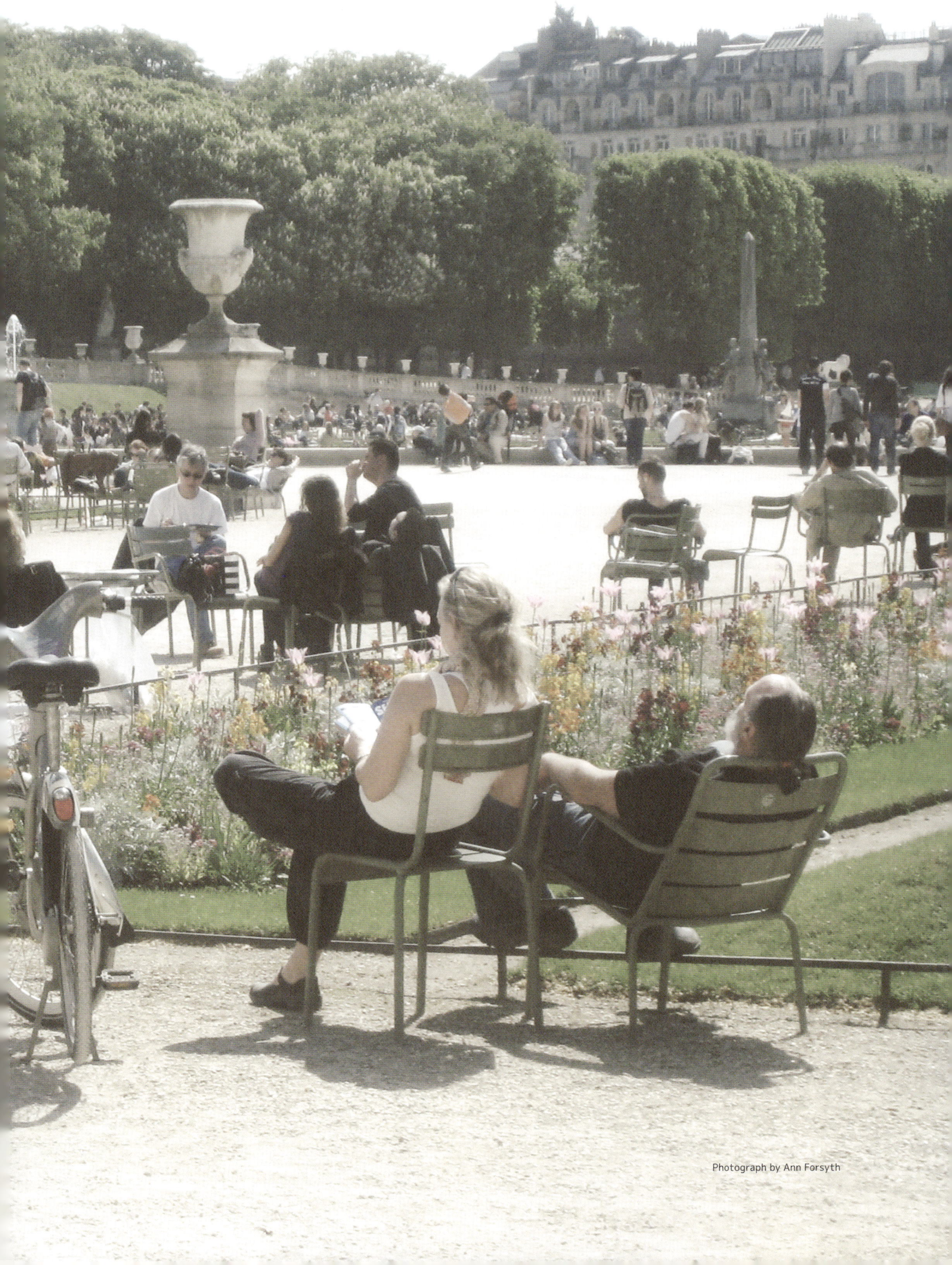

Photograph by Ann Forsyth

Prototypes Design Research Team

Design Coordinators:
Leire Asensio Villoria
David Syn Chee Mah

Team:
Justin Kollar
Xinhui Li
Leo Miller
Yannis Orfanos
Bingjie Shi
Weishun Xu
Han Yang
Yujun Yin
Elizabeth Wu

Upper Level Graduate Option Studio: Life-Styled – China-Town

Studio Instructors:
Leire Asensio Villoria
David Syn Chee Mah

Students:
Whitney Hansley (M'Arch 1)
Ali Karimi (M'Arch 1)
Justin Kollar (M'Arch 1)
Alejandro Lara (MAUD)
Yi Li (M'Arch 1)
Wei Lin (MAUD)
Zhe Peng (M'ARCH2)
Dima Rachid (MLA2)
Won Joon Seol (MLAUD/MLA1)
Rituparna Simlai (MLA1)
Clayton Strange Lee (MAUD)
Wen Wen (M'Arch 1)
Yujun Yin (M'ARCH2/MLA1)

Editors

David Syn Chee Mah:
David Mah has been a lecturer in landscape architecture at Harvard's Graduate School of Design since 2010. Previous to Harvard, he has taught at Cornell University's departments of Architecture as well as City and Regional Planning from 2007 till 2010. David has also taught within the postgraduate design, Landscape Urbanism program at the Architectural Association in London from 2004 till 2007.

Leire Asensio Villoria:
Leire Asensio-Villoria is a registered architect in Spain and studied architecture at the ETSASS and the Architectural Association (AA). She received her diploma in architecture (with honors) from the AA. She has been a lecturer in architecture and landscape architecture at Harvard's Graduate School of Design since 2011. Asensio-Villoria was a design studio instructor in graduate design school at the AA from 2004 to 2007 and a Visiting Lecturer in Architecture at Cornell from 2006 to 2010.

Both Leire and David have been design research coordinators for the prototypes design research team of Harvard University's Health and Places Initiative (a collaboration between the Graduate school of Design and the TH Chan School of Public Health) from 2014 till 2016.

Contributing Authors

Dr. Gary Evans:
Dr. Gary Evans is the Elizabeth Lee Vincent professor at the College of Human Ecology at Cornell University in Ithaca, New York. He is an environmental and developmental psychologist interested in how the physical environment affects human health and well-being among children. Evans' specific areas of expertise include children's environments, the environment of childhood poverty, cumulative risk and child development, environmental stressors, and the development of children's environmental attitudes and behaviors.

Ann Forsyth:
Trained in planning and architecture, Ann Forsyth is a professor of urban planning at the Harvard Graduate School of Design. From 2007-2012 she was a professor of city and regional planning at Cornell. She taught previously at the University of Minnesota, directing the Metropolitan Design Center (2002-2007), Harvard (1999-2002), and the University of Massachusetts (1993-1999) where she was co-director of a small community design center, the Urban Places Project.

Har Ye Kan:
Har Ye Kan is a Research Associate and Post-Doctoral Fellow at the Graduate School of Design, Harvard University, where she recently completed her doctoral degree. The author of several articles and book chapters dealing primarily with Chinese urbanism, she also served as an instructor with Peter Rowe in a graduate seminar on housing.

Ichiro Kawachi:
Ichiro Kawachi, MB.ChB., Ph.D., is the John L. Loeb and Frances Lehman Loeb Professor of Social Epidemiology, and Chair of the Department of Social and Behavioral Sciences at the Harvard School of Public Health. Dr Kawachi received both his medical degree and Ph.D. (in epidemiology) from the University of Otago, New Zealand. He has taught at the Harvard School of Public Health since 1992.

Peter G. Rowe:
Peter G. Rowe is the Raymond Garbe Professor of Architecture and Urban Design and a Harvard University Distinguished Service Professor at Harvard University where he has taught since 1985 and served as Dean of the Graduate School of Design between 1992 and 2004. He is an author or editor of numerous books, several of which deal with housing, including Making a Middle Landscape, Modernity and Housing, and Modern Housing in China, 1840-2000.

Laura Smead:
Laura Smead is a research associate in urban planning for the Health and Places Initiative at Harvard's Graduate School of Design. With master's degrees in both urban planning and psychology, Ms. Smead has specialized knowledge on health, aging, climate change, and sustainable urban planning. Her contributions to the Health and Places Initiative include being the primary author of research briefs on health and place, contributing to the development of a new suite of health impact assessment tools for planners, and co-authoring a guidelines book on creating healthy neighborhoods.

Yu Yifan:
Yu Yifan, Ph.D (EHESS, France, 2003), has been a professor at the Urban Planning Department of Tongji University since 1996. She has been a research fellow at Harvard University Graduate School of Design and Sorbonne University in Paris. She also serves as Vice President of Shanghai Urban Planning Association, Deputy Secretary General of the China Real Estate Research Association, and Deputy President of Sino-francophone Scholars Association (SORSA). Yu's practice and research focus on urban housing and city renovation, and she has published more than 40 articles and has authored three books: Urban Habitation Morphology, Urban Design Project and Atlas de Shanghai (with UNESCO).

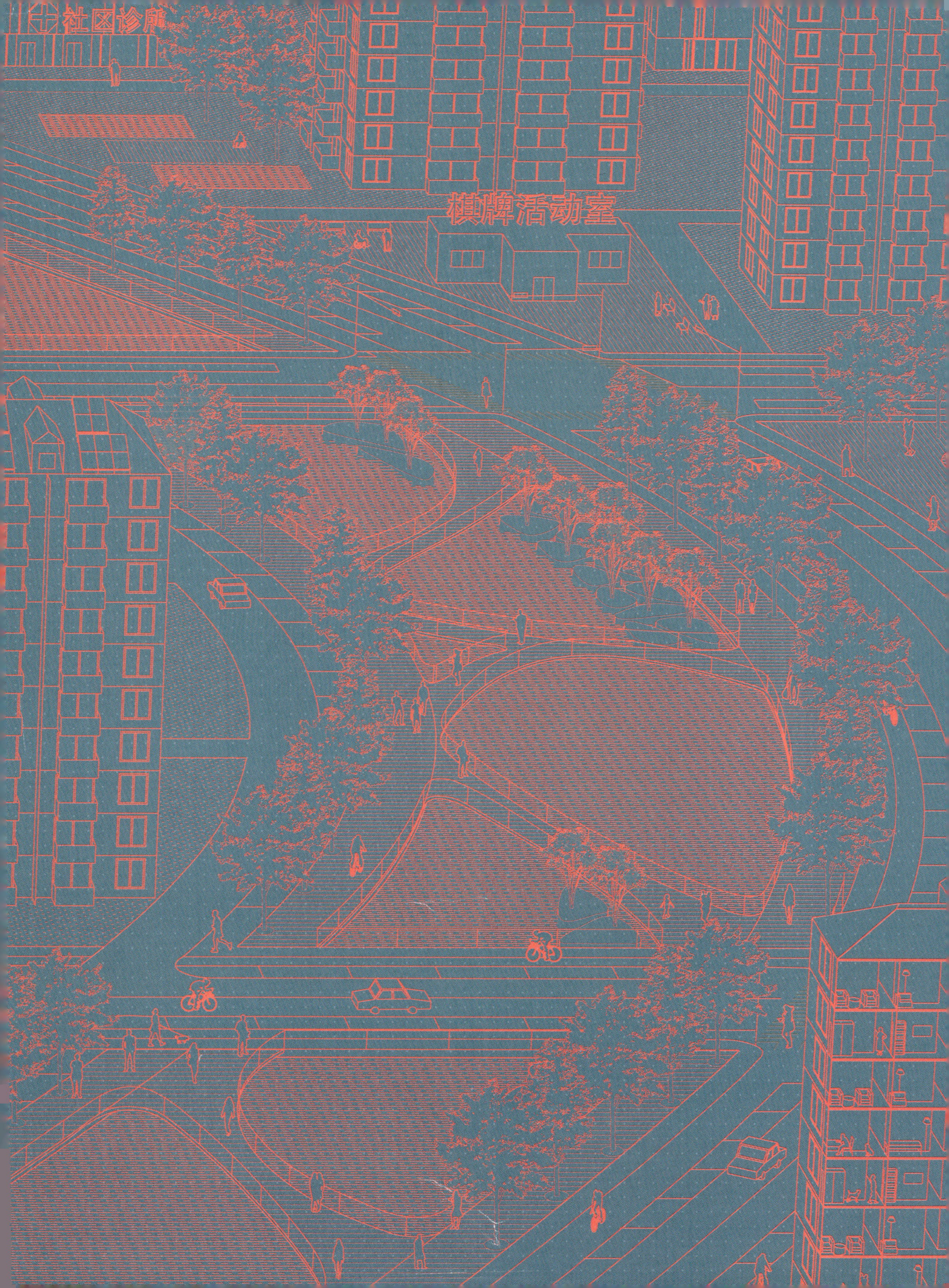
社区诊所
棋牌活动室